Clinical Endocrinology of Companion Animals

Clinical Endocrinology of Companion Animals

C.B. CHASTAIN, DVM, MS

Associate Professor, S.A. Medicine
College of Veterinary Medicine
University of Missouri—Columbia
Veterinary Teaching Hospital
Columbia, Missouri

V.K. GANJAM, BVSc, MS, PhD

Professor, Veterinary Physiology
Department of Biomedical Sciences
College of Veterinary Medicine
University of Missouri
Columbia, Missouri

LEA & FEBIGER   1986   *Philadelphia*

Lea & Febiger
600 Washington Square
Philadelphia, PA 19106-4198
U.S.A.
(215) 922-1330

The authors, editors, and publisher have taken meticulous care to insure the accuracy of the drugs, dosages, and schedules recommended in this book. Since the law requires that information about changes in accepted indications and methods of drug use be printed in the package insert, the reader is advised to consult this document before using a drug. He then can be certain that new data have not led to altered instructions. The reader is also advised to interpret the results of laboratory tests by using the laboratory's normals, not the approximate normals found in this book.

Library of Congress Cataloging-in-Publication Data

Chastain, C.B.
    Clinical endocrinology of companion animals.

    Includes bibliographies and index.
    1. Veterinary endocrinology.   2. Pets—Diseases.
I. Ganjam, V.K.   II. Title.   [DNLM: 1. Endocrine
Diseases—veterinary.   2. Endocrine Glands.   3. Veterinary Medicine.
SF 768.3 C489c]
SF768.3.C47   1986   636.089'64   85-18159
ISBN 0-8121-1017-X

PRINTED IN THE UNITED STATES OF AMERICA

Print No.   4   3   2   1

DEDICATION

To our teachers and colleagues, who have helped us to investigate; to our students, who have helped us to clarify; to our patients, who have taught us to be rational and practical; and to our families, who have shared us with our profession.

PREFACE

We are a veterinary internist (C.B.C.) and a veterinary physiologist (V.K.G.). Both as individuals and as a team, we have realized that there is a need for an introductory textbook, written for students of veterinary internal medicine, on the clinical endocrinology of companion animals. As a clinical endocrinology text, the book should also function as a procedural guide in diagnosis and treatments for veterinarians in clinical practice. This textbook is our attempt to answer the needs of both students and practitioners of veterinary internal medicine.

Clinical endocrinology depends upon interrelated activities: history-taking, physical examinations, laboratory determinations, treatment, and follow-up examinations. Each is equally important. Because hormones modify the rate of activity of target organs, endocrine disorders are often mistaken for primary diseases of the target organ system. Without adequate consideration, endocrinopathies can easily be overlooked. The purposes of this textbook are to help the reader become more aware of the possibility of endocrine disorders in companion animals, to review briefly the physiology of major endocrine organs, to describe presenting complaints and physical findings of endocrinopathies, and to recommend current diagnostic protocols and treatments.

Wishing to be pragmatic in our approach to the diagnosis and management of each endocrinopathy, we have integrated and consolidated the recommendations of our colleagues with our own experience, using the combined material to suggest an apparent best method. We have tried to point out controversial means of diagnosis and management, but for the sake of clarity we have avoided in-depth descriptions of alternative methods. More information on other diagnostic or therapeutic procedures can be found in the references.

We have tried to make this textbook readable and easily examined for review. Most illustrations are original line drawings. Photographs have been limited to examples of case subjects, radiographs, and gross pathology. Microphotographs of histopathology have generally been excluded. Simple tables of listed data and italicized key words in the text have been used to facilitate rapid reference or review.

Columbia, Missouri

C.B. Chastain
V.K. Ganjam

vii

ACKNOWLEDGMENTS

Much of the work in preparing a manuscript such as this goes beyond the literature searches, case reviews, and initial compositions. Our secretaries, particularly Brenda John, Sandy Popelka, and Jo Ann Hartsell, carefully and tirelessly aided in the preparation of its various stages and drafts. Nearly all the artwork are original drawings provided by artists of the University of Missouri's Academic Support Center and Iowa State University's Media Resources Center, We also appreciate the enthusiastic encouragement of Mr. Christian C. Febiger Spahr, Jr., of Lea & Febiger.

CONTENTS

Section I

INTRODUCTION

1

Clinical Endocrinology of Companion Animals

Two words of Greek origin, endocrine and hormone, describe the endocrine system. The term *endocrine* literally means "to separate within," which refers to the wide separation of the organs of the endocrine system throughout the body. The term *hormone* is translated as "I excite." Although in many cases endocrine glands are separated by considerable distances, they function together to give the body the ability to adjust to external and internal hormonal demands (the adaptive action is usually accomplished by the stimulation of the endocrine glands' target cells). The signals for adaptation are carried by the endocrine glands' secretions, which are transported in circulating body fluids without the aid of a duct system of their own.

In Far Eastern philosophy there is the concept that all forces in nature are perfectly balanced by counteropposition. Natural forces are called Yin or Yang, whose symbol is a circle divided by two contiguous, comma-shaped figures that appear as if in motion, but in balance. Forces of Yin are earthly, female, dark, passive, absorbing, evenly numbered, and of the lowlands; they are represented by the tiger, the color orange, or a broken line. Yang is heavenly, male, light, active, penetrating, odd numbered, and of the mountains; it is represented by the dragon, the color azure, or an unbroken line. If Yin changes, Yang changes correspondingly to reestablish harmony. With regard to endocrine secretions, a parallel to Yin and Yang can be seen. Each hormonal secretion is normally regulated by its effect on the body. As a hormone creates a greater effect, that effect causes an adjustment, called *feedback,* in the secretion of the hormone. The study of clinical endocrinology consists of the study and practice of detecting and correcting the cause or effect of imbalances in endocrine secretions.

More than any other branch of internal medicine, clinical endocrinology affects other medical subspecialties. Every system of the body is influenced by or exists as a part of the endocrine system. Signs of endocrine diseases generally present as an illness of a hormone's target organ. For example, deficiencies in mineralocorticoids and glucocorticoids occur in patients with a history of gastrointestinal disturbances. Laboratory findings mimic those of kidney disease. Other examples of presenting signs of endocrine diseases are listed in Table 1–1.

Unless clinicians maintain their suspicion that endocrine disease may be responsible for causing the illness, they can easily be mislead into thinking that the cause of the disease's clinical signs always lies within the system

Table 1–1. Presenting Signs of Endocrine Disorders

Weight loss and weakness
 Diabetes mellitus
 Thyrotoxicosis
 Pheochromocytoma
 Hypoadrenocorticism

Anorexia
 Ketoacidotic diabetes mellitus
 Hypoadrenocorticism
 Primary hyperparathyroidism or
  pseudohyperparathyroidism
 Gastrinoma

Increased appetite
 Diabetes mellitus
 Hypothalamic disease
 Thyrotoxicosis
 Insulinomas
 Growth hormone excess

Obesity
 Hypothalamic disease
 Hyperadrenocorticism
 Hypothyroidism
 Insulinomas

Mental disturbances
 Hyperthyroidism
 Hypoparathyroidism
 Hypothalamic disease
 Pituitary lesions
 Hypoadrenocorticism
 Hyperadrenocorticism
 Primary hyperparathyroidism and
  pseudohyperparathyroidism
 Ovarian endocrine dysfunction
 Feminizing testicular tumors
 Hypothyroidism

Inappropriate galactorrhea
 Pseudocyesis
 Growth hormone excess
 Prolactin-secreting pituitary tumor
 Estrogen-producing adrenal tumors
 Cystic corpora lutea

Pathologic fractures
 Secondary hyperparathyroidism
 Primary hyperparathyroidism
 Hyperadrenocorticism

Delayed puberty
 Hypothalamic disease
 Pituitary disorders
 Primary hypogonadism
 Hypothyroidism
 Hyperadrenocorticism

Recurrent urinary calculi
 Primary hyperparathyroidism
 Hypervitaminosis D

Polyuria and polydipsia
 Diabetes mellitus
 Diabetes insipidus
 Primary hyperparathyroidism and
  pseudohyperparathyroidism
 Hyperadrenocorticism
 Hyperthyroidism

Tetany, muscle spasms and muscle
  cramps
 Hypoparathyroidism
 Hyperadrenocorticism
 Hypothyroidism

Dwarfism
 Hypothyroidism
 Hyperadrenocorticism
 Growth hormone deficiency
 Primary hypogonadism

Alopecia
 Hypothyroidism
 Hyperadrenocorticism
 Ovarian endocrine dysfunction
 Feminizing testicular tumors

Gynecomastia
 Feminizing testicular tumors
 Feminizing adrenal tumors
 Thyrotoxicosis
 Iatrogenic estrogens, progestogens, or
  androgens
 Hypothyroidism

Persistant anestrus, impotency, or
  decreased libido
 Hypothalamic disease
 Hypopituitarism
 Hypothyroidism
 Hypoadrenocorticism
 Hyperadrenocorticism
 Primary hypogonadism
 Thyrotoxicosis
 Feminizing testicular tumors
 Adrenal feminizing tumor

showing the signs. No other medical specialty, with the possible exception of hematology, depends as much as endocrinology does on data from the examination room and laboratory. The elusiveness of endocrinologic diagnoses adds to the clinical interest of the specialty.

Our knowledge of endocrine disorders has multiplied severalfold over the last 20 years because of the refinement and availability of endocrine assays. An expanding interest in veterinary endocrinology suggests that the rate of accumulation of this knowledge will increase in the near future. Clinical endocrinology in veterinary medicine, especially nonreproductive endocrinology, was based on studies of the dog; however, the increasing popularity of cats as companion pets has brought about studies increasing our understanding of their endocrine disorders. Much less is known of the spontaneous endocrine disorders affecting the less common companion pets, such as avians, rodents, and amphibians.

HISTORICAL LANDMARKS IN CLINICAL ENDOCRINOLOGY

The first recorded suggestion of chemical messengers in body fluids has been credited to Hippocrates in about 400 B.C. He described four "humors"—blood, phlegm, black bile, and yellow bile whose balance was necessary to good health. Aristotle, about the same time, described the effects of castration on men and birds, but he did not attribute the cause to loss of humoral substances. In the first century A.D., Celsus (10 A.D.) and Aretaeus (100 A.D.) described the clinical signs of diabetes mellitus.

Little else occurred in endocrinology until after 1000. In 1170, an Italian surgeon, Roger of Palermo, recommended seaweed in the treatment of goiter. In 1564 Eustachus, also an Italian, first described the adrenal glands. In the Netherlands, Graaf described the structure of the testes in 1668 and the vesicular sacs of the ovary in 1672.

Willus, an Englishman, is credited with first noting that urine from patients with diabetes mellitus is sweet. In 1656, Wharton, also from England, described and named the thyroid glands. In 1759, in Germany, Wolff described the mesonephric ducts that form male internal reproductive organs. In France, acromegaly was first described by Saucerotte in 1772, and in 1775 Bordeu realized that the testes secreted substances into the blood, causing male behavior. Bordeu was the first to suggest the presence of endocrine secretions.

Medical advances remained slow between 1800 and 1850. In 1815, Chevreul, a Frenchman, discovered that the sweet material in diabetic urine is glucose. In 1819, Elliotson was the first to use iodine to treat goiter in England. In 1825, Muller, a German anatomist, described the ducts that become female oviducts, uterus, and vagina.

Progress in the understanding of the endocrine system improved rapidly after 1850. When, in 1849, the German Berthold reimplanted the testes of a rooster into the body cavity, reversing the expected atrophy of the rooster's comb, this finding was largely ignored for several years. Also in 1849,

Addison presented a lecture to London physicians describing the progression of signs he attributed to destruction of the adrenals. In the 1850s, the French physiologist Bernard first introduced the idea that the internal secretion of organs affected other parts of the body. In 1850, Curling in England accurately described the clinical signs of cretinism, suspecting that the changes were due to a decrease in the thyroid's function. Also in 1850, the German Leydig described interstitial cells and indicated that he suspected they secrete a substance causing male behavior. In 1857, Petters found acetone in the urine of a diabetic in Prague.

Langerhans, a German histologist, described the pancreatic islets in 1869. In 1871, dwarfism with sexual and mental infantilism was reported by Lorain in France. In England in 1874, Gull was able to attribute the cause of myxedema to atrophy of the thyroid. The same year in Germany, Kussmaul reported "air hunger," i.e., labored respiration caused by metabolic acidosis, in diabetes mellitus. In 1880, the parathyroids were discovered by Sandstrom from Sweden. More than 100 years after its first description in France, acromegaly was described and given its name by another Frenchman, Marie, in 1886, but it was a Russian, Minkowski, who in 1887 linked a pituitary tumor to the development of acromegaly.

In 1889, von Mering and Minkowski showed that the removal of the pancreas in a dog caused diabetes mellitus. In 1891, Gley in France expanded Sandstrom's description of the parathyroids, showing that they are essential to life. In England, Murry in 1891 used injections of thyroid extracts taken from sheep to successfully treat myxedema in humans. In 1894, Oliver and Sharpey-Schafer discovered a vasopressor substance originating in the adrenals. An American, Magnus-Levy, found in 1895 that desiccated thyroid products could be used to treat thyroid deficiency. In Germany, Reidel first described chronic thyroiditis in 1896. In the United States, epinephrine was isolated by Takamine and Abel and named by Abel in 1897.

A prominent French physician, Brown-Sequard, reported in 1899 that he had been rejuvenated by self-injection of aqueous testicular extracts from dogs. Although the extracts were probably inactive, Brown-Sequard's story received much attention and intensified interest in endocrinology. In the United States in 1901, Frohlich described adipogenital dystrophy resulting from hypothalamic disease, Opie linked degenerative changes in the islets with diabetes mellitus, and Aldrich elucidated the chemical structure of epinephrine. Askanazy, a German, associated parathyroid tumors with osteitis fibrosa cystica in 1904.

The term "hormone" was first applied by Bayliss and Starling in 1905 to a gastrointestinal substance, secretin, that caused secretion of pancreatic juice. In 1908, the German Zuelzer first isolated a crude form of insulin. This discovery was followed in a year by MacCallum's finding that the islets of Langerhans are the source of insulin within the pancreas. That same year Pende, an Italian physician, introduced the term "endocrinology." Soon after, Aschner and Crow hypophysectomized dogs and reported their growth and sexual development were arrested. Following Biedl from Czechoslovakia, who discovered in 1910 that the adrenal cortex is necessary for life, Waterhouse in 1911 and Friderichsen in 1918 described acute collapse associated with adrenal hemorrhage.

Other landmarks occurring during the period of 1910 to 1920 include Frank's discovery in 1912 that the neurohypophysis produces an antidiuretic hormone. In 1914, Allen promoted a starvation diet to treat diabetes mellitus in the United States. In Germany, Simmonds described cachexia caused by hypopituitarism in 1914. Kendall, later famous for his work with the adrenal cortex, first isolated and produced a crystalline form of thyroxine. In 1915, the American Cannon found that dogs' and cats' endocrine glands are affected by emotions. In 1918, Mellanby recognized that vitamin D deficiency is the cause of rickets.

During the years before World War II, discoveries in endocrinology were numerous. In Canada, Banting and Best isolated therapeutically effective insulin in 1922. In America, Hanson isolated parathyroid hormone in 1923, while the next year in Toronto Collip reported that parathyroid gland extracts can raise serum calcium levels. Collip soon after became the first to treat tetany with parathyroid extracts. Also in 1924, Steenbock in the United States synthesized vitamin D. Gastrin was first identified by the American Ivy in 1925. In 1926, Abel first prepared crystalline insulin. In 1926, ovarian extracts were found to cause dilatation of the symphysis pubis in guinea pigs. Hisaw, who discovered this, called the substance *relaxin*.

In 1926 Harrington synthesized thyroxine and also elucidated its structure in England. In America, Smith found in 1927 that adenohypophyseal implants could cause precocious sexual maturity in young mice. The same year, Aschheim and Zondek described a method of detecting pregnancy in women by injecting immature mice with the woman's urine and noting the effects on the mice ovaries. The Swiss veterinarians Strike and Gruter reported that pituitary extracts stimulate lactation in 1928. The same year investigators at Parke Davis Laboratories found that two separate substances originating in the neurohypophysis caused antidiuretic and oxytocic effects in 1928. In 1929, Allen discovered progesterone, and Rogoff used adrenocortical extracts for the treatment of adrenal insufficiency.

Spectacular growth in endocrine knowledge occurred in the 1930s. In 1930 the Argentinian, Houssay, reported that hypophysectomy decreased the severity of diabetes mellitus in pancreatomized dogs. Also in 1930, Doisy isolated the first estrogen, estrone, in the United States. In 1931, Riddle used the term *prolactin* to describe the substance in pituitary extracts that causes crop milk to be secreted.

In 1932 a Boston surgeon, Cushing, reported a link between basophil adenomas of the adenohypophysis and bilateral adrenocortical hyperplasia. In France the same year, Lacassagne reported that mammary carcinomas could be produced in animals with estrone benzoate. Collip, who had worked earlier with parathyroid hormone, extracted adrenocorticotropic hormone (ACTH) in 1933. After his work with thyroxine, Kendall isolated ACTH at the Mayo Clinic in 1934. Testosterone was synthesized by Butenandt in Germany in 1935. In 1936, Kerr and Hagedorn made insulin therapy more practical by finding that zinc and protamine, respectively, retard injected insulin absorption. Also in 1936, MacCorquodale isolated estradiol. One year later Young produced diabetes mellitus with adenohypophyseal extracts. In 1938, the American Turner described a syndrome in which retarded sexual development was caused by genetic effects on endocrinologic functions. In 1939, diabetes insipidus was experimentally produced by injuring the hypothalamus.

With the exception of research on the adrenocortical hormones, the Second World War caused most endocrine research to stop during the 1940s. Research efforts continued as a result of a rumor among Allied countries that German pilots were being administered adrenocortical extracts to enable them to perform better in combat. Then in 1950 Kendall, along with Hench and Reichstein, shared the Nobel prize for medicine for work with adrenocortical hormones.

Investigations in the 1950s led to Sanger's description of the structure of insulin and du Vigneaud's description of the structure of oxytocin and antidiuretic hormone (ADH). In 1953, Simpson and Tait identified aldosterone. In 1954, Conn recognized that some adrenocortical tumors were a remediable cause for hypertension in humans. Glucagon was isolated by Staub in 1955.

Hormones are secreted in extremely minute quantities. Until 1960, further advances in endocrinology had been hampered by the inaccuracies of crude biochemical assays and bioassays. In 1960, Berson and Yalow initiated a revolution in diagnostic and investigative endocrinology by reporting a new method of assaying insulin, the radioimmunoassay, which is capable of accurately measuring very small quantities of hormones. Other advances during the 1960s included the discovery of calcitonin in Vancouver by Copp; the synthesis of insulin by investigative teams in the United States, China, and Germany; the description of calcitonin's structure by Potts; and the identification of the structure of thyrotropin-releasing hormone (TRH) by Schally and Guillemin in 1969.

In 1971, Holick and DeLuca described 1,25-dihydroxy D_3. Also in 1971, Schally identified the structure of gonadotropin-releasing hormone (GnRH). Guillemin reported somatostatin's structure in 1973.

The radioimmunoassay technique continues to supply new data on clinical endocrinology, and a revolution is just beginning in endocrinous therapies. Genetic engineering with recombinant DNA has made it feasible to produce hormones with bacteria in mass quantities. The first of these, human insulin, was released for commercial use in 1983. Others, such as human growth hormone, will follow soon. The clinical treatment of companion animals should benefit indirectly by the lower cost and greater availability of these hormones, even though they are synthesized human hormones in structure.

Veterinary endocrinology has always received attention because of interest in the reproduction of food-producing animals and the use of animal models to study human disease, but until the mid-1970s not much work had been done on the clinical endocrinology of companion animals (before that time sources of information included only occasional chapters on endocrinology in various textbooks on veterinary medicine and scattered articles in journals). In 1977, Dr. E.T. Siegel, a pioneer in the study of the clinical endocrinology of companion animals, authored the first textbook on this subject *Endocrine Diseases of the Dog*.[7] Partly because of his book, the clinical endocrinology of companion animals is becoming a separate specialty of veterinary internal medicine.

Credit for the original information consolidated in this book belongs to many other authors: Capen, Kaneko, Belshaw, Rijnberk, and others listed in references at the end of each chapter. See also references 6 and 8.

INCIDENCE OF ENDOCRINE DISORDERS

The organs generally considered part of the endocrine system are listed in Table 1–2, and possible disorders that could affect each endocrine system are listed in Table 1–3. The thymus and pineal body are considered by some to be endocrine organs, but they have not been listed because they currently lack clinical significance as endocrine organs.

The incidence of endocrine disorders reflects our present ability to diagnose and understand endocrine disorders.[5] The diagnosis of endocrine disorders is hampered by several factors, including the interrelationships occurring among endocrine glands and compensatory mechanisms. Other factors that may make diagnosis difficult include the following: the effects produced by tumorous endocrine disorders are often not proportionate to the size of the tumor; physiologic adaptation is frequently difficult to differentiate from endocrine disease; endocrine disorders can occur as multiple concurrent disorders; and, finally, laboratory tests may be unavailable and insensitivity and errors can occur.

Estimates of the relative incidence of major endocrine disorders in dogs and cats are shown in Tables 1–4, 1–5, and 1–6. Based on data taken from the American Veterinary Data Program, female dogs more frequently develop diabetes mellitus, hyperadrenocorticism, hypoadrenocorticism, adrenocortical tumors and hypoparathyroidism than do male dogs. Male dogs seem more predisposed to hyperparathyroidism, diabetes insipidus, and pheochromocytomas.

Although feline hyperthyroidism ranked second in occurrence in the survey shown in Table 1–5, it is now the most frequently diagnosed endocrine disorder. It was virtually unknown until 1975. Older house cats are more likely to present with diabetes mellitus. They are usually neutered, a

Table 1–2.   Endocrine Organs and Their Major Endocrine Secretions

Hypothalamus
  Thyrotropin-releasing hormone
  Prolactin-inhibiting hormone (dopamine)
  Gonadotropin-releasing hormone
  Corticotropin-releasing hormone
  Growth-hormone-releasing hormone
  Growth-hormone-inhibiting hormone (somatostatin)
  Antidiuretic hormone
  Oxytocin

Hypophysis
  Thyrotropin (thyroid-stimulating hormone [TSH])
  Corticotropin (adrenocorticotropic hormone [ACTH])
  Follicle-stimulating hormone
  Luteinizing hormone
  Prolactin
  Growth hormone

Thyroids
  Thyroxine (T_4)
  Triiodothyronine (T_3)
  Calcitonin

Parathyroids
  Parathyroid hormone

Pancreatic islets and gastrointestinal tract
  Insulin
  Glucagon
  Gastrin
  Somatostatin
  Secretin
  Cholecystokinin-pancreozymin
  Gastric inhibitory peptide
  Vasoactive intestinal peptide
  Glucagon-like immunoreactivity

Adrenals
  Cortisol
  Aldosterone
  Adrenal androgens
  Epinephrine
  Norepinephrine

Gonads
  Testosterone
  Estrogens
  Progesterone

Kidney
  1,25 dihydroxycholecalciferol
  Renal erythropoietic factor

Placenta
  Chorionic gonadotropin*
  Chorionic somatomammotropin*

* Suspected but not proven placental secretions in dogs and cats.

Table 1–3. Possible Endocrine Disorders

Possible causes of hyperfunction
Neoplasia
Hyperplasia
Hypersecretion
Ectopic production

Possible causes of hypofunction or nonfunction
Abnormal development
Infarction
Atrophy
Fibrosis
Cyst
Neoplasia
Inflammation
Production of abnormal hormone
Unresponsive target organ
Abnormal blood transport

fact explaining the high incidence of diabetes in sexually neutered cats. Male cats may be affected more frequently than expected.

The observations of several veterinary teaching hospitals indicate that endocrine disorders are involved in 10% to 20% of the medical diseases of dogs. In comparison, occurrence of clinical endocrinologic diagnoses in cats

Table 1–4. The Relative Diagnostic Incidence of
Endocrine Disorders in Dogs*

Disorder	Neutered		Sexually Intact		Total
	Male	Female	Male	Female	
Hypothyroidism and thyroiditis	59	284	452	273	1068
Diabetes mellitus	24	178	121	143	466
Hyperadrenocorticism	33	156	164	108	461
Hypoadrenocorticism	18	102	67	64	251
Thyroid tumors	8	39	46	26	119
Hyperparathyroidism	4	16	36	14	70
Adrenocortical tumors	3	17	19	16	55
Hypophyseal tumors	3	13	21	8	45
Diabetes insipidus	1	8	26	8	43
Insulinomas	0	13	13	4	30
Hyperthyroidism	3	9	7	10	29
Pheochromocytoma	0	5	16	0	21
Hypoparathyroidism	1	8	2	4	15

* Data obtained from the American Veterinary Data Program. Incidence of endocrine disorders is taken from data on dogs in 20 contributing institutions from January 1977 to December 1979. Gender distribution for population at risk was as follows: neutered males, 5%; neutered females, 21%; males, 44%; and females, 30%.

is about 10% that of dogs. At present, endocrine diagnoses in other companion animals are even less common.

Many endocrinopathies are subclinical and are not included in Tables 1–4, 1–5, 1–6. For example, each time glucocorticoids are administered to an animal with a functional hypothalamic-hypophyseal-adrenocortical axis, production of endogenous cortisol diminishes or ceases. However, if it is assumed that the dose of administered glucocorticoids is near physiologic or replacement levels, no adverse effects are noted clinically unless the suppression of exogenous hormones is long-term and withdrawal of exogenous glucocorticoids is abrupt.

The incidence of endocrine disorders can be affected by the breeding of animals with inheritable defects and by environmental factors, particularly dietary imbalances or deficiencies. Endocrine disorders with a known or probable genetic base are listed in Table 1–7.[2,3] Certain breeds seem to be predisposed to different endocrinopathies (breed predispositions will be described in following chapters concerned with endocrinopathies). It is possible that at least some of these apparent predispositions are genetically based, but sufficient proof is lacking at present.

Some genetically based endocrine disorders can be identified by chromosomal studies. For example, Turner's syndrome, the result of several chromosomal anomalies, causes gonadal dysgenesis and estrogen deficiency in humans and animals. The most common chromosomal anomaly in Turn-

Table 1–5. The Relative Diagnostic Incidence of
Endocrine Disorders in Cats*

Disorder	Neutered		Sexually Intact		Total
	Male	Female	Male	Female	
Diabetes mellitus	31	25	5	3	64
Hyperthyroidism (thyroid adenomas and adenocarcinomas)	6	5	2	2	15
Secondary hyperparathyroidism	3	3	2	4	12
Hypothyroidism (thyroid atrophy and thyroiditis)	3	0	1	3	7
Hyperadrenocorticism, adrenocortical adenomas, and adenocarcinomas	4	2	1	0	7
Hypoadrenocorticism and congenital hypoplasia of adrenals	1	2	0	2	5
Diabetes insipidus	1	1	0	2	4

* Data obtained from the American Veterinary Data Program. Incidence of endocrine disorders is taken from data on cats presented to 20 contributing institutions from January 1977 to December 1979. Gender distribution for population at risk was neutered males, 24%; neutered females, 25%; males, 26%; and females, 25%.

Table 1–6. The Relative Diagnostic Incidence of Gonadal
Disorders Capable of Causing Endocrine Disorders
in Dogs and Cats*

Disorder	Sex	Dog	Cat
Seminoma	M	184	0
Sertoli cell tumor	M	177	0
Interstitial cell tumor	M	154	0
Ovarian hypofunction	F	24	1
Hypogonadism	M	14	0
Granulosa cell tumor	F	14	15
Ovarian adenocarcinoma	F	13	1
Ectopic testes	M	11	0
Ovarian cystadenoma	F	10	1
Ovarian hyperfunction	F	8	3

* Data obtained from the American Veterinary Data Program. Incidence of gonadal disorders is taken from data on dogs and cats in 20 contributing institutions from January 1977 to December 1979. Gender distribution for canine population at risk was as follows: 59% for sexually intact males and 41% for sexually intact females. For felines, the gender distribution for the population at risk was as follows: 51% for sexually intact males and 49% for sexually intact females.

er's syndrome is XO, which is identifiable by chromosomal analysis. Other diseases, like diabetes mellitus in humans, may be linked to particular leukocyte antigens. Perhaps in the future chromosomal analyses and histocompatibility testing of leukocyte antigens may become more commonplace in veterinary medicine and will provide valuable data on genetically based endocrine diseases.

Aging and nutrition also influence the incidence of endocrine disorders. Nutritionally based endocrine disorders are listed in Table 1–8. Examples of the incidence of common endocrinopathies in dogs and cats are shown according to age in Table 1–9 (most endocrinopathies affect dogs and cats after they reach 5 years of age). Serum levels of some hormones normally change with aging (for example, a gradual decrease in serum thyroxine levels is associated with aging in dogs). Changes associated with aging should not be misinterpreted as a sign of disease.

Table 1–7. Known and Probable Genetically Based
Endocrine Disorders in Dogs

Disorder	Breeds Affected
Pituitary dwarfism	German shepherds Carelian bear-dogs
Diabetes mellitus	Keeshounds
Hypothyroidism and thyroiditis	Beagles
Goiter	Wirehaired fox terriers

Table 1–8.   Nutritionally Based Endocrine Disorders

Nutritionally induced secondary hyperparathyroidism
Nutritionally induced hypercalcitoninism
Goiter resulting from iodine deficiency or excess
Hypervitaminosis D
Various endocrine deficiencies associated with starvation

BASIC CAUSES OF ENDOCRINE DISEASE

There are eight basic causes of endocrine disease in companion animals. Examples of each cause are listed in Table 1–10.

1. PRIMARY HYPERFUNCTION.   Normally the rate of secretion of a hormone is counterbalanced by stimulating or inhibitory influences that result from the hormone's effects on the body. *Autonomy* occurs when a hormone is produced in amounts exceeding normal production because it is no longer inhibited by feedback mechanisms. Autonomous hyperfunction is usually caused by neoplasia, but hyperplasia can also cause autonomous hyperfunction.

Table 1–9.   Incidence of Common Endocrinopathies According to Age

Age Range	Disorders
0 to 1 years	Familial diabetes mellitus Pituitary dwarfism Cretinism Nutritionally reduced secondary hyperparathyroidism Hypervitaminosis D Secondary hyperparathyroidism resulting from congenital renal disease
1 to 5 years	Hypoadrenocorticism Pseudohyperparathyroidism resulting from lymphosarcoma Hypoparathyroidism Hypothyroidism
5 to 10 years	Hypothyroidism Diabetes mellitus Hyperadrenocorticism Insulinomas Secondary hyperparathyroidism resulting from acquired renal disease Feminizing testicular tumors Ovarian endocrine dysfunctions
10 years and older	Diabetes insipidus Primary hyperparathyroidism Pseudohyperparathyroidism resulting from apocrine gland anal sac tumors Secondary hyperparathyroidism resulting from acquired renal disease Feminizing testicular tumors Ovarian endocrine dysfunctions

Table 1-10.   Causes and Examples of Endocrine Disorders

Primary hyperfunction
    Hyperthyroidism from thyroid follicular cell neoplasia
    Hypercalcitoninism from a medullary carcinoma of the thyroid
    Primary hyperparathyroidism
    Insulinoma
    Gastrinoma
    ACTH-secreting chromophobe adenoma of the pituitary
    Male feminizing testicular tumors
    Hyperestrogenism from ovarian neoplasia
    Hyperadrenocorticism from adrenocortical neoplasia

Secondary hyperfunction
    Hyperadrenocorticism from bilateral adrenocortical hyperplasia
    Secondary hyperparathyroidism

Primary hypofunction
    Primary congenital or acquired hypothyroidism
    Hypoparathyroidism from lymphocytic parathyroiditis
    Spontaneous hypoadrenocorticism
    Hypopituitarism from cystic malformation of the adenohypophysis
    Insulin-dependent diabetes mellitus

Secondary hypofunction
    Secondary hypothyroidism, hypoadrenocorticism, or hypogonadism resulting from
      hypopituitarism

Ectopic hypersecretion of hormones or hormone-like substances
    Pseudohyperparathyroidism
    Hyperadrenocorticism resulting from ectopic hypersecretion of ACTH

Failure of target cell response
    Testicular feminization syndrome of humans
    Insulin-independent diabetes mellitus
    Pseudohypoparathyroidism of humans

Abnormal degradation of a hormone
    Feminization resulting from chronic liver disease
    Hypercalcemia secondary to primary renal disease

Iatrogenic hormone excess
    Iatrogenic hyperadrenocorticism
    Iatrogenic thyrotoxicity
    Hypervitaminosis D
    Progestogen-induced acromegaly and hypoadrenocorticism
    Estrogen toxicity in dogs
    Hepatotoxicity of iatrogenically administered androgenic steroids

2. SECONDARY HYPERFUNCTION.   Occasionally, hypersecretion of a hormone results from overstimulation of its organ of production by a tropic hormone or persistent metabolic stimulus.

3. PRIMARY HYPOFUNCTION.   Failure of proper development or destructive processes in an endocrine gland can render it unable to secrete normal amounts of hormone. Failures in development can be structural or biochemical, that is, caused by deficiencies in enzymes necessary for hormone synthesis. Destructive processes are often related to a breakdown in immunity, but trauma, drug-induction, and neoplasia can also impair endocrine gland function.

4. SECONDARY HYPOFUNCTION. Deficiency of a tropic (stimulatory) hormone will impair the target endocrine gland's ability to produce normal quantities of its secretory product.

5. ECTOPIC HYPERSECRETION OF HORMONES OR HORMONE-LIKE SUBSTANCES. When neoplasms occur in non-endocrine glands, sometimes the glands gain the ability to synthesize hormones, especially peptide hormones. The abnormal secretion may be excessive and cause a syndrome of mimicking that of primary hyperfunction in an endocrine organ. Sometimes the secretion may only cause subclinical effects (subclinical secretion of an ectopically produced hormone has been used as a diagnostic marker in humans for the presence of early developing tumors, and tumor metastasis, and as a means of monitoring the patient's response to tumor treatment).

6. FAILURE OF TARGET CELL RESPONSE. Hormones mediate their effects on target organs by attaching to receptors and modifying intracellular activities. The failure of a hormone to produce a normal effect can result from a lack in the quantity or quality of target cell receptors, or from a failure in the target cell's intracellular response.

7. ABNORMAL DEGRADATION OF A HORMONE. Disorders of organs necessary for degradation and elimination of hormones can lead to excessive accumulation of hormone levels. Some drugs are known to decrease the degradation of hormones, whereas other drugs can induce an increased rate of hormone degradation.

8. IATROGENIC HORMONE EXCESS. When endocrine drugs are administered for any reason other than replacement of that hormone's endogenous deficiency, hormones reach excessive levels. Administration of hormones for purposes beyond their replacement for deficiency should be reduced to the minimally necessary dose for the minimally necessary time to produce the desired pharmacologic effect.

In humans and ruminants, it is well established that there is a close interrelationship between the fetal and maternal endocrine systems. Failure of fetal endocrine function is considered a cause of endocrine disease in these species. Failure of fetal endocrine function in companion animals could presumably be a cause or result of endocrine disease, although proof is currently lacking.

See reference 1.

REFERENCES

1. Capen, C.C.: Mechanisms of endocrine disease in animals. Proceedings of the 6th Kal Kan Symposium. Columbus, OH, 1982, pp. 31–43.
2. Foley, C.M., Lasley J.F., and Osweiler, G.D.: Abnormalities of Companion Animals: Analysis of Heritability. Ames, Iowa, Iowa State University Press, 1979.
3. Merton, D.A.: Selective breeding in the dog and cat. Part II. Known and suspected genetic diseases. Compendium on Continuing Educ. for the Practicing Vet., 4:332, 1982.

4. Meyer, D.J.: Clinical manifestation associated with endocrine disorders. Vet. Clin. North Am., 7:433, 1977.
5. Fausner, D.G., et al.: Endocrine disorders in dogs (panel report). Mod. Vet. Pract., 62:891, 1981.
6. Schmidt, J.E.: Medical Discoveries: Who and When. Springfield, Illinois, Charles C Thomas, 1959.
7. Siegel, E.T.: Endocrine Diseases of the Dog. Philadelphia, Lea & Febiger, 1977.
8. Tausk, M.: Pharmacology of Hormones. Chicago, Year Book Medical Publishers, 1975.
9. Weller, R.E.: Paraneoplastic disorders in companion animals. Compendium on Continuing Educ. for the Practicing Vet., 4:423, 1982.

2

Control Mechanisms, Actions, and Measurements
of Hormones

The effects created by hormones depend on many factors. Among these factors are the hormones' chemical structure; concentration in the bloodstream; method of transport in the bloodstream; quantity of unbound target cell receptors; integrity of the target cell's post-receptor, hormone-induced functions; and the rate of degradation and elimination. At present, the clinical diagnosis of endocrinopathies is predominantly based on the measurements of total hormone concentrations in the bloodstream.

TYPES OF HORMONES

Endocrine glands produce four categories of hormones based on their chemical structure: peptides, steroids, catecholamines, and iodothyronines (Table 2–1). Some endocrine organs produce more than one category of hormone—for example, the thyroid produces iodothyronines in the form of thyroxine and peptides in the form of calcitonin. However, most only produce one type.

Peptides are composed of three or more amino acids. They are not administered orally because they would be destroyed by the digestive tract. Steroids contain a hydrogenated cyclopentanophenanthrene-ring. Because they resist digestion, they can be administered orally. Catecholamines have an aromatic portion, which is a benzene (catechol), and an aliphatic portion, which is an amine. Catecholamines are not effective when given orally because of digestive destruction, plus oxidation and conjugation in the liver. Iodothyronines are iodinated derivatives of tyrosine. Even though they are partially destroyed by digestive processes, iodothyronines can be effective when given orally. Doses must be great enough to compensate for the partial destruction.

Prostaglandins, histamine, serotonin, and kinins are considered *autacoids* (Gr., self remedy). Autacoids are sometimes referred to as "local hormones" because they primarily affect surrounding tissue. They are not accepted as true hormones, but they do have an effect on endocrine glands' functioning.

CONCENTRATION OF HORMONES IN THE BLOODSTREAM

The concentration of a hormone in the bloodstream is affected by its rate of secretion. Most hormones are secreted continuously, with severalfold

Table 2-1.   Types of Hormones and Their Sources

Peptides
  Hypothalamus
  Hypophysis
  Parathyroid glands
  Gastrointestinal tract
  Pancreas
  Thyroid (parafollicular cells)
  Placenta

Steroids
  Adrenal cortices
  Testes
  Ovaries
  Kidney
  Placenta

Catecholamines
  Hypothalamus
  Adrenal medulla

Iodothyronines
  Thyroids

increases possible when appropriate stimuli are present. In some cases, the suppressive factors of a hormone, rather than its stimuli, may be more important in altering the hormone's secretory rate; consequently, the secretory rate of an endocrine gland is governed by tonic stimulation or suppression. Reciprocal modifications in the concentrations of hormones in the bloodstream, which correspond in intensity to the hormones' stimuli and suppressive factors, form loops that are termed *feedback loops*. For example, cortisol secretion is stimulated by increasing the serum concentration of adrenocorticotropic hormone (ACTH). Increasing the serum concentration of cortisol suppresses secretion of ACTH (Fig. 2-1).

Three factors determine the secretory rates of the endocrine gland: (1) humoral feedback loops, which can influence the endocrine secretory rate in the form of another hormone, an electrolyte, or a metabolic substance such as glucose or arginine; (2) neurologic stimulation or suppression; and (3) genetic influence.

The speed at which the blood concentrations of a hormone can change depends somewhat on how much preformed hormone is available for release. Peptide hormones and catecholamines are uniquely stored as preformed hormone in cytoplasmic secretory granules. Their release rates can change rapidly. Precursors of active thyroid hormones are stored in the follicles' colloid before their release into the bloodstream as triiodothyronine (T_3) and thyroxine (T_4). Steroid hormones are released as soon as they are formed. The release rates of thyroid and steroid hormones are slow in comparison to peptide hormones.

Many hormones, such as cortisol and growth hormone (GH), fluctuate in concentration at rhythmic intervals each day. These daily rhythmic changes

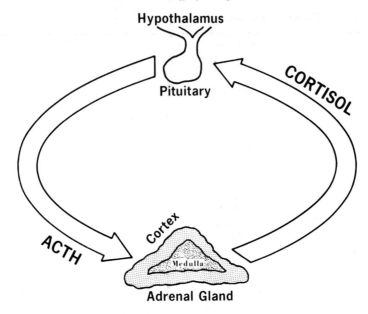

Fig. 2–1.   Normal feedback between the central nervous system and adrenal hormones.

are called *circadian* (Lat., about a day) *variations*. Some refer to daily rhythmic changes as *diurnal* (Lat., day) *rhythms*. Many of these rhythms are coordinated by the suprachiasmatic nuclei of the hypothalamus.[9] Other hormones, the gonadotropins and gonadal hormones, are produced in female dogs in rhythmic biannual intervals or in female cats in weekly intervals during certain seasons. These weekly or biannual changes in gonadotropins and gonadal hormones in female animals are called the *estral* or *estrous* cycle.

Minute-to-minute variations in concentrations of hormone occur. Provided there are no strong stimulatory or suppressive influences, the degree of variation is affected by the sensitivity of the assays being used and the rate of hormone turnover by the body. The hormone turnover rate, *serum half-life,* is a function of the rate of a hormone's degradation. In general, serum half-lives for catecholamines are less than 2 minutes, polypeptide hormones are less than 60 minutes, steroid hormones are several hours, and iodothyronines are several hours to several days, depending on the species.

Normal concentrations of various hormones are usually reported in units permitting single- or double-digit numbers and no more than single- to double-digit decimal numbers (examples of reporting units for concentrations of hormones are shown in Table 2–2). Some laboratories, particularly in Europe, report values in micromoles (μmol) per liter. Other less common units of hormone measurement and their abbreviations can be found in the appendices.

Table 2–2. Common Reporting Units for Hormone Concentrations in Serum or Plasma

Unit	Size	Hormone	Per dl or ml
Microgram (μg)	10^{-6} g	Cortisol	dl
		T_4	dl
		Testosterone	dl
Nanogram (ng)	10^{-9} g	T_3	dl
		Progesterone	ml
Picograms (pg)	10^{-12} g	Estrogen	ml

HORMONE TRANSPORT IN THE BLOODSTREAM

Hormones may or may not be bound to plasma proteins while transported in the bloodstream. Peptide hormones and catecholamines are water-soluble and do not bind to specific plasma proteins. Steroid hormones are lipid-soluble and reversibly bind to specific binding plasma proteins such as cortisol-binding globulin and sex-hormone-binding globulin. Iodothyronines are water-soluble but bind to plasma proteins that prolong their plasma half-life.

With hormones that bind to plasma proteins, small percentages of the total amount of the hormone in the bloodstream are not protein bound. This unbound portion is called *free hormone*. Free hormones are generally thought to be the only portion in circulation capable of binding cell receptors and producing the cell effects expected of the hormone. Binding proteins probably modulate the effects of fluctuations in secretory rates by providing a ready source of free hormone when needed.

Drugs can affect the hormone-binding affinity or the quantity of a specific hormone-binding plasma protein. Changes in the amount of available hormone-binding plasma proteins or their hormone affinity affect the hormone's total levels in circulation, but do not necessarily influence the hormone's effects in target cells. For example, estrogen increases cortisol-binding globulin, which in turn increases the amount of total plasma cortisol, but since the concentration of free hormone is unaffected, the biologic effects are unchanged. Phenytoin displaces T_4 from T_4-binding proteins. As a result, the adenohypophysis rapidly adjusts secretion of thyroid-stimulating hormone (TSH) to enable the thyroid to secrete only enough T_4 to maintain normal levels of free T_4. Again, the concentration of total hormone is altered, but because free hormone levels are normal, the biologic effects are normal.

Blood concentrations of active peptide hormones and catecholamines may be difficult to measure accurately. All have very short half-lives in the bloodstream. Peptide hormones also may have prohormones or hormone fragments in the bloodstream that can interfere with assays for the active hormone.

HORMONE RECEPTORS AND MECHANISMS OF HORMONAL ACTION

Only appropriate target cells are affected by all the various hormones in the bloodstream. Target cells have hormone-specific receptors, and these bind circulating hormones that are not bound to plasma proteins. The binding of a hormone to its target cell receptor initiates the intracellular events leading to the final effect characteristic of the hormone on that target organ. The various actions of one hormone, like glucocorticoids, are possible because of the variety of glucocorticoid receptors. Generally, receptors are very hormone-specific, but to a limited extent other hormones or drugs with structures similar to a hormone may bind to receptors. For example, progesterone can occupy glucocorticoid receptors and cause some glucocorticoid-like effects.

Hormone receptors occur in different cell locations, depending on the class of hormone they bind. Receptors for peptide hormones, as well as catecholamines, are on the external surface of the target cell's membrane. Steroid hormone receptors occur in the target cell's cytoplasm. The thyroid hormone receptors are found in the chromatin of the nucleus of target cells.

See reference 2.

Mechanisms of Peptide Hormones and Catecholamine Action

After a catecholamine or peptide hormone attaches to a cell membrane receptor, many but not all activate the enzyme *adenyl cyclase*. The hormone-receptor complex may activate adenyl cyclase through a regulatory protein, called *guanine nucleotide regulatory protein,* which is found in the cell membranes. Activated adenyl cyclase stimulates conversion of adenosine triphosphate (ATP) to cyclic adenosine-3′,5′ monophosphate (cAMP). Cyclic AMP is often referred to as the *second messenger,* and the hormone is the first. Cyclic AMP stimulates the activation of cAMP-dependent protein kinases, which facilitate the phosphorylation of some protein products of the target cell. Phosphodiesterase, which inactivates cAMP (Fig. 2–2), can be inhibited by xanthines such as caffeine and theophylline to prolong hormone-induced effects on cells. Examples of those peptide hormones and catecholamines that stimulate production of adenyl cyclase (and those peptide hormones that do not) are shown in Table 2–3.

Peptide hormones that do not activate cAMP may activate another enzyme like guanylate cyclase or regulate the intracellular concentration of calcium. Guanylate cyclase activates cyclic guanosine monophosphate (cGMP), which, like cAMP, can also stimulate protein kinase activity. Intracellular calcium is known to activate glycogen phosphorylase kinase, cAMP phosphodiesterase, and other hormones after binding to a protein called *calmodulin*. Gastrin, oxytocin, cholecystokinin (CCK), angiotensin, and α-adrenergic catecholamines use calmodulin as their second messenger.

Originally it was thought that peptide hormones and catecholamines did not enter cells, but now it is known that at least some do. The cell mem-

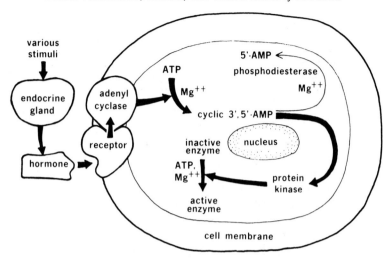

Fig. 2–2. Proposed action of peptide hormones.

brane invaginates and engulfs the hormone-receptor complex in a process called *internalization*. In some cases, it seems that polypeptide hormones may bind to intracellular receptors. The significance of intracellular binding is not yet known.

Table 2–3. Peptide and Catecholamine Hormones Capable and Incapable of Stimulating Adenyl Cyclase

Hormones Capable of Stimulating Adenyl Cyclase	Hormones Incapable of Stimulating Adenyl Cyclase
ACTH	Angiotensin
Calcitonin	Alpha-adrenergic catecholamines
Beta-adrenergic catecholamines	Chorionic somatomammotropin
Chorionic gonadotropin	GH
FSH	Insulin
Glucagon	Oxytocin
LH	Prolactin
Lipotropin	Somatomedin
MSH	Somatostatin
PTH	Gastrin
TRH	CCK
ADH	
TSH	

Modified from Baxter, J.D., and Funder, J.W.: Hormone receptors. N. Engl. J. Med., *301:*1149, 1979.

ACTH = adrenocorticotropic hormone; FSH = follicle-stimulating hormone; LH = luteinizing hormone; MSH = melanocyte-stimulating hormone; PTH = parathyroid hormone; TRH = thyroid releasing hormone; ADH = antidiuretic hormone; TSH = thyroid-stimulating hormone; GH = growth hormone; and CCK = cholecystokinin.

Mechanism of Steroid Action

Steroid hormones are able to pass through target cell membranes by passive diffusion to combine with cytoplasmic hormone receptors. The hormone-receptor complex then moves into the nucleus to bind with the nuclear chromatin. The intranuclear effects regulate specific messenger RNAs (mRNA) by activation or derepression of genes. In turn, mRNAs regulate the rate of target cell protein synthesis (Fig. 2–3).

Mechanism of Thyroid Hormones' Action

Thyroid hormones readily pass into a target cell's cytoplasm and nucleus to bind with receptors in the chromatin. The predominant nuclear receptor for thyroid hormones is for T_3. In fact, most of the T_4 presented to the target cell is converted to T_3 before nuclear binding. Nuclear binding causes changes in the concentrations of specific mRNAs, and by means of these mRNAs hormones mediate the synthesis of target cells' protein products (Fig. 2–4).

Factors That Influence the Number or Affinity of Hormone Receptors

The number of hormone receptors bound with hormones does not necessarily parallel the effects produced. For most steroid and thyroid hormones there is a direct relationship between receptor occupancy and magnitude of response; however, for peptide hormones and catecholamines there are spare receptors at the time of maximum response. The limiting factor in the magnitude of response for peptide hormones and catecholamines seems to be concentrations of protein kinase. "Spare" receptors enhance the speed of the target cell's hormonal response and the cell's sensitivity to low concentrations of the hormone.

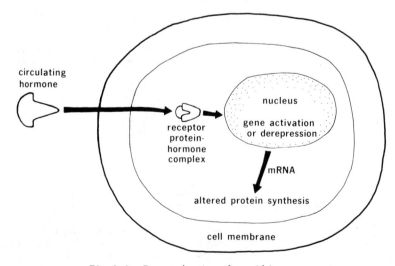

Fig. 2–3. Proposed action of steroid hormones.

Receptors' affinity for a hormone and receptor numbers are not static. The concentration of hormone receptors is affected by genetics, the stage of growth, the stage of the target cell's cycle, and the degree of the target cell's differentiation or transformation. The hormone affinity of target cell receptors is influenced by ionic balance and temperature. Receptors' concentration and affinity are affected by the homologous hormone, heterologous hormones, and antibodies against the receptor.

Frequently, the concentration of a homologous hormone and the concentration of its receptor are in an inverse relationship. When a target cell is exposed to high concentrations of its homologous hormone, it decreases the concentration of its receptors. This is called *down regulation*. In some cases, the desensitivity may be caused by limited post-receptor events. On the other hand, prolactin, gonadotropin-releasing hormone (GnRH), and angiotensin II increase the number of their own receptors. At least one reason why certain hormones must be present to permit another hormone to affect the target cell (the *permissive effect*) is that heterologous hormones can regulate receptor concentrations for other hormones. For example, estrogens increase the receptors for progesterone.

Hormone antagonists are molecules capable of binding to a hormone receptor but incapable of initiating hormone-mediated events. Antagonists do not cause down regulation; therefore, when antagonists are present the hormone response is diminished, but when the antagonist is withdrawn, target cells may be hypersensitive to its primary hormone's induced effects. Some antagonists are actually partial agonists since they produce a hormone-like effect, but the effect is weak in comparison to the normal response to hormone-receptor binding. For example, clomiphene is a weak

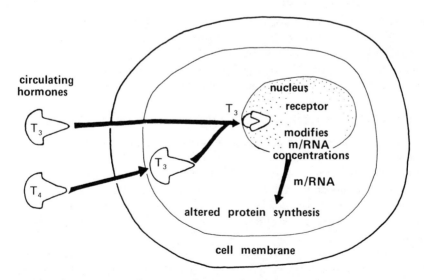

Fig. 2–4. Proposed action of thyroid hormones.

synthetic estrogen that binds to estrogen receptors without causing percep-
tible estrogen-like effects.

It is not known how commonly antibodies are produced against hormone
receptors. Receptors are primarily protein and potentially antigenic. In
humans, there is a rare form of insulin-resistant diabetes mellitus that seems
to be caused by anti-insulin-receptor antibodies. Not all antireceptor antibodies reduce a hormone's effects. In humans, there can also be antibodies
produced against TSH receptors that mimic the effects of TSH-receptor
binding.

The structure of thyroid hormones, catecholamines, and steroid hormones does not vary among mammals, but the structures of peptide hormones do. Usually a peptide hormone's structure, even when the hormone
comes from a different species, is similar enough to bind the recipient's
receptors and produce the same effect as a homologous-source hormone;
however, the difference in structure is often sufficient to cause the heter-
ologous-source hormone to be antigenic to the recipient. To illustrate, the
administration of parenteral bovine GH to dogs causes GH effects, but
repeated administration can cause antibovine GH antibodies. These antibodies may cause inactivation of the administered hormone and local or
systemic adverse reactions.

DEGRADATION AND ELIMINATION OF HORMONES

Hormones may or may not be degraded before their elimination from the
body. Some metabolites of degraded hormones are metabolically active.
Others are inactive. Degradation of hormones may be carried out by serum
proteases, peripheral target cells, the liver, or the kidneys. Some hormones
are eliminated unchanged into the bile or urine. There are also differences
in a hormone's degradation and elimination in different species. In most
species studied, glucocorticoids are mostly degraded to inactive metabolites
before they are eliminated in the urine; however, dogs reduce their urinary
metabolites of glucocorticoids to a greater extent than do humans, and cats
are thought to eliminate glucocorticoids primarily in their bile.

MEASUREMENT OF A HORMONE'S CONCENTRATION

The diagnosis of a clinical endocrinopathy is usually based on finding an
abnormal concentration of a hormone in the bloodstream or urine. Endocrinopathies caused by defective synthesis of hormones, abnormal plasma
protein binding, abnormal concentration of receptors or abnormal hormonal affinity, and post-receptor dysfunction in hormone-mediated events
are generally diagnosed by elimination of more common possibilities and by
deduction.

The ideal endocrine assay does not exist. If it did, it would be inexpensive, simple, rapid, extremely specific for only the hormone in question,
and sensitive to infinitely small concentrations. Fortunately, all the ideal

qualities for an assay are not absolutely necessary to arrive at reliable and useful data for diagnostic purposes.

There are three types of assays for hormones and their metabolites: biologic, chemical, and displacement. *Bioassays* are the oldest, least sensitive, and least specific method. They depend on the evaluation of a response of a living tissue or animal to a hormone-containing substance. Bioassays are often difficult to do, time-consuming, and expensive. An example of a bioassay is the assay of human urinary gonadotropins, in which extracts of urine are injected into female mice. Changes in the uterine weights of the mice are measured to evaluate the quantity of gonadotropins in the urine sample. Because of the complexity of their structure, peptide hormone concentrations could be determined only by bioassays until the 1960s.

Chemical assays became possible for hormones with more simple structures (the steroids, catecholamines, and thyroid hormones) as their structures were elucidated. Chemical methods were usually more specific, more sensitive, quicker, and less expensive than bioassays. Catecholamine metabolites in the urine are still determined by a chemical assay, fluorometry, for the diagnosis of functional neoplasia of the adrenal medulla. Another chemical method, chromatography, serves to validate many immunologic assays for hormones.

Displacement assays are the most sensitive and specific assays known since 1960. Radioimmunoassays (RIAs) have replaced virtually all the older bioassays and most of the chemical assays. Other displacement or immunologic assays now used less commonly than RIAs are the competitive protein binding assay, the enzyme-linked immunoabsorbent assay (ELISA), the enzyme-multiplied immunoassay (EMIT), the magnetic antibody immunoassay (MAIA), and the radioreceptor assay.[3, 12, 13] Displacement tests using radiolabeled hormone to evaluate binding ability to specific binding antibodies, proteins, or receptors are called *radioligand assays*.

Radioimmunoassay

The RIA, which measures a hormone's concentration in the blood, urine, or other body fluids, is done by allowing an unknown concentration of hormone from a patient to compete for binding sites on a specific antibody with a known concentration of a radioisotope-tagged hormone. The measurements are based on changes in radioactive counts measured by a gamma spectrometer. Four elements are required for RIAs: a highly specific antibody against the hormone to be measured, a radiolabeled hormone, a purified hormone to be used as a standard, and a means of separating the bound and free hormone.

Antibodies against hormones are obtained by sensitizing laboratory animals such as rabbits or guinea pigs with repeated injections of the pure hormone. Some hormones, such as steroids, with small molecular structures must be combined with a large protein to be made antigenic. Adjuvants are used to delay absorption of the injection and intensify the response. A desirable antibody has good binding affinity, is specific for the hormone to be tested, and can displace bound radiolabeled hormone with unlabeled hormone.

Radiolabeled hormones are usually tagged with radioactive iodine (^{125}I) or tritium. Oxidizers, chloramine T or lactoperoxidase, are used to label hormones with ^{125}I. ^{131}I is less desirable than ^{125}I because the half-life of ^{131}I is shorter. The labeled hormone is purified by chromatography and frozen with a protective protein for storage.

Standards should be highly purified hormones. It is preferable that the standard comes from the species being tested, particularly if the hormone is a peptide, but if cross-reactivity is sufficient, a hormone from another species may be used. Standards should be prepared in hormone-free serum from the species being tested, so that binding can be compared more effectively with that from unknown samples.

Bound hormone can be separated from free hormone in various ways. Dextran-coated charcoal and double antibody techniques are most common. Dextran-coated charcoal adsorbs only the free hormone. The double antibody technique depends on an anti-gamma globulin antibody to precipitate the antibody (gamma globulin)-bound hormone. Sometimes ammonium sulfate, dioxane, or polyethylene glycol are used to precipitate bound hormone. Talc may be used in a manner similar to dextran-coated charcoal. Chromatographic columns will also separate bound from unbound radiolabeled hormone.

Dilutions of antibody and labeled hormone are incubated with unlabeled hormone standard or fluid with an unknown concentration of hormone from the patient in RIA tubes. The volumes of antibody, standard, labeled hormone, and test fluid are kept constant. Since all four components are not added to all the tubes, the volume of each tube is made equal by the addition of a buffer such as phosphate, tris buffer, or barbital. Duplicate samples with only the antibody and labeled hormone are tested for nonspecific binding. The mixtures are incubated for 1 to 18 hours at 4°C to 22°C, depending on the test and antibody used.

After the bound from the free hormone has been separated, the percentage of bound hormone is determined by counting the bound hormone's radioactivity and subtracting counts of nonspecific binding. Then, the counts bound are divided by the counts added, and the result multiplied by 100. The resulting percentages of bound labeled hormone from known concentrations are plotted on a standard curve (Fig. 2–5). The concentration of hormone in the unknown sample is determined by plotting its counts of radioactivity on the standard curve. Lower counts of radioactivity indicate that greater amounts of unlabeled hormone were present to displace labeled hormone from the antibody.

Competitive protein binding (CPB) and radioreceptor assays are radioligand assays similar to RIAs. They also use displacement of radioactivity to

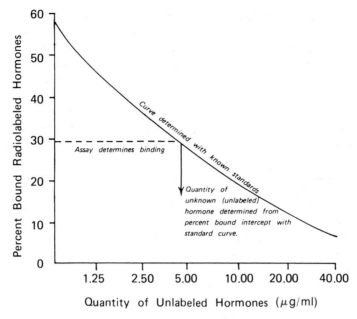

Fig. 2–5. An example of a standard curve for radioimmunoassay.

measure the concentration of a hormone. In place of an RIA antibody, CPB uses a binding protein with high affinity and specificity for the hormone to be measured, and the radioreceptor assay uses hormone receptors in place of an RIA antibody. Radioreceptor assays identify biologically active hormone concentrations, whereas the RIA and CPB methods measure hormones or hormone-like substances that may or may not be biologically active.

See references 5 to 7.

Validation of Assay Methods

An RIA that is valid for one species may not be valid enough to be clinically useful for another species. Some species have interfering substances—that is, nonspecific displacing contaminants—in their serum that affect certain RIA procedures. Multiple forms of the hormone, such as prohormones, active hormones, inactive hormones, and degradation products, may be detected and assumed to be only one form of the hormone. Other species have hormone concentrations that are not within the range of reasonable sensitivity for certain RIA procedures. All RIA procedures should be validated for the hormone to be assayed and the species being assayed.

The quality of an RIA is determined by its precision, accuracy, sensitivity, and specificity (PASS). *Precision* is the degree, based on the coefficient of variation, to which repeated test results on the same sample agree with each other within one assay batch and among other assay batches. Quality control samples should also agree with detected assay results. *Accuracy* is the degree of agreement between the amount of hormone measured and the concentration that was determined by other means considered accurate, such as biologic, competitive protein binding (CPB), fluorometric, or double isotope derivative assays. Accuracy is also evaluated by adding various quantities of pure hormone to test samples and plotting the recovery rates by the assay method. *Sensitivity* records how small the first detectable concentration is above 0.

Specificity is the degree to which the assay measures the hormone desired without detecting similar substances by cross reaction. Specificity can be evaluated by inhibiting the binding of radiolabeled hormone with dilutions of patient samples and known standards in order to compare the slopes produced on the Scatchard plot analysis. Specificity produces parallel slopes. Specificity can also be evaluated by determining the concentrations of known similar substances necessary to inhibit radiolabeled binding by 50%, and by showing that concentrations are affected appropriately by the administration of a known stimulant and inhibitor for the hormone's secretion to a test subject. Specificity is usually most affected by impurities in the radiolabeled hormone or the hormone used to produce antihormone antibodies.

If a clinician wishes to check the validity of a laboratory's endocrine assays, he may ask for data on the precision, accuracy, sensitivity, and specificity for the assay. Alternatively, he may submit dilutions of serum samples, send portions of the same sample coded as if they were separate samples, and send portions of one sample on different days. Other means of assessing the quality of a laboratory assay include submitting samples from a test subject that should be elevated by the administration of a stimulating substance or depressed by an inhibitory substance. Pure hormone or possible interfering substances with similar structures may be added to some samples.

These methods of validating an outside laboratory's assays are time-consuming and expensive. Most laboratories are willing to provide information on request. Those that are not are best avoided. The instructional staff at the teaching hospital of a university can usually direct practitioners to a laboratory that provides validated assays for the hormone desired.

Concern for the validity of an assay within a species or among different species should be greatest when one is attempting to assay the larger peptide hormones or employing the CPB method. The probability of cross-reactivity within a species is greatest when polypeptides are being assayed, because of the structural similarities of other peptide hormones. It is also true that the possibility that an antibody produced against one species of polypeptide hormone will not bind the comparable polypeptide hormone from a different species is greatest during the assay of polypeptides. For example, the structure of TSH is very similar to follicle-stimulating hormone (FSH) and luteinizing hormone (LH). The beta subunit of TSH in dogs is different from that of humans. Antibodies produced against human TSH are very likely to cross-react with FSH and LH in dogs if the antibodies are being used to detect canine TSH. Another possibility is that the antibodies produced against human TSH will not detect canine TSH, LH, or FSH.

Competitive protein binding uses a specific hormone-binding protein. Unfortunately, the specificity and degree of hormone binding with proteins varies among species. Hormone-specific antibodies, if available, are preferable to a CPB assay method.

The validity of an assay depends on the care taken in collecting, storing, and transporting the sample to the laboratory.[11] Common guidelines for the collection, storage, and transport of samples for endocrine assays are found in the appendices.

Although reasonable accuracy is the most important criterion in selecting a laboratory to do clinical endocrine assays, it is by no means the only desirable quality. Clinical endocrine assays are a means to an end, not an end in themselves. Laboratories should be rapid and reliable in reporting results. Costs should be reasonable. Requested sample sizes should be minimal. Laboratory personnel may help only in general interpretations of the results; the clinical diagnosis for a particular patient is the responsibility of the attending clinician. Laboratory reports may include interpretative guidelines, but these should not be thought to indicate conclusively the clinical diagnosis of a patient.

Finally, because all urine, serum, and plasma samples sent to a reference laboratory are subject to leaking in transit, being lost, and other misfortunes, clinicians should routinely freeze and store duplicates or aliquots of samples sent to the laboratory until results are received.

See references 4, 8, and 10.

Stimulation and Suppression Tests

Measurement of the serum or plasma *baseline (resting) levels* of hormones cannot always separate normal subjects from those with an endocrinopathy. Baseline blood levels can fluctuate in response to environmental, psychic, circadian, and drug-induced elements and can also be influenced by age, breed, and other factors. A random blood sample for baseline hormone levels may not be representative of the levels generally present. Urine samples obtained from 24-hour collections are not affected by sudden transient fluctuations of blood hormone levels, but 24-hour urine collections are difficult to obtain from house-trained pets. In addition, production levels of many hormones cannot be assessed by urine samples.

Rather than taking multiple baseline samples to determine the mean level of a hormone, the clinician can use stimuli or suppressants of an endocrine organ's hormones to evaluate whether the response and the degree of the response are within normal limits. Suppression tests can help show whether

Table 2–4. Example Stimulation and Suppression Tests

Hormone	Stimulation Test	Suppression Test
ACTH	Metyrapone ADH Insulin infusion	Dexamethasone
ADH	Dehydration Saline infusion	Water loading
Calcitonin	Pentagastrin Calcium infusion	EDTA infusion
Catecholamines	Glucagon Tyramine	Phentolamine
Cortisol	ACTH	Dexamethasone
Estrogen	FSH	Testosterone
FSH/LH	Clomiphene GnRH	Estrogen Testosterone
GH	Insulin infusion Clonidine Arginine L-Dopa	Glucose
Glucagon	Arginine Alanine	Glucose
Insulin	Glucose Tolbutamine Glucagon Arginine	Fasting
Prolactin	TRH Perphenazine	L-Dopa
PTH	EDTA infusion Phosphate infusion	Calcium infusion Thiazide
Renin	Furosemide	Saline infusion
T_4/T_3	TSH	T_4 or T_3
Testosterone	LH (ICSH)	Estrogen
TSH	TRH	T_4 or T_3

ACTH = adrenocorticotropic hormone; ADH = antidiuretic hormone; FSH = follicle-stimulating hormone; LH = luteinizing hormone; GnRH = gonadotropin-releasing hormone; GH = growth hormone; TRH = thyroid-releasing hormone; PTH = parathyroid hormone; T_4 = thyroxine; T_3 = triiodothyronine; TSH = thyroid-stimulating hormone; ICSH = interstitial cell-stimulating hormone.

partial or complete autonomy is present in hyperfunctional endocrinopathies. Stimulation tests can help confirm the diagnosis of a hypofunctional endocrinopathy and assess the degree of hypofunction. Examples of stimulation and suppression tests are given in Table 2–4.

See reference 1.

Inappropriate Hormone Levels

Stimulation and suppression of endocrine organs occur continuously in vivo. When the level of the primary endogenous stimulus or suppressant can be measured along with the level of the affected hormone, a comparison of the two values can be of diagnostic value. For example, high plasma levels of parathyroid hormone (PTH) are inappropriate if the serum calcium level is high. In addition, serum glucose-to-insulin ratios are used to diagnose insulin-secreting tumors when insulin levels are inappropriately high in comparison to serum glucose levels.

REFERENCES

1. Alsever, R.N., and Gotlin, R.W.: Handbook of Endocrine Tests in Adults and Children. 2nd Ed. Chicago, Year Book Medical Publishers, 1978.
2. Baxter, J.D., and Funder, J.W.: Hormone receptors. N. Engl. J. Med., *301:*1149, 1979.
3. Donne, C.S., and Wildgoose, W.H.: Magnetic antibody immunoassay thyroid function tests in general practice. Vet. Rec., *115:*79, 1984.
4. Hafs, H.D., et al.: Guidelines for radioimmunoassays. J. Anim. Sci., *46:*927, 1977.
5. Jaffe, B.M., and Behrman, H.R.: Methods of Hormone Radioimmunoassay. 2nd Ed. New York, Academic Press/Grune & Stratton, 1978.
6. Jubiz, W.: Endocrinology. A Logical Approach for Clinicians. New York, McGraw-Hill, 1979.
7. Korenman, S.G., Granner, D.K., and Sherman, B.M.: Endocrine Disease (Practical Diagnosis). Boston, Houghton Mifflin, 1978.
8. Malecki, J.C.: Radioimmunoassay of equine serum for thyroxine: reference values (a selected report) (Letter). Am. J. Vet. Res., *40:*455, 1979.
9. Moore-Ede, M.C., Czeisler, C.A., and Richardson, G.S.: Circadian timekeeping in health and disease. Part 1. Basic properties of circadian pacemakers. N. Engl. J. Med., *309:*469, 1983.
10. Reimers, T.J., et al.: Validation of radioimmunoassays for triiodothyronine, thyroxine, and hydrocortisone (cortisol) in canine, feline, and equine sera. Am. J. Vet. Res., *42:*2106, 1981.
11. Reimers, T.J., et al.: Effects of storage, hemolysis, and freezing and thawing on concentrations of thyroxine, cortisol and insulin in blood samples. Proc. Soc. Exp. Biol. Med., *170:*509, 1982.
12. Voller, A., Bidwell, D.E., and Bartlett, A.: Enzyme immunoassays in diagnostic medicine. Theory and practice. Bull. W.H.O., *53:*55, 1976.
13. Watts, N.B., and Keffer, J.H.: Practical Endocrine Diagnosis. 2nd Ed. Philadelphia, Lea & Febiger, 1978.

Section II

THE ENDOCRINE BRAIN

3

The Endocrine Brain and Clinical Tests of Its Function

The body's ability to adapt to changes in its internal and external environment depends on the functional integrity of the nervous and endocrine systems. These two systems respond to many environmental stimuli by means of coordinated responses. Nowhere else in the body is the interrelationship between the nervous and endocrine systems more anatomically or functionally intimate than in "the endocrine brain," consisting of the hypothalamus, adenohypophysis, neurohypophysis, and pineal body.

REGIONAL ANATOMY

The *hypothalamus* (Lat., below the inner chamber) consists of the rostral portion of the diencephalon and is divided by the third ventricle. It lies just cranial to the interpeduncular nuclei, mammillary bodies, and foramen of Monro. The optic chiasm is ventral to the cranial portion of the hypothalamus.

The *neurohypophysis* (Lat., innervated lower growth) is a ventral extension of the hypothalamus. Attached to the neurohypophysis is the *adenohypophysis* (Lat., glandular lower growth), which has the epithelium of the oral cavity as its origin. The adenohypophysis and neurohypophysis are collectively termed the *hypophysis* (Lat., lower growth), or more commonly by clinicians, the *pituitary* (Lat., secreting mucus—the name was derived from the theory that the pituitary drained waste material from the brain into the nasopharynx).

The *pineal* (Lat., shaped like a pine cone) or epiphysis is a protuberance from the caudal commissure and habenular commissure, which form part of the roof of the third ventricle. It lies ventral to the corpus callosum and caudal to the interthalamic adhesion. The pituitary-midbrain relationships are illustrated in Figures 3–1, 3–2, and 3–3.

DEVELOPMENT OF THE ENDOCRINE BRAIN

The Hypothalamus

The hypothalamus develops from the alar plates of the ventrolateral walls of the diencephalon. Both clearly delineated and ill-defined nuclei arise and become centers that regulate visceral functions.

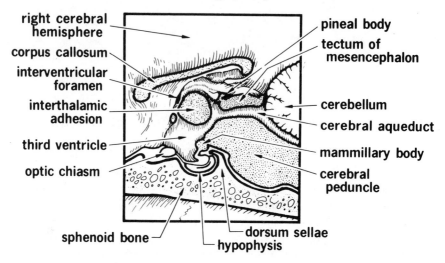

right cerebral hemisphere
corpus callosum
interventricular foramen
interthalamic adhesion
third ventricle
optic chiasm

pineal body
tectum of mesencephalon
cerebellum
cerebral aqueduct
mammillary body
cerebral peduncle

sphenoid bone
dorsum sellae
hypophysis

Fig. 3–1. Pituitary-midbrain relationships. (Adapted from Evans, H.E., and Christiansen, G.C.: Miller's Anatomy of the Dog. 2nd Ed. Philadelphia, W.B. Saunders Co., 1979.)

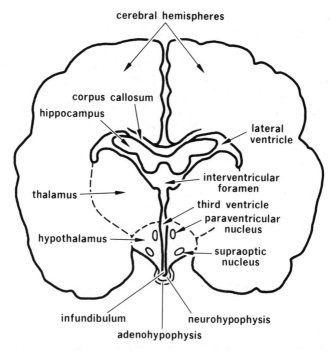

cerebral hemispheres

corpus callosum
hippocampus

lateral ventricle

thalamus

interventricular foramen
third ventricle
paraventricular nucleus

hypothalamus

supraoptic nucleus

infundibulum
adenohypophysis
neurohypophysis

Fig. 3–2. Diagrammatic transverse view of the brain through the hypothalamus and pituitary.

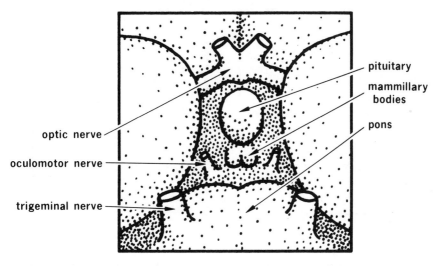

Fig. 3–3. Ventral-dorsal view of the pituitary.

The Pituitary

The pituitary is a fusion of the adenohypophysis and neurohypophysis. The neurohypophysis develops as a ventral evagination of the diencephalon, while the adenohypophysis begins as a dorsal pouch of the oral cavity, *Rathke's pouch*. The adenohypophysis migrates dorsally through the mesoderm of what becomes the sphenoid bone to partially surround the neurohypophysis (Fig. 3–4). Its relationship to the neurohypophysis is like a fist (the neurohypophysis) pushed into a balloon (the adenohypophysis); therefore, the anterior and posterior pituitary are somewhat inappropriate terms for the dog's and cat's adenohypophysis and neurohypophysis. The sphenoid cavity, which contains the adult pituitary, is called the *sella turcica* (Lat., turkish saddle). Its caudal lip over the pituitary is called the *dorsum sellae* (Fig. 3–5).

See reference 61.

The Pineal

The pineal body develops from the caudal portion of the roof plate of the diencephalon. It is large in young animals, but involutes before puberty.

DEVELOPMENTAL ANOMALIES OF THE ENDOCRINE BRAIN

Developmental anomalies, particularly cystic Rathke's pouch or patent hypophyseal ducts, are rather common. Approximately 70% of brachycephalic dogs have patent hypophyseal ducts (pharyngeal hypophysis). Clinical disorders stemming from these anomalies are infrequent. Occasionally cysts are very large, producing adenohypophyseal, neurohypophyseal, or even hypothalamic deficiency disorders by compression. An enlarging

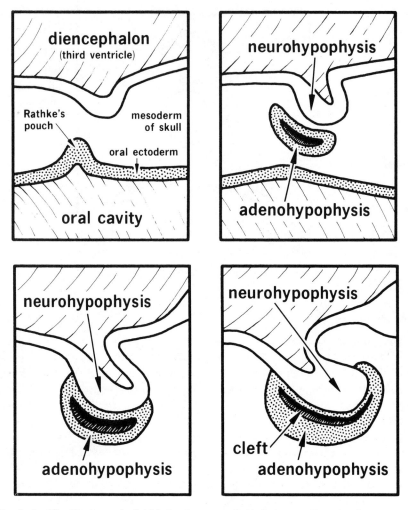

Fig. 3–4. The Pituitary. *A*, Initial development. *B*, Early-intermediate development. *C*, Late-intermediate development. *D*, Completed development.

cystic mass may be caused by a neoplastic proliferation, craniopharyngioma, arising from primordial pituitary structures. Craniopharyngiomas may be intrasellar or suprasellar.

See references 1, 60, and 84.

STRUCTURE AND FUNCTION OF THE ENDOCRINE BRAIN

The Hypothalamus

The hypothalamus has three general functions: (1) the production of hormones to be transferred to the neurohypophysis for release into the general circulatory system; (2) the production of releasing and inhibiting

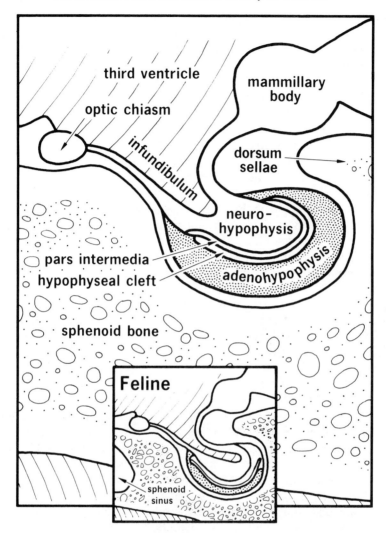

Fig. 3–5. The normal canine pituitary.

factors (hormones) for the regulation of adenohypophyseal activity; and (3) a group of visceral function regulatory activities only indirectly related to the endocrine system. There are at least 14 known neural pathways to and 14 known regulatory functions of the hypothalamus.[38]

Several pathways link the hypothalamus to the limbic system, which encompasses the amygdala, hippocampus, and septal nuclei. Together they are concerned with sexual behavior, motivation, and the emotions of rage and fear. Autonomic responses are indirectly affected by limbic-hypothalamic activity such as changes in heart rate, pupil size, and urinary and gastrointestinal sphincter function.

Only two nuclei, the supraoptic and paraventricular, are well demarcated with routine stains. Other nuclei and activity centers are less clearly delineated, although immunohistochemistry has allowed centers of other activities to be discovered. Axons from the supraoptic and paraventricular nuclei extend down to the neurohypophysis. These axons are called the *hypothalamohypophyseal tract* and transport the hormones *oxytocin* (Lat., rapid birth) and *antidiuretic hormone* (ADH) (vasopressin).

In addition to oxytocin and ADH, the hypothalamus produces at least seven hormones (factors) that stimulate or inhibit the release of adenohypophyseal hormones. Hypothalamic hormones that control adenohypophyseal functions are listed in Table 3–1. Hypothalamic releasing and inhibiting hormones are transported from the *median eminence* of the ventral hypothalamus to the adenohypophysis by the *portal hypophyseal vessels,* which begin and end with fenestrated capillary beds (Fig. 3–6). The median eminence is outside the blood-brain barrier.

Certain biogenic amines (dopamine, norepinephrine, epinephrine, serotonin, and histamine) and others (acetylcholine and substance P) are neurotransmitters that influence hypothalamic releasing and inhibiting hormones. Dopamine is not only a neurotransmitter, but also a hormone inhibiting the release of prolactin. Higher and lower centers in the brain can modify the secretion of hypothalamic releasing and inhibiting hormones for the adenohypophysis by neurotransmission.

Several hormones found in the hypothalamus are found throughout the brain, spinal cord, and elsewhere in the body. For instance, thyrotropin-releasing hormone (TRH), bombesin, secretin, somatostatin, substance P, cholecystokinin-pancreozymin (CCK-PZ), vasoactive intestinal peptide (VIP), and insulin are also found in the pancreatic islets or small intestines. In the retina are found TRH, somatostatin, GnRH, VIP, CCK-PZ, substance P, and glucagon. Visceral functions regulated by the hypothalamus include parasympathetic and sympathetic responses, sleep, circadian rhythms, hunger, thirst, and regulation of temperature.

Some clinicians think that the cranial hypothalamus has a parasympathetic center; however, the only parasympathetic response that can be unquestionably attributed to the hypothalamus is contraction of the urinary bladder.[38] The lateral portions of the hypothalamus seem to affect the sym-

Table 3–1. Hypothalamic Hormones Controlling the Adenohypophysis

---

Corticotropin-releasing hormone (CRH)
Thyrotropin-releasing hormone (TRH)
Growth hormone-releasing hormone (GH-RH, GRH)
Growth hormone-inhibiting hormone (GH-IH, somatostatin)
Gonadotropin-releasing hormone (GnRH, LHRH*)
Prolactin-releasing hormone (PRH)
Prolactin-inhibiting hormone (PIH, dopamine)

---

* LHRH = luteinizing-hormone-releasing hormone.

pathetic responses of increased blood pressure, piloerection, and pupillary dilatation. Neural pathways from the cerebral cortex, which cause cholinergic sympathetic vasodilatation, pass through the hypothalamus. The dorsomedial and caudal areas of the hypothalamus can increase the release of catecholamines from the adrenal medulla.

Lesions of the caudal hypothalamus can cause prolonged sleep; however, dysfunction of the dorsal hypothalamus will induce sleep. These effects occur because fibers from the reticular activating system pass through the hypothalamus to reach the thalamus and cerebral cortex.

The *suprachiasmatic nuclei* in the cranioventral hypothalamus control most of the circadian (nyctohemeral) and seasonal rhythms, especially secretions of ACTH and gonadotropins.[72] Light-dark cycles are the best understood stimuli for programming circadian and seasonal rhythms.[91] The suprachiasmatic nuclei receive light-dark information from the eyes via the retinohypothalamic fibers.

The lateral hypothalamus contains the *feeding center,* which stimulates eating, and in the ventromedial nucleus of the hypothalamus is the *satiety center,* which produces the feeling of dietary sufficiency. Destruction of the feeding center causes anorexia, whereas destruction of the satiety center causes hypothalamic obesity. Lesions of the amygdaloid nuclei can also

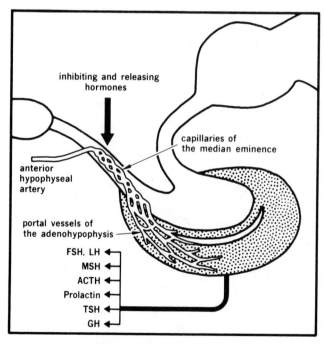

Fig. 3–6. Transport of hypothalamic control hormones for the adenohypophysis. FSH = follicle-stimulating hormone; LH = luteinizing hormone; MSH = melanocyte-stimulating hormone; ACTH = adrenocorticotropic hormone; TSH = thyroid-stimulating hormone; GH = growth hormone.

produce hyperphagia. The satiety center is thought to monitor blood glucose levels with specialized cells, called *glucostats,* which are unique brain cells that require insulin to permit the entrance of glucose.

The center for thirst is caudolateral to the paraventricular nuclei. It may be stimulated by angiotensin II, a hormone generated in response to hypovolemia, and by *osmoreceptors,* cells in the hypothalamus activated by hyperosmolality of the plasma. Lesions of the thirst center cause adipsia, leading to dehydration and hypernatremia.

The cranial portion of the hypothalamus can elevate the body's temperature and activate normal responses to heat such as panting. The caudal aspect of the hypothalamus can lower the body's temperature and activate normal responses to cold such as shivering. Miscellaneous functions of the hypothalamus are illustrated in Figure 3–7.

See references 31, 38, and 85.

The Neurohypophysis

The neurohypophysis, also called the *pars nervosa* of the pituitary, is a storage area for ADH and oxytocin received from the hypothalamus by axon flow. The bulk of the neurohypophysis consists of pituiticytes, a special form of microglial cells. The neurohypophysis is supplied with an independent network of capillaries into which ADH and oxytocin are released by appropriate stimuli.

See reference 38.

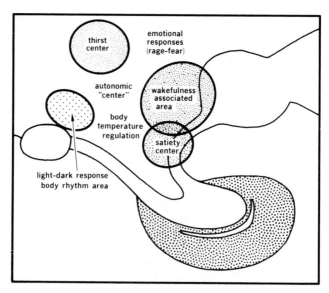

Fig. 3–7.   Miscellaneous functions of the hypothalamus.

The Adenohypophysis

The adenohypophysis is composed of three portions: the *pars tuberalis* (stalk portion), *pars intermedia* (intermediate lobe fused to the neurohypophysis), and *pars distalis* (the bulk of the glandular pituitary). The cells of the adenohypophysis are arranged in interlacing cords separated by profuse sinusoidal fenestrated capillaries.

Although the adenohypophysis may produce more than 14 active substances, 6 hormones, including growth hormone (GH), thyroid-stimulating hormone (TSH), luteinizing hormone (LH), follicle-stimulating hormone (FSH), prolactin, and adrenocorticotropic hormone (ACTH), are the most important (those discussed in this chapter are listed in Table 3–2). The cell types have been classically identified by light microscopy and staining characteristics with acidic and basic dyes. Acidophils secrete either GH or prolactin. Those that secrete GH stain with eosin or Orange G, and those that secrete prolactin stain with erythrosin or carbimoisine. Basophils that stain with periodic acid-Schiff (PAS) and aldehyde thionin (or alcian blue) secrete FSH, LH, TSH, β-lipotropin (β-LPH), and ACTH. Cells secreting ACTH stain best with PAS, TSH-secreting cells stain best with aldehyde thionin, and gonadotropin-secreting cells stain an intermediate color. Chromophobes, which do not stain with acidic or basic dyes, secrete ACTH and β-LPH.

In humans, 40% of the adenohypophyseal cells are acidophils, 10% are basophils, and 50% are chromophobes. Today, five different adenohypophyseal cells can be identified by immunohistochemistry and electron microscopy[24–28, 43, 89] (these are listed in Table 3–3). TSH, LH, and FSH are glycoproteins—that is, they contain a carbohydrate. The others are simple polypeptides. TSH, LH, FSH, and ACTH regulate target organs whose secretions feed back to the pituitary and hypothalamus to suppress the tropic hormone's secretion. GH and prolactin are under tonic inhibition from the hypothalamus, and their cells of origin do not receive negative feedback from their target cells. The function of β-LPH is not known, but it is a precursor of endorphins, natural analgesics produced by the brain, and enkephalins, a form of neurotransmitter substances.

See references 6, 17, 38, 40 and 74.

Table 3–2. Adenohypophyseal Hormones

Thyroid-stimulating hormone (TSH, thyrotropin)
Adrenocorticotropic hormone (ACTH, corticotropin)
Growth hormone (GH, somatotropin, STH)
Follicle-stimulating hormone (FSH)
Luteinizing hormone (LH, interstitial cell-stimulating hormone [ICSH])
Prolactin (mammotropin)
Lipotropin (LPH)—β, γ
β-endorphin
Melanocyte-stimulating hormone (MSH)—α, β, γ

Table 3–3.   Adenohypophyseal Cells and Their Hormones

Cells	Hormones Produced
Thyrotrope	TSH
Corticotrope	ACTH and β-LPH
Gonadotrope	FSH and LH
Mammotrope	Prolactin
Somatotrope	GH

TSH = thyroid-stimulating hormone; ACTH = adrenocorticotropic hormone; β-LPH = lipotropin hormone; FSH = follicle-stimulating hormone; LH = luteinizing hormone; and GH = growth hormone.

The Pineal Body

The pineal is made up predominantly of pinealocytes that contain norepinephrine and serotonin. Pinealocytes are surrounded and supported by astrocytes. The significance of the pineal body, thought by Descartes to be the seat of the soul, even now is unknown for mammals. It receives neurotransmissions from the retina and the suprachiasmatic nucleus of the hypothalamus, and it produces gonadotropin-inhibiting substances. The pineal body atrophies before puberty, but the cause and reason for its atrophy are not known.

Melatonin, N-acetyl-5-methoxytryptamine, is an indole produced by the pineal when stimulated by a dark environment. Its levels are in a circadian rhythm entrained to the light-dark cycle. Synthesis of melatonin from tryptophan via serotonin and melatonin's secretion are also increased by norepinephrine. Melatonin lightens the skin of larval amphibians by causing aggregation of melanophore granules. Mammals do not have melanophores, and melatonin has no known effect in mammals.

See reference 38.

HORMONES PRODUCED BY THE HYPOTHALAMUS FOR RELEASE BY THE NEUROHYPOPHYSIS

Oxytocin and ADH are octapeptides (nonapeptides, if each half cystine is counted as one amino acid) produced by paraventricular nuclei and supraoptic nuclei (Fig. 3–8). Most oxytocin comes from the paraventricular nuclei, and most ADH comes from the supraoptic nuclei. ADH, its neurophysin, and a glycopeptide are produced from *prepropressophysin*. Oxytocin and its neurophysin are produced from *preprooxyphysin*. After production, oxytocin and ADH move down the axons of the hypothalamo-hypophyseal tract, bound to polypeptides with a molecular weight of about 10,000 called *neurophysins*, which are also produced by the supraoptic and paraventricular nuclei. Neurophysin complexes of oxytocin or ADH can be stained with Gomori stain. The granules apparent with this staining are called *Herring bodies*. Neurophysins are released into the general circulation with oxytocin and ADH from the neurohypophysis.

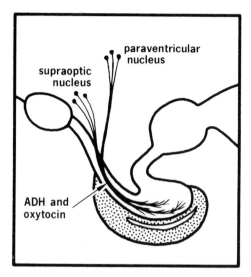

Fig. 3–8. Hormone transport to the neurohypophysis.

Oxytocin

After stimulation by a neuroendocrine reflex initiated by suckling of the mammae, oxytocin causes contraction of the myoepithelial cells of the mammae to cause ejection of preformed milk. It also causes contraction of the uterus if the uterus has been preconditioned by estrogens. Oxytocin effects on the uterus are inhibited by progesterone. Dilatation of the cervix during early parturition causes secretion of oxytocin and subsequent enhanced uterine contractions.

Natural and synthetic oxytocin is commercially available as injections (Pitocin, Syntocinon, Oxytocin Injection, and P.O.P.) or nasal spray (Syntocinon Nasal Spray).

Antidiuretic Hormone (Vasopressin)

ADH, whose molecular weight is about 1080, inhibits diuresis by increasing the permeability of the distal convoluted tubule and collecting ducts of the kidney so that water (up to 20% of the glomerular filtration rate [GFR]) is reabsorbed into the hypertonic interstitium of the kidney. Without ADH, or its effects, the urine produced is voluminous and hypotonic to the plasma (hyposthenuric polyuria). This condition is called *diabetes insipidus*.

Stimuli and inhibitors of ADH secretion are presented in Table 3–4. Drugs stimulating secretion of ADH include nicotine, morphine, barbiturates, and chlorpropamide. Drugs inhibiting secretion of ADH include alcohol, phenytoin, and opiate antagonists (butorphanol and oxilorphan). In large amounts, ADH stimulates secretion of ACTH. An ADH response test using changes produced in serum cortisol levels has been recom-

Table 3–4.   Factors Affecting Secretion of Antidiuretic Hormone

Stimuli	Inhibitors
Increased plasma osmolality	Exposure to cold temperature
Hypovolemia	Decreased plasma osmolality
Pain	Hypervolemia
Exercise	Drugs*
Drugs*	

* For further discussion, see p. 47.

mended as a test of hypothalamic-pituitary function. An increase in serum cortisol after administration of ADH indicates normal adenohypophyseal function.

Hypovolemia-hypotension and plasma hyperosmolality are the primary causes of the secretion of ADH. Osmolality of the plasma is monitored by osmoreceptors in the hypothalamus associated with the thirst center. Hypovolemia-hypotension is monitored by low-pressure receptors in the pulmonary vessels, great veins, and atria of the heart. Hypovolemia-hypotension also causes increases in the levels of angiotensin II, and these increased levels can directly stimulate the paraventricular and supraoptic nuclei to produce ADH. Plasma concentrations of ADH in dogs under normal conditions are about 0.5 to 4 pg/ml. Its serum half-life is 5 to 10 minutes, and it is not bound to plasma proteins. Some ADH is excreted unchanged in the urine.

Natural and synthetic ADH is available commercially for the diagnosis and treatment of diabetes insipidus. Natural ADH (Pitressin) from cows and pigs is available as a water-soluble extract or a tannate in oil for injection. Dogs, cats, horses, and humans produce arginine-ADH, whereas pigs produce lysine ADH; therefore, natural ADH of porcine origin is more foreign antigenically than a source of arginine ADH. Synthetic lysine-ADH (Diapid), dD-arginine vasopressin, and desmopressin acetate (DDAVP) are commercially available as nasal sprays for humans.

HORMONES PRODUCED BY THE HYPOTHALAMUS TO MODIFY ADENOHYPOPHYSEAL SECRETION

The chemical substances produced by the hypothalamus to modify the secretion of the adenohypophysis have been called factors because their actions were recognized before their structures were known. The structure of six of these factors—growth-hormone-releasing hormone (GRH), corticotropin-releasing hormone (CRH), thyrotropin-releasing hormone (TRH), gonadotropin-releasing hormone (GnRH), prolactin-inhibiting hormone (PIH), and growth hormone-inhibiting hormone (GH-IH) are now known and generally referred to as hormones (to prevent confusion, all hypothalamic releasing and inhibiting factors in this chapter will be referred to as hormones).

See references 64 and 65.

Thyrotropin-Releasing Hormone

TRH was the first hypothalamic releasing hormone to be synthesized. It is a tripeptide, pyroglutamyl-histidyl-proline. About 75% of the hormone occurs outside the hypothalamus, particularly in the gastrointestinal tract, spinal cord, retina, pancreatic islets, reproductive tract, and placenta, but hypothalamic concentrations of TRH are greater than elsewhere in the body. Produced in the cranial aspects of the median eminence near the dorsomedial nuclei, TRH causes release of TSH and can cause the release of prolactin. There is some evidence that it has therapeutic effects when used for spinal trauma. It has antidepressant effects, but they are only transient and partial.

Some opiate peptides' action seem to be blocked by TRH. The hormone's action on the adenohypophysis is blocked by pharmacologic doses of glucocorticoids. Secretion of TRH is increased by dopamine, norepinephrine, histamine, and serotonin. High serum levels of T_3 and T_4 inhibit the release of TRH. Protirelin (Thypinone) is a synthetic form of TRH used to assess pituitary-thyroid function.

Gonadotropin-Releasing Hormone

The structure of GnRH, a decapeptide, was elucidated soon after the synthesis of TRH. It originates from the cranial hypothalamus and is found in and near the preoptic area. FSH and LH are released by GnRH. Endogenous secretion of GnRH is pulsatile. Intermittent stimulation by GnRH seems more effective in eliciting secretion of gonadotropins from the adenohypophysis than are persistently elevated blood levels of GnRH. The secretion of GnRH is affected by circadian and seasonal rhythms that vary with species. Secretion of GnRH is increased by dopamine, norepinephrine, and epinephrine. Serotonin decreases the secretion of GnRH. The cause for the initial increase in secretion of GnRH associated with the onset of puberty is not known. The hypothalamus may be genetically coded to detect a certain body weight or body composition to initiate puberty.

Gonadorelin (Cystorelin) is a synthetic GnRH used in cattle for the treatment of cystic ovaries. Although its effectiveness is no greater than LH for the treatment of cystic ovaries, administration of GnRH is less likely to induce antibody formation. In other instances, the induction of GnRH antibodies against endogenous GnRH is being attempted in the hope of producing a safe injectable contraceptive.

See references 7, 8, 53, 54, 66, and 71.

Somatostatin (Growth Hormone-Inhibiting Hormone)

Somatostatin, like TRH, is found throughout the brain and spinal cord. It is also located in the D cells of pancreatic islets in concentrations that equal those of the hypothalamus, but some is present in the peripheral ganglia, stomach, small intestines, and parafollicular cells of the thyroid. Somatostatin is a tetradecapeptide with a disulfide bridge. It is the growth hormone-inhibiting hormone. It is found throughout the brain, spinal cord, and gastrointestinal tract. In the gastrointestinal system it inhibits insulin, gastrin, secretin, VIP, motilin, glucagon, and pancreatic polypeptide. Its primary function in the pancreas seems to be the paracrine inhibition of glucagon secretion.

Somatostatin can inhibit the secretion of other peptide hormones such as TSH and ACTH. Its biologic half-life is about 1 minute. Hypothalamic secretion of somatostatin occurs predominantly in the cranial hypothalamus above the optic chiasm. Dopamine and serotonin may inhibit secretion of somatostatin in the hypothalamus. Somatomedin C (insulin-like growth factor I) stimulates the secretion of hypothalamic somatostatin.

See references 86 and 87.

Corticotropin-Releasing Hormone

CRH was identified in 1981.[97] It is a polypeptide with 41 amino acids secreted by the paraventricular nuclei. Its secretion is pulsatile, with a circadian rhythm that depends on the hours of wakefulness characteristic of the species and the individual. In dogs, CRH seems to be secreted in the hours immediately before awakening. Its secretion is stimulated by ADH, epinephrine, and serotonin, and may be inhibited by the serotonin antagonist, cyproheptadine. CRH secretion is also inhibited by cortisol and other glucocorticoids. However, the stresses of trauma, pain, apprehension, nausea, fever, or hypoglycemia can override negative feedback suppression of CRH-ACTH by glucocorticoids. CRH stimulates ACTH and β-lipotropic hormone (β-LPH) secretion from the pars distalis.

See references 38 and 47.

Growth Hormone-Releasing Hormone

GRH is a polypeptide containing 44 amino acids. Its secretion is stimulated by hypoglycemia, amino acids, dopamine, serotonin, melatonin, norepinephrine, and epinephrine. The primary site of hypothalamic secretion of GRH is not known.

See references 38 and 47.

Dopamine (Prolactin-Inhibiting Hormone)

The neurotransmitter-catecholamine, dopamine, is PIH. It is found in the brain, sympathetic ganglion, and adrenal medulla. In the hypothalamus, most dopamine comes from the arcuate nuclei. Dopamine secretion is inhibited by chlorpromazine and reserpine and is stimulated by serotonin. Ergot derivatives such as bromocryptine are agonists of dopamine receptors that mimic dopamine's effects.

See also reference 38.

Prolactin-Releasing Hormone

The structure of PRH is not known. Its secretion seems to be stimulated by serotonin.

See reference 38.

HORMONES FROM THE ADENOHYPOPHYSIS

Nine well established hormones are produced by the pars distalis and pars intermedia of the adenohypophysis (Table 3–2). All are polypeptides. Three (TSH, FSH, LH) are glycoproteins, carbohydrate-containing polypeptides. The carbohydrate portions increase the activity of TSH, LH, and FSH because their degradation is slowed. Adenohypophyseal hormones are referred to as -tropic (Gr., turning) or -trophic (Gr., nourishing) hormones because they stimulate the secretory activities of target organs to attain and maintain normal fertility, growth, milk production, response to stress, and various aspects of energy balance and metabolism. Deficiencies of tropic hormones are called *secondary hypofunctions*.

Thyroid-Stimulating Hormone

A glycoprotein with 211 amino acid residues, plus carbohydrates produced by thyrotropes, TSH has a molecular weight of about 28,000. It has two subunits, α and β. The α-subunit of TSH has amino acid components identical to those of FSH and LH, but the carbohydrate portions differ. The β-subunit's structure is all that is necessary for the normal biological effects of TSH, but the β-subunit's structure varies among species. For example, the TSH of monkeys is not immunologically similar to human TSH. Although bovine TSH is biologically effective in all domestic animals, human assays of TSH by RIA may not be valid for assaying canine or feline TSH.[9, 67] However, one assay of TSH using antihuman TSH antibodies has been reported valid for the measurement of canine TSH.[59]

The biologic half-life of TSH is about 60 minutes in humans. It is secreted in bursts that decline in amount throughout the daytime. The mean secretion of TSH is stimulated by TRH and inhibited by T_3, T_4, glucocorticoids, dopamine, somatostatin, and stress. TSH is eliminated primarily by the kidney. The placenta in humans produces a TSH-like substance now thought to be chorionic gonadotropin, a glycoprotein with a structure similar to TSH. The follicular cells of the thyroid are the target cells for TSH. Thyroid secretions and thyroid growth are stimulated by TSH. Bovine origin TSH (Thyropar, Dermathycin) is commercially available for diagnostic purposes.

See reference 38.

Adrenocorticotropic Hormone

A polypeptide of 39 amino acids with a molecular weight of about 4500, ACTH is hydrolyzed from a prohormone, *pro-opiomelanocortin* (POMC), in the corticotropes (Fig. 3–9). Beta-LPH, γ-melanocyte-stimulating hormone (MSH), and an N-terminal peptide are also produced as a result of the hydrolysis of POMC. Beta-LPH is a large polypeptide with 91 amino acid residues that can be degraded to γ-LPH and β-endorphin. Beta-MSH is a fragment of γ-LPH, and met-enkephalin, a neurotransmitter, is a fragment of β-endorphin. In the pars intermedia, ACTH can fragment into α-MSH and corticotropin-like intermediate lobe peptide (CLIP). Like α-MSH, ACTH can stimulate melanin synthesis, but its effectiveness is only one thirtieth as effective as that of α-MSH. The melanocyte-stimulating effect of ACTH is the cause of pigmentation of scars in dogs, which may occur in response to the discontinuation of glucocorticoid therapy. Circulating ACTH is primarily produced in the pars distalis. Beta-MSH, CLIP, γ-LPH, and β-endorphins are produced in and primarily secreted from the pars intermedia. Their secretion from the pars intermedia is controlled by serotoninergic and dopaminergic fibers from the hypothalamus. The pro-hormone POMC is also produced in the hypothalamus and other portions of the nervous system.

The first (N-terminal) 23 amino acids of ACTH produce all its biologic effects. These 23 amino acids are the same in humans, cattle, pigs, and sheep. Presumably it is the same in all companion animals. The sequence of the remaining 16 amino acids vary among species. The serum half-life of ACTH is about 10 minutes.

The secretion of ACTH is pulsatile. In dogs, its mean level is highest in the early morning hours, and in cats, levels of ACTH are greatest in the evening hours. The circadian rhythm is not as pronounced in dogs and cats as it is in humans. Circadian fluctuations of ACTH are governed by the suprachiasmatic nuclei. Stimuli for the secretion of ACTH are stress-related emotions via the limbic system (amygdaloid nuclei), trauma via the spino-thalamic tracts, and circadian rhythmic stimuli from the suprachiasmatic nuclei, each of which is mediated through the increased release of CRH. Secretion of ACTH from the pars intermedia is stimulated by serotoninergic

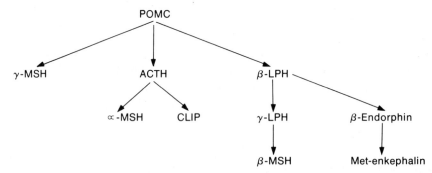

Fig. 3–9. Fragmentation of pro-opiomelanocortin. POMC = pro-opiomelanocortin; MSH = melanocyte-stimulating hormone; ACTH = adrenocorticotropic hormone; LPH = lipotropin; CLIP = corticotropin-like intermediate lobe peptide.

and dopaminergic innervation. Low blood levels of glucocorticoids result in an increase in the release of ACTH by the absence of glucocorticoid's inhibitory influence on the hypothalamus and the adenohypophysis.

The secretion of ACTH is inhibited by elevated blood levels of glucocorticoids and by the baroreceptors via the nucleus of the tractus solitarus and the medial lemniscus. Negative feedback on the secretion of ACTH by glucocorticoids can be overridden by various stresses. The cells of the adrenal cortex's zona fasciculata and reticularis are the primary target cells for ACTH, which stimulates the growth and secretion of the adrenal cortex. Secretion of adrenocortical glucocorticoids, androgens, and estrogens are nonselectively increased by ACTH. Natural water-soluble ACTH (Acthar), natural ACTH in gel (Adrenomone, Cortrophin Gel, and Cortrophin Zinc, HP Acthar Gel), and synthetic ACTH (Cortrosyn) are commercially available for diagnostic and therapeutic uses. "Repository" preparations of ACTH exert effects on the adrenal cortex for 12 to 48 hours.

See references 38, 39, and 43.

Growth Hormone

Produced by the somatotropes, GH is a large polypeptide hormone with about 190 amino acid residues, 2 to 4 disulfide bridges, and a molecular weight of more than 20,000 (depending on the species). Its structure, which is similar to that of prolactin and chorionic somatomammotropin, varies enough among different species that many species' GH will not have GH-like effects in other species. For example, bovine GH and porcine GH do not affect growth in humans even though they are somewhat diabetogenic in people. The plasma half-life of GH is about 20 minutes.

GH stimulates chondrogenesis in the cartilaginous epiphyseal plate of prepubescent animals, producing growth of the long bones and the production of bone matrix. Although plasma levels of GH are somewhat higher before puberty than after, there is no spurt in the secretion of GH that would explain the rapid growth of adolescence. This growth instead seems to be the result of increased androgen production, which occurs at puberty. Chondrogenesis and the other effects of GH are listed in Table 3–5. The effects of GH are to promote growth and to provide a ready source of energy during fasting.

Table 3–5. Effects of Growth Hormone

Accelerates chondrogenesis in epiphyseal plates
Facilitates entry of amino acids into cells
Stimulates erythrogenesis
Increases gastrointestinal absorption of calcium
Decreases blood urea nitrogen
Increases urinary hydroxyproline
Reduces excretion of sodium and potassium in urine
Sensitizes β cells of the pancreas to glucose
Releases free fatty acids (which produce ketones)

The action of GH on bones is indirect—that is, its action is mediated via other polypeptides called *somatomedins*.[80, 81] Somatomedins are a family of peptides with a molecular weight of 5,000 to 10,000. They are produced in the liver and, to a lesser degree, in other tissues. They circulate bound-to-carrier plasma proteins. The best-known somatomedins are somatomedin A, somatomedin C (insulin-like growth factor I), insulin-like growth factor (IGF) II, multiplication-stimulating activity, epidermal growth factor, nerve growth factor, ovarian growth factor, fibroblast growth factor, and thymosin.

The structures of somatomedin C and IGF II are very similar to proinsulin. Most somatomedins have some insulin-like effects. They are anabolic and enhance proliferation of cartilage. Somatomedin C seems to inhibit the adenohypophyseal secretion of GH. Not all effects of GH, such as lipolysis, stimulation of erythrogenesis, increased pancreatic B cell sensitivity to glucose, and facilitated cellular uptake of amino acids, are mediated by somatomedins. Similarly, GH is not the only stimulus for the secretion of somatomedin. Insulin and increased dietary protein are also stimuli for at least some somatomedins. Inhibition of the production of somatomedin is caused by estrogens and glucocorticoids. Normal plasma levels of somatomedin C in dogs parallel body size.[23] For example, plasma levels of somatomedin C in cocker spaniels are about 5 to 90 ng/ml, whereas in German shepherd dogs levels are about 230 to 330 ng/ml.

Secretion of GH varies throughout the day, depending on stimulative and inhibiting influences. After puberty, secretion continues in levels that are lower but not dissimilar to those recorded before puberty. Major physiologic factors stimulating secretion of GH include non-rapid eye movement (REM) sleep, hypoglycemia and fasting, increased plasma levels of certain amino acids such as arginine, and stress, presumably via GRH. Between 20% to 40% of the daily secretion of GH occurs in the first 90 minutes of sleep. Glucagon, dopamine, norepinephrine, clonidine, xylazine, serotonin, megestrol acetate, medroxyprogesterone acetate, and apomorphine also stimulate secretion of GH. Thyroid hormone is necessary for normal secretion of GH and is required for the normal action of GH on cells. Glucose, glucocorticoids, free fatty acids (FFAs), REM sleep, serotonin antagonists, and GH itself will inhibit GH's secretion, probably via somatostatin. All cells in the body are directly or indirectly targets for GH. The role of GH in adults is unknown. GH from human pituitaries (Asellacrin, Crescormon) is now available, and a form produced by genetically engineered bacteria should be available soon.

See references 20 and 38.

Follicle-Stimulating Hormone and Luteinizing Hormone (the Gonadotropins)

FSH (follitropin) and LH (lutropin) are glycoprotein polypeptides produced by the gonadotropes. They contain 204 amino acids in humans (89 in the α-chain; 115 in the β-chain), and approximately one fourth of their structures is carbohydrates. The molecular weight of FSH is about 32,000, and that of LH is about 30,000. The serum half-lives of FSH and LH in humans are about 3 hours and 1 hour, respectively. Both are released by GnRH, if the stimulation by GnRH is not prolonged (GnRH is normally produced in bursts). If GnRH's stimulation of the gonadotropes is prolonged, down regulation of their receptors occurs. Secretion of FSH is stimulated by GnRH in estrous and seasonal cycles innate to the species. Secretion of LH is stimulated by declining estrogen levels in dogs and facilitated by rising progesterone levels.[13]

In cats, secretion of LH must be stimulated by afferent stimuli associated with copulation stimuli received by the genitalia, eyes, ears, and nose.[92, 100] Ovulation of the follicular contents is induced by LH. Cats and ferrets are *induced or reflex ovulators,* while dogs and mares are *spontaneous ovulators.* The secretion of FSH and LH is inhibited by persistent estrogen feedback on the hypothalamus or adenohypophysis.

In addition to estrogens, secretion of FSH can be inhibited by *inhibin,* a peptide with a molecular weight of more than 10,000. Inhibin is produced by the ovarian follicles or the Sertoli cells of the testes. In addition to estrogens, LH is inhibited by testosterone, via aromatization to estrogens, and persistent high serum levels of progesterone. The target organs for FSH are the ovarian follicles in the female and the seminiferous tubules in the male, where it stimulates ovarian follicle growth and spermatogenesis, respectively. In females, LH stimulates ovulation and formation and main-

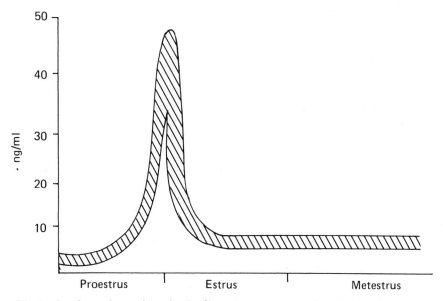

Fig. 3–10. Approximate plasma levels of luteinizing hormone in sexually intact female dogs.

tenance of the corpus luteum and in males secretion of testosterone by the interstitial cells of the testes. Approximate normal plasma levels of LH and FSH in bitches are illustrated in Figures 3–10 and 3–11.[88]

FSH is commercially available (FSH-P) for the induction of ovarian follicular growth in females and the stimulation of spermatogenesis in males. Pregnant mare's serum (PMS) has predominant FSH activity. Clinically FSH is used to aid in the development of follicles and enhance LH-induced ovulation. LH is commercially available (P.L.H.) for the stimulation of follicle maturation and ovulation in females and for the production of testosterone in males. Human chorionic gonadotropin (A.P.L., Follutein, Glukor, Profasi HP, and Chorionic Gonadotropin) has predominant LH activity. It is used clinically to induce ovulation, to treat cystic ovaries, or to induce descent of cryptorchid testes.

FSH and LH from equine pituitaries (A.P. Godin-5, Gonadotropin, and Gonadovet) are used to induce estrus and ovulation in females or to treat secondary hypogonadism in males. Equal amounts of FSH and LH are available in extracts of urine from postmenopausal women (Pergonal) to induce estrus and ovulation.

See also references 12, 15, 16, 25, 29, 30, 33, 34, 38, 42, 52, 77, 79, 93, 94, 98, 101, and 102.

Prolactin

Prolactin is a polypeptide hormone with 198 amino acid residues and three disulfide bridges (in humans) produced by the mammotropes. Its molecular weight is about 22,500, and its structure is very similar to GH.

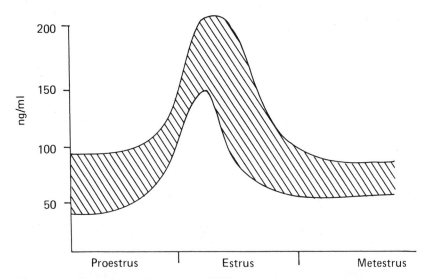

Fig. 3–11. Approximate plasma levels of follicle-stimulating hormone in sexually intact female dogs.

The term *luteotropic hormone* (LTH) has been used synonymously with prolactin. LTH is an inappropriate name for prolactin in companion animals because it does not maintain the structure and function of the corpus luteum in all species. In females, prolactin causes milk secretion after priming of the mammae by estrogen and progesterone. In males, it may cause prostatic growth. Prolactin is secreted persistently, but is tonically inhibited by dopamine. Normal plasma levels of prolactin in bitches are depicted in Figure 3–12. Male dogs' plasma levels of prolactin range from about 7 to 10 ng/ml. Prolactin can inhibit its own releasing factors from the hypothalamus. Prolactin secretion is increased by stimulation of the nipple, mammary gland trauma, exercise, sleep, pregnancy, hypothyroidism, estrogens, renal failure, and certain stresses. Estrogens aid prolactin and progesterone to promote development of mammary tissue, but withdrawal of estrogen initiates lactation, and serum progesterone levels are generally in an inverse relationship with plasma prolactin levels. TRH stimulates secretion of prolactin as well as secretion of TSH. Dopamine receptors can be stimulated by the administration of bromocriptine and apomorphine, resulting in decreased release of prolactin. Tranquilizers deriving from promazine block dopamine receptors, causing the increased release of prolactin.

Prolactin is not commercially available for diagnostic or therapeutic purposes.

See references 36 and 38.

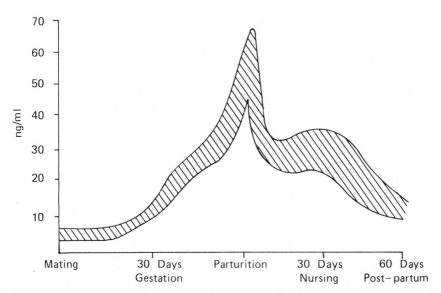

Fig. 3–12. Approximate plasma levels of prolactin in female dogs during gestation and lactation.

Melanocyte-Stimulating Hormone

There are three MSHs: α-MSH is the first 13 amino acids of the ACTH molecule, β-MSH is the last 18 amino acids of the γ-LPH molecule, and γ-MSH is a fragment of the POMC molecule, the precursor to ACTH. All three forms of MSH are produced primarily in the pars intermedia; some are produced in the pars distalis. The stimulus for secretion of MSH is exposure of the body to ultraviolet light. Neural regulation via hypothalamic fibers extending into the pars intermedia may also affect secretion of MSH. MSHs stimulate melanocytes to synthesize melanin. They are not commercially available for diagnostic or therapeutic uses.

TESTS OF ENDOCRINE BRAIN FUNCTION

Assessments of possible early hypothalamic-hypophyseal diseases are difficult. Severe hypothalamic-hypophyseal diseases cause confusing complexes of clinical signs and laboratory evaluations. Clinical neurologic evaluations, special radiographic examinations of the skull, and endocrine assays for hypophyseal hormones or assessment of target cell effects may aid in the clinical determination of hypothalamic-hypophyseal disease. Known pineal diseases are limited to rare incidences of neoplasia.

Clinical Neurologic Evaluations

Headaches and sleep disturbances may occur because of increased intracranial pressure. Headaches are thought the cause of head pressing against stationary objects and one of the causes of behavioral changes, nausea and vomiting, and apparent depressed level in consciousness.

Visual disturbances may result from pressure on the hypothalamus, optic chiasm, or optic nerves. These disturbances can take the form of anisocoria, amaurosis, strabismus, or ocular paresis. Other neurologic abnormalities that may be evident in the history or physical examination include thirst disorders, appetite disorders, abnormal body temperature, anosmia, or hyposomia. Cytologic evaluation of the cerebrospinal fluid and measurement of cerebrospinal pressures may be helpful in diagnosing severe hypothalamic-hypophyseal disease caused by space-occupying lesions.

Radiographic Examination of the Skull

Plain radiographs of the skull are not helpful in assessing possible hypothalamic-hypophyseal diseases, but tomography (CT scans) can be helpful in the diagnosis of hypothalamic tumors of compression[70] (Fig. 3–13). Using radiographic studies to evaluate hypophyseal diseases is less effective in companion animals than in humans because the dorsum sellae of the dog and cat is incomplete, allowing dorsal expansion into the hypothalamus rather than erosion of the sella turcica. Cerebral angiography might be useful in detecting vascular abnormalities of the hypothalamic-hypophyseal area.[10]

More practical than tomography, scintigraphy,[21,58] CT scans,[70] and cerebral angiography[10] in dogs with suspected hypothalamic-hypophyseal diseases is *cranial sinus venography*.[68,75] This procedure is done by injecting contrast media into the angularis oculi vein on the maxilla ventral to the eye (Fig. 3–14). The contrast media then fills the venous plexus surrounding the hypophysis. Space-occupying lesions visibly compress the veins, impeding their ability to fill with contrast media (Figs. 3–15 and 3–16).

Endocrine Evaluations

Even though RIAs have been developed for research purposes for some hypothalamic releasing and inhibiting hormones, they are not of clinical value. Concentrations in the general circulation are too minute. Direct assays of hypophyseal hormones could be of considerable clinical value, but technical obstacles and cost have severely limited their clinical use.

See reference 2.

GROWTH HORMONE.   A homologous RIA has been developed for canine GH. Assays for feline GH have been done also, but to a lesser extent.[37] Baseline levels (0 to 4 ng/ml) are usually near the lower limits of sensitivity, so stimulation tests are necessary to evaluate for possible deficiency of GH. Stimulation tests for GH include clonidine, xylazine, arginine, insulin-induced hypoglycemia, and L-dopa response tests. The *xylazine response test*

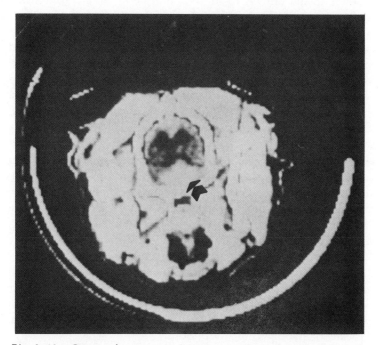

Fig. 3–13. Computed tomograph after the intravenous administration of contrast media showing a chromophobe adenoma (*arrow*) of the adenohypophysis. (From Mandelker, L.: Using a computed brain and orbital tomography to diagnose a brain tumor in a dog. VM/SAC, 76:1164, 1981.)

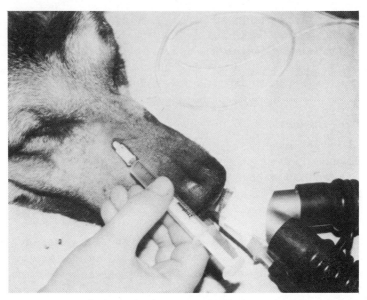

Fig. 3-14.   Injection of radiopaque contrast media into the angulus oculi vein.

is preferable to the others; 15 to 30 minutes after an intravenous dose of 100 μg/kg of xylazine is given, the plasma values of GH in dogs increase to approximately 50 to 70 ng/ml.

Baseline levels of GH are likely to be diagnostic if an excess of GH exists. If baseline plasma GH levels are equivocal for abnormal elevation, a glucose suppression test should be performed. The glucose suppression test, which uses an oral dose of 2.2 g/kg body weight of glucose, should show marked suppression of GH secretion in 1 hour in normal dogs. Lack of GH suppression following glucose challenge substantiates excessive GH secretion.

Assays for GH are not readily available for companion animals. There are no commercial reference laboratories offering the test for dogs or cats. When arrangements for a homologous assay of GH cannot be made with a research laboratory, an indirect evaluation of GH secretion, the *insulin-tolerance test,* can be used. It is based on the relative ease with which hypoglycemia develops in response to small intravenous doses of crystalline insulin (0.05 U/kg body weight) when secretion of GH is deficient. If the blood glucose drops to 50% or less of the baseline levels, levels of GH are probably deficient. It is essential to have first established that secretion of ACTH is normal by measuring serum levels of cortisol or by ACTH assay. A 50% glucose solution for intravenous infusion should be available if clinical signs of hypoglycemia develop.

Levels of somatomedin C in plasma vary according to the size of the breed of dogs but parallel the secretion of GH. When normal values are established for a particular breed and species of companion animal, levels of

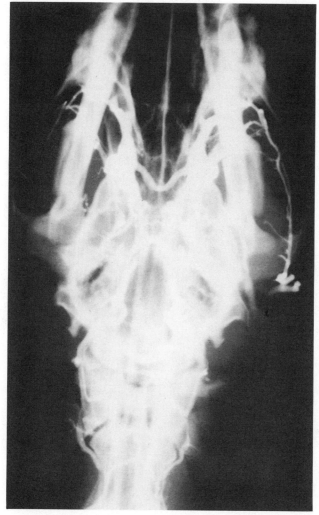

Fig. 3–15. Normal venogram of the cavernous venous sinuses of the ventral aspect of the cranial vault.

somatomedin C in plasma can be used to indirectly assess secretion of GH. Somatomedin C is bound to plasma proteins, and its levels do not fluctuate as rapidly as do levels of GH.

See references 11, 22, 23, 44–46, 96, and 99.

PROLACTIN.   Although RIAs for prolactin have been developed for research purposes for the dog, horse, and cat, none is commercially available. Normal baseline levels reported in dogs and horses are about 1 to 4 ng/ml. Values in cats are very similar.[3] Female animals have higher levels than male animals, especially near the end of metestrus and parturition-lactation (Fig. 3–12).[18,41] Levels of prolactin exist in inverse relationship to levels of

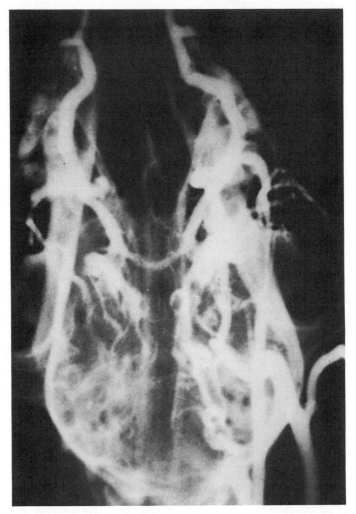

Fig. 3–16. Compression of the venous sinuses by a chromophobe adenoma of the adenohypophysis. (From Chastain, C.B., Riedesel, D.H., and Graham, C.L.: Secondary hypothyroidism in a dog. Canine Pract., 6:59, 1979.)

testosterone and to progesterone. They rise mildly at the end of metestrus in nonpregnant bitches, presumably from decreased progesterone production. In addition to baseline plasma levels, secretion of prolactin can be evaluated further in humans with suppression by L-dopa, stimulation by TRH, and stimulation tests with perphenazine or chlorpromazine. Some of these response tests will probably be helpful in assessing pituitary disease in companion animals when prolactin assays are more readily available and more cost effective.

See references 3, 18, 41, 56, 57, 62, 63, 76, 88, and 90.

ADRENOCORTICOTROPIC HORMONE. Commercial RIAs for ACTH, which detect the N-terminal 24 amino acids of ACTH, can be adapted to the dog and probably the cat because the structure of that portion of the molecule is identical in all species studied so far. Normal baseline plasma levels of ACTH reported in dogs are about 20 to 100 pg/ml. Plasma levels of ACTH in cats and horses are similar. Assessment of ACTH reserve can be done by the insulin-induced hypoglycemia test, the ADH response test, or the metyrapone response test. Metyrapone is an inhibitor of the 11-hydroxylation of adrenal steroids, which precedes synthesis of cortisol. Since production of cortisol is inhibited, plasma levels of ACTH should rise within a few hours after the administration of metyrapone. More recently, a radioreceptor assay more sensitive than the RIA for ACTH has been developed, but it is also more expensive. Levels of β-LPH in plasma are about 20 to 80 pg/ml in dogs and parallel changes in plasma levels of ACTH.[78]

Indirect evaluations of the production of ACTH are used more frequently than RIAs for ACTH. The RIA for ACTH is available at only a few laboratories, is expensive, and requires very careful handling (refrigerated centrifugation, plastic syringe and tubes, and transport in the frozen state). Indirect evaluations of ACTH secretion include measuring the baseline values of serum cortisol, and the serum levels of cortisol following stimulation of ACTH or ADH, and doing the dexamethasone suppression test to measure serum levels of cortisol, as well as insulin sensitivity tests, urinary cortisol assays, and the metyrapone response test with plasma 11-deoxycortisol determinations or urinary 17-ketogenic steroid assays.

See references 35 and 83.

THYROID-STIMULATING HORMONE. A homologous canine RIA for TSH has been developed for research.[82] Normal values reported were about 3 to 8 ng/ml.[82] Slightly lower values (2 to 4 ng/ml) have been detected by an RIA using antihuman TSH antibody.[59] Slightly higher values (8 to 12 ng/ml) have been reported in normal horses.[95] Valid RIAs for canine and feline TSH are not available from commercial reference laboratories. When commercially available, homologous canine and feline RIAs for TSH should be interpreted along with the measurement of a serum T_4 level from the same sample. A stimulation test using TRH has been used to measure the ability of the adenohypophysis to secrete TSH. Ideally, RIAs for TSH should be used to evaluate the response to TRH, but serum T_4 levels have been used as a less direct, but more readily available means of evaluating the effects of TRH in dogs. Six hours after an intravenous dose of 0.1 mg/kg body weight of TRH has been given, serum T_4 levels should increase 50% from the baseline level.[69] The TRH response tests, which use serum T_4 levels to monitor the response, are employed very little in companion animals because of the variable response in normal dogs and the current expense of TRH.

Secretion of TSH is more commonly assessed by indirect means. Serum T_4 levels, the serum T_4 response to TSH, and thyroid biopsies can yield evidence that the secretion of TSH is adequate. Deficiency of TSH causes atrophy of the thyroid, which is characterized by cuboidal follicular cells and few colloid vacuoles. Secondary hypothyroidism will respond with increased serum T_4 levels if multiple (three to seven) daily injections of TSH are given. Primary hypothyroidism cannot respond even to multiple injections of TSH.

See references 9 and 67.

FOLLICLE-STIMULATING HORMONE AND LUTEINIZING HORMONE. Although RIAs for FSH and LH for the dog and cat have been developed and are being used for research purposes, none is commercially available from laboratories. Normal levels of FSH in dogs are about 40 to 70 ng/ml, with higher levels expected in female dogs in proestrus (Fig. 3–11).[33, 88] In one laboratory, normal levels of LH reported in dogs were as follows: about 0 to 3 ng/ml in male dogs, 6 to 10 ng/ml in female dogs in estrus, less than 2 ng/ml in female dogs in metestrus and anestrus, and 3 to 10 ng/ml in neutered dogs. In females, levels of LH peak at estrus (Fig. 3–10).[15, 55, 73] Higher values have been reported in cats,[8, 16] but values for both dogs and cats vary among laboratories and according to the methods used. Serum levels of LH in male dogs may vary with different seasons of the year.[32] Whenever these assays are possible, the measurement of levels of FSH and LH should be interpreted along with determinations of testosterone, estrogen, and progesterone levels taken from the same sample. To stimulate the secretion of FSH and LH, GnRH can be administered and the adequacy of the response evaluated. Clomiphene is a synthetic analogue of chlorotrianisene with weak estrogenic effects that can be used to block estrogen receptors in order to stimulate the release of gonadotropins.

Indirect evaluation of the secretion of gonadotropin is currently more practical. With prior evidence of hypogonadism, if the administration of FSH or LH achieves a therapeutic response, such a response is indirect evidence of gonadotropin deficiency. For example, if testosterone deficiency is established by an RIA for serum testosterone, and serum levels of testosterone at least double after 3 days of injections of HCG, it is assumed the deficiency in testosterone is caused by a deficiency in gonadotropin.

See references 4, 5, 8, 15, 19, 32, 49–51, 55, 73, 88, and 100.

ANTIDIURETIC HORMONE AND OXYTOCIN. Plasma ADH has been assayed in dogs and reported to be about 1 to 4 pg/ml in anesthetized subjects. Clinical evaluations of the secretion of ADH are usually done by indirect assessments—that is, by the water deprivation test and the ADH response test. Deficiencies or excesses of oxytocin have not been described in companion animals, but a deficiency in oxytocin is sometimes suspected in cases of idiopathic agalactia or dystocia responsive to injections of oxytocin.

See reference 83.

REFERENCES

1. Alexander, J.E.: Anomaly of cranio-pharyngeal duct and hypophysis. Can. Vet. J., *3:*83, 1962.

2. Alsever, R.N., and Gotlin, R.W.: Handbook of Endocrine Tests in Adults and Children. 2nd Ed. Chicago, Year Book Medical Publishers, 1978.
3. Banks, D.R., Paape, S.R., and Stabenfeldt, G.H.: Prolactin in the cat. I. Pseudopregnancy, pregnancy and lactation. Biol. Reprod., 28:923, 1983.
4. Bell, E.T., Parkes, M.F., and Christie, D.W.: Gonadotrophin excretion in ovariectomized bitches. J. Reprod. Fertil., 27:83, 1971.
5. Boyns, A.R., et al.: Development of a radioimmunoassay for canine luteinizing hormone. J. Endocrinol., 55:279, 1972.
6. Carlon, N.: Cytologie due lobe anterieur de l'hypopphyse du chien. Z. Zellforsch., 78:76, 1967.
7. Chakraborty, P.K., and Fletcher, W.S.: Responsiveness of anestrous Labrador bitches to GnRH. Proc. Soc. Exp. Biol. Med., 154:125, 1977.
8. Chakraborty, P.K., Wildt, D.E., and Seager, W.J.: Serum luteinizing hormone and ovulatory response to luteinizing hormone-releasing hormone in the estrous and anestrous domestic cat. Lab. Anim. Sci., 29:338, 1979.
9. Chastain, C.B.: Human thyroid stimulating hormone radioimmunoassay in the dog. J. Am. Anim. Hosp. Assoc., 14:368, 1978.
10. Clarkson, T.B., Netsky, M.G., and de la Torre, E.: Chromophobe adenoma in a dog: angiographic and anatomic study. J. Neuropathol. Exp. Neurol., 18:559, 1959.
11. Cocola, F., et al.: A rapid radioimmunoassay method of growth hormone in dog plasma. Proc. Soc. Exp. Biol. Med., 151:140, 1976.
12. Concannon, P.: Effects of hypophysectomy on luteal phase plasma progesterone levels in the beagle bitch. J. Reprod. Fertil., 58:407, 1980.
13. Concannon, P., Cowan, R., and Hansel, W.: LH release in ovariectomized dogs in response to estrogen withdrawal and its facilitation by progesterone. Biol. Reprod., 20:523, 1979.
14. Concannon, P., Hansel, W., and McEntee, K.: Changes in LH, progesterone and sexual behavior associated with preovulatory luteinization in the bitch. Biol. Reprod., 17:604, 1977.
15. Concannon, P.W., Hansel, W., and Visek, J.: The ovarian cycle of the bitch: plasma estrogen, LH, and progesterone. Biol. Reprod., 13:112, 1975.
16. Concannon, P., Hodgson, B., and Lein, D.: Reflex LH release in estrous cats following single and multiple copulations. Biol. Reprod., 23:111, 1980.
17. Dammrich, K.: Die morphologische und funktionelle Pathologie der Geschwulste der Adenohypoophyse bei Hunden. Zentralbl. Veterinarmed., 14A:137, 1967.
18. DeCoster, R., et al.: A homologous radioimmunoassay for canine prolactin: plasma levels during the reproductive cycle. Acta Endocrinol., 103:473, 1983.
19. DePalatis, L., Moore, J., and Falvo, R.E.: Plasma concentrations of testosterone and LH in the male dog. J. Reprod. Fertil., 53:201, 1978.
20. Dorsa, D.M., and Connors, M.H.: Serotoninergic control of growth hormone (GH) secretion in dogs as measured by dose responsiveness. Life Sci., 22:1391, 1978.
21. Dijkshoorn, N., and Rijnberk, A.: Detection of brain tumors in dogs by scintigraphy. J. Am. Vet. Radiol. Soc., 18:147, 1977.
22. Eigenmann, J.E., and Eigenmann, R.Y.: Radioimmunoassay of canine growth hormone. Acta Endocrinol., 98:514, 1981.
23. Eigenmann, J.E., Patterson, D.F., and Froesch, E.R.: Body size parallels insulin-like growth factor I levels but not growth hormone secretory capacity. Acta Endocrinol., 106:448, 1984.
24. El Etreby, M.F., and Dubois, M.P.: The utility of antisera to different synthetic adrenocorticotrophins (ACTH) and melanotrophins (MSH) for immunocytochemical staining of the dog pituitary gland. Histochemistry, 66:245, 1980.
25. El Etreby, M.F., and Fath El Bab, M.R.: Effect of $^{17}\beta$-estradiol on cells stained for FSH β and/or LH β in the dog pituitary gland. Cell Tissue Res., 193:211, 1978.
26. El Etreby, M.R., and Fath El Bab, M.R.: Localization of gonadotrophic hormones in the dog pituitary gland. A study using immunoenzyme histochemistry and chemical staining. Cell Tissue Res., 183:167, 1977.
27. El Etreby, M.F., and Fath El Bab, M.R.: Localization of thyrotropin (TSH) in the dog pituitary gland. Cell Tissue Res., 186:399, 1978.
28. El Etreby, M.R., and Fath El Bab, M.R.: Utility of antisera to canine growth hormone and canine prolactin for immunocytochemical staining of dog pituitary gland. Histochemistry, 53:1, 1977.

29. El Etreby, M.F., et al.: Evaluation of effects of sexual steroids on the hypothalamic-pituitary system of animals and man. Arch. Toxicol. [Suppl.], *2:*11, 1979a.
30. El Etreby, M.F., et al.: Effect of $^{17}\beta$-estradiol on cells of the pars distalis of the adenohypophysis in the beagle bitch. Endokrinologie, *69:*202, 1977.
31. Ezrin, C., Kovacs, K., and Horvath, E.: A functional anatomy of the endocrine hypothalamus and hypophysis. Med. Clin. North Am., *62:*229, 1978.
32. Falvo, R.E., et al.: Annual variations in plasma levels of testosterone and luteinizing hormone in the laboratory male mongrel dog. J. Endocrinol., *86:*425, 1980.
33. Falvo, R.E., and Vincent, D.L.: Testosterone regulation of follicle-stimulating hormone secretion in the male dog. J. Andrology, *1:*197, 1980.
34. Falvo, R.E., et al.: Effects of testosterone and testosterone propionate administration on luteinizing hormone secretion in the male mongrel dog. Biol. Reprod., *21:*807, 1979.
35. Feldman, E.C., Bohannon, N.V., and Tyrrell, J.B.: Plasma adrenocorticotropin levels in normal dogs. Am. J. Vet. Res., *38:*1643, 1977.
36. Frantz, A.G.: Prolactin. N. Engl. J. Med., *298:*201, 1978.
37. French, E.D., Garcia, J.F., and George, R.: Acute and chronic morphine effects on plasma corticosteroids and growth hormone in the cat. Psychoneuroendocrinology, *3:*237, 1979.
38. Ganong, W.F.: Review of Medical Physiology. 11th Ed. Los Altos, California, Lange Medical Publications, 1983.
39. Ganong, W.F., Alpert, L.C., and Lee, T.C.: ACTH and the regulation of adrenocortical secretion. N. Engl. J. Med., *290:*1006, 1974.
40. Goldberg, R.C., and Chaikoff, I.L.: On the occurrence of six cell types in the dog anterior pituitary. Anat. Rec., *112:*265, 1952.
41. Graf, K-J., et al.: Homologous radioimmunoassay for canine prolactin and its application in various physiological states. J. Endocrinol., *75:*93, 1977.
42. Hall, A., and Dale, H.E.: The effect of gonadotrophic hormones and progesterone on the estrous cycle of the female dog. Vet. Med. Small Anim. Clin., *59:*852, 1964.
43. Halmi, N.S., et al.: Pituitary intermediate lobe in dog: two cell types and high bioactive adrenocorticotropin content. Science, *211:*72, 1981.
44. Hampshire, J., and Altszuler, N.: Clonidine or xylazine as provocative tests for growth hormone secretion in the dog. Am. J. Vet. Res., *42:*1073, 1981.
45. Hampshire, J., et al.: Radioimmunoassay of canine growth hormone: enzymatic radio-iodination. Endocrinology, *96:*822, 1975.
46. Hashimoto, C., Irie, M., and Matsuzaki, F.: Purification and characterization of growth hormone from dog pituitary glands. Endocrinology, *88:*881, 1971.
47. Holland, F.J., et al.: The role of biogenic amines in the regulation of growth hormone and corticotropin secretion in the trained conscious dog. Endocrinology, *102:*1452, 1978.
48. Jackson, I.M.D.: Thyrotropin-releasing hormone. N. Engl. J. Med., *306:*145, 1982.
49. James, R.W., Crook, D., and Heywood, R.: Canine pituitary testicular function in relation to toxicity testing. Toxicology, *13:*237, 1979.
50. Johnson, L.M., and Gay, V.L.: Luteinizing hormone in the cat. I. Tonic secretion. Endocrinology, *109:*240, 1981.
51. Johnson, L.M., and Gay, V.L.: Luteinizing hormone in the cat. II. Mating-induced secretion. Endocrinology, *109:*247, 1981.
52. Jones, G.E., Boyns, A.R., and Cameron, E.H.: Plasma estradiol, luteinizing hormone, and progesterone during pregnancy in the Beagle bitch. J. Reprod. Fertil., *35:*187, 1973.
53. Jones, G.E., et al.: Effect of luteinizing hormone releasing hormone on plasma levels of luteinizing hormone, oestradiol and testosterone in the male dog. J. Endocrinol., *68:*469, 1976.
54. Jones, G.E., and Boyns, A.R.: Effect of gonadal steroids on the pituitary responsiveness to synthetic luteinizing hormone releasing hormone in the male dog. J. Endocrinol., *61:*123, 1974.
55. Jones, G.E., et al.: Immunoreactive luteinizing hormone and progesterone during pregnancy and following gonadotrophin administration in beagle bitches. Acta Endocrinol., *72:*573, 1973.
56. Jones, G.E., Brownstone, A.D., and Boyns, A.R.: Isolation of canine prolactin by polyacrylamide gel electrophoresis. Acta Endocrinol., *82:*691, 1976.
57. Jones, G.E., Stockell Hartree, A., and Boyns, A.R.: Comparative immunological studies between canine prolactin and prolactin from other species. Acta Endocrinol., *82:*475, 1976.

58. Kallfelz, F.A., de Lahunta, A., and Allhands, R.V.: Scintigraphic diagnosis of brain lesions in the dog and cat. J. Am. Vet. Med. Assoc., *172:*589, 1978.

59. Kaufman, J., et al.: Serum concentrations of thyroxine, 3,5,3'-triiodothyronine, thyrotropin, and prolactin in dogs before and after thyrotropin-releasing hormone administration. Am. J. Vet. Res., *46:*486, 1985.

60. Kingsbury, B.F.: The pharyngeal hypophysis of the dog. Anat. Rec., *82:*39, 1942.

61. Kingsbury, B.F., and Roemer, F.J.: The development of the hypophysis of the dog. Am. J. Anat., *66:*449, 1940.

62. Knight, P.J., Hamilton, J.M., and Scanes, C.G.: Homologous radioimmunoassay for canine prolactin. Acta Endocrinol., *85:*765, 1977.

63. Knight, P.J., Hamilton, J.M., and Hiddleston, W.A.: Serum prolactin during pregnancy and lactation in the beagle bitch. Vet. Rec., *101:*202, 1977.

64. Krieger, D.T., and Martin, J.B.: Brain peptides. Part 1. N. Engl. J. Med., *304:*876, 1981.

65. Krieger, D.T., and Martin, J.B.: Brain peptides. Part 2. N. Engl. J. Med., *304:*944, 1981.

66. Kumar, M.S.A., Chen, C.L., and Kalra, S.P.: Distribution of luteinizing hormone releasing hormone in the canine hypothalamus: effect of castration and exogenous gonadal steroids. Am. J. Vet. Res., *41:*1304, 1980.

67. Larsson, M.: Evaluation of a human TSH radioimmunassay as a diagnostic test for canine primary hypothyroidism. Acta Vet. Scand., *22:*589, 1981.

68. Lee, R., and Griffiths, I.R.: A comparison of cerebral arteriography and cavernous sinus venography in the dog. J. Small Anim. Pract., *13:*225, 1972.

69. Lothrop, C.D., Jr., Tamas, P.M., and Fadok, V.A.: Canine and feline thyroid function assessment with the thyrotropin-releasing hormone response test. Am. J. Vet Res., *45:*2310, 1984.

70. Mandelker, L.: Using a computed brain and orbital tomography to diagnose a brain tumor in a dog. Vet. Med. Small Anim. Clin., *76:*1164, 1981.

71. McCann, S.M.: Luteinizing-hormone-releasing hormone. N. Engl. J. Med., *296:*797, 1977.

72. Moore-Ede, M.C., Czeisler, C.A., and Richardson, G.S.: Circadian timekeeping in health and disease. Part 1. Basic properties of circadian pacemakers. N. Engl. J. Med., *309:*469, 1983.

73. Nett, T.M., et al.: Levels of luteinizing hormone, estradiol and progesterone in serum during estrous cycle and pregnancy in the Beagle. Proc. Soc. Exp. Biol. Med., *148:*134, 1975.

74. Mikami, S., and Ono, K.: Cytological studies of the dog anterior pituitary and special reference to its staining properties. Acta Anat., *2:*440, 1956.

75. Oliver, J.E., Jr.: Cranial sinus venography in the dog. J. Am. Vet. Rad., *15:*66, 1969.

76. Papkoff, H.: Canine Pituitary Prolactin: isolation and partial characterization. Proc. Soc. Exp. Biol. Med., *153:*498, 1976.

77. Paisley, L.G., and Fahning, M.L.: Effects of exogenous follicle-stimulating hormone and luteinizing hormone in bitches. J. Am. Vet. Med. Assoc., *171:*181, 1977.

78. Peterson, M.E., Drucker, W.D., and Orth, D.N.: Immunoreactive ACTH and β-lipotropin in spontaneous canine Cushing's and Addison's disease. Clin. Res., *28:*762A, 1980.

79. Post, K.: Effects of human chorionic gonadotrophin and castration on plasma gonadal steroid hormones of the dog. Can. Vet. J., *23:*98, 1982.

80. Phillips, L.S., and Vassilopoulou-Sellin, R.: Somatomedins. Part 1. N. Engl. J. Med., *302:*371, 1980.

81. Phillips, L.S., and Vassilopoulou-Sellin, R.: Somatomedins. Part 2. N. Engl. J. Med., *302:*438, 1980.

82. Quinlan, W.J., and Michaelson, S.: Homologous radioimmunoassay for canine thyrotropin: response of normal and x-irradiated dogs to propylthiouracil. Endocrinology, *108:*937, 1981.

83. Raff, H., et al.: Vasopressin, ACTH, and corticosteroids during hypercapnia and graded hypoxia in dogs. Am. J. Physiol., *244:*E453, 1983.

84. Rao, R.R., and Bhat, N.G.: Incidence of cysts in pars distalis of mongrel dogs. Indian Vet. J., *48:*128, 1971.

85. Reichlin, S.: Regulation of the endocrine hypothalamus. Med. Clin. North Am., *62:*235, 1978.

86. Reichlin, S.: Somatostatin. Part I. N. Engl. J. Med., *309:*1495, 1983.

87. Reichlin, S.: Somatostatin. Part II. N. Engl. J. Med., *309:*1556, 1983.

88. Reimers, T.J., Phemister, R.D., and Niswender, G.D.: Radioimmunological measure-

ment of follicle stimulating hormone and prolactin in the dog. Biol. Reprod., *19:*673, 1978.
89. Sandusky, G.E., Jr., and Wightman, K.A.: Application of the peroxidase-antiperoxidase procedure to the localization of pituitary hormones and calcitonin in various domestic animals and human beings. Am. J. Vet. Res., *46:*739, 1985.
90. Saluja, P.G., and Kwa, H.G.: Some immunological properties of canine prolactin. Eur. J. Cancer, *8:*579, 1972.
91. Scott, P.P., and Lloyd-Jacob, M.A.: Reduction in the anestrus period of laboratory cats by increased illumination. Nature, *184:*2022, 1959.
92. Shille, V.M., et al.: Ovarian and endocrine responses in the cat after coitus. J. Reprod. Fertil., *68:*29, 1983.
93. Shille, V.M., and Stabenfeldt, G.H.: Luteal function in the domestic cat during pseudopregnancy and after treatment with prostaglandin $F_{2\alpha}$. Biol. Reprod., *21:*1217, 1979.
94. Smith, M.J., and McDonald, L.E.: Serum levels of luteinizing hormones and progesterone during the estrous cycle, pseudopregnancy and pregnancy in the dog. Endocrinology, *94:*404, 1974.
95. Thompson, D.L., Jr., and Nett, T.M.: Thyroid stimulating hormone and prolactin secretion after thyrotropin releasing hormone administration to mares: dose response during anestrus in winter and during estrus in summer. Dom. Anim. Endocrinol., *1:*263, 1984.
96. Tsushima, T., Irie, M., and Sakuma, M.: Radioimmunoassay for canine growth hormone. Endocrinology, *89:*685, 1971.
97. Vale, W., et al.: Characterization of 41-residue ovine hypothalamic peptide that stimulates secretion of corticotrophin and β-endorphin. Science, *213:*1394, 1981.
98. Vincent, D.L., et al.: Testosterone regulation of luteinizing hormone secretion in the male dog. Int. J. Androl., *2:*241, 1979.
99. Wilhelmi, A.E.: Canine growth hormone. Yale J. Biol. Med., *41:*199, 1968.
100. Wildt, D.E., Seager, S.W.J., and Chakraborty, P.K.: Effect of copulatory stimuli on incidence of ovulation and on serum luteinizing hormone in the cat. Endocrinology, *107:*1212, 1980.
101. Wildt, D.E., et al.: Ovarian activity, circulatory hormones, and sexual behavior in the cat. I. Relationships during the coitus-induced luteal phase and the estrous period without mating. Biol. Reprod., *25:*15, 1981.
102. Worgul, T.J., Santen, R.J., and Samojlik, E.: Evidence that brain aromatization regulates LH secretion in the male dog. Am. J. Physiol., *241:*E246, 1981.

4

Disorders of Hypothalamic and Adenohypophyseal Function

Generally, only severe hypothalamic and adenohypophyseal diseases are recognized in veterinary medicine. The diencephalon is rather inaccessible to examination except by expensive and sophisticated techniques. Our current understanding of hypothalamic and adenohypophyseal diseases in animals is primarily based on necropsy surveys, comparative disorders in humans, and a few clinical reports of affected companion animals. The clinical incidence of hypothalamic and adenohypophyseal diseases is not known, but the reported incidence is no doubt much less than the true incidence.

Disorders of the adenophypophysis are more common than hypothalamic disorders. Hypothalamic disorders are usually manifested by concurrent neurologic disturbances, but hypothalamic endocrine disorders may not be suspected until signs of an excess or deficiency of hypophyseal hormones appear. In many cases both areas may be involved in the same disease process, such as enlarging space-occupying lesions extending from the adenohypophysis into the hypothalamus.

The most commonly recognized hypothalamic-adenohypophyseal disorders in dogs are pituitary dwarfism, pituitary-dependent hyperadenocorticism, acromegaly, and diabetes insipidus. Cats are rarely affected by hypothalamic or adenohypophyseal disorders. Older horses and budgerigars are occasionally affected by adenohypophyseal tumors. Cardinal signs of hypothalamic and adenohypophyseal (pituitary) disorders are illustrated in Figure 4–1.

HYPOTHALAMIC DISORDERS

Clinical disorders of the hypothalamus are uncommon in comparison to other endocrine disorders. Potential lesions of the hypothalamus include aberrant parasite migration, craniopharyngiomas,[78] dermoid cysts, granulomas, traumatic lesions, encephalitis, hamartoma,[17] and various metastatic neoplasia (Fig. 4–2).[24, 65, 79, 92] Among hypothalamic disorders, deficiencies of single releasing or inhibiting hormones seem particularly rare. By the time a hypothalamic disease becomes clinical, multiple disorders of hypothalamic function occur.

Disorders of hypothalamic function may be neurologic, endocrine, or metabolic. Usually some disorders in each category are evident. Deficiencies of hypothalamic releasing hormones are called *tertiary hypofunctions*. Signs of hypothalamic disease in humans are listed in Table 4–1. Although

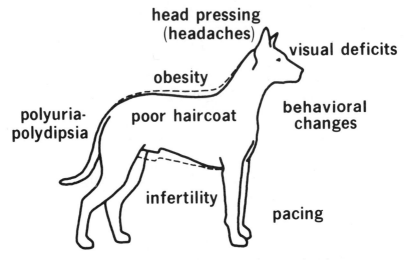

Fig. 4–1. Cardinal signs of hypothalamic-pituitary disorders.

the cases reported in companion animals are few, information is sufficient to indicate that the frequency and order of signs of hypothalamic disease in animals are similar to those observed in humans.

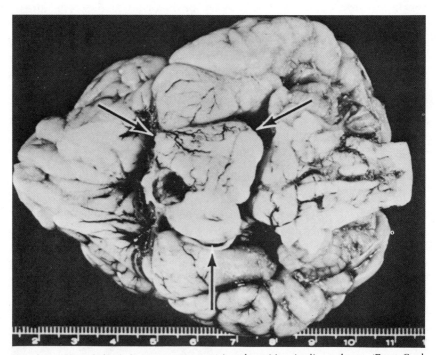

Fig. 4–2. Hypothalamic hamartoma (*arrows*) in a dog with episodic weakness. (From Cook, R.W.: Hypothalamic hamartoma in a dog. Vet. Pathol., *14:*138, 1977.)

Table 4–1. Signs of Hypothalamic Disease in Humans in Decreasing Order of Occurrence

Disturbances of vision
Sensory deficits
Headache
Vomiting
Precocious puberty
Disorders of behavior
Diabetes insipidus
Tertiary hypogonadism
Somnolence
Obesity
Hyperthermia or hypothermia
Emaciation
Convulsions
Polyphagia
Anorexia

Evidence is accumulating that some idiopathic adenohypophyseal disorders are in fact hypothalamic in origin. Many cases of pituitary-dependent hyperadrenocorticism may be caused by hypothalamic dysfunction leading to excesses of corticotropin-releasing hormone (CRH). Such cases have been effectively treated with drugs that modify hypothalamic neurotransmission. More recently, it has been proposed that cystic ovary syndrome may be caused by desynchronized hypothalamic control of luteinizing hormone (LH) released from the adenohypophysis. In humans, an inherited gonadotropin-releasing hormone (GnRH) deficiency, Kallman's syndrome, has been described.

The most common cause for hypothalamic disorders is suprasellar craniopharyngiomas (Figs. 4–3 and 4–4). Craniopharyngiomas are benign solid or cystic neoplasms of the remnants of Rathke's pouch. Adenohypophyseal adenomas frequently extend into or compress the hypothalamus in dogs and cats because their dorsum sellae is incomplete.

Some common signs of hypothalamic disease are more subtle than others. Visual disturbances often occur with hypothalamic space-occupying disease.[44] The optic chiasm lies just below the cranial aspect of the hypothalamus, and oculomotor nerve tracts are closely associated with the hypothalamus. Although loss of peripheral vision may occur with compression of the optic chiasm (Fig. 4–5), abnormalities in pupillary light reflexes are more likely to be first noted in companion animals with hypothalamic disease. Headaches cannot be verified in animals, but presumably headaches are the cause of head pressing and pacing seen in animals affected with hypothalamic disease. Obviously, sensory deficits cannot be detected until they are severe, since animals cannot relate to us their lack of many sensations.

Hypothalamic disorders are usually diagnosed by clinical signs of combined neurologic, endocrine, and metabolic dysfunction referrable to the hypothalamus; however, involvement of the hypothalamus might be con-

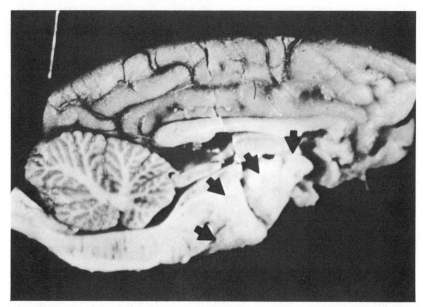

Fig. 4–3. Craniopharyngioma (*arrows*) in a dog with hypothalamic diabetes insipidus and secondary hypothyroidism. (From Neer, T.M., and Reavis, D.U.: Craniopharyngioma and associated central diabetes insipidus and hypothyroidism in a dog. J. Am. Vet. Med. Assoc., *182:*519, 1983.)

firmed by one or more of several diagnostic examinations. Routine skull radiographs may show calcification in the hypothalamus if a suprasellar craniopharyngioma is present. If available, computed tomography scans may be helpful. Attempts can be made to show the patient's lack of response to GnRH or thyrotropin-releasing hormone (TRH) in comparison to the response of control subjects. A normal indirect response to TRH in dogs has been reported to be an increase of at least 1 μg/dl in serum levels of thyroxine (T_4) 4 hours after an intravenous dose of 0.2 mg of TRH has been administered, or a 50% rise in serum T_4 6 hours after the administration of an intravenous dose of 0.1 mg/kg body weight of TRH. Plasma levels of LH may be directly assayed by RIA, or testosterone levels in intact male animals could be monitored for elevations following the administration of GnRH. Findings suggestive of hypothalamic disease would be subnormal baseline plasma levels of T_4 or testosterone (or LH), and a significant improvement in T_4 or testosterone (or LH) levels following the administration of TRH and GnRH, respectively.

ADENOHYPOPHYSEAL INSUFFICIENCY

Insufficiencies of adenohypophyseal hormones are rarely singular. A deficiency in only one adenohypophyseal hormone is called *monotropic hypopituitarism.* It is suspected that most cases of monotropic hypopituitar-

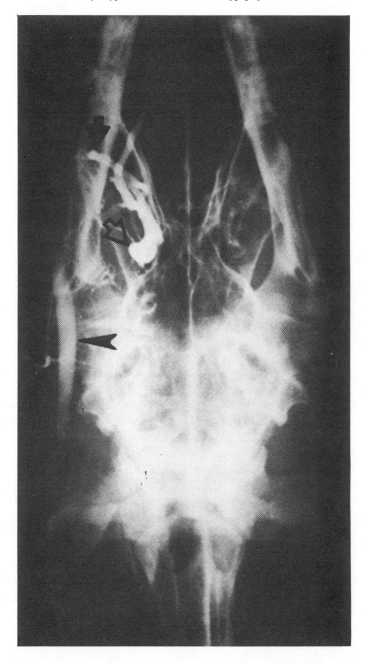

Fig. 4–4. Obstructed flow of contrast media caused by a craniopharyngioma noted during a cranial sinus venogram. Obstruction is caudal to the globe of the eye (*open arrow*). The facial vein (*arrowhead*) and angularis oculi vein (*solid arrow*) are also evident. (From Neer, T.M., and Reavis, D.U.: Craniopharyngioma and associated central diabetes insipidus and hypothyroidism in a dog. J. Am. Vet. Med. Assoc., *182:*519, 1983.)

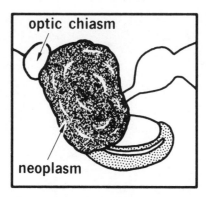

Fig. 4–5. Compression of the optic tract by hypothalamic-pituitary space-occupying lesions.

ism are actually caused by deficiencies of hypothalamic releasing hormones. While multiple insufficiencies are the rule rather than the exception, the combination of adenohypophyseal hormone insufficiencies varies considerably. The usual order of insufficiencies in adenohypophyseal hormones is growth hormone (GH), first followed by follicle-stimulating hormone (FSH)-LH, then thyroid-stimulating hormone (TSH), and, finally, adrenocorticotropic hormone (ACTH). Clinical and experimental investigations have shown that at least 70% of the adenohypophysis must be destroyed before an insufficiency in GH is meaningful, 90% destruction is required for loss of FSH-LH, 95% for TSH, and 98% for ACTH.[36] Deficiencies in FSH-LH, TSH, and ACTH are called *secondary hypogonadism, hypothyroidism,* and *hypoadrenocorticism,* respectively. Secondary hypofunction of the thyroids or adrenal cortices causes less severe signs than primary hypofunction. Possible endocrine deficiencies produced by discrete pituitary and hypothalamic lesions are illustrated in Figure 4–6.

Possible causes of pituitary insufficiency include congenital hypoplasia,[7, 43] destructive lesions (infections, lymphocytic hypophysitis, infiltrative diseases, trauma, tumors, adenohypophyseal adenomas, craniopharyngiomas[64]), and vascular lesions. The most common known cause of pituitary insufficiency in humans is Sheehan's syndrome, which results from postparturient ischemic necrosis. It has not been reported in companion animals. The most common known cause of pituitary insufficiency in prepuberal dogs is cysts affecting Rathke's pouch. In adult dogs, the most common cause is compression by adenohypophyseal tumors.

See references 55 and 60.

Growth Hormone Deficiency (Pituitary Dwarfism)

Pituitary dwarfism has often been reported in dogs, but only rarely in cats. The result of a deficiency in GH, it usually occurs with deficiencies in other adenohypophyseal hormones. The most frequently recognized cause of GH deficiency in the dog is a cystic Rathke's pouch.

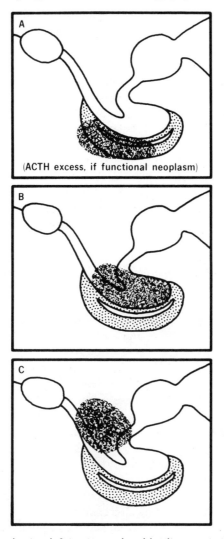

(ACTH excess, if functional neoplasm)

Fig. 4–6. Possible endocrine deficiencies produced by discrete pituitary and hypothalamic lesions. *A,* Deficiencies of gonadotropins, thyroid-stimulating hormone, and adrenocorticotropic hormone. *B,* Antidiuretic (and oxytocin) hormone deficiency. *C,* Hypothalamic inhibitory and releasing factor deficiencies. (Antidiuretic hormone deficiency, obesity, somnolence, behavior changes, abnormal body temperature, and visual disturbances are possible.) ACTH= adrenocorticotropic hormone.

Canine pituitary dwarfism was first reported in Germany in about 1940. Many breeds, such as the German shepherd, toy pinscher, Weimaraner, spitz, and Carelian bear-dog, have since been reported as having the condition. In German shepherds and a related breed, Carelian bear-dogs, it has been established that pituitary dwarfism can be transmitted as an autosomal recessive trait.[3–5, 66] There is no predisposition for sex.

Clinical signs of pituitary dwarfism in dogs first become apparent at 2 to 3 months of age. Possible clinical signs of pituitary dwarfism are listed in Table 4–2. Signs of adenohypophyseal deficiency may become worse with age because secretions into the pituitary cysts may cause continuing enlargements with compression of surrounding adenohypophyseal cells. Cysts of Rathke's pouch can become large enough to occlude partially the nasal pharynx and cause dyspnea.[84] As proportional dwarfism is caused by GH deficiency, the affected animal becomes a miniature of its littermates (Fig. 4–7).

Deficiency in GH alone does not lead to below average intelligence; however, most affected dogs have behavioral abnormalities such as fear biting and aggressiveness. Some of these animals are also deficient in TSH, which causes concurrent cretinism. Others may develop belligerent behavior as a separately inherited trait or as a result of socialization with much larger animals.

When affected dogs grow older, prognathism, delayed dentition, and haircoat abnormalities become evident. Haircoat abnormalities that can be seen include the animal's failure to develop primary hairs to replace the soft wooly (lanugo) haircoat of a puppy at the time of normal puberty. Alopecia and hyperpigmentation eventually appear on the perineum, tail, medial-caudal thighs, ventral abdomen, and collar area of the neck. In addition to becoming hyperpigmented, the skin of pituitary dwarfs is thin, because of decreased dermal collagen, and stains poorly for dermal elastin. Comedones may be present. Some canine pituitary dwarfs have also had patent ductus arteriosus, cryptorchidism, and megaesophagus. In GH-deficient Weimaraners, hypoplasia of the thymus with aplasia of the thymic cortex occurs.[68, 77] Affected Weimaraners have depressed lymphocytic blastogenesis on exposure to phytohemagglutinin.[76] Often what results is a wasting syndrome that resembles a condition in Ames or Snell-Bagg immunodeficient dwarf mice.

Radiographs can provide further evidence of GH deficiency. There is delayed closure of growth plates, particularly in the vertebral bodies. Those animals with TSH deficiency may also exhibit epiphyseal dysgenesis. Eruption of the permanent teeth is delayed, and the os penis may not mineralize at the time of puberty. A deficiency in GH may also cause a smaller than usual heart, liver, and kidneys.

Differential diagnoses for dwarfism in dogs include malnutrition, congenital hypothyroidism, juvenile diabetes mellitus, gonadal dysgenesis, se-

Table 4–2.   Possible Clinical Signs of Pituitary Dwarfism in Dogs

Proportional (limb-trunk) dwarfism
Normal or subnormal mentality
Prognathism
Delayed eruption of permanent teeth
Retained puppy coat leading to eventual alopecia
Suppressed immune responses

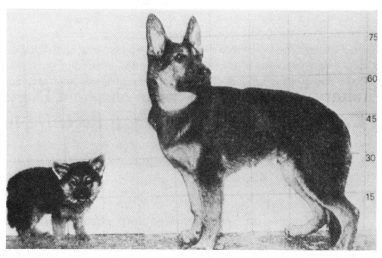

Fig. 4–7. Pituitary dwarfism in a 5½-month-old German shepherd dog (*left*). Dog on right is the affected dog's littermate. (From Andresen, E., and Willeberg, P.: Pituitary dwarfism in German shepherd dogs: additional evidence of simple, autosomal recessive inheritance. Nord. Vet. Med., 23:481, 1976.)

vere metabolic diseases (portal caval shunts, congenital renal diseases, congenital heart defects), and skeletal dysplasias (chondrodysplasia in Alaskan malamutes, pseudoachondroplastic dysplasia in miniature poodles, mucopolysaccharidosis). Some instances of canine dwarfism may be the result of idiopathic constitutional delayed growth. In humans, less than 2% of abnormal short stature is due to GH deficiency, although more than 2% do respond to administration of GH. Some responders may have GH dyshormonogenesis.

Routine hemograms, serum chemistries, and urinalyses are usually normal with pituitary dwarfism, with the possible exception of hypophosphatemia due to GH deficiency. If levels of TSH are deficient, serum cholesterol levels may be elevated, and if levels of ACTH are deficient, there may be anemia and fasting hypoglycemia. Increased insulin sensitivity may be shown by administering an intravenous dose of 0.025–0.05 U/kg body weight of crystalline insulin and monitoring the degree of decline in blood glucose in comparison to that of a control subject. If levels of GH are deficient, blood glucose levels may decrease to less than half their original values.

The definitive diagnosis of pituitary dwarfism requires measurement of GH before and 15 minutes after stimulation with xylazine (Rompun) in an intravenous dose of 100 μg/kg body weight or clonidine (Catapres) in an intravenous dose of 16.5 μg/kg body weight.[40] Other stimuli such as arginine or insulin-induced hypoglycemia may be used but are not generally necessary. Normal baseline levels of canine GH are about 0 to 4 ng/ml.

A deficiency in GH is indicated by the patient's failure to respond to stimulation. The possibilities of hyperadrenocorticism or hypothyroidism should be excluded first because an excess of glucocorticoids[70] or a deficiency of thyroid hormone impairs the secretion of GH. Other possible suppressors of GH are obesity, primary hypogonadism, and pregnancy.

Low plasma levels of somatomedins have been assayed in pituitary dwarf dogs.[30, 95] Normal plasma levels of canine somatomedins have been reported to be more than 0.90 U/ml or 5 ng/ml. Heterozygous carriers have somatomedin levels that are intermediate between normal levels and those of pituitary dwarfs. Assays for both somatomedins and GH are useful in determining the cause of pituitary dwarfism. For example, human Laron dwarfs have normal levels of GH, but either biologically inactive GH is produced (Laron type I) or somatomedin levels are decreased in response to a decrease in GH receptors in the liver (Laron type II). In African human pygmies, levels of GH are normal and GH receptors seem normal, but levels of somatomedin C are decreased, whereas other somatomedin levels remain normal.

Treatment of pituitary dwarfism in dogs is often not attempted because of the difficulty in obtaining GH; however, when available, porcine GH is the preferred treatment. Human GH from recombinant DNA synthesis by genetically engineered bacteria may soon be commercially available in large quantities. Since human GH is effective in dogs, it will permit more frequent treatment of pituitary dwarfs. The recommended dosage of porcine GH in dogs is 0.1 U/kg body weight, subcutaneously, three times per week for 4 to 6 weeks. If gonadotropins are present and puberty has occurred, the growth plates will close and no significant increase in height will occur during treatment with GH. The possibility of using other adenohypophyseal hormones, especially ACTH and TSH, should be investigated. If levels of TSH and ACTH are deficient, glucocorticoids should always be given before treatment with thyroid hormone.

Owners should be informed of the cost and difficulties in treatment. The risk of hypersensitivity reactions to GH or inducing diabetes mellitus should also be mentioned.

See references 1, 13, 20, 21, 48, 54, 61–63, 75, and 81.

Growth Hormone-Responsive Alopecia in Dogs

Although secretion of GH continues in adulthood, its purpose and necessity are not clear. Problems resulting from GH deficiency have not been reported in postpubertal humans; however, a GH-responsive alopecia has been reported in dogs. Young (1- to 2-year-old) male dogs are primarily at risk. Breeds reported to have been affected are the chow chow, Samoyed, Pomeranian, miniature poodle, and keeshond.

Clinical signs are limited to the abnormal haircoat (Fig. 4–8). A bilateral symmetrical alopecia affecting the trunk of the body, collar area of neck, tail, and medial thighs develops with hyperpigmentation of the skin. Biopsy

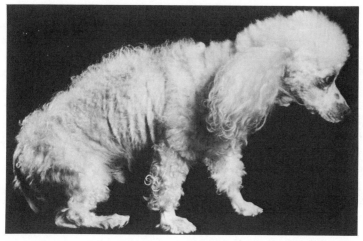

Fig. 4–8. Growth-hormone-responsive alopecia in a male miniature poodle.

of the skin usually shows a decrease in dermal collagen and elastin. The dermatologic appearance somewhat resembles that of hyperadrenocorticism, leading to the term "pseudo-Cushings syndrome."

A few assays for GH have been reported in affected dogs. Some are deficient in GH. Other possible causes include GH dyshormonogenesis, deficient or abnormal receptors of GH, or abnormal synthesis of somatomedin. At present, the diagnosis of GH-responsive alopecia is most frequently based on eliminating other possible causes of endocrine-related alopecia, finding decreased dermal elastin in a skin biopsy, and recording a favorable response to treatments with GH.

Although not commercially available, treatment with either bovine or, preferably, porcine GH has been advocated in a dose of 5 to 10 U, subcutaneously, every other day. Five to 15 injections are necessary. Response should be evident in 1 to 3 months. A favorable response will last 6 months to more than 3 years after the treatment series. The owner should be informed that hypersensitivity reactions are possible, as well as the induction of diabetes mellitus.

An enigma, GH-responsive alopecia has no precedent in any other species. A definitive diagnostic test is not readily available. And, finally, there is no adequate explanation why effects resulting from treatment with GH should persist for periods as long as 3 years. Until more information about the pathophysiology and hazards of therapy with GH becomes available, clinicians should be cautious in diagnosing this condition and advocating treatments with GH.

See references 25, 69, and 83.

Gonadotropin Deficiencies

After GH, gonadotropins (FSH and LH) are the most likely hormones to be deficient in animals with adenohypophyseal insufficiency. However, GH deficiency does not have to be associated with deficiencies in gonadotropins. Subjects with prepubertal GH deficiency with normal sexual function are called *sexual ateliotic dwarfs*; however, it should be remembered that monotropic gonadotropin deficiency has been reported in some humans as a familial trait called Kallman's syndrome. Deficiencies in gonadotropins cause secondary hypogonadism, that is, testicular hypoplasia or atrophy in males, or persistent anestrus in females.

With secondary hypogonadism, plasma levels of LH, FSH, estrogen, and testosterone should be decreased, and there should be no rise in any of these values following intramuscular injections of GnRH in doses of 25 μg for cats, and 50 μg for dogs. Repeated injections of gonadotropins should cause an increase in serum levels of estrogen or testosterone. Responses to the administration of gonadotropin in cats and dogs have not been consistent, but an intramuscular injection of FSH-P in a dose of 0.75 mg/kg body weight/day for up to 10 days (5 days in the cat), followed by one or two intramuscular injections of 500 U of human chorionic gonadotropin (HCG) in 48 hours, should increase serum levels of estrogen and progesterone in female dogs and cats with secondary hypogonadism.[8, 14, 68, 82, 85, 90, 93, 94, 96]

Care to prevent overstimulation with FSH should be taken. Overstimulation can cause cystic ovaries or vaginal prolapse. Response to follicle stimulation can be monitored by vaginal cytology to detect the release of estrogen or by assays for serum estrogen levels. Repeated intramuscular injections of 500 U of HCG for 3 days should increase serum testosterone levels in male dogs or cats with secondary hypogonadism.

In few clinical situations is the induction of estrus by the administration of gonadotropins justified. If companion animals used for breeding purposes do not have normal estrous cycles, the cause of the abnormality should be determined and, if possible, corrected. For example, malnutrition, overcrowding, hypothyroidism, persistent corpora lutea, and drugs are only a few of the causes for abnormal estrous cycles or persistent anestrus. It would be inappropriate with these conditions to overlook or ignore their cause and attempt to induce an estrous cycle with exogenous gonadotropins. Ramifications and potential hazards (cystic ovaries, superovulation, and prolapsed vagina) of treatment with exogenous gonadotropins should be discussed with owners of companion animals who are interested in inducement of estrous cycles.

Thyroid-Stimulating Hormone Deficiency

After the deficiencies in GH and the gonadotropins, TSH deficiency is the most common adenohypophyseal hormone deficiency caused by destructive lesions of the pituitary. The clinical signs of secondary hypothyroidism are similar to, but less obvious than, those of primary hypothyroidism.[15, 64] Elevated levels of serum cholesterol with hypogonadism or signs of hypothalamic disease may be the first indication of possible secondary hypothyroidism. If the baseline T_4 deficiency is established, there should be an eventual response in the production of T_4 if repeated (three to seven) daily injections of 5 to 10 U of TSH are administered. With primary hypothyroidism there is no improvement in the production of T_4 following repeated injections of TSH.

With secondary hypothyroidism, the uptake of radioactive iodine is subnormal, uptake may approach or reach normal values if a later study of radioactive iodine uptake is preceded by repeated injections of TSH. When TRH is administered, levels of T_4 are determined in 4 hours, and there should be an increase in levels of T_4—at least 1 μg/dl above the baseline value if the adenohypophysis is capable of secreting TSH. Signs of hypothalamic dysfunction, combined with subnormal baseline levels of T_4 and a normal response to TRH, suggest tertiary hypothyroidism rather than secondary hypothyroidism. When there is a deficiency in TSH, biopsy of the thyroid should show atrophic follicles, cuboidal follicular cells, and decreased colloid vacuoles.

Treatment of secondary hypothyroidism entails attempts to correct the cause, if possible, and supplementation of thyroid hormones. Supplementation of thyroid hormones can precipitate an acute hypoadrenocortical crisis if there is concurrent hypoadrenocorticism. The possibility of secondary hypoadrenocorticism (ACTH deficiency) or primary hypoadrenocorticism should be investigated and, if present, treated before supplementing thyroid hormones in secondary hypothyroidism.

Adrenocorticotropic Hormone Deficiency

Most ACTH deficiencies result from the administration of glucocorticoids. Within 1 hour secretion of ACTH will cease and production of cortisol will significantly decrease in normal dogs given as little as 0.01 mg/kg body weight of dexamethasone. Secretion of ACTH seems to occur again promptly if administration of glucocorticoids consists of infrequent, low-dose administration of a short- or intermediate-acting glucocorticoid (given no longer than 2 weeks).

Clinical signs of secondary hypoadrenocorticism are nonspecific. Deficiency resulting from the administration of glucocorticoids and adrenal androgens causes depression, anorexia, weight loss, and, possibly, hypotensive shock when the subject is acutely stressed by illness or injury. Fasting hypoglycemia is possible. Nonregenerative anemia may develop. Serum concentrations of sodium and potassium remain normal since the secretion of aldosterone is not affected by the lack of ACTH.

Cysts of Rathke's pouch, adenohypophyseal tumors, and other less common destructive processes in the adenohypophysis can cause ACTH deficiency. Plasma levels of ACTH may be determined by an RIA in the dog and probably the cat by using antibody against the N-terminal 24 amino acids. Since plasma levels of ACTH should be very low in animals with secondary hypoadrenocorticism, a metyrapone response test may be useful in evaluating the production capability of reserve ACTH. If the serum cortisol level is very low and plasma levels of ACTH are simultaneously low, secondary hypoadrenocorticism is the most probable cause. A RIA for ACTH may not be convenient or affordable. Repeated daily injections of ACTH for 3 to 7 days should raise the serum cortisol from subnormal to normal (or above) levels if secondary hypoadrenocorticism is present.

Prolactin Deficiency

Only rarely does a deficiency in prolactin cause clinical signs of disease. Agalactia can be caused by a deficiency in prolactin. However, female dogs or cats with an adenohypophyseal disorder severe enough to cause a deficiency in prolactin are unlikely to become pregnant and have cause to lactate.

Panhypopituitarism

The term *panhypopituitarism* is used to describe deficiency in all adenohypophyseal hormones. Conditions that cause panhypopituitarism usually also cause a deficiency in ADH. Paradoxically, if panhypopituitarism exists concomitantly with diabetes insipidus or diabetes mellitus, the severity of the latter two diseases is decreased. Deficiencies of GH, TSH, and ACTH decrease the production of osmoles, which results from catabolism. Decreased glomerular filtration decreases the excessive urine volume caused by diabetes insipidus. ACTH (cortisol), TSH (T_4), and GH also have insulin-antagonistic actions. Deficiency of these adenohypophyseal hormones ameliorates concurrent diabetes mellitus by increasing insulin sensitivity. In fact, deficiencies of GH and ACTH can lead to hypoglycemia during fasting in nondiabetic subjects. Possible clinical signs and laboratory findings of panhypopituitarism are summarized in Table 4–3.

Definitive diagnosis requires the demonstration of deficient secretion of gonadotropin, TSH, and ACTH. Direct assays for LH, TSH, and ACTH may be done before and after injections of GnRH (for LH), TRH (for TSH), and metyrapone (for ACTH). Evidence for secondary hypofunction of the gonad, thyroid, and adrenal glands can also be gathered by repeated injections of tropic hormones and the finding of increased target organ function. Deficiencies in GH and prolactin may also be verified by direct

Table 4–3.   Possible Signs of Panhypopituitarism

Anemia
Alopecia
Hypogonadism and sexual dysfunction
Fasting hypoglycemia
Polyuria-polydipsia
Recurrent infections
Microcardia and hypotension
Muscular weakness

assays, when available. Reserves of GH should be measured by xylazine or clonidine stimulation tests.

Treatment of panhypopituitarism consists of replacing the hormones missing in adenohypophyseal target organs. Continuous replacement of the deficient adenohypophyseal hormones is not practical because of the expense, the necessity for parenteral administration, the hormones' short-lived actions, and possible induction of antibodies against the hormones. Replacement of GH should not be necessary in mature animals with panhypopituitarism. Prolactin and the gonadotropins are also not necessary to maintain normal health, but a deficiency in thyroid hormones and glucocorticoids can be life-threatening. Glucocorticoids should be administered to replace the deficiency in cortisol before thyroid hormones are administered. Otherwise, there is the danger of precipitating a hypoadrenocortical collapse.

ADENOHYPOPHYSEAL HORMONE EXCESSES

Among the six major adenohypophyseal hormones, GH and ACTH are the most commonly involved in disorders of excessive adenohypophyseal function. An excess in ACTH may be caused by hypothalamic dysfunction in the regulation of CRH production or by adenohypophyseal adenomas. An excess in GH can be induced in dogs by chronic stimulation of progesterone or progestogen and, possibly, by the presence of adenohypophyseal adenomas.

See reference 60.

Growth Hormone Excess

Excess GH causes *gigantism* if the excess is present before the epiphyses close at puberty. Postpubertal excess of GH causes *acromegaly* (Gr., great extremity).[72] Acromegaly is an insidious condition characterized by the slow (months to years) development of enlarged extremities and other clinical signs of disease (Table 4–4, Figs. 4–9, 4–10, and 4–11). Visual distur-

Table 4–4. Possible Clinical Signs of Acromegaly in Dogs and Cats

Enlarged paws and skull
Prognathism
Widening of the interdigital spaces
Inspiratory stridor
Myxedematous thickening of the skin
Hypertrichosis
Lethargy
Enlarged abdomen (hepatomegaly)
Cardiomegaly
Degenerative arthritis
Galactorrhea
Polyuria-polydipsia-polyphagia (diabetes mellitus)

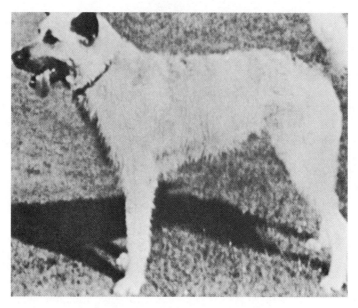

Fig. 4–9.   A mixed-breed bitch at the age of 3 years before the development of acromegaly. (From Rijnberk, A., et al.: Acromegaly associated with transient overproduction of growth hormone in a dog. J. Am. Vet. Med. Assoc., *177:*534, 1980.)

bances and signs suggestive of headaches are possible if the excess in GH is caused by an enlarging adenohypophyseal adenoma.

An excess in GH may play a role in the development of some canine mammary tumors.[6, 34] An increase in the number and size of somatotropes in the dorsal portion of the pars distalis has been found in association with spontaneous and progestogen-induced canine mammary tumors.

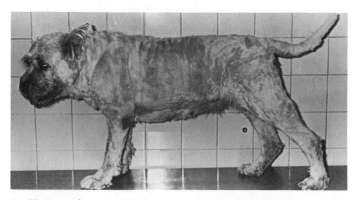

Fig. 4–10.   The same dog as seen in Figure 4–9, 2 years later, after clipping of the haircoat. Acromegalic features, such as enlargement of the extremities and increased skin folds, are evident. (From Rijnberk, A., et al.: Acromegaly associated with transient overproduction of growth hormone in a dog. J. Am. Vet. Med. Assoc., *177:*534, 1980.)

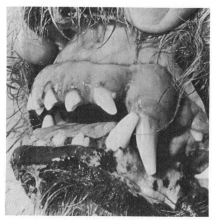

Fig. 4–11. Enlarged interdental spaces also occurred in the dog seen in Figures 4–9 and 4–10 as part of its acromegaly. (From Rijnberk, A., et al.: Acromegaly associated with transient overproduction of growth hormone in a dog. J. Am. Vet. Med. Assoc., *177:*534, 1980.)

Acromegaly has been caused by eosinophilic adenoma of the pars distalis, eosinophilic hyperplasia of the pars distalis, metestrus in the sexually intact bitch, and progesterone or progestogens in dogs.[16, 22, 23, 26, 27, 29, 32, 73, 80] In humans, acromegaly or gigantism is caused 20% of the time by acidophil adenomas and 80% of the time by chromophobe adenomas of the adenohypophysis. Acromegaly has been reported in cats with tumors of the pars distalis.[28] Study of affected dogs has not shown a predisposition for breed or age. Most cases of acromegaly have occurred in female dogs, and are probably related to conditions causing metestrus and to treatments with progestogen.

There are often no laboratory findings suggestive of GH excess. Overt diabetes mellitus may occur, but glucose intolerance without fasting hyperglycemia is more common. Even glucose intolerance is not always present. Serum levels of inorganic phosphorus and alkaline phosphatase may be elevated, the hematocrit decreased, and the concentration of calcium in the urine increased. Radiographs of phalanges may show widening, and the vertebrae may enlarge.

Since the clinical signs are eventually very impressive and laboratory findings are not consistent or specific for an excess of GH, it is the clinical appearance that leads a clinician to suspect acromegaly or gigantism. Definitive diagnosis is best based on plasma GH assays and the failure of plasma GH to be suppressed by a glucose suppression test (using an intravenous dose of 1 g/kg body weight). Baseline levels of GH may be extremely and consistently high, reaching levels higher than 1000 ng/ml, and therefore diagnostic in themselves. Because there are several stimuli for the increased secretion of GH, and because these stimuli may be present at the time of sampling, a single baseline measurement of plasma GH levels is usually meaningless. Levels of somatomedin C (IGF-I) should also be consistently elevated in animals with gigantism and acromegaly. Levels of somatomedin C do not fluctuate as rapidly as do plasma levels of GH. Normal levels of somatomedin C in plasma vary with species and breeds. However, plasma levels above 300 ng/ml in dogs are probably excessively high.[31] Insulin resistance may be verified by administering an intravenous dose of 0.3 U/kg body weight of crystalline insulin and monitoring the decrease in blood glucose in comparison to a control subject's response.

The appropriate treatment for the condition of GH excess depends on the cause. In the case of GH excess induced by exogenous administration of progestogens, cessation of drug treatment will lead to remission. If the excess in GH is caused by metestrus, an ovariohysterectomy is the preferred treatment. Adenohypophyseal "hyperplasia" or adenomas may be suppressed by the administration of bromocryptine mesylate, an ergot derivative.[86] Treatment with bromocryptine is effective in 10% to 30% of acromegalic humans. Other treatments found effective in humans with GH-secreting adenohypophyseal adenomas are teletherapy of the hypophysis with cobalt 60 or Cesium 137 linear accelerators, implants of yttrium, and hypophysectomy. Signs of improvement after the irradiation of the pituitary may not be apparent for 6 months. Hypophysectomy can result in panhypopituitarism.[45]

See reference 19.

Adrenocorticotropic Hormone Excess

An excess of ACTH causes bilateral hyperplasia and hypersecretion of the adrenal cortices. The hyperplastic adrenal cortices produce excessive quantities of cortisol and, to a lesser extent, adrenal androgens. Hypercortisolemia resulting from an excess of adenohypophyseal ACTH is called *pituitary-dependent hyperadrenocorticism.* Because in 1932 Dr. Harvey Cushing, a Boston surgeon, first described the syndrome caused by hypercortisolemia, pituitary-dependent hyperadrenocorticism is frequently referred to as Cushing's syndrome (*Cushing's-like syndrome* in dogs). Pituitary-dependent hyperadrenocorticism caused by an adenohypophyseal adenoma is also called *Cushing's-like disease* (Fig. 4–12). Most (85%) cases of spontaneous hyperadrenocorticism in the dog are caused by an excess of adenohypophyseal ACTH. Rarely, excessive levels of ACTH are caused by the synthesis of ACTH by an nonadenohypophyseal malignant neoplasm. Hyperadrenocorticism resulting from a neoplasm occurring outside the adenohypophysis is called the *ectopic ACTH syndrome.* Ectopic excesses of ACTH have been reported in dogs with lymphosarcoma and bronchial carcinomas.

Pituitary-dependent hyperadrenocorticism is the most frequently recognized disorder of the canine hypophysis. It may be associated with a chromophobe adenoma or, rarely, a carcinoma or a basophil adenoma of the adenohypophysis. However, most cases of pituitary-dependent hyperadrenocorticism in dogs are not associated with a morphologic change in the adenohypophysis. The number of reports of no morphologic change in the

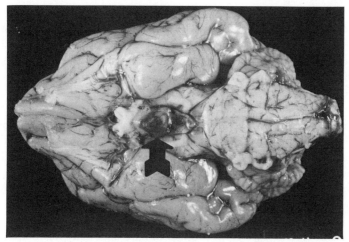

Fig. 4–12. Adenohypophyseal adenoma in a dog with Cushing's-like disease.

adenohypophysis varies among institutions. Many cases of pituitary-dependent hyperadrenocorticism thought morphologically normal may in fact be caused by microadenomas, which are easily overlooked. Some researchers have proposed that the cause of pituitary-dependent hyperadrenocorticism, in subjects without pituitary tumors or in some with ACTH-secreting microadenomas, is a disorder of the hypothalamic-adenophypophyseal feedback and the regulation of the release of CRH from the hypothalamus.[52] Pituitary-dependent hyperadrenocorticism in horses is usually caused by an adenoma of the pars intermedia.

The hallmark of hyperadrenocorticism in dogs, regardless of the initiating cause, is a triad of signs: alopecia, polyuria-polydipsia, and pendulous abdomen. The clinical signs and laboratory findings of hyperadrenocorticism and causes of the condition other than the excessive secretion of ACTH are described in more detail in a later chapter. Horses affected with hyperadrenocorticism have physical and laboratory findings similar to those of dogs, with the exception that horses develop long curly coats of hair rather than alopecia.

Definitive diagnosis of pituitary-dependent hyperadrenocorticism is attempted after confirming the diagnosis of hyperadrenocorticism. Hyperadrenocorticism is diagnosed by finding persistently elevated baseline plasma levels of cortisol, an exaggerated adrenocortical response (as determined by elevated plasma cortisols) to injections of exogenous ACTH or ADH, persistently elevated plasma levels of ACTH concurrent with elevated baseline plasma levels of cortisol, or the subject's failure to suppress plasma levels of ACTH and cortisol after receiving a low intravenous dose (0.01 mg/kg body weight) of dexamethasone. Pituitary-dependent hyperadrenocorticism is characterized by the suppression of plasma levels of ACTH and cortisol in response to a high intravenous dose (0.1 mg/kg body weight, or more) of dexamethasone; however, even large doses of dexamethasone may not inhibit large pars distalis tumors or tumors of the pars intermedia. Gamma camera imaging of the adrenal cortices using [131]I-19-iodocholesterol will show symmetrically enlarged adrenal cortices. Images of the adrenal cortices are produced by detecting emitted gamma irradiation with a high energy collimator and transforming the collected energy to an image on an oscilloscope.

Treatment of excessive levels of ACTH may be aimed at the adenohypophysis or the adrenal cortices. In dogs, it is more economical and practical to suppress adrenocortical hyperactivity. The most commonly used method is pharmacologic control with the drug mitotane (Lysodren). Chronic suppression of hypercortisolemia with metyrapone or aminoglutethiamide has been less successful than treatment with mitotane. Bilateral adrenalectomy is still used if problems develop with the use of mitotane. Sudden reduction of the hypercortisolemia resulting from bilateral adrenalectomy has been associated with rapid enlargement of ACTH-secreting adrenohypophyseal adenomas, a condition called *Nelson's syndrome.*

Treatment designed to lower levels of ACTH and correct pituitary-dependent hyperadrenocorticism include hypophysectomy, irradiation of the pituitary, and drug therapy. Hypophysectomy has been successfully used on affected dogs. Successful irradiation of the pituitary to treat affected companion animals has not been reported. Drug therapy has involved cyproheptadine (Periactin), bromocryptine mesylate (Parlodel), and sodium valproate.[88] Cyproheptadine, a serotonin antagonist, and bromocryptine, a dopamine agonist, are thought to suppress the release of CRH, but direct inhibition of the adenohypophysis is also possible. Sodium valproate is a gamma-aminobutyric acid transaminase inhibitor that has reduced plasma levels of ACTH in Nelson's syndrome in humans.

See also references 10, 53, 58, 59, and 71.

Prolactin Excess

An excess of prolactin in the plasma is an important marker for adenohypophyseal tumors and an important cause of infertility in humans.[50, 51] About 70% of all human pituitary tumors are associated with hyperprolactinemia. The same may be true in companion animals, but proof is lacking because of the unavailability of commercial prolactin assays for the dog and cat. Pathologic causes for hyperprolactinemia are listed in Table 4–5.

Table 4–5. Pathologic Causes for Hyperprolactinemia

Prolactin-secreting adenohypophyseal adenomas
Adenohypophyseal or hypothalamic disease suppressing dopamine
Ectopic prolactin production by malignant tumors
Acromegaly
Primary hypothyroidism
Chronic renal disease

Clinical signs of hyperprolactinemia in humans, rats, and presumably companion animals are persistent anestrus in females and lack of libido and impotence in males. Prolactin may affect gonadotropin activity by inhibiting GnRH, desensitizing the response of the adenohypophysis to GnRH, or interfering with gonadotropin-induced synthesis of steroids in the gonads. Hyperprolactinemia will also cause *galactorrhea* (any persistent white discharge from the mammae) in the patients whose mammae have been adequately sensitized by estrogens and progesterone. Galactorrhea is likely only in females that have had at least one normal estrus period before developing hyperprolactinemia, but males may occasionally lactate if hyperprolactinemic.

The diagnosis of hyperprolactinemia requires valid assays for plasma levels of prolactin for the species involved. In humans, baseline plasma levels are similar to reported plasma levels in dogs. The persistent report of plasma levels of prolactin in excess of 300 ng/ml is diagnostic of an excess of prolactin in humans and presumably dogs. Plasma levels of prolactin between 100 and 300 ng/ml suggest the hypersecretion of prolactin. In equivocal cases the diagnosis may be confirmed by exaggerated production of prolactin in response to phenothiazine, chlorpromazine, or perphenazine.[44]

Treatment of hyperprolactinemia depends on its cause. If the cause is adenohypophyseal or hypothalamic in origin, the safest, most economical therapy for short-term control is suppression of the production of prolactin with bromocryptine. Even the size of prolactin-secreting tumors can be reduced by treatment with bromocryptine. Hypophysectomy or irradiation of the pituitary can be effective treatments for adenohypophyseal tumors. The possibility of other causal conditions should be investigated and corrected if discovered.

Overt pseudopregnancy may be caused by prolactin. Clinical signs in dogs include mothering of inanimate objects, enlarged mammary glands, behavior abnormalities such as reclusiveness or aggression, lactation, and self-nursing. Clinical signs can be suppressed by administering estrogens, androgens, or progestins. Androgenic drugs are the safest treatment in affected dogs.

Excesses of Other Adenohypophyseal Hormones

It is rare for TSH or the gonadotropins to be produced in excess, except in subjects with primary hypothyroidism or sexual neutering, respectively. Microadenomas secreting TSH have been reported in children affected with untreated hypothyroidism of long duration. Gonadotropin-secreting microadenomas have been found in castrated males. The possibility for gonadotropin-secreting microadenomas in companion animals is great since they are so frequently sexually neutered.

TUMORS OF THE ADENOHYPOPHYSIS

Older companion animals, especially dogs, are often affected by tumors of the adenohypophysis. In fact, more than 10% of all primary brain tumors in the dog are adenohypophyseal tumors. These are the most common acquired disorder of the pituitary, and because of suprasellar extension, they are also the most commonly acquired disease of the hypothalamus.

See also references 2, 9, 11, 18, 33, 35, 38, 41, 42, 56, and 67.

Tumor Types

Primary tumors of the adenohypophysis are infrasellar craniopharyngiomas and adenomas of chromophobes, acidophils,[12, 47] or basophils. Adenohypophyseal carcinomas are rare.[18, 74] Primary adenomas are generally slow-growing and may secrete excesses of hormones, whereas primary carcinomas usually do not produce hormones, grow rapidly, and severely compress surrounding tissue.

Chromophobe adenomas are the most common primary adenohypophyseal tumor in companion animals. In dogs, they comprise 75% to 80% of all adenohypophyseal tumors. Acidophil adenomas are second in rate of occurrence. Basophil adenomas are the least common adenoma of the adenohypophysis.

Secondary tumors in the adenohypophysis can reach the pituitary by metastasis or by extension. Examples of metastasis include lymphosarcoma, malignant melanomas, malignant transmissible veneral tumor,[87] and carcinomas of the mammary gland. Tumors originating from nearby bone, meninges, or brain can extend into the sella and compress the pituitary.

Developmental (congenital) cysts of the adenohypophysis may be located in the sella or the nasopharynx. Pharyngeal cysts may become large enough or, after rupturing, may induce enough of an inflammatory response to impede normal respiration via the nares. Large pharyngeal adenohypophyseal cysts may be palpable through the oral pharynx and the soft palate.[88]

Tumor Location and Behavior

Primary tumors of the adenohypophysis may occur in the pars distalis or pars intermedia. Most tumors found in the dog occur in the pars distalis. There is no predilection for sex, but the dachshund, boxer, and Boston terrier are predisposed. Most chromophobe adenomas of the pars distalis in the dog secrete excess ACTH, causing pituitary-dependent hyperadrenocorticism. In humans, chromophobe adenomas more often secrete excessive amounts of GH. If GH- and ACTH-secreting adenohypophyseal adenomas are excluded, 70% of the remaining adenomas in humans produce excessive amounts of prolactin, either autonomously or as a result of the deprivation of dopamine's inhibiting effects. The association of hyperprolactinemia and pituitary tumors in companion animals is not known. Investigations have been hampered by the lack of a clinically accessible assay for prolactin. Adenomas of the pars distalis are usually solid tumors that compress surrounding adenohypophyseal cells, the neurohypophysis, and, occasionally, the hypothalamus. Clinical signs may be produced from the excessive secretion of adenohypophyseal hormones, adenohypophyseal insufficiencies, or both. Extension into the hypothalamus may cause cranial pain and a wide variety of signs of hypothalamic dysfunction. The size of the tumor does not correlate well with the degree of clinical signs of disease. Microadenomas may produce excessive amounts of ACTH, GH, or prolactin, leading to marked clinical abnormalities, whereas relatively large tumors may go undetected until discovery at postmortem examination.

Tumors of the pars intermedia are less frequent in dogs than are adenomas of the pars distalis. Two thirds of canine pituitary tumors are found in the pars distalis and one third in the pars intermedia. Adenomas (cystadenomas) of the pars intermedia are slow-growing cystic tumors that usually do not compress the neurohypophysis or hypothalamus. In dogs, there is no predisposition for breed or sex, but the occurrence is greater in nonbrachycephalic breeds. Equine adenohypophyseal adenomas generally occur in the pars intermedia. Cystadenomas of the pars intermedia will compress the pars distalis and may or may not secrete excessive amounts of ACTH. Those that secrete ACTH may be poorly suppressed by dexamethasone, stimulated by TRH or GnRH,[88] and inhibited by cyproheptadine or bromocryptine. Diabetes insipidus will result if the neurohypophysis is compressed.

Adenohypophyseal tumors are much less common in cats than in dogs.[37, 97] Their biologic behavior is similar to that in dogs. Adenohypophyseal tumors in horses are often associated with diabetes mellitus, hyperhidrosis, laminitis, hirsutism, and diabetes insipidus.[46, 49] Presumably, the excessive production of ACTH or, possibly, GH causes diabetes mellitus. Excessive amounts of ACTH could produce an excess of adrenal androgens, causing hirsutism and hyperhidrosis, and neurohypophyseal compression causes diabetes insipidus. Chromophobe adenomas in budgerigars can cause seizures, proptosis, impaired vision, and polyuria-polydipsia.[57]

Associated Tumors

When adenohypophyseal tumors are found, the presence of tumors of the pancreatic islets and parathyroid glands should be considered. Adenohypophyseal adenomas can develop concurrently with adenomas of the pancreatic islets and parathyroid glands in humans affected with an inherited disorder, *multiple endocrine adenomatosis, Type I* (Wermer's syndrome). The pituitary adenoma usually does not secrete hormones, but the parathyroids often produce excessive amounts of parathyroid hormone, and the pancreatic islet adenoma may secrete excessive amounts of insulin or gastrin.

Multiple endocrine adenomatosis, Type I, is one of several types of multiple tumor combinations that are related developmentally and functionally. The tumors are called *APUDomas* (the abbreviation "APUD" stands for amine precursor uptake and decarboxylation). They share several common characteristics: the synthesis of aromatic amines or polypeptides, decarbox-

Table 4–6. Amine Precursor Uptake and Decarboxylation Cells

Adenohypophysis
Adrenal medulla and paraganglia
Parafollicular cells of the thyroid
Parathyroids
Pancreatic islets
Some bronchial cells and some gastrointestinal mucosal cells
Thymus
Melanocytes ·
Chemoreceptors in carotid and aortic bodies

---

ylation and storage of aromatic amine precursors, a high concentration of esterases, and the secretion of similar hormones. These tumors develop simultaneously with other tumors of the endocrine organs. They originate in the endoderm or oral ectoderm. All are thought to have components that came from the neural crest. In Table 4–6, APUD cells are listed.

See also reference 91.

REFERENCES

1. Allan, G.S., et al.: Pituitary dwarfism in German Shepherd dogs. J. Small Anim. Pract., *19:*711, 1978.
2. Allison, R.M.M., Watson, A.D.J., and Church, D.B.: Pituitary tumour causing neurological and endocrine disturbances in a dog. J. Small Anim. Pract., *24:*229, 1983.
3. Andresen, V.E., and Willeberg, P.: Pituitary dwarfism in German Shepherd dogs: additional evidence of simple autosomal recessive inheritance. Nord. Vet. Med., *28:*481, 1976.
4. Andresen, V.E., and Willeberg, P.: Pituitary dwarfism in Carelian bear-dogs: evidence of simple autosomal recessive inheritance. Hereditas, *84:*232, 1976.
5. Andresen, V.E., Willeberg, P., and Rasmussen, P.G.: Pituitary dwarfism in German shepherd dogs—genetic investigations. Nord. Vet. Med., *26:*692, 1974.
6. Attia, M.A.: Cytological study on the anterior pituitary of senile untreated Beagle bitches with spontaneous mammary tumours. Arch. Toxicol., *50:*35, 1982.
7. Baker, E.: Congenital hypoplasia of the pituitary and pancreas glands in the dog. J. Am. Vet. Med. Assoc., *126:*468, 1955.
8. Bardens, J.W.: Hormonal therapy for ovarian and testicular dysfunction in the dog. J. Am. Vet. Med. Assoc., *159:*1405, 1971.
9. Capen, C.C., and Koestner, A.: Functional chromophobe adenomas of the canine adenohypophysis. Pathol. Vet., *4:*326, 1967.
10. Capen, C.C., and Martin, S.L.: Hyperadrenocorticism (Cushing's-like syndrome and disease) in dogs. Am. J. Pathol., *81:*459, 1975.
11. Capen, C.C., Martin, S.L., and Koestner, A.: Neoplasms in the adenohypophysis of dogs. Pathol. Vet., *4:*301, 1967.
12. Capen, C.C., Martin, S.L., and Koestner, A.: The ultrastructure and histiopathology of an acidophil adenoma of the canine adenohypophysis. Pathol. Vet., *4:*348, 1967.
13. Cassel, S.E.: Ovarian imbalance in a German shepherd dwarf. Vet. Med. Small Anim. Clin., *73:*162, 1978.
14. Chakraborty, P.K., Wildt, D.E., and Seager, S.W.J.: Induction of estrus and ovulation in the cat and dog. Vet. Clin. North Am., *12:*85, 1982.
15. Chastain, C.B., Riedesel, D.H., and Graham, C.L.: Secondary hypothyroidism in a dog. Canine Pract., *6:*59, 1979.
16. Concannon, P., et al.: Growth hormone, prolactin, and cortisol in dogs developing mammary nodules and an acromegaly-like appearance during treatment with medroxyprogesterone acetate. Endocrinology, *106:*1173, 1980.
17. Cook, R.W.: Hypothalamic hamartoma in a dog. Vet. Pathol., *14:*138, 1977.

18. Dammrich, K.: Die morphologische und funktionelle Pathologie der Geschwulste der Adenohypophyse bei Hunden. Zentralbl. Veterinarmed., *14A:*137, 1967.
19. Eigenmann, J.E.: Acromegaly in the dog. Vet. Clin. North Am., Small Anim. Pract., *14:*827, 1984.
20. Eigenmann, J.E.: Diagnosis and treatment of dwarfism in a German shepherd dog. J. Am. Anim. Hosp. Assoc., *17:*798, 1981.
21. Eigenmann, J.E.: Diagnosis and treatment of pituitary dwarfism in dogs. Proceedings of the 6th Kal Kan Symposium. Columbus, OH, 1982, p. 107.
22. Eigenmann, J.E.: Naturally occurring and iatrogenic acromegaly in the dog. Proceedings of the 6th Kal Kan Symposium. Columbus, OH, 1982, p. 81.
23. Eigenmann, J.E., and Eigenmann, R.Y.: Influence of medroxyprogesterone acetate (provera) on plasma growth hormones levels and on carbohydrate metabolism. II. Studies in the ovariohysterectomized, oestradiol-primed bitch. Acta Endocrinol., *98:*603, 1981.
24. Eigenmann, J.E., Lubberink, A.A.M.E., and Koemann, J.P.: Panhypopituitarism caused by a suprasellar tumor in a dog. J. Am. Anim. Hosp. Assoc., *19:*377, 1983.
25. Eigenmann, J.E., and Patterson, D.F.: Growth hormone deficiency in the mature dog. J. Am. Anim. Hosp. Assoc., *20:*741, 1984.
26. Eigenmann, J.E., and Rijnberk, A.: Influence of medroxyprogesterone acetate (provera) on plasma growth hormone levels and on carbohydrate metabolism I. Studies in the ovariohysterectomized bitch. Acta Endocrinol., *98:*599, 1981.
27. Eigenmann, J.E., and Venker-van Haagen, A.J.: Progestogen-induced and spontaneous canine acromegaly due to reversible growth hormone overproduction: clinical picture and pathogenesis. J. Am. Anim. Hosp. Assoc., *17:*813, 1981.
28. Eigenmann, J.E., Wortman, J.A., and Haskins, M.E.: Elevated growth hormone levels and diabetes mellitus in a cat with acromegalic features. J. Am. Anim. Hosp. Assoc., *20:*747, 1984.
29. Eigenmann, J.E., et al.: Progesterone-controlled growth hormone overproduction and naturally occurring canine diabetes and acromegaly. Acta Endocrinol., *104:*167, 1983.
30. Eigenmann, J.E., et al.: Growth hormone and insulin-like growth factor I in German shepherd dwarf dogs. Acta Endocrinol., *105:*289, 1984.
31. Eigenmann, J.E., et al.: Insulin-like growth factor I in the dog: a study in different dog breeds and in dogs with growth hormone elevation. Acta Endocrinol., *105:*294, 1984.
32. El Etreby, M.F., Fath, E.L., and Bab, M.R.: Effects of cyproterone acetate, d-norgestrel and progesterone on cells of the pars distalis of the adenohypophysis in the beagle bitch. Cell Tissue Res., *191:*205, 1978.
33. El Etreby, M.F., et al.: Functional morphology of spontaneous hyperplasia and neoplasia in the canine pituitary gland. Vet. Pathol., *17:*109, 1980.
34. El Etreby, M.F., et al.: The role of the pituitary gland in spontaneous canine mammary tumorigenesis. Vet. Pathol., *17:*2, 1980.
35. Farrow, B.R.H.: Chromophobe adenoma of the pituitary in a dog. Vet. Rec., *84:*609, 1969.
36. Ganong, W.F., and Hume, D.M.: The effect of graded hypophysectomy on thyroid, gonadal, and adrenocortical function in the dog. Endocrinology, *59:*293, 1956.
37. Gembardt, C., and Loppnow, H.: To the pathogenesis of the spontaneous diabetes mellitus in cats. Part II. Acidophilic adenomas of the pituitary gland and diabetes mellitus in two cases. Berl. Munch. Tierarztl. Wochenschr., *89:*336, 1976.
38. Gilbert, G.J., and Willey, E.N.: Pituitary chromophobe adenoma in the bulldog. J. Am. Vet. Med. Assoc., *154:*1071, 1969.
39. Graf, K-J., and El Etreby, M.R.: The role of the anterior pituitary gland in progestagen-induced proliferative mammary gland changes in the beagle. Drug. Res., *23:*54, 1978.
40. Hampshire, J., and Altszuler, N.: Clonidine or xylazine as provocative tests for growth hormone secretion in the dog. Am. J. Vet. Res., *42:*1073, 1981.
41. Hare, T.: Chromophobe cell adenoma of the pituitary gland associated with dystrophia adiposogenitalis in a maiden bitch. Proc. R. Soc. Med., *25:*1493, 1935.
42. Hartigan, P.J.: A chromophobe adenoma of the pituitary gland in a dog. Ir. Vet. J., *31:*57, 1977.
43. Hartigan, P.J., and McGilligan, C.A.: Piperazine neurotoxicity in a pituitary dwarf cat. Ir. Vet. J., *30:*188, 1976.
44. Heavner, J.E., and Dice, P.F.: Pituitary tumor as a cause of blindness in a dog. Vet. Med. Small Anim. Clin., *72:*873, 1977.

45. Henry, R.W., et al.: Transoral hypophysectomy with mandibular symphsiotomy in the dog. Am. J. Vet. Res., *43:*1825, 1982.
46. Holscher, M.A., et al.: Adenoma of the pars intermedia and hirsutism in a pony. Vet. Med. Smalll Anim. Clin., *73:*1197, 1978.
47. Hottendorf, G.H., Nielsen, S.W., and Lieberman, L.L.: Acidophil adenoma of the pituitary gland and other neoplasms in a boxer. J. Am. Vet. Med. Assoc., *148:*1046, 1966.
48. Jensen, E.C.: Hypopituitarism associated with cystic Rathke's cleft in a dog. J. Am. Vet. Med. Assoc., *135:*572, 1959.
49. King, J.M., Kavanaugh, J.F., and Bentinck-Smith, J.: Diabetes mellitus with pituitary neoplasms in a horse and a dog. Cornell Vet., *52:*133, 1962.
50. Kleinberg, D.L., Noel, G.L., and Frantz, A.G.: Galactorrhea: study of 235 cases, including 48 with pituitary tumors. N. Engl. J. Med., *296:*589, 1977.
51. Kirby, R.W., Kotchen, T.A., and Rees, E.D.: Hyperprolactinemia—a review of recent clinical advances. Arch. Intern. Med., *139:*1415, 1979.
52. Krieger, D.T.: The central nervous system and Cushing's disease. Med. Clin. North Am., *62:*261, 1978.
53. Krieger, D.T.: Physiopathology of Cushing's disease. Endocr. Rev., *4:*22, 1983.
54. Lund-Larsen, T.R., and Grondalen, J.: Ateliotic dwarfism in the German shepherd dog. Acta Vet. Scand., *17:*293, 1976.
55. Mach, R., and Haase, G.: Hypofunktion der Adenohypophyse eines Hundes. Tierarztl. Umschan., *8:*242, 1953.
56. Madewell, B.R., and Mulnix, A.: Neoplasms of endocrine glands. Vet. Clin. North Am., *7:*195, 1977.
57. Martin, S.L.: Diagnosis and management of common endocrine and metabolic diseases of pet birds. Proceedings of the 6th Kal Kan Symposium. Columbus, OH, 1982, p. 25.
58. McNichol, A.M., Thomson, H., and Stewart, C.J.R.: The corticotrophic cells of the canine pituitary gland in pituitary-dependent hyperadrenocorticism. J. Endocrinol., *96:*303, 1983.
59. Meijer, J.C., et al.: Hypothalamic catecholamine levels in dogs with spontaneous hyperadrenocorticism. Neuroendocrinology, *32:*197, 1981.
60. Morrow, L.B.: Clinical evaluation of pituitary adenomas. Postgrad. Med. J., *68:*155, 1980.
61. Muller, G.H.: Pituitary dwarfism. Vet. Clin. North Am., *9:*41, 1979.
62. Muller, G.H., and Jones, S.R.: Pituitary dwarfism and alopecia in a German shepherd with a cystic Rathke's cleft. J. Am. Anim. Hosp. Assoc., *9:*567, 1973.
63. Muller-Peddinghaus, R., et al.: Pituitary dwarfism in a German shepherd dog. Vet. Pathol., *17:*406, 1980.
64. Neer, T.M., and Reavis, D.U.: Craniopharyngioma and associated central diabetes insipidus and hypothyroidism in a dog. J. Am. Vet. Med. Assoc., *182:*519, 1983.
65. Nelson, R.W., et al.: Diencephalic syndrome secondary to intracranial astrocytoma in a dog. J. Am. Vet. Med. Assoc., *179:*1004, 1981.
66. Nicholas, F.: Pituitary dwarfism in German shepherd dogs: a genetic analysis of some Australian data. J. Small Anim. Pract., *19:*167, 1978.
67. Osborne, J.C., and Harris, J.E.: Chromophobe adenoma in a dog. Vet. Med. Small Anim. Clin., *65:*1079, 1970.
68. Paisley, L.G., and Fahning, M.L.: Effects of exogenous follicle-stimulating hormone and luteinizing hormone in bitches. J. Am. Vet. Med. Assoc., *171:*181, 1977.
69. Parker, W.M., and Scott, D.W.: Growth hormone responsive alopecia in the mature dog: a discussion of 13 cases. J. Am. Anim. Hosp. Assoc., *16:*824, 1980.
70. Peterson, M.E., and Altszuler, N.: Suppression of growth hormone secretion in spontaneous canine hyperadrenocorticism and its reversal after treatment. Am. J. Vet. Res., *42:*1881, 1981.
71. Peterson, M.E., et al.: Immunocytochemical study of the hypophysis in 25 dogs with pituitary-dependent hyperadrenocorticism. Acta Endocrinol., *101:*15, 1982.
72. Putman, T.J., Benedict, F.B., and Teel, H.M.: Studies in acromegaly VIII. Experimental canine acromegaly produced by injection of anterior lobe pituitary extract. Arch. Surg., *18:*1708, 1929.
73. Rijnberk, A., et al.: Acromegaly associated with transient overproduction of growth hormone in a dog. J. Am. Vet. Med. Assoc., *177:*534, 1980.
74. Ringheim, H.P.: Pituitary adenocarcinoma in a dog. Mod. Vet. Pract., *53:*41, 1972.
75. Roberg, J.W.: Dwarfism in the German shepherd. Canine Pract., *6:*42, 1979.

76. Roth, J.A., et al.: Thymic abnormalities and growth hormone deficiency in dogs. Am. J. Vet. Res., *41:*1256, 1980.

77. Roth, J.A., et al.: Improvement in clinical condition and thymus morphologic features associated with growth hormone treatment of immunodeficient dwarf dogs. Am. J. Vet. Res., *45:*1151, 1984.

78. Saunders, L.Z., and Richard, C.G.: Craniopharyngioma in a dog with apparent adiposo-genital syndrome and diabetes insipidus. Cornell Vet., *42:*490, 1952.

79. Saunders, L.A., Stephenson, H.C., and McEntee, K.: Diabetes insipidus and adiposogeni-tal syndrome in a dog due to an infundibuloma. Cornell Vet., *41:*445, 1951.

80. Scott, D.W., and Concannon, P.W.: Gross and microscopic changes in the skin of dogs with progestagen-induced acromegaly and elevated growth hormone levels. J. Am. Anim. Hosp. Assoc., *19:*523, 1983.

81. Scott, D.W., et al.: Clinicopathological findings in a German shepherd with pituitary dwarfism. J. Am. Anim. Hosp. Assoc., *14:*183, 1978.

82. Scrogie, N.J.: The treatment of sterility in the bitch by the use of gonadotrophic hor-mones. Vet. Rec., *51:*265, 1939.

83. Siegel, E.T.: Endocrine Diseases of the Dog. Philadelphia, Lea & Febiger, 1977.

84. Slatter, D.H., Schirmer, R.G., and Krehbiel, J.D.: Surgical correction of cystic Rathke's cleft in a dog. J. Am. Anim. Hosp. Assoc., *12:*641, 1976.

85. Sokolowski, J.H., Medernach, R.W., and Helper, L.C.: Exogenous hormone therapy to control the estrous cycle of the bitch. J. Am. Vet. Med. Assoc., *153:*425, 1968.

86. Spark, R.F., et al.: Bromocriptine reduces pituitary tumor size and hypersecretion. J. Am. Vet. Med. Assoc., *247:*311, 1982.

87. Spence, J.A., et al.: Metastasis of a transmissible venereal tumor to the pituitary. J. Small Anim. Pract., *19:*175, 1978.

88. Stolp, R., Croughs, R.J., and Rijnberk, A.: Results of cyproheptadine treatment in dogs with pituitary-dependent hyperadrenocorticism. J. Endocrinol., *101:*311, 1984.

89. Stolp, R., et al.: Plasma cortisol response to thyrotrophin releasing hormone and luteinizing hormone releasing hormone in healthy kennel dogs and in dogs with pituitary-dependent hyperadrenocorticism. J. Endocrinol., *93:*365, 1982.

90. Thun, R., Watson, P., and Jackson, G.L.: Induction of estrus and ovulation in the bitch, using exogenous gonadotropins. Am. J. Vet. Res., *38:*483, 1977.

91. Tischler, A.S., et al.: Neuroendocrine neoplasms and their cells of origin. N. Engl. J. Med., *296:*919, 1977.

92. White, E.G.: A suprasellar tumor in a dog. J. Pathol. Bacteriol., *47:*323, 1938.

93. Wildt, D.E., and Seager, S.W.J.: Ovarian response in the estrual cat receiving varying dosages of HCG. Horm. Res., *9:*144, 1978.

94. Wildt, D.E., Kinney, G.M., and Seager, S.W.J.: Gonadotropin-induced reproductive cyclicity in the domestic cat. Lab. Anim. Sci., *28:*301, 1978.

95. Willeberg, P., Kastrup, K.W., and Andresen, E.: Pituitary dwarfism in German shepherd dogs: studies on somatomedin activity. Nord. Vet. Med., *27:*448, 1975.

96. Wright, P.J.: The induction of oestrus and ovulation in the bitch using pregnant mare serum gonadotrophin and human chorionic gonadotrophin. Aust. Vet. J., *56:*137, 1980.

97. Zaki, F.A., and Leu, S.K.: Pituitary chromophobe adenoma in a cat. Vet. Pathol., *10:*232, 1973.

5

Disorders of Hypothalamic
and Neurohypophyseal Function

The neurohypophysis does not produce any hormone, but it does store antidiuretic hormone (ADH) and oxytocin for release into the systemic circulation. ADH and oxytocin are produced by hypothalamic nuclei, the supraoptic and paraventricular. Both hormones are transported to nerve endings in the neurohypophysis by nerve fibers, originating from the nuclei. The supraoptic and paraventricular nuclei, hypothalamohypophyseal nerve fibers, and neurohypophyseal nerve endings are anatomically and functionally one unit. ADH permits passive reabsorption of water from the distal convoluted tubules and collecting ducts into the hypertonic interstitium of the kidneys (Fig. 5–1). Oxytocin causes uterine contraction and myoepithelial contraction in the mammae.

Recognized clinical disorders of the hypothalamic-neurohypophyseal unit only involve effects resulting from an excess or deficiency in ADH. Deficiencies or noniatrogenic excesses of oxytocin action have not been recognized in any species, including humans. An excess of ADH causes water intoxication, which can be iatrogenic or spontaneous. When levels of ADH spontaneously develop an inappropriate excess, the condition is called the *syndrome of inappropriate ADH* (SIADH). SIADH has been reported in humans and a dog. The action of deficient ADH causes uncontrolled water loss in the urine, and persistent thirst develops to compensate the water loss. This is called *diabetes insipidus,* which has been recognized for many years in dogs, cats, horses, budgerigars, and humans, among other species. Deficient ADH action may be due to deficient levels of ADH or due to an inability of ADH to mediate its usual effects on the renal tubules.

SYNDROME OF INAPPROPRIATE ANTIDIURETIC HORMONE
(Schwartz-Bartter-like syndrome)

Causes

Normally secretion of ADH decreases if plasma osmolality decreases or if high pressure receptors in the aorta or carotid body are stimulated. Factors known to promote secretion of ADH inappropriate to plasma osmolality and blood pressure are listed in Table 5–1. Drugs that are known to cause SIADH are chlorpropamide, vincristine, cyclophosphamide, potassium-wasting diuretics, barbiturates, morphine, and carbamazepine. Central

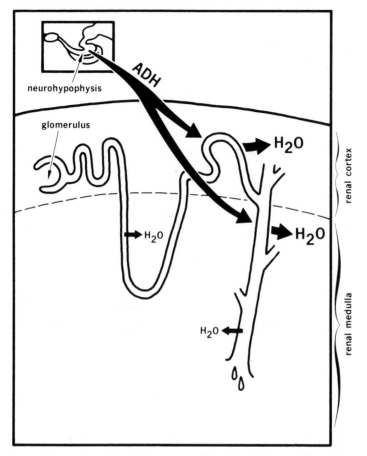

Fig. 5-1. Effects of antidiuretic hormone on kidneys. ADH = antidiuretic hormone.

nervous system diseases that have caused SIADH in humans are encephalitis, cerebral thrombosis or hemorrhage, and intracranial neoplasia. Neoplasms, especially bronchogenic carcinomas, in humans have produced ectopic ADH. Other neoplasms that have produced ectopic ADH are pancreatic carcinoma, duodenal carcinoma, and lymphosarcoma. Non-neoplastic intrathoracic diseases may produce SIADH by interfering with vagal afferent nerves from pressure receptors in the atria and great veins. Examples in humans have included tuberculosis pneumonia, aspergillosis, and lung abscesses. In one case, SIADH has been associated with dirofilariasis in a dog.[7]

Clinical Signs and Laboratory Findings

The clinical signs found in subjects with SIADH depend on the cause of the syndrome and on the concentration of serum sodium. Signs of a central nervous system disease, pulmonary disorder, surgical or traumatic stress, or

Table 5-1.   Possible Causes of the Syndrome of Inappropriate
Antidiuretic Hormone

Neopiasia (ectopic production of antidiuretic hormone)
Non-neoplastic intrathoracic diseases
Central nervous system disorders
Surgical or traumatic stress
Various drugs (see text)

---

drug intoxication may overshadow signs of SIADH. This may account for
its currently rare recognition in companion animals. Regardless of its cause,
if the serum sodium is severely decreased (less than 120 mEq/L) signs of
hyponatremia may prevail (Table 5-2).

The outstanding initial abnormal laboratory finding is usually hyponatremia. The hyponatremia is caused by the dilutional effects of retained water
and urinary losses of sodium. Sodium is lost in the urine despite hyponatremia because the secretion of aldosterone is inhibited by hypervolemia
caused by water retention. An increase in prostaglandin E, a natriuretic
paracrine secretion stimulated by an expanded extracellular fluid volume, is
also possible. Clinical features characteristic of SIADH are summarized in
Table 5-3. Even though water is retained, edema usually does not develop
due to continuing natriuresis (loss of sodium in the urine). The degree of
natriuresis is quite variable, being dependent on the quantity of ingested
dietary sodium.

Other serum constitutent concentrations, such as potassium and chloride,
may also be diluted. Hypochloridemia may be severe enough to cause metabolic alkalosis. Serum urate concentrations are decreased by dilution and
other unexplained reasons. Decreased serum urate levels in humans with
SIADH help to differentiate SIADH from other causes for hyponatremia.[2]

Diagnosis

The clinical features of SIADH are most easily confused with those of
primary hypoadrenocorticism. It differs from primary hypoadrenocorticism
in having normal to low levels of blood urea nitrogen and serum concentrations of potassium. Primary hypoadrenocorticism is associated with azote-

Table 5-2.   Clinical Signs of the Syndrome of Inappropriate
Antidiuretic Hormone Related to Hyponatremia

Nausea
Anorexia
Emesis
Irritable behavior
Confusion
Head pressing
Seizures
Cardiac arrhythmias

Table 5–3. Characteristic Clinical Features of the Syndrome of Inappropriate Antidiuretic Hormone

Hyponatremia with natriuresis
Hypo-osmolality of plasma
Urine osmolality exceeds plasma osmolality
Normal renal and adrenal function
Improvement after restricted consumption of water

mia and hyperkalemia. Other differential diagnoses for hyponatremia include congestive heart failure, nephrosis, severe liver disease, hyperglycemia, and hyperlipidemia.

A clinical diagnosis can be based on finding the characteristic clinical features of SIADH (Table 5–3) and the exclusion of other causes of hyponatremia. Plasma concentrations of ADH can be directly measured, but collection and assay are difficult, requiring an ice bath, refrigerated centrifugation, and transport in the frozen state. The lack of assay availability and the expenses involved also contribute to the difficulty. Plasma levels of ADH should be inappropriate for the concurrent measurement of plasma osmolality. Normal plasma levels in dogs given free access to water are usually less than 5 pg/ml.[42, 46]

Treatment

When possible, the cause for SIADH should be determined and corrected. Mild cases may only require restricted access to water. Hypertonic (3%) saline can be slowly given in an intravenous dose over 2 to 4 hours if neurologic signs are thought to be due to severe hyponatremia. Improvement would be temporary because of continuing natriuresis. Although risks of volume overload are great, volume overload may be corrected with furosemide. If the cause is not the secretion of ectopic ADH, the anticonvulsant phenytoin or narcotic antagonists, butorphanol or oxilorphan, can inhibit the secretion of ADH. A tetracycline, demeclocycline, inhibits the action of ADH on the renal tubules. It has been effective in treating humans with SIADH caused by excessive secretion from hypothalamic nuclei or by the secretion of ectopic ADH.[10, 14, 15, 19] Lithium will also inhibit the action of ADH on the renal tubules, but its potential use is precluded by its toxicity relative to that of demeclocycline. If sodium and potassium are sufficiently supplemented, low-dose furosemide can be effective in correcting SIADH by inhibiting the reabsorption of free water in the renal tubules.[13]

DIABETES INSIPIDUS

Causes

Diabetes insipidus (Gr., tasteless diuresis) has a variety of causes, but the most frequently recognized cause in companion animals is primary neoplasia of the hypothalamus or tumors extending into the hypothalamus. There are two major types of causes for diabetes insipidus—an insufficiency or deficiency of ADH (hypothalamic diabetes insipidus) and *nephrogenic* causes (Fig. 5–2). Examples of various types of causes are given in Table 5–4.[4, 29, 32, 35, 38, 48, 49, 52]

Familial diabetes insipidus has not been reported in companion animals. In humans, familial hypothalamic diabetes insipidus is an autosomal dominant inherited trait causing abnormal development of the ADH-producing nuclei. Familial nephrogenic diabetes insipidus in humans is an X-linked recessive trait. Congenital hypothalamic diabetes insipidus has been noted

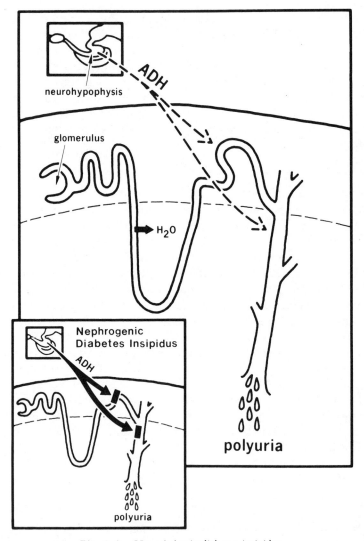

Fig. 5–2. Hypothalamic diabetes insipidus.

Table 5-4.   Types and Possible Causes for Diabetes Insipidus

Hypothalamic—insufficiency or deficiency of antidiuretic hormone
Primary or metastatic tumor
Infection
Granulomatous lesions
Trauma or surgery
Vascular lesions
Familial
Idiopathic
"High-set osmoreceptors"

Nephrogenic—insensitivity of antidiuretic hormone
Congenital (familial)
Acquired
Pathologic
Pyelonephritis
Hypokalemic nephropathy
Hypercalcemic nephropathy
Renal amyloidosis
Drug-induced
Demeclocycline
Lithium
Methoxyflurane

by the authors and reported by others in dogs[22] and cats.[51] Congenital nephrogenic diabetes insipidus has also been reported in dogs,[8,35,38] but familial defects in the supraoptic nuclei or ADH receptors without other lesions in the kidneys have not been reported in either dogs or cats.

Plasma osmolality is normally regulated within a range of 280 to 310 mOsm/kg body weight in dogs and cats, and a range of 270 to 300 mOsm/kg body weight in the horse.[20] Osmolality of the plasma is continuously monitored by osmoreceptors in or near the supraoptic and paraventricular nuclei. As little as 1 mOsm/L change in plasma osmolality affects the secretion of ADH. An increase of 1 mOsm/L causes an increase of about 0.3 pg/ml in the secretion of ADH, which leads to an increase of 85 mOsm/kg body weight in urine osmolality. Defective ("high-set") osmoreceptors may cause diabetes insipidus, even though the subject's ability to secrete ADH remains when stimulated by greater-than-usual increases in plasma osmolality or by nonosmolar stimuli such as nicotine. In subjects with "high-set" osmoreceptor diabetes insipidus, thirst is stimulated and water is ingested before ADH is secreted to retain the ingested water.

Lesions of the nearby thirst center will result in severe dehydration and hypernatremia, a condition called *essential hypernatremia.*[12,23,33] Congenital essential hypernatremia has been reported in the miniature schnauzer. The secretion of ADH remains intact, responsive to plasma osmolality, and effective in its action on renal tubules.

Lesions of the distal neurohypophysis do not cause permanent diabetes insipidus, but levels of ADH may be deficient for about 2 weeks. Experimentally, damage to the stalk proximal to the hypothalamus can produce diabetes insipidus for a few days, followed by a short-lived remission, after which normality, then permanent diabetes insipidus, results. The worsening of the condition is caused by retrograde degeneration of the nerve fibers.

See references 5, 8, 9, 11, 16, 18, 21, 37, and 47.

Clinical Signs

The first signs of diabetes insipidus are excessive thirst (more than 100 ml/kg body weight/day) and great volumes of water-clear voided urine (more than 50 ml/kg body weight/day).[17] The severity of clinical signs varies since diabetes insipidus may result from either complete or partial insufficiency on the part of ADH action. Its onset may be insidious or abrupt, depending on the initiating cause. Most cases have an abrupt onset. Its duration may be temporary or permanent. Latent diabetes occurs if glomerular filtration is reduced by adenohypophyseal insufficiency or hypoadrenocorticism. It is unmasked by treatment with glucocorticoids.

The range of manifest clinical signs is also affected by the cause. Concomitant signs of other hypothalamic dysfunctions or adenohypophyseal hormone excesses or insufficiencies are possible, especially if the cause is intracranial vascular disease, trauma, granulomas, infection, or tumor. Acquired nephrogenic diabetes insipidus may be associated with concomitant signs of hyperkalemia, hypercalcemia, amyloidosis, pyelonephritis, or drug toxicities. Familial or idiopathic causes are usually not associated with signs of disease other than diabetes insipidus.

When severe polyuria resulting from diabetes insipidus occurs, it is unrelenting; however, dehydration should not occur if the patient has free access to water at all times, and the thirst center and osmoreceptors are normal. With severe polyuria, nocturia (excessive voiding of urine at night) takes place because the bladder is distended. Drinking even becomes necessary during periods when sleep would be expected.

If the patient is given a choice, he may have an inexplicable preference for ice water. Distention of the stomach may cause vomiting. Weight loss is common, resulting from either the patient's preoccupation with drinking or from underlying hypothalamic disease. Causes of inadequate ingestion of water such as restricted access to water, coma, paralysis, or other reasons may cause severe dehydration, coma, and then death within a few hours. Despite dehydration, polyuria persists.

The amount of urine voided does not always reflect the true severity of the patient's illness. The amount of urine not reabsorbed in the collecting ducts and distal convoluted tubules depends, in part, on the glomerular filtration rate (GFR). A decreased GFR resulting from adenohypophyseal insufficiency, adrenocortical insufficiency, or cardiovascular disease will cause a decrease in the degree of polyuria caused by a lack of ADH or its action on the renal tubules. Still, the volume of urine voided is generally three to ten times the normal amount. Other factors contributing to the patient's inability to concentrate urine include impaired urea synthesis caused by protein malnutrition or severe liver disease and renal medullary "washout" resulting from severe polyuria of any cause.

Laboratory Findings and Diagnosis

If diabetes insipidus is not complicated by the presence of other diseases, it does not produce any abnormalities in blood counts or chemistries. Urinalysis shows that the urine is persistently dilute (hyposthenuric), often with a specific gravity and osmolality of less than 1.006 and 200 mOsm/kg body weight, respectively. Random urinalyses done in normal dogs and cats generally have shown an osmolality in excess of 400 mOsm/kg body weight and a specific gravity of more than 1.015. Plasma osmolality is nearly identical to serum osmolality if heparinized blood is used. Sodium EDTA adds 5 to 20 mOsm/kg body weight to actual plasma osmolality.

Many other diseases cause polyuria and polydipsia. The most common are diabetes mellitus, hyperadrenocorticism, hyperthyroidism, severe liver disease, pyometra, and end-stage renal disease.[1, 25, 36] Each causes marked abnormalities in the hemogram or serum chemistries. Psychogenic polydipsia (potomania), a rare disorder reported in some dogs and humans, can be easily confused with diabetes insipidus.[25] Most cases in dogs have been recognized in young large breeds, especially German shepherd dogs 6 to 12 months of age. The presenting signs of psychogenic polydipsia are similar to those of diabetes insipidus, although the patient's behavior may be more excitable and nocturia is rare. Hemograms and serum chemistries are normal, and the urine is hyposthenuric. In subjects with psychogenic polydipsia the serum osmolality is usually decreased; in subjects with diabetes insipidus plasma osmolality is normal or increased.

Once a patient with polyuria and polydipsia has been screened with routine baseline laboratory examinations (Table 5–5) and diabetes insipidus is still suspected, a water deprivation test may be considered. Before a water deprivation test is done in some patients, liver function tests, determination of levels of serum cortisol, creatinine clearance tests, or radiographic examinations may be necessary to rule out causes of polyuria and polydipsia in addition to diabetes insipidus. The purpose of water deprivation test is to stimulate endogenous secretion of ADH to determine if the secretion of ADH and the means to respond to ADH are present. The water deprivation test is unnecessary and contraindicated if dehydration or plasma

Table 5–5. Suggested Baseline Laboratory Data for Polyuria-Polydipsia

Hemogram
Blood urea nitrogen
Serum creatinine
Blood glucose
Serum alkaline phosphatase
Serum alanine aminotransferase
Urinalysis

hyperosmolality are already present (the procedures of the water deprivation test are outlined in Table 5–6). If an osmometer is not available, urine osmolality can be estimated by multiplying the last 2 digits of the specific gravity by 36.[31] For example, a specific gravity of 1.020 would be calculated as 720 mOsm/kg body weight. Close supervision is advisable since patients with complete hypothalamic or nephrogenic diabetes insipidus may lose more than 5% of their body weight in voided urine and have cardiovascular collapse within 4 hours of water deprivation.

When normal dogs are deprived of water, peak levels of urine osmolality are not reached for about 42 hours. Laboratory dogs and cats can concentrate urine to 2400 mOsm/kg body weight and 2800 mOsm/kg weight,

Table 5–6. Recommended Procedure for the Water Deprivation and Antidiuretic Hormone Response Tests

Step	Procedure
1	Review history, physical, and laboratory data to exclude other possible causes for polyuria-polydipsia.
2	Verify presence and severity of polyuria and polydipsia by measuring consumption of water over 24 hours and volume of urine voided for 2 or more days.
3	If polyuria has been severe, or low urea nitrogen or low serum sodium is present, reduce access to water 10% per day for 3 to 5 days, but do not limit access to less than 100 ml/kg body weight/day. Also administer 1 to 3 g of enteric-coated sodium chloride per day and feed high-protein meals for 3 to 5 days.
4	Withhold food for 12 hours.
5	Empty the urinary bladder, collect urine in a clean dry pan, then determine and record patient's Body weight Serum urea nitrogen Serum and urine osmolality Specific gravity of urine
6	If patient's hydration is normal, begin complete deprivation of water and continue to withhold food.
7	Every 2 hours repeat step No. 5 and weigh any eliminated feces.
8	Discontinue total water deprivation whenever any of the following occur: 5% of the initial body weight minus eliminated feces that has been lost. Urine osmolality fails to increase more than 30 mOsm/kg body weight and 3% of the body weight has been lost. Urine specific gravity fails to increase more than 0.001 and 3% of the body weight has been lost. Serum urea nitrogen exceeds 30 mg/dl.
9	Assuming inadequate urine concentration occurred after water deprivation, administer 2 to 5 U of aqueous antidiuretic hormone in an intramuscular injection, empty the urinary bladder, and provide limited access to water (20 ml/kg body weight).
10	Repeat step No. 5 two hours later.

respectively. Because of the clinical variations in the patients' dietary protein, as well as advanced age, prolonged polyuria, and other unassessable factors, urinary concentrations of 900 mOsm/kg body weight and a specific gravity of 1.025 are considered adequate responses to water deprivation in dogs. A specific gravity of 1.030 and a urinary concentration of 1000 mOsm/kg body weight after water deprivation are the responses considered adequate in the cat.

Urine osmolality to plasma osmolality ratios, determined after water deprivation, may be used to evaluate the patient's ability to concentrate urine. A ratio of less than 1:1 is characteristic of diabetes insipidus. Ratios of more than 3:1 are normal. Partial diabetes insipidus, renal medullary washout, nephrogenic diabetes insipidus, and severe dehydration in conjunction with complete hypothalamic diabetes insipidus can produce values of 1:1 to 3:1.

Urine osmolality may slightly exceed that of the glomerular filtrate, even in the absence of ADH or its effects. This occurs when there is a severe decrease (more than 50%) in the glomerular filtration rate, resulting in increased reabsorption of sodium chloride and water in the proximal convoluted tubule. Such severe decreases are unlikely to occur in a dog with diabetes insipidus, except when extreme dehydration is allowed to occur.

Partial deprivation of water for 3 days is recommended in cases of severe polyuria, hyponatremia, or abnormally decreased concentrations of serum urea nitrogen since renal medullary hypertonicity may have been compromised. Renal medullary "washout" can impair concentration of the urine in

Table 5-7. Typical Responses to Water Deprivation and Exogenous Administration of Antidiuretic Hormone

	After Water Deprivation			Two Hours After ADH Administration*
	Plasma Osmolality	Urine Osmolality	Urine Specific Gravity	Percent Increase in Urine Osmolality
Normal	280–310	>900	>1.025	<5
Hypothalamic diabetes insipidus				
Complete	>310	<200	<1.008	>100
Partial	>300	<900	<1.025	5–100
High-set osmoreceptor	>310	>900	>1.025	<5
Nephrogenic diabetes insipidus	>310	<450	<1.012	<5
Psychogenic polydipsia	<300	>900	>1.025	<5

* 2 to 5 U of aqueous ADH in an intramuscular dose. ADH = antidiuretic hormone.

cases of psychogenic polydipsia even though endogenous secretion of ADH and mechanisms of ADH action are normal.

Failure to concentrate urine adequately after a properly conducted water deprivation test is diagnostic for diabetes insipidus. To differentiate the type of diabetes insipidus, an exogenous aqueous *ADH response test,* using an intramuscular dose of 2 to 5 U of Vasopressin, should be done at the completion of the water deprivation procedure. Response is evaluated by determining the percentage of increase in urine osmolality compared to the values obtained at the end of the period of water deprivation (Table 5–7).

Normally, if water is deprived to the point that 3% to 5% of the body weight is lost, or the urine osmolality reaches a plateau, the maximum endogenous secretion of ADH should have been attained. If exogenous ADH is administered to a normal patient at this point, urine osmolality will not increase more than 5%; however, if the renal tubules are capable of responding to ADH and the endogenous concentration of ADH is insufficient to stimulate all the available ADH receptors in the tubules, an increase in urine osmolality will exceed 5% within 2 hours of administration of ADH. In subjects with nephrogenic diabetes insipidus the response to water deprivation and to exogenous ADH is inadequate. If the patient is normal, or has psychogenic polydipsia or nephrogenic diabetes insipidus, plasma osmolality changes little (if at all) after the administration of exogenous ADH. Plasma osmolality will decrease after the administration of ADH in patients with hypothalamic diabetes insipidus.

Other tests are rarely necessary for the diagnosis and differentiation of diabetes insipidus. In comparison to the water deprivation test, the hypertonic (3%) saline infusion test (Hickey Hare test) may be done in a shorter period of time (1 hour), and decreased renal medullary hypertonicity may be simultaneously corrected. However, the risks of volume overload and cellular dehydration with saline infusion make the water deprivation test preferable. A nicotine response test, using an intramuscular dose of 1 mg has been used in humans to stimulate the secretion of ADH independently, without the concomitant stimulation of osmoreceptors. The test may be helpful in verifying high-set osmoreceptor diabetes insipidus, but its safety in companion animals has not been established. ADH mediates its effects through cyclic adenosine monophosphate (AMP). In humans, the concentration of cyclic AMP increases in the urine after the administration of ADH. Although the failure to increase urinary cyclic AMP with the administration of ADH is considered diagnostic of nephrogenic diabetes insipidus, this test has not been evaluated in companion animals. The RIA for ADH should show very high plasma levels after water deprivation, if nephrogenic diabetes insipidus is present, and low plasma levels if hypothalamic diabetes insipidus is the cause of polyuria and polydipsia.[43, 53]

A review of the patient's history and a physical examination are warranted if the diagnosis of diabetes insipidus is made. If the diagnosis is hypothalamic diabetes insipidus, the clinician should conduct an examination to rule out the possibility of a primary intracranial tumor or intracranial metastasis from likely distal sites such as the mammae. If the diagnosis is nephrogenic diabetes insipidus, the possibility of primary renal diseases or the administration of drugs that impair ADH's action should be reinvestigated.

See references 3, 6, 25–28, 34, 40, 41, 44, 45, and 50.

Treatment

Companion animals capable of ingesting enough water to compensate for urinary water loss may not require any treatment other than ensuring access to sufficient drinking water. In most cases nocturia, urination in the owner's living quarters, vomiting, weight loss, or the owner's apprehension dictate that additional treatment is necessary.

Hypothalamic diabetes insipidus caused by insufficiency or deficiency of ADH is most effectively treated with exogenous ADH (Pitressin tannate in oil), given in an intramuscular injection of 1.25 to 5 U (0.25 to 1 ml) every 1 to 3 days. Very small patients should receive a dose of 0.2 U/kg body weight. The duration of treatment is based on the amount of time the urine osmolality of concentrated urine has remained above 300 mOsm/kg body weight or the specific gravity has remained above 1.010. Injections are given in the evenings to prevent nocturia for as long as possible. Care must be taken to warm the vial by holding it in the hand until it reaches body temperature and mix the vial to suspend the hormone, which appears as brown particles in the oil.

An overdose of ADH can cause water intoxication and retention of nitrogenous waste products. Its use requires particular care in patients with congestive heart failure or azotemia. The repeated use of ADH can cause hypersensitivity reactions such as urticaria in some cases.

While ADH can be absorbed from mucous membranes, it cannot be given orally without destruction by digestion. Crude extracts of ADH given intranasally often lead to nasal and bronchial hypersensitivity. In comparison to the crude extracts, a synthetic lysine ADH, lypressin (Diapid Nasal Spray), is not as sensitizing, but the short duration (4 hours) of its effect is not desirable. A synthetic arginine ADH for intranasal use, desmopressin (DDAVP) has the least potential for sensitization and pressor effects. Because its structure is more resistant to degradation by peptidases, the frequency of administration (one drop one to three times per day in a nostril or conjunctival sac) is not as high as that required for lypressin. Its use is currently limited by its expense.[22]

Some drugs stimulate the secretion of ADH and may be useful in treating subjects with ADH insufficiency. Clofibrate (Atromid-S), a blood lipid lowering agent, and carbamazine (Tegretol), an anticonvulsant, have been used successfully in humans with partial hypothalamic diabetes insipidus. Appropriate dosages are not known for companion animals. Chlorpropamide (Diabinese) is a sulfonylurea used to lower blood glucose levels in human insulin-independent diabetics (patients with diabetes mellitus). It not only stimulates secretion of ADH, but also sensitizes the renal tubules to ADH. To treat diabetes insipidus, chlorpropamide has been used in average-sized dogs in doses of 50 to 250 mg[23] per day and cats in doses of about 50 mg per day.[11,48] Major potential adverse reactions are hypoglycemia, nausea, and skin eruptions.

The only treatment available for nephrogenic diabetes insipidus, assuming the cause cannot be eliminated, is a twice-daily dose of 10 to 20 mg/kg body weight of chlorothiazide (Diuril) or a twice-daily dose of 2 to 4 mg/kg body weight of hydrochlorothiazide (Hydrodiuril) and a low-salt diet. Thiazide diuretics have a paradoxical effect on the polyuria-polydipsia of diabetes insipidus. By decreasing the GFR, thiazide diuretics can indirectly cause increased reabsorption of sodium in the proximal convuluted tubule. This decreases the volume of water presented to the loop of Henle and distal convoluted tubules. The volume of polyuria may be reduced 50% by thiazide diuretics and low-sodium diets. Treatment with supplements of potassium may be necessary to prevent hypokalemia.

See reference 28.

REFERENCES

1. Asheim, A.: Pathogenesis of renal damage and polydipsia in dogs with pyometra. J. Am. Vet. Med. Assoc., *147:*736, 1965.
2. Beck, L.H.: Hypouricemia in the syndrome of inappropriate secretion of antidiuretic hormone. N. Engl. J. Med., *301:*528, 1979.
3. Belshaw, B.E.: Differential diagnosis of polyuria and polydipsia in dogs. Proceedings of the 6th Kal Kan Symposium. Columbus, OH, 1982, p. 1.
4. Bennett, C.M.: Urine concentration and dilution in hypokalemic and hypercalcemic dogs. J. Clin. Invest., *49:*1447, 1970.
5. Bovee, K.C.: Diabetes insipidus. Vet. Clin. North Am., *7:*603, 1977.
6. Breitswerdt, E.B.: Clinical abnormalities of urine concentration and dilution. Compend. Contin. Ed., *3:*414, 1981.
7. Breitswerdt, E.B., and Root, C.R.: Inappropriate secretion of antidiuretic hormone in a dog. J. Am. Vet. Med. Assoc., *175:*181, 1979.
8. Breitswerdt, E.B., Verlander, J.W., and Hribernik, T.N.: Nephrogenic diabetes insipidus in three dogs. J. Am. Vet. Med. Assoc., *179:*235, 1981.
9. Burnie, A.G., and Dunn, J.K.: A case of central diabetes in the cat: diagnosis and treatment. J. Small Anim. Pract., *23:*237, 1982.
10. Cherrill, D.A., Stote, R.M., and Birge, J.R.: Demeclocycline treatment in the syndrome of inappropriate antidiuretic hormone secretion. Ann. Intern. Med., *83:*654, 1975.
11. Court, M.H., and Watson, A.D.J.: Idiopathic neurogenic diabetes insipidus in a cat. Aust. Vet. J., *60:*245, 1983.
12. Crawford, M.A., Kittleson, M.D., and Fink, G.D.: Hypernatremia and adipsia in a dog. J. Am. Vet. Med. Assoc., *184:*818, 1984.
13. Decaus, G., et al.: Treatment of the syndrome of inappropriate secretion of antidiuretic hormone with furosemide. N. Engl. J. Med., *304:*329, 1981.
14. DeTroyer, A., and Demanet, J.C.: Correction of antidiuresis by demeclocycline. N. Engl. J. Med., *293:*915, 1975.
15. Dousa, T.P., and Wilson, D.M.: Effects of demethylchlortetracycline on cellular action of antidiuretic hormone in vitro. Kidney Int., *5:*279, 1974.
16. Edwards, D.F., Richardson, D.C., and Russel, R.G.: Hypernatremic, hypertonic dehydration in a dog with diabetes insipidus and gastric dilatation-volvulus. J. Am. Vet. Med. Assoc., *182:*973, 1983.
17. English, P.B., and Filippich, L.J.: Measurement of daily water intake in the dog. J. Small Anim. Pract., *21:*189, 1980.
18. Feldman, E.C.: Central diabetes insipidus in a dog. Mod. Vet. Pract., *60:*615, 1979.

19. Forrest, J.N., Cox, M., and Hong, C.: Superiority of demeclocycline over lithium in the treatment of chronic syndrome of inappropriate secretion of antidiuretic hormone. N. Engl. J. Med., *298:*173, 1978.
20. Green, R.A.: Perspectives of clinical osmometry. Vet. Clin. North Am., *8:*287, 1978.
21. Green, R.A., and Farrow, C.S.: Diabetes insipidus in a cat. J. Am. Vet. Med. Assoc., *164:*524, 1974.
22. Greene, C.E., Wong, P.E., and Finco, D.R.: Diagnosis and treatment of diabetes insipidus in two dogs using two synthetic analogs of antidiuretic hormone. J. Am. Anim. Hosp. Assoc., *15:*371, 1979.
23. Hall, E.J.: Hypernatremia and adipsia in a dog (Letter). J. Am. Vet. Med. Assoc., *185:*4, 1984.
24. Hankinson, R.K.: Diabetes insipidus treatment. Vet. Rec., *100:*477, 1977.
25. Hardy, R.M.: Disorders of water metabolism. Vet. Clin. North Am., *12:*353, 1982.
26. Hardy, R.M., and Osborne, C.A.: Water deprivation test in the dog: maximal normal values. J. Am. Vet. Med. Assoc., *174:*479, 1979.
27. Hardy, R.M., and Osborne, C.A.: Aqueous vasopressin response test in clinically normal dogs undergoing water diuresis: techniques and results. Am. J. Vet. Res., *43:*1987, 1982.
28. Hardy, R.M., and Osborne, C.A.: Repositol vasopressin response test in clinically normal dogs undergoing water diuresis: technique and results. Am. J. Vet. Res., *43:*1991, 1982.
29. Hayek, A., and Ramirez, J.: Demeclocycline-induced diabetes insipidus. J. Am. Med. Assoc., *229:*676, 1974.
30. Hays, R.M.: Antidiuretic hormone. N. Engl. J. Med., *295:*659, 1976.
31. Hendriks, H.J., DeBruijne, J.J., and Van Den Brom, W.E.: The clinical refractometer: a useful tool for the determination of specific gravity and osmolality in canine urine. Tijdschr. Diergeneeskd., *103:*1065, 1978.
32. Henry, W.B., and Sieber, S.E.: Traumatic diabetes insipidus in a dog. J. Am. Vet. Med. Assoc., *146:*1317, 1965.
33. Hoskins, J.D., and Rothschmitt, J.: Hypernatremic thirst deficiency in a dog. Vet. Med., *79:*489, 1984.
34. Jamison, R.L., and Maffly, R.H.: The urinary concentrating mechanism. N. Engl. J. Med., *294:*1059, 1976.
35. Joles, J.A., and Gruys, E.: Nephrogenic diabetes in a dog with renal medullary lesions. J. Am. Vet. Med. Assoc., *174:*830, 1976.
36. Joles, J.A., et al.: Studies on the mechanism of polyuria induced by cortisol excess in the dog. Vet. Quart., *2:*199, 1980.
37. Koestner, A., and Capen, C.C.: Ultrastructural evaluation of the canine hypothalamic-neurohypophyseal system in diabetes insipidus associated with pituitary neoplasms. Vet. Pathol., *4:*513, 1967.
38. Lage, A.L.: Nephrogenic diabetes insipidus in a dog. J. Am. Vet. Med. Assoc., *163:*251, 1973.
39. Lieberman, L.L., Kircher, C.H., and Lein, D.H.: Polyuria and polydipsia associated with pituitary visceral larva migrans in a dog. J. Am. Anim. Hosp. Assoc., *15:*237, 1979.
40. Lorenz, M.D., and Cornelius, L.M.: Laboratory diagnosis of endocrinological disease. Vet. Clin. North Am., *6:*687, 1976.
41. Madewell, B.R., Osborne, C.A., and Norrdin, R.A.: Clinicopathologic aspects of diabetes insipidus in the dog. J. Am. Anim. Hosp. Assoc., *11:*497, 1975.
42. Malayan, S.A., et al.: Effects of increases in plasma vasopressin concentration and plasma renin activity, blood pressure, heart rate, and plasma corticosteroid concentration in conscious dogs. Endocrinology, *107:*1899, 1980.
43. Morton, J.J., Padfield, P.L., and Forsling, M.L.: A radioimmunoassay for plasma arginine-vasopressin in man and dog: application to physiological and pathological states. J. Endocrinol., *65:*411, 1975.
44. Mulnix, J.A., Rijnberk, A., and Hendriks, J.: Evaluation of a modified water-deprivation test for diagnosis of polyuric disorders in dogs. J. Am. Vet. Med. Assoc., *169:*1327, 1976.
45. Oliver, R.E., and Jamison, R.L.: Diabetes insipidus: a physiologic approach to diagnosis. Postgrad. Med. J., *68:*120, 1980.
46. Raff, H., et al.: Vasopressin, ACTH, and corticosteroids during hypercapnia and graded hypoxia in dogs. Am. J. Physiol., *244:*E453, 1983.
47. Richards, M.A., and Sloper, J.C.: Diabetes insipidus—the complexity of the syndrome. Acta Endocrinol., *62:*627, 1969.

48. Rogers, W.A., Valdez, H., and Anderson, B.C.: Partial deficiency of antidiuretic hormone in a cat. J. Am. Vet. Med. Assoc., *170:*545, 1977.
49. Singer, I., and Rotenberg, D.: Demeclocycline-induced nephrogenic diabetes insipidus. Ann. Intern. Med., *79:*679, 1973.
50. Swartz, S.L.: Solving antidiuretic hormone puzzles. Patient Care, *16:*114, 1982.
51. Winterbotham, J., and Mason, K.V.: Congenital diabetes insipidus in a kitten. J. Small Anim. Pract., *24:*569, 1983.
52. Zaki, F., Harris, J., and Budzilovich, G.: Cystic pituicytoma of the neurohypophysis in a Siamese cat. J. Comp. Pathol., *85:*467, 1975.
53. Zerbe, R.L., and Robertson, G.L.: A comparison of plasma vasopressin measurements with a standard indirect test in the differential diagnosis of polyuria. N. Engl. J. Med., *305:*1539, 1981.

Section III

THE THYROID

6

The Normal Thyroid and Clinical Tests of Its Function

The thyroid (Gr., shield-shaped) is the largest of the wholly endocrine organs. The thyroid of the dog and cat is bilobed and situated in the neck on the ventrolateral side of the trachea. Its lobes extend craniad to the caudal border of the larynx. Caudally, the lobes extend to the fifth to eighth tracheal ring (Fig. 6–1). Laterally and ventrally they are covered by the sternocephalicus muscles. Immediately dorsal lie the carotid artery, vago-sympathetic trunk, internal jugular veins, and recurrent laryngeal nerve. The size and weight vary with the animal's general body size. The thyroid lobes' combined weight is about 0.01% of the body weight or about 0.1 g/kg body weight. A lobe's size in a 10- to 15-kg dog is about $2 \times 1.5 \times 0.5$ cm.

The thyroids are not normally palpable. Palpable enlargements are called *goiter*. An isthmus may exist in adult brachycephalic dogs or in adult cats, but an isthmus is rare. Parathyroids, which originate from the third pharyngeal pouch (parathyroids III), are located craniolaterally to the thyroids, whereas parathyroids from the fourth pharyngeal pouch (parathyroids IV) are located medially or within the thyroids.

Thyroid hormones have wide-ranging and vital effects. They maintain optimal function of virtually all other organs, including other endocrine organs. Consumption of oxygen is stimulated in target cells, lipid and carbohydrate metabolism is regulated, and normal growth and maturation are promoted.

DEVELOPMENT OF THE THYROID

The thyroid gland is the first of the endocrine glands to develop in the embryo. It begins as a bilobed bud on the ventral aspect of the primitive pharynx between the first and second pharyngeal (branchial) pouches (Fig. 6–2). The bud is attached to the pharyngeal pouch epithelium by a stalk, the *thyroglossal duct*. As the thyroid bud develops, it eventually detaches from the pharynx by involution of the thyroglossal duct. The thyroids become functional midway in gestation. The isthmus joining the two glands also disappears.

During development, the thyroid becomes incorporated with the ultimobranchial bodies from the last (fifth) pharyngeal pouch. The ultimobranchial bodies are the precursors to the parafollicular (C) cells, which produce

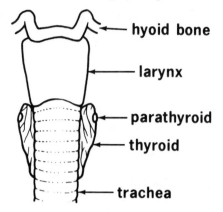

Fig. 6–1. Normal canine thyroid.

calcitonin to maintain calcium's homeostasis. Parafollicular cells originate from the neural crest before infiltrating the ultimobranchial bodies.

See reference 6.

ANOMALIES OF THE THYROID

Persistent thyroglossal ducts occasionally occur, causing cystic enlargements in the midventral neck. They can be found anywhere from the caudal origin of the tongue to the normal position of the thyroids caudal to the larynx. If thyroglossal cysts rupture to the surface of the skin, they form thyroglossal fistulas. Ultimobranchial cysts also occur rarely in the ventrolateral neck area.

A more frequent anomaly of development is the occurrence of ectopic thyroid tissue, which is often displaced by migration of the aortic sac. Small (1 to 2 mm) aberrant thyroid tissue may be present in as much as 50% of

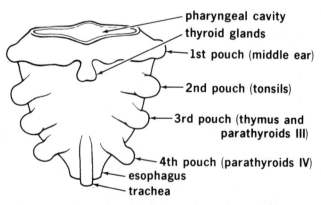

Fig. 6–2. Development of the thyroids and parathyroids. (Adapted from Netter, F.H.: Endocrine system and selected metabolic diseases. *In* The CIBA Collection of Medical Illustrations. Vol. 4. Summit, NJ, CIBA, 1965.)

the canine population, occurring within "aortic fat bodies" at the intrapericardial base of the aorta.[45] Other locations may be found anywhere in the ventral neck or thoracic regions. Even abdominal ectopic thyroid tissue has been reported. Parafollicular cells do not occur in ectopic thyroid tissue, but ectopic parafollicular cells may occur in the parathyroids, thymus, or adrenal medulla. Ectopic thyroid tissue is clinically important if it becomes neoplastic, in which case a thyroidectomy is considered.[22]

STRUCTURE AND FUNCTION OF THE THYROID GLAND

Microstructure of the Thyroid

The thyroid is a very vascular organ composed of colloid-filled follicles. It has one of the greatest blood flow rates per gram of tissue in the body. The follicles are normally lined with cuboidal or columnar epithelial cells that produce and release components of colloid. The cell surface of the follicular cells on the colloid side are lined with microvilli that project into the colloid. The follicular cell functions are to collect and transport iodide, synthesize and secrete thyroglobulin, and remove and secrete triiodothyronine (T_3) and thyroxine (T_4). Between the follicles are connective tissue, blood vessels, and parafollicular cells. The function of the parafollicular cells is to produce calcitonin.

Control of Thyroid Secretion

The activity of the follicular thyroid cells is indirectly dependent on stimulation by thyroid-releasing hormone (TRH) from the hypothalamus and directly dependent on thyroid-stimulating hormone (TSH) released from the adenohypophysis. All major steps in the synthesis and release of thyroid hormones are stimulated by TSH. Circadian rhythmic secretion of thyroid hormones does not seem to occur in dogs.[53] The adult canine and adult feline have a greater metabolic rate than does the human adult. Likewise, their rate of production of thyroid follicular hormones is more than double that of humans.

Follicular hormones released into the circulation are either bound to plasma proteins and incapable of attaching to cell receptors, or unbound and capable of binding to cell receptors. Unbound follicular hormones depress the production of TSH and probably TRH, so that a deficiency of unbound hormones stimulates the production of TSH and probably TRH (Fig. 6–3). The production of TSH is also depressed by stress and warmth. Exposure to cold temperatures increases the secretion of TSH. Euthyroid goiters or goiters incapable of producing sufficient follicular hormones can result from the compensatory increased production of TSH in response to dietary iodine deficiency, goitrogenic drugs, or dyshormonogenesis.

Synthesis of Thyroid Hormones

Iodide uptake is an active process that concentrates iodides, resulting in levels that are 10 to 200 times that of serum. After uptake, iodide is trans-

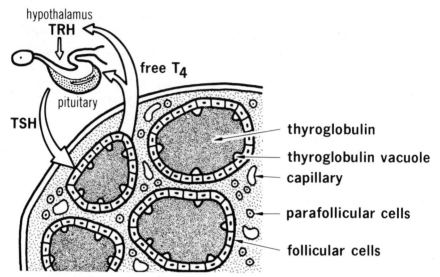

Fig. 6–3. Regulation of thyroid secretion. TRH = thyrotropin-releasing hormone; T_4 = thyroxine.

ported across the follicular cell and oxidized by peroxidase to iodine. Iodine is organically bound to the amino acid tyrosine in the thyroglobulin by a process called organification, forming monoiodotyrosine (MIT). Transfollicular migration is competitively inhibited by other monovalent anions such as perchlorate. Oxidative organification can be blocked by thiourea derivatives such as propylthiouracil or methimazole. Even excessive circulating iodide can transiently block organification, a phenomenon called the Wolff-Chaikoff effect. Two MITs are then iodinated to form diiodotyrosine (DIT). From MIT and DIT the principal thyroid hormones, 3,5,3′,5′-*tetraiodothyronine* (T_4) and 3,5,3′-*triiodothyronine* (T_3) are produced by coupling (oxidative condensation). The combination of MIT plus DIT yields T_3 and DIT plus DIT yields T_4.

Trace amounts of *"reverse T_3"* (3,3′,5′-triiodothyronine) (rT_3), which is inactive, are formed by combining DIT plus MIT. The normal proportion of iodinated tyrosine products are approximately as follows: MIT, 23%; DIT, 33%; T_4, 35%; T_3, 7%; and rT_3, 2%. The T_3 and T_4 remain bound with a peptide link to thyroglobulin until the microvilli of the follicular cells ingest colloid by endocytosis and proteolytic enzymes from lysosomes of the follicular cells release T_4 and T_3 by proteolysis into the thyroid capillaries, leaving scalloped colloidal vacuoles called *reabsorption lacunae* (Fig. 6–4). Reabsorption lacunae are actually artifacts of the fixation process, but they only occur at sites of the recent resorption of colloid. Although MIT and DIT are also ingested by endocytosis of the colloid, only small amounts of DIT are released into the circulation. Most of the DIT is deiodinated by iodotyrosine dehalogenase, and the iodine is returned to the colloid in a process called the "intrathyroidal iodine cycle." T_3 is secreted preferentially

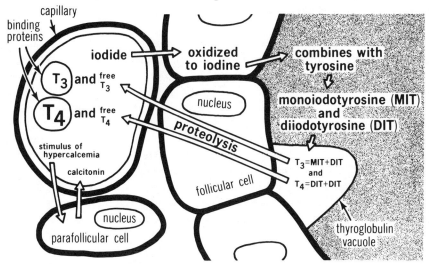

Fig. 6–4. Formation, release, and transport of thyroid hormones. T_3 = triiodothyronine; T_4 = thyroxine.

in greater amounts in response to dietary iodine deficiency and developing hypothyroidism.

The production rate of T_3 and T_4 is much greater in dogs and cats than in humans. In the dog, T_3 and T_4 are produced at 0.8 to 1.5 and 2.5 to 3.2 μg/kg body weight/day, respectively. The thyroid releases T_4 in greater amounts than T_3—the ratio is approximately 4:1. In various species, the secretion rate of thyroid hormones exists in an inverse ratio to their body size. For example, the dog produces twice as much T_4 and more than three times as much T_3 per kg than do humans.

For further information on the structure and function of the thyroid gland, see references 6, 88, 89, and 90.

TRANSPORT AND ACTION OF THYROID FOLLICULAR HORMONES

Transport in the Circulation

More than 99% of the T_3 and T_4 released by the thyroid's follicular cells into the circulation is bound to plasma proteins. The proteins that are bound and the strength of the bond vary among species. In the dog, T_4 binds to three globulins and albumin, and T_3 binds to one globulin and albumin. In humans, most of the circulating T_4 and T_3 binds to an alpha globulin with a high affinity for T_4 and T_3 called *thyroxine-binding globulin* (TBG). TBG occurs in smaller quantities in the dog than humans. Albumin does not bind thyroid hormones well because of its poor affinity, but the amount bound is important due to the great concentration of albumin normally present in the circulation. In the cat, no binding globulins for thyroid hormones have yet been found. The horse is thought to bind T_4, mostly to an alpha globulin.

Only the unbound (free) hormones enter target cells and bind to nuclear receptors. The term *euthyroid* describes that normal amounts of free thyroid hormones are available to target cell receptors. Total serum thyroid hormones may be high or low. Free T_4 and T_3 are approximately 0.15% and 0.25% of the total serum T_4 and T_3, respectively. T_3 does not bind as well to plasma proteins, especially TBG, as does T_4. Total serum concentrations of T_4 and T_3 in the dog, cat, horse, and budgerigar are similar: approximately 1 to 4 μg/dl for T_4, and 50 to 150 ng/dl for T_3; however, their total serum T_4 is considerably less than that measured in humans (about 8 to 9 μg/dl). This difference presumably occurs because of the relative lack of TBG in domestic species. Serum T_3, which does not bind as well to TBG, is found in about the same concentration in domestic animals as in humans. Free serum concentrations of T_4 are essentially the same (about 0.7 to 2 ng/dl) in dogs as in humans.

Protein-bound thyroid hormones serve as a readily available reservoir for physiologically active, free thyroid hormones. There is considerable flexibility in the ability of animals to bind thyroid hormones. Under normal conditions only 1% to 30% of available plasma protein binding sites for T_4 are occupied. Protein binding prolongs the half-life of T_3 and T_4 in the serum, which, in part, explains why the serum half-life of T_4 is about 7 days and the half-life of T_3 is 1 day in humans, and why the serum half-life of T_4 is between 12 and 24 hours and that of T_3 is 5 to 6 hours in dogs. In fact, in dogs more than 100% of extrathyroidal T_4 is replaced daily, and more than 200% of extrathyroidal T_3 is replaced daily.

See references 6, 9, 19, 25, 36, 37, 41, 72, 73, 86, 96, and 97.

Peripheral Metabolism and Effects of Thyroid Hormones

Although the ratio of the production of T_4 to the production of T_3 is 4:1, the serum concentration ratio of T_4 to T_3 is 20:1 (2 μg/dl; 100 ng/dl). Reasons for this difference include a smaller amount of the plasma protein binding of T_3 compared to that of T_4 and a greater intracellular compartment for extrathyroidal T_3—90% compared to 60% for T_4. Thirty percent of the extrathyroidal T_4 is stored in the liver and can be rapidly diffused into the serum. In addition, the serum half-life of T_3 in the dog is about 6 hours, less than half that of T_4.

There are more T_3 receptors in the nuclei of target cells than T_4 receptors. On a molar basis, T_3 is three to four times more potent than T_4. For these reasons, T_4 is thought to serve primarily as a prohormone for T_3. About one third of serum T_4 is converted to T_3 by the monodeiodination of the outer ring. Thirty-three and a third percent to forty-five percent of serum T_4 is converted to rT_3 by monodeiodination of the inner ring in peripheral tissues. Normal serum concentrations of T_3 and rT_3 in dogs is each about 100 ng/dl. The conversion of T_4 to T_3 is done by *thyroxine 5'-*

deiodinase. The conversion of T_4 to rT_3 is done by *thyroxine 5-deiodinase.* Approximately 60% to 80% of serum T_3 concentrations is produced by the peripheral deiodination of T_4.

Reverse T_3 is metabolically inactive. Its structure may prevent T_3 receptor binding. A beneficial change shifting production of T_3 away from the deiodination of T_4 occurs during periods of catabolism such as starvation, anorexia of 3 or more days' duration, or debilitating illnesses. The T_4 deiodination shifts toward metabolically inactive rT_3. Secretion of TSH can be inhibited, and in severe cases total serum levels of T_4 may decrease (this beneficial adaptation to catabolic influences is called the *euthyroid sick syndrome*). Conversely, overfeeding generally increases the T_3 pathway and decreases rT_3.

The exact means by which thyroid hormones alter the target cell's metabolism is still a matter of speculation. It is known that the hormones stimulate protein synthesis by cells and increase cellular oxygen consumption—possibly this is done by increasing the activity of cells' "sodium pump" (sodium-potassium ATPase). The general effects of thyroid hormones are listed in Table 6–1. Consumption of cellular oxygen is increased in all tissues except the adenohypophysis, adult brain (T_4 does not normally enter the cerebrospinal fluid), testes, uterus, spleen, and lymph nodes. Thyroid hormones are required for normal maturation of red blood cells and the conversion of carotene to vitamin A (this conversion does not occur in cats with or without the aid of thyroid hormones). Some effects of thyroid hormones, such as stimulation of the nervous and cardiovascular systems, are mediated by an increased sensitivity to the catecholamines, epinephrine and norepinephrine.

The Metabolic Cycle of Iodine

Thyroid follicular hormones are iodinated amino acids. T_4 is 64.3% iodine by weight. T_3 and T_4 are formed by the follicular cells of the thyroid and stored as a colloid, thyroglobulin. A glycoprotein with a molecular weight of 660,000, thyroglobulin is composed of 2 subunits. Ingested iodine is converted to iodide and absorbed from the gastrointestinal tract. Several organs other than the thyroid also take up iodide, including the parotid salivary glands, gastric mucosa, placenta, ciliary body of the eye, choroid plexus, and mammary glands. These usually rapidly return iodide to the circulation. Their uptake of iodine is not affected by TSH.

Table 6–1. Effects of Thyroid Follicular Hormones

Stimulates consumption of cellular oxygen
Promotes general growth and maturation
Regulates lipid metabolism
Promotes intestinal absorption of carbohydrates
Increases red blood cells' 2,3-DPG (oxygen-release capability)

Mammary glands are unique among these organs in that they can bind iodide to form DIT.

Not all the circulating iodine is incorporated in thyroid hormone molecules. In the dog, about one half of the protein-bound iodine is nonhormonal. The absolute concentration and percentage of inorganic iodine in the serum of dogs is much greater than that in humans. Absolute serum protein-bound iodine values in cats are generally the same as those in humans.

Iodinated amino acids are metabolized by one of four processes. One process is their conjugation in the liver to sulfates and glucuronides and their excretion in the bile, where some of the amino acids are hydrolyzed in the intestine and reabsorbed, thus completing the enterohepatic cycle. Most of the conjugated thyroid hormones in the dog pass out in the feces. Slightly more than 50% of circulating T_4 and 30% of T_3 is eventually removed by biliary excretion in the dog.

The second possible metabolic degradation process is by deamination and decarboxylation. Deamination and decarboxylation produce pyruvic and acetic acid analogues with weak residual T_4-T_3 effects. The third method of degradation is deiodination by various organs of T_4 to T_3 and T_3 to DIT. In the dog, almost 50% of circulating T_4 and 70% of T_3 is removed from circulation by deiodination. The last method involves a small portion of the total serum iodinated amino acids. The urinary excretion of T_4 and T_3 enables most of the T_4 and T_3 in the glomerular filtrate to be reabsorbed by the renal tubules.

For more information on the transport and action of thyroid follicular hormones, see references 6, 19, 25, 36, 37, 41, 72, 73, 86, and 97. For more information on the metabolic cycle of iodines, see references 7, 75, and 77.

PHARMACOLOGIC PREPARATIONS OF THYROID HORMONE

Several preparations of thyroid hormones are available (Table 6–2). Indications for the administration of thyroid hormone are only two: the replacement of thyroid hormone in deficiencies and suppression of the release of TSH to manage some thyroid tumors. Some preparations of thyroid hormones are synthetic, and some are by-products of animal slaughter. Sodium levothyroxine, a synthetic form of T_4, is preferred for the replacement of thyroid hormone in deficiencies or suppression of the secretion of TSH because of its inexpensiveness, long serum half-life, and ready conversion to T_3. Serum T_4 and T_3 levels can be measured to evaluate the absorption and duration of thyroid hormone preparations in patients on sodium levothyroxine. All thyroid hormone preparations are produced for oral administration. To treat myxedema coma, sodium levothyroxine is also available for parenteral administration.

An analogue of T_4, D-thyroxine (Choloxin) is available for the control of

Table 6-2.   Thyroid Hormone Preparations

Preparation	$T_4:T_3*$ (Weight:Weight Ratio)	Source	Equivalent Effects
Dessicated thyroid USP	Beef 4:1 Hog 2:1	Natural	1 gr
Thyroglobulin	2:1	Natural	1 gr
Levothyroxine	All T_4	Synthetic	0.1 mg
Liothyronine	All T_3	Synthetic	0.025 mg
Liotrix	4:1	Synthetic	T_4—0.06 mg T_3—0.015 mg

* T_3 = triiodothyronine; T_4 = thyroxine.

certain forms of hyperlipidemia. It has little effect on the basal metabolic rate and consumption of cellular oxygen.

CALCITONIN AND THE PARAFOLLICULAR CELLS

The thyroid not only produces the hormones T_4 and T_3 from the follicles, but its parafollicular (clear or C-) cells also produce a polypeptide hormone with a straight chain of 32 amino acid residues called *calcitonin* (thyrocalcitonin). Its structure differs among species studied, with the exception of nine amino acids (numbers 1, 3–7, 9, 28, and 32). The first 25 amino acids are essential for its activity. The plasma half-life is 5 to 15 minutes. Some calcitonin is stored within the parafollicular cells. Its mechanism of action is primarily on bone with lesser effects on the kidneys and gastrointestinal tract. Calcitonin can also be produced, in lesser amounts, by the thymus, parathyroids, or ectopic cervical C- cells.

The function of calcitonin is primarily to decrease serum calcium and phosphate. It also inhibits the osteoclastic resorption of bone and decreases the renal activation of vitamin D. Calcitonin blocks renal reabsorption of phosphorus and calcium and, to a lesser extent, sodium, magnesium, chloride, and potassium. The renal action of parathyroid hormone (PTH) in decreasing phosphorus reabsorption is synergistic with that of calcitonin. Secretion of sodium, potassium, chloride, and water in the small intestine is increased by calcitonin. Elevated levels of serum calcium or magnesium stimulate the secretion of calcitonin beyond the normal basal secretion rate. There is also evidence that factors from the gastrointestinal tract, possibly gastrin and others, stimulate the release of calcitonin before the serum calcium levels become elevated. Pentagastrin (Peptavlon) can be used as a stimulant to test for hypercalcitoninism. Calcitonin is thought to act as a protective mechanism to prevent hypercalcemia after the excessive ingestion of calcium and to help protect the maternal skeleton from excessive demineralization during pregnancy.

Parafollicular (solid or C-) cell thyroid tumors are usually rich in calcitonin, and hypocalcemia associated with hypercalcitoninism resulting from functional neoplasia has been recognized in some dogs developing this tumor. Hypercalcitoninemia may also be caused by gastrinomas. A syndrome of hypocalcitoninism has not been recognized.

Salmon calcitonin (Calcimar) is commercially available. Compared on the basis of effect by weight, salmon calcitonin is five to ten times more potent than mammalian calcitonin. It may be of value in the treatment of hyperparathyroidism-induced osteopenia or in the emergency treatment of hypercalcemia. Its expense, the necessity of parenteral administration, and the hazard of hypersensitization limit its potential value.

See also reference 4.

CLINICAL TESTS OF THYROID FUNCTION

Insensitive and Antiquated Tests

More tests have been developed for the assessment of thyroid function than for any other endocrine organ. Virtually all of the older tests have been replaced by radioligand assays. Most older tests were indirect or insensitive assays for total T_4. Examples of antiquated tests are the protein-bound iodine (PBI) test, the butanol-extractable iodine test, and the T_4 iodine test measured by column chromatography. T_3-*uptake* (by resin or red blood cell) *tests* are still frequently used in humans to determine qualitatively the degree of plasma protein binding.[14, 15, 42, 47, 57, 64] Currently, the T_3-uptake test is considered an insensitive test of plasma protein binding in companion animals because companion animals bind T_4 and T_3 to TBG less avidly than do humans. Normal T_3 uptake in the dog is about 40% to 60%.

The *free thyroxine index* (FTI, T7) is the product of multiplying the total serum T_4 level by the percentage of the T_3 uptake. The result is an indirect index of free T_4. Because of the insensitivity of the T_3-uptake test, the FTI rarely yields more information than the total serum T_4 level in companion animals.

Levels of TBG in the serum can be determined by a radioimmunoassay for TBG. Since very little T_4 binds to canine TBG, and apparently no T_4 in cats binds to alpha globulins, this determination is not considered to be of value in companion animals. Its usefulness in horses has not been investigated.

See references 65, 70, 84, and 94.

Radioimmunoassays for Serum (plasma) T_4

Measuring T_4 by RIA has been modified and validated for companion animals. Blood levels of T_4, as measured by radioimmunoassay, are the sole basis for the diagnosis of hypothyroidism or hyperthyroidism in companion animals. Since normal serum levels of T_4 in adult companion animals are lower than levels in humans (Table 6-3), commercial RIA kits for T_4 and reference laboratories (which measure human samples) often do not have

Table 6–3. Approximate Normal Serum T_4 Values Determined by Radioimmunoassay in Adults

Species	T_4 (μg/dl)
Dog	1.0–4.0
Cat	1.5–5.0
Horse	1.0–3.5
Budgerigar*	2.5–4.5
Human	5–12

* Mean serum T_4 values in other psittacine birds are reported to vary from 0.13 to 1.36 μg/dl.[68]

the necessary accuracy to separate low normal from abnormally low levels in companion animals.

Total serum levels of T_4 are higher in young animals than adults, and serum levels decrease gradually throughout life.[12, 98] For example, total serum levels of T_4 in puppies during the first 3 months after birth are 2 to 5 times greater than the concentrations of the normal adult. In dogs, total levels of T_4 decline about 0.07 μg/dl/year from young adult levels. Serum levels of T_3 do not decline.

Unless otherwise specified, RIAs for T_4 report total (plasma protein bound and free) hormone. Since more than 99% of the total T_4 is bound to plasma proteins, and it is only the remaining percentage (less than 1%) of total T_4 that affects target cells, knowing what can alter plasma protein levels and their affinity for T_4 is important for the proper interpretation of total serum T_4 levels.

Total levels of T_4 have been measured by T_4-CPB (competitive protein binding) (also known as the Murphy-Pattee method).[39] With the development of an RIA for T_4, the T_4-CPB is being abandoned. One reason why the T_4-RIA is superior to the T_4-CPB is that the T_4-CPB can be falsely elevated by the release of serum fatty acids if blood samples are left at room temperature for more than 1 day. The results of measuring serum T_4 by RIA are not affected under such conditions.

Conditions that can increase total levels of T_4 while free concentrations of T_4 remain normal do so by inducing the increased synthesis of T_4-binding globulins. Effects on the synthesis of TBG are best known. Conditions that can increase the synthesis of TBG, and presumably other T_4-binding globulins, are listed in Table 6–4.[54, 102]

Total levels of T_4 may be low while levels of free T_4 are normal. Conditions such as these are due either to the decreased quantity of T_4-binding plasma proteins or a decreased binding affinity for T_4. Possible causes are listed in Table 6–5.[86, 95] Severe illnesses may also cause transiently depressed serum levels of T_4 by impairing the secretion of TSH.

Baseline levels of T_4 are frequently diagnostic for hyperthyroidism, but they are often not abnormally low in patients with hypothyroidism. In

Table 6–4. Conditions or Drugs That May Increase T₄-Binding to Plasma Proteins

Administration of Estrogen
Pregnancy or progestins
Methadone
Tranquilizers
Clofibrate

humans, there is considerable (10% to 20%) overlapping of baseline serum levels of T_4 between normal persons and persons with developing hypothyroidism. In dogs, overlapping may occur in up to 50% of cases of hypothyroidism because of breed differences, individual differences, serum protein binding, assay specificity, and other unknown reasons.

If baseline serum T_4 concentrations are in the low normal range, a *TSH-stimulation test* should be done.[40, 67] The purpose of the TSH-stimulation test is to assess the thyroid's reserve capacity to form and release T_4 while under maximum stimulation. This assessment is most accurate when based on the maximum concentration of serum T_4 attained.

A popular misconception of the TSH-stimulation test in dogs is that serum T_4 should double in 4 hours after the intravenous administration of TSH.[78] This concept ignores the knowledge that serum T_4 does not reach peak concentrations until 8 hours after the intravenous administration of TSH. The 4-hour intravenous TSH-stimulation test also makes allowance for the possibility that a euthyroid dog, with a normal thyroid baseline T_4 sampled near peak natural production of T_4, might not have doubled serum

Table 6–5. Conditions or Drugs That May Decrease Total Serum T₄ Levels While Free T₄ Remains Normal

Those conditions or drugs decreasing binding proteins
Glucocorticoids
Androgens
Antiestrogens
L-asparaginase
Nephrotic syndrome
Protein-losing enteropathies
Severe malnutrition
Chronic hepatitis
Ovariectomy
Those conditions or drugs decreasing T_4 binding
Salicylates
Chlorpropamide
Phenytoin
Tolbutamide
Mitotane
5-Fluorouracil
Glucocorticoids
Phenylbutazone

levels of T_4 after stimulation with TSH. It is also possible that a hypothyroid dog's baseline level of T_4, sampled while serum concentrations of T_4 were low or subnormal, could double even though total reserve capacity was abnormally low.

Interpretation of the adequacy of response to TSH depends on the amount of TSH used and the length of the interval before levels of T_4 are sampled after stimulation. Normal dogs and cats, given 10 and 5 U, respectively, should produce serum T_4 concentrations in excess of 4 $\mu g/dl$. Usually, they are in excess of 5 $\mu g/dl$ when the peak concentration is attained.[34, 35, 46,] ̣ ̣seline levels of T_4 in horses double or nearly double 4 to 5 hours after the administration of an intravenous dose of 5 U of TSH.[29, 74] Psittacine birds generally double their baseline levels of T_4 4 to 6 hours after the intramuscular administration of 1 to 2 U of TSH.[68] Stimulation with TSH does not cause signs of hyperthyroidism since the elevated concentrations of T_4 are mostly bound to plasma proteins as soon as the T_4 is released. Free T_4 concentrations change little with administration of TSH. The ACTH-stimulation test does not interfere with TSH-stimulation tests done the same day.[85]

See references 1–3, 8, 10, 11, 20, 21, 23, 28, 30, 33, 38, 49, 50, 59, 71, 87, 91, and 92.

Radioimmunoassays for Thyroid-stimulating Hormone

A RIA for TSH would be of tremendous benefit in properly interpreting baseline serum levels of T_4 and in differentiating primary from secondary hypothyroidism and secondary from tertiary hypothyroidism. Unfortunately, attempts to use commercial reference laboratories and RIA kits designed to detect human TSH have generally been unsuccessful in dogs. One such test met the criteria for validation, but detected a small (less than double) increase in TSH following TRH stimulation.[48] It seems that a homologous anti-TSH antibody is necessary for each companion species. A homologous RIA for TSH has been developed for research in the dog, but the assay is not commercially available for clinical purposes.[81]

See also references 17, 48, 58, 81, and 99.

Stimulation with Thyrotropin-releasing Hormone

TRH (Thypinone) may be administered to elevate the ability of the adenohypophysis to secrete TSH. Since direct assays for TSH are not yet clinically available for companion animals, the response is indirectly evaluated by monitoring serum levels of T_4. Four hours after an intravenous dose of 0.2 mg of TRH, the serum T_4 should increase at least 1 $\mu g/dl$ if the adenohypophysis and the thyroid are normal. Another method is to administer an intravenous dose of 0.1 mg/kg body weight. A response considered normal would be an increase in serum T_4 by at least 50% above the baseline level 6 hours after the administration of TRH. Glucocorticoids inhibit TRH-induced TSH release. Insufficient responses should be re-evaluated. See also references 56, 69, 93, and 100.

Serum (plasma) Levels of Free T₄

Free T_4 is permeable to diffusion through membranes that will not permit diffusion of protein-bound T_4. After the free T_4 has been microdialyzed, its concentration can be determined by highly sensitive RIA methods. The concentration of free T_4 measured by microdialysis is about 0.7 to 2 ng/dl in dogs and humans. Because microdialysis is difficult and expensive, its use is currently limited to clinical research. Other means of determining free T_4 concentrations are considered inferior to microdialysis.

Serum (plasma) Levels of T₃

Levels of T_3 in the serum or plasma are very similar in dogs and humans, being about 50 to 150 ng/dl in both. Cats have lower serum T_3 levels (15 to 60 ng/dl).

A serum T_3 assay is a poor measure of decreased thyroid function. Serum T_3 will decrease in severe hypothyroidism, but lowered serum T_3 concentrations are more often caused by nonthyroidal illnesses. While 100% of serum T_4 results from secretion of the thyroid, only about 30% of serum T_3 originates directly from the thyroid. Approximately 60% to 80% of serum T_3 is produced by the peripheral deiodination of serum T_4 by T_4-5'-deiodinase. About one third of all T_4 produced is converted to T_3. Since T_3 has three to four times the effect per μg of T_4, it is estimated that only 10% to 15% of the cellular effects of thyroid hormones are due directly to T_4. A failing thyroid preferentially produces T_3, apparently because of the intracellular importance of T_3 and the economy of synthesizing its more simple structure. The result is that serum T_4 drops before serum T_3 does as hypothyroidism develops.

In contrast, serum T_3 concentrations often drop due to a wide variety of nonthyroidal disease as a beneficial adaptation to illness or starvation. Inappropriately large concentrations of thyroid hormones are catabolic. If the body is in a state of negative nitrogen balance (a condition caused by acute starvation, chronic caloric deprivation, hepatic cirrhosis, renal failure, surgical stress, chronic illness, or glucocorticoid therapy), the deiodination of T_4 to T_3 is suppressed. The deiodination of T_4 to rT_3, which is metabolically inactive, is favored. This process, called the low T_3 syndrome or euthyroid sick syndrome, occurs in about 50% of all hospitalized human patients.[18, 24, 102] The shift from deiodination of T_4 to T_3 to the deiodination of T_4 to rT_3 also occurs in normal neonates and normal geriatric patients.[18]

Elevated levels of serum T_3 can preceed serum T_4 elevations, or exceed elevations of T_4, or persist as the exclusive excessive thyroid hormone in hyperthyroidism. An RIA for serum T_3 should be done in every case of suspected hyperthyroidism.

See also references 8, 16, 26, and 60–63.

Reverse Triiodothyronine

The measurement of rT_3 levels in the serum has limited diagnostic value. More than 90% of serum rT_3 results from the peripheral deiodination of serum T_4. Serum rT_3 and T_3 levels are similar in normal dogs (T_3, 50 to 150 ng/dl; rT_3, 50 to 150 ng/dl), although during catabolic illness or malnutrition they tend to occur in an inverse relationship—that is, T_3 levels decrease and rT_3 levels increase.[80] Most surgical procedures cause such a shift toward production of rT_3 for up to 2 days after surgery.[55] Elevated serum rT_3 levels would eliminate the diagnosis of hypothyroidism even if baseline levels of serum T_3 and T_4 are low, since serum rT_3 is a deiodination product of T_4.

Antithyroid Antibodies

Antithyroid antibodies can develop in reaction to several thyroidal antigens: thyroglobulin, a second colloid antigen not containing iodine, follicular cell cytoplasmic microsomes, and a cell surface antigen. Antithyroglobulin antibodies can be detected by passive hemagglutination, anticytoplasmic (microsomal) antibodies by complement fixation, and other unidentified colloidal protein antibodies by indirect fluorescent antibody tests.

General antithyroid antibodies can be detected by a double diffusion technique. About one half of clinically hypothyroid dogs have significant antithyroid antibodies as measured by a chromic chloride passive hemagglutination or an antithyroglobulin enzyme-linked immunosorbent assay (ELISA). Probably many of the dogs without antibodies may have had elevated levels of antithyroid antibodies before the thyroid was immunologically destroyed and antigenic stimulation ceased. Antithyroid antibody tests may be of clinical value in detecting family members who could develop hypothyroidism from severe lymphocytic thyroiditis and in differentiating the diagnosis of patients with primary hypothyroidism (who may have high antithyroid antibody titers) from that of patients with secondary or tertiary hypothyroidism (which does not cause antithyroid antibodies). However, antithyroid antibody assays are not commercially available for companion animals. One study, using the ELISA method, reported antithyroglobulin antibodies in 13% of the general canine population. The greatest incidence was found in Old English sheepdogs, Irish setters, and Great Danes. There seemed to be a familial incidence in some Great Danes.[27]

Serum Thyroglobulin

Trace amounts of thyroglobulin are often found in normal human serum. In people with well-differentiated carcinoma of the thyroid, serum thyroglobulin levels are elevated. Although the detection of elevated serum thyroglobulin is not diagnostic of thyroid carcinoma, serial measurements of serum thyroglobulin before and after treatment of the carcinoma can act as a tumor recurrence marker. The clinical usefulness of serum thyroglobulins' determination in companion animals has not been investigated.

Diagnostic Nuclear Medicine

In a thyroid scan, radioisotopes are temporarily concentrated in the thyroid so that images of the thyroid can be produced, and the ability of the thyroid to take up iodine can be measured in a radioactive iodine uptake test.

Thyroid scans (scintigraphy, imaging) are used to discern the size, shape, and location of the thyroid (Fig. 6–5).[5] Sodium pertechnetate (^{99m}Tc), ^{123}I, and ^{131}I can be used, but ^{99m}Tc is the most commonly used radioisotope employed in thyroid scanning because it has a short half-life (6 hours), is inexpensive, does not emit β particles, allows scans to be done about 20 minutes after the administration of ^{99m}Tc, and requires a short period of

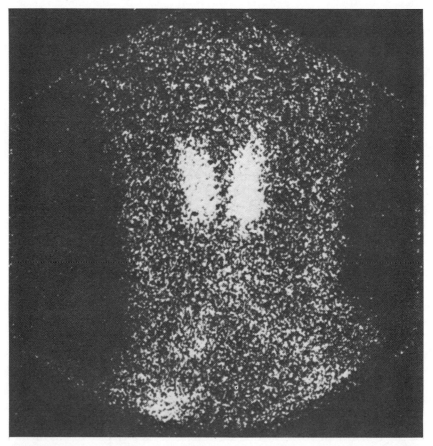

Fig. 6–5. Normal thyroid scan of a cat. (From Peterson, M.E., et al.: Feline hyperthyroidism: pretreatment clinical and laboratory evaluation of 131 cases. J. Am. Vet. Med. Assoc., *183:*103, 1983.)

restraint (about 1 minute). [99m]Tc is trapped by the thyroid-like iodine, but it is not organically bound to tyrosine in colloid. Thyroid scans with ^{99m}Tc are not affected by treatment with prophylthiouracil or methimazole.

Images in dogs and cats are usually recorded by a gamma camera and pinhole collimator (rather than a rectilinear scanner) 30 minutes after an intravenous dose of 0.5 to 2 mCi of [99m]Tc. Horses require 35 mCi of ^{99m}Tc for thyroid scans. Thyroid scans can be useful in investigating the possible presence of thyroid tumors, evaluating the thyroid's response to TSH, differentiating hypothyroidism from drug-induced serum T_4 depression, and evaluating a patient's recovery from a partial thyroidectomy.

A *radioactive iodine uptake* study is used to determine the thyroid's functional ability to take up iodine against a gradient and organify it. Radioactive tracers that can be used include ^{123}I, ^{125}I, or [131]I. [123]I is generally preferred due to its lower radiation hazard. In dogs and cats, approximately 24 to 72 hours after the administration of ^{123}I in an intravenous dose of 10 to 20 μCi or an oral dose of 10 to 50 μCi in capsule form, radioactivity counts are taken over the thyroid and background counts are taken over the thigh area. Hyperthyroidism will cause the uptake to peak earlier than usual. Values for uptake are reported as a percentage of the administered dose. Normal values in dogs and cats are about 10% to 40%, but results can be influenced significantly by several factors (Table 6–6).

Radioactive iodine uptake is an expensive, time-consuming test not available to many veterinary practitioners. Uptake of iodine is usually decreased in thyroiditis or hypothyroidism and increased in hyperthyroidism, but results often overlap normal ranges. Repeated measurements of the uptake of iodine before and after 1 week of T_3 administration can also help verify an autonomous functional thyroid tumor.

Monovalent hydrated anions such as thiocyanate and perchlorate can competitively inhibit organification of iodide. Perchlorate is most often used for diagnostic purposes in the perchlorate discharge test. Normally, if

Table 6–6.   Factors Affecting Uptake of Radioactive Iodine

Increased uptake
  Low dietary intake of iodine
  Pregnancy
  Rebound after discontinuation of antithyroid drugs
  Loss of iodine from nephrosis or diarrhea

Decreased uptake
  Antithyroid drugs
  High dietary intake of iodine
  Decreased excretion of iodine resulting from renal
    failure or cardiac failure
  Recent use of iodine-containing drugs or radio-
    contrast media
  Breed differences (basenji)

perchlorate is administered after there has been sufficient time (24 hours) for the thyroid to take up the radioactive iodine, less than 10% of the uptake will be discharged in 1 hour. The determination that a greater than normal amount of iodine has been discharged indicates the failure of the thyroid to organify the iodine.

See references 6, 13, and 101.

Echography Scan

The usefulness of echography in evaluating the thyroid is very limited. Scanning thyroid tumors with echography is a noninvasive means of detecting the rare cyst that is greater than 1 cm in diameter. Cystic tumors of the thyroid are usually benign.

Thyroid Biopsy

Although biopsies have no place in establishing the diagnosis of hypothyroidism, they can help differentiate the cause of hypothyroidism. Secondary hypothyroidism is characterized by flattened follicular cells and the relative absence of colloid vacuoles caused by recent proteolysis.

Thyroid biopsies are always indicated for thyroid tumors. A fine needle aspiration biopsy may be sufficient if the presence of malignancy is definite on cytologic examination. If the cytologic results of the fine needle biopsy are equivocal or suspect, they should be substantiated or clarified by a core biopsy taken with a special biopsy needle, or by excision of the tumor, or by wedge section. Initial fixation in formalin can distort biopsies of the thyroid, so it is recommended to first fix thyroid biopsies in Bouin's solution for 4 to 6 hours, cut the sample in thin slices, fix the sample in Bouin's solution for another 1 to 2 hours, and then place it in 10% buffered formalin.

Radioimmunoassay for Plasma Calcitonin

Medullary carcinoma of the thyroid elevates plasma calcitonin levels. Normal fasting levels in dogs are less than 2.5 pg-eq/ml. Elevated plasma calcitonin levels also occur in subjects with acute pancreatitis, renal failure, gastrinomas, and during pregnancy, lactation, and subacute thyroiditis. If plasma levels of calcitonin are equivocal for diagnosis, an intravenous dose of calcium or, preferably, pentagastrin can be administered to evaluate the response.

For further data on clinical tests of thyroid function, see references 6, 30–32, 44, 51, 66, 76, 82, and 83.

REFERENCES

1. Afifi, A., and Kraft, W.: Influence of dexamethasone, triamcinolone acetonide and estradiol benzoate on thyroid function tests in the dog. Zentralbl. Veterinarmed., 24:856, 1977.
2. Anderson, J.H., and Brown, R.W.: Serum thyroxine (T_4) and triiodothyronine (T_3) uptake values in normal adult cats as determined by radioimmunoassay. Am. J. Vet. Res., 40:1493, 1979.

3. Anderson, J.J.B., and Dorner, J.L.: Total serum thyroxine in thyroidectomized beagles, using ^{125}I-labeled thyroxine, and comparison of T_3 and T_4 tests. J. Am. Vet. Med. Assoc., *159:*760, 1971.
4. Austin, L.A., and Heath, H.: Calcitonin physiology and pathophysiology. N. Engl. J. Med., *304:*269, 1981.
5. Beck, K.A., Hornof, W.J., and Feldman, E.C.: The normal feline thyroid: technetium pertechnetate imaging and determination of thyroid to salivary gland radioactivity ratios in 10 normal cats. Vet. Radiol., *26:*35, 1985.
6. Belshaw, B.E.: Thyroid disease. *In* Textbook of Veterinary Internal Medicine. Diseases of the Dog and Cat. Edited by Ettinger, S.J. 2nd Ed. Philadelphia, W.B. Saunders, 1983, p. 1592.
7. Belshaw, B.E., et al.: A model of iodine kinetics in the dog. Endocrinology, *95:*1078, 1974.
8. Belshaw, B.E. and Rijnberk, A.: Radioimmunoassay of plasma T_4 and T_3 in the diagnosis of primary hypothyroidism in dogs. J. Am. Anim. Hosp. Assoc., *15:*17, 1979.
9. Bigler, B.: Thyroxinbindende Serumproteine bei der Katze in Vergleich zu Hund und Mensch. Schweiz. Arch. Tierheilkd., *118:*559, 1976.
10. Blackmore, D.J., Greenwood, R.E.S., and Johnson, C.: Observations on thyroid hormones in the blood of thoroughbreds. Res. Vet. Sci., *25:*294, 1978.
11. Blake, S., and Lapinski, A.: Hypothyroidism in different breeds. Canine Pract., *7:*48, 1980.
12. Book, S.A.: Age related changes in serum thyroxine and ^{125}I-triiodothyronine resin sponge uptake in the young dog. Lab. Anim. Sci., *27:*646, 1977.
13. Branam, J.E., Leighton, R.L., and Hornof, W.J.: Radioisotope imaging for the evaluation of thyroid neoplasia and hypothyroidism in a dog. J. Am. Vet. Med. Assoc., *180:*1077, 1982.
14. Bullock, L.: Protein bound iodine determination as a diagnostic aid for canine hypothyroidism. J. Am. Vet. Med. Assoc., *156:*892, 1970.
15. Bush, B.M.: Thyroid function tests in a group of euthyroid dogs. Res. Vet. Sci., *13:*177, 1972.
16. Center, S.A., et al.: Effects of propranolol on thyroid function in the dog. Am. J. Vet. Res., *45:*109, 1984.
17. Chastain, C.B.: Human thyroid stimulating hormone radioimmunoassay in the dog. J. Am. Anim. Hosp. Assoc., *14:*368, 1978.
18. Chastain, C.B., and Zenoble, R.D.: Hypothyroidism—possible cause of disk disease (Letter). J. Am. Anim. Hosp. Assoc., *15:*533, 1979.
19. Chen, C.L., and Riley, A.M.: Serum thyroxine and triiodothyronine concentrations in neonatal foals and mature horses. Am. J. Vet. Res., *42:*1415, 1981.
20. Chester, D.K., et al.: T_4, T_3 uptake, T_7 and cholesterol values in radiothyroidectomized beagles. Southwest. Vet., *27:*183, 1974.
21. Davis, P.J., and Handwerger, B.S.: Thyroid hormone binding in dog plasma. Endocrinology, *93:*1445, 1973.
22. DiScala, V.A., Lippe, R.D., and Segal, R.L.: A simple reliable method for producing hypothyroidism in the dog and thyroid function tests in normal and hypothyroid dogs. Endocrinology, *88:*504, 1971.
23. Eckersall, P.D., and Williams, M.E.: Thyroid function tests in dogs using radioimmunoassay kits. J. Small Anim. Pract., *24:*525, 1983.
24. Ferguson, D.: Canine hypothyroidism (Letter). J. Am. Vet. Med. Assoc., *178:*1028, 1981.
25. Furth, E.D., et al.: Thyroxine metabolism in the dog. Endocrinology, *82:*976, 1968.
26. Gharib, H.: Triiodothyronine. Physiology and clinical significance. J. Am. Vet. Med. Assoc., *227:*302, 1974.
27. Haines, D.M., Lording, P.M., and Penhale, W.J.: Survey of thyroglobulin autoantibodies in dogs. Am. J. Vet. Res., *45:*1493, 1983.
28. Harless, S.J., Kullenberg, W., and Lloyd, W.E.: Use of a modified-RIA test kit to detect hypothyroidism in dogs. Vet. Med. Small Anim. Clin., *76:*1454, 1981.
29. Held, J.P., and Oliver, J.W.: A sampling protocol for the thyrotropin-stimulation test in the horse. J. Am. Vet. Med. Assoc., *184:*326, 1984.
30. Hightower, D., Kyzar, J.R. and Chester, D.K.: Hypothyroid test results in normal dogs. Southwest. Vet., *27:*155, 1969.

31. Hightower, D., and Miller, L.F.: Thyroid function tests in veterinary medicine. Part I. A review. Southwest. Vet., *22:*200, 1969.
32. Hightower, D., Miller, L.F., and Kyzar, J.R.: Thyroid function tests in veterinary medicine. Part II. Results and applications. Southwest. Vet., *23:*15, 1969.
33. Hightower, D., Miller, L., and Kyzar, J.R.: Comparison of serum and plasma thyroxine determinations in horses. J. Am. Vet. Med. Assoc., *159:*449, 1971.
34. Hoenig, M., and Ferguson, D.C.: Assessment of thyroid functional reserve in the cat by the thyrotropin-stimulation test. Am. J. Vet. Res., *44:*1229, 1983.
35. Hoge, W.R., Lund, J.E., and Blakemore, J.C.: Response to thyrotropin as a diagnostic aid for canine hypothyroidism. J. Am. Anim. Hosp. Assoc., *10:*167, 1974.
36. Irvine, C.H.G.: Thyroid function in the horse. Proc. Am. Assoc. Equine Pract., *12:*197, 1966.
37. Irvine, C.H.G., and Evans, M.J.: Post-natal changes in total and free thyroxine and triiodothyroxine in foal serum. J. Reprod. Fertil., (Suppl.) *23:*709, 1975.
38. Kallfelz, F.A.: Comparison of the ^{125}T-3 and ^{125}T-4 tests in the diagnosis of thyroid gland function in the dog. J. Am. Vet. Med. Assoc., *154:*22, 1969.
39. Kallfelz, F.A.: Determination of total serum thyroxine in the dog by competitive protein binding of labeled thyroxine. Am. J. Vet. Res., *30:*929, 1969.
40. Kallfelz, F.A.: Observations on thyroid gland function in dogs: response to thyrotropin and thyroidectomy and determination of thyroxine secretion rate. Am. J. Vet. Res., *34:*535, 1973.
41. Kallfelz, F.A.: Thyroid function in the dog. Vet. Clin. North Am., *7:*497, 1977.
42. Kallfelz, F.A.: The triiodothyronine ^{131}I resin sponge uptake test as an indicator of thyroid function in dogs. J. Am. Vet. Med. Assoc., *152:*1647, 1968.
43. Kallfelz, F.A., and Erali, R.P.: Thyroid function tests in domesticated animals: free thyroxine index. Am. J. Vet. Res., *34:*1449, 1973.
44. Kallfelz, F.A., and Lowe, J.E.: Some normal values of thyroid function in horses. J. Am. Vet. Med. Assoc., *156:*1888, 1970.
45. Kameda, Y.: The assessory thyroid gland of the dog around the intrapericardial aorta. Arch. Histol. Jpn., *34:*375, 1972.
46. Kaneko, J.J., Comer, K.M., and Ling, G.V.: Thyroxine levels by radioimmunoassay (T$_4$-RIA) and the thyroid stimulating hormone response test in normal dogs. Calif. Vet., *Jan.:*9, 1978.
47. Kaneko, J.J., et al.: Clinical applications of the thyroidal I^{131} uptake test in the dog. J. Am. Vet. Med. Assoc., *135:*516, 1959.
48. Kaufman, J., et al.: Serum concentrations of thyroxine, 3, 5, 3'-triiodothyronine, thyrotropin, and prolactin in dogs before and after thyrotropin-releasing hormone administration. Am. J. Vet. Res., *46:*486, 1985.
49. Kelley, S.T., and Oehme, F.W.: Circulating thyroid levels in dogs, horses, and cattle. Vet. Med. Small Anim. Clin., *69:*1531, 1974.
50. Kelley, S.T., Oehme, F.W., and Brandt, G.W.: Measurement of thyroid gland function during the estrous cycle of nine mares. Am. J. Vet. Res., *35:*657, 1974.
51. Kelley, S.T., Oehme, F.W., and Hoffman, S.B.: Evaluation of selected commercial thyroid function tests in dogs. Am. J. Vet. Res., *35:*733, 1974.
52. Kemppainen, R.J., Mansfield, P.D., and Sartin, J.L.: Endocrine responses of normal cats to TSH and synthetic ACTH administration. J. Am. Anim. Hosp. Assoc., *20:*737, 1984.
53. Kemppainen, R.J., and Sartin, J.L.: Evidence for episodic but not circadian activity in plasma concentrations of adrenocorticotrophin, cortisol and thyroxine in dogs. J. Endocrinol., *103:*219, 1984.
54. Kemppainen, R.J., et al.: Effects of prednisone on thyroid and gonadal function in dogs. J. Endocrinol., *96:*293, 1983.
55. Kemppainen, R.J., et al.: Effect of surgery on levels of cortisol and thyroid hormones in dogs. Proceedings of Am. Coll. Vet. Intern. Med. 1984, p. 42.
56. Kraft, W., and Gerbig, T.: Experiments with the TRH-stimulation test in the dog. Dtsch. Tierarztl. Wochensch., *84:*185, 1977.
57. Kyzar, J.R., Chester, D.K., and Hightower, D.: Comparison of T-3, T-4 tests and radioactive iodine uptake determinations in the dog. Vet. Med. Small Anim. Clin., *67:*321, 1972.
58. Larsson, M.: Evaluation of a human TSH radioimmunoassay as a diagnostic test for canine primary hypothyroidism. Acta Vet. Scand., *22:*589, 1981.

59. Larsson, M., and Lumsden, J.H.: Evaluation of an enzyme linked immunosorbent assay (ELISA) for determination of plasma thyroxine in dogs. Zentralbl. Veterinarmed., *27:*9, 1980.

60. Laurberg, P.: Iodothyronine release from the perfused canine thyroid. Acta Endocrinol., *94*(Suppl. 236);1, 1980.

61. Laurberg, P.: Non-parallel variations in the preferential secretion of 3,5,3'-triiodothyronine (T₃) and 3,3',5',-triiodothyronine (rT₃) from dog thyroid. Endocrinology, *102:*757, 1978.

62. Laurberg, P.: Selective inhibition of the secretion of triiodothyronines from the perfused canine thyroid by prophylthiouracil. Endocrinology, *103:*900, 1978.

63. Laurberg, P.: T₄ and T₃ release from the perfused canine thyroid isolation *in situ.* Acta Endocrinol. (Copenh.), *83:*105, 1976.

64. Ling, G.V., Lowenstine, L.J., and Kaneko, J.J.: Serum thyroxine (T₄) and triiodothyronine (T₃) uptake values in normal adult cats. Am. J. Vet. Res., *35:*1247, 1974.

65. Lombardi, M.H., Comar, C.L., and Kirk, R.W.: Diagnosis of thyroid gland function in the dog. Am. J. Vet. Res., *23:*412, 1962.

66. Lorenz, M.D., and Cornelius, L.M.: Laboratory diagnosis of endocrinological disease. Vet. Clin. North Am., *6:*687, 1976.

67. Lorenz, M.D., and Stiff, M.E.: Serum thyroxine content before and after thyrotropin stimulation in dogs with suspected hypothyroidism. J. Am. Vet. Med. Assoc., *177:*78, 1980.

68. Lothrop, C.D., Loomis, M.R., and Olsen, J.H.: Thyrotropin stimulation test for evaluation of thyroid function in psittacine birds. J. Am. Vet. Med. Assoc., *186:*47, 1985.

69. Lothrop, C.D., Tamas, P.M., and Fadok, V.A.: Canine and feline thyroid function assessment with the thyrotropin-releasing hormone response test. Am. J. Vet. Res., *45:*2310, 1984.

70. Mallo, G.L., and Harris, A.L.: I¹³¹-triiodothyronine resin uptake, serum PBI and serum cholesterol tests in normal dogs. Vet. Med., *62:*533, 1967.

71. Mincey, E.K.: Direct determination of free thyroxine in canine serum using single tube radioimmunoassay. Vet. Clin. Pathol., *10:*25, 1981.

72. Mitin, V., and Kallfelz, F.A.: Partial purification of thyroid hormone binding proteins from dog serum by affinity chromatography and DEAE sephadex chromatography. Vet. Arh., *46:*123, 1976.

73. Monty, D.E., Wilson, O., and Stone, J.M.: Thyroid studies in pregnant and newborn beagles, using ¹²⁵I. Am. J. Vet. Res., *40:*1249, 1979.

74. Morris, D.D., and Garcia, M.: Thyroid-stimulating hormone: response test in healthy horses, and effect of phenylbutazone on equine thyroid hormones. Am. J. Vet. Res., *44:*503, 1983.

75. Norris, W.P., Fritz, T.E., and Taylor, J.A.: Cycle of accommodation to restricted dietary iodide in the thyroid gland of the beagle dog. Am. J. Vet. Res., *31:*21, 1970.

76. Nunez, E.A., et al.: Breed differences and similarities in thyroid function in purebred dogs. Am. J. Physiol., *218:*1337, 1970.

77. Oliver, J.W., and Waldrop, M.S.: Sampling protocol for the thyrotropin stimulation test in the dog. J. Am. Vet. Med. Assoc., *182:*486, 1983.

78. Olson, W.G., Stevens, J.B., and Haggard, D.W.: Iodine: a review of dietary requirements, therapeutic properties and assessment of potential toxicity. Compend. Contin. Ed., *2:*164, 1980.

79. Peterson, S.L., and Yoshioka, M.M.: The use of technetium 99m pertechnetate for thyroid imaging in a case of feline hyperthyroidism. J. Am. Anim. Hosp. Assoc., *19:*1015, 1983.

80. Premachandra, B.N., and Lang, S.: Circulating reverse triiodothyronine (rT₃) in the dog. Life Sci., *20:*1449, 1977.

81. Quinlan, W.J., and Michaelson, S.: Homologous radioimmunoassay for canine thyrotropin: response of normal and X-irradiated dogs to propylthiouracil. Endocrinology, *108:*937, 1981.

82. Reap, M., Cass, C., and Hightower, D.: Thyroxine and tri-iodothyronine levels in ten species of animals. Southwest. Vet., *31:*31, 1978.

83. Refetoff, S., Robin, N.I., and Fang, V.S.: Parameters of thyroid function in serum of 16 selected vertebrate species: a study of PBI, serum T₄, free T₄, and the pattern of T₄ and T₃ binding to serum proteins. Endocrinology, *86:*793, 1970.

84. Reid, C.F.: Thyroid function tests in the dog. J. Am. Vet. Med. Assoc., *155:*1571, 1969.

85. Reimers, T.J., Concannon, P.W., and Cowan, R.G.: Changes in serum thyroxine and cortisol in dogs after simultaneous injection of TSH and ACTH. J. Am. Anim. Hosp. Assoc., *18:*923, 1982.
86. Reimers, T.J., et al.: Effects of reproductive state on concentrations of thyroxine, 3,5,3'-triiodothyronine and cortisol in serum of dogs. Biol. Reprod., *31:*148, 1984.
87. Rosskopf, W.J., et al.: Normal thyroid values for common pet birds. Vet. Med. Small Anim. Clin., *77:*409, 1982.
88. Shively, J.N., Phemister, R.D., and Epling, G.P.: Fine structure of thyroid epithelium of young dogs treated with thyrotropin. Am. J. Vet. Res., *30:*229, 1969.
89. Sterling, K.: Thyroid hormone action at the cell level. Part I. N. Engl. J. Med., *300:*117, 1979.
90. Sterling, K.: Thyroid hormone action at the cell level. Part II. N. Engl. J. Med., *300:*173, 1979.
91. Thoday, K.L., Seth, J., and Elton, R.A.: Radioimmunoassay of serum total thyroxine and triiodothyronine in healthy cats: assay methodology and effects of age, sex, breed, heredity, and environment. J. Small Anim. Pract., *25:*457, 1984.
92. Thomas, C.L., and Adams, J.C.: Radioimmunoassay of equine serum for thyroxine: reference values. Am. J. Vet. Res., *39:*1239, 1978.
93. Thompson, D.L., Jr., and Nett, T.M.: Thyroid stimulating hormone and prolactin secretion after thyrotropin releasing hormone administration to mares: dose response during anestrus in winter and during estrus in summer. Dom. Anim. Endocrinol., *1:*263, 1984.
94. Thomson, R.A.E., and Michaelson, S.M.: A source of false iodine-[131] uptake and protein bound iodine values in dogs. Am. J. Vet. Res., *28:*1623, 1967.
95. Van der Walt, J.A., Van der Walt, L.A., and LeRoux, P.H.: Functional endocrine modification of the thyroid following ovariectomy in the canine. J. S. Afr. Vet. Assoc., *54:*225, 1983.
96. Van Herle, A.J., Vassart, G., and Dumont, J.E.: Control of thyroglobulin synthesis and secretion. Part I. N. Engl. J. Med., *301:*239, 1979.
97. Van Herle, A.J., Vassart, G., and Dumont, J.E.: Control of thyroglobulin synthesis and secretion. Part II. N. Engl. J. Med., *301:*307, 1979.
98. Weller, R.E., et al.: Basal serum thyroxine concentration and its response to thyroid stimulating hormone administration decreases with chronologic age in beagle dogs. New York, Proceeding of Am. Coll. Vet. Intern. Med., 1983, p. 38.
99. Weller, R.E., et al.: Serum thyroid-stimulating hormone (TSH) concentration in euthyroid, hypothyroid and aged dogs. Proceedings of Am. Coll. Vet. Intern. Med., 1984, p. 31.
100. Wheeler, S.L., Olson, P.N., and Husted, P.W.: Concentrations of thyroxine (T_4) and 3,5,3'-triiodothyronine (T_3) in canine serum before and after intravenous and intramuscular thyrotropin administration. Proceedings of Am. Coll. Vet. Intern. Med., 1984, p. 31.
101. Wilson, O., Stone, J.M., and Monty, D.E.: Long-term study of thyroid function in healthy beagle dogs, using [125]I. Am. J. Vet. Res., *44:*1392, 1983.
102. Woltz, H.H., et al.: Effect of prednisone on thyroid gland morphology and plasma thyroxine and triiodothyronine concentrations in the dog. Am. J. Vet. Res., *44:*2000, 1983.

7

Hypothyroidism and Thyroiditis

Thyroiditis and hypothyroidism are common endocrinologic diseases in dogs. Neither disease is often diagnosed in other companion animals. Thyroiditis is any inflammatory disorder of the thyroid. Hypothyroidism is a deficiency of the thyroid follicular cell hormones thyroxine (T_4) and triiodothyronine (T_3). Thyroiditis may or may not lead to sufficient thyroidal destruction to cause hypothyroidism. The two conditions may occur concurrently or separately. Deficiencies of calcitonin, the thyroid's parafollicular hormone, are not known to cause any discernible clinical abnormality.

HYPOTHYROIDISM

Hypothyroidism is the most frequently diagnosed endocrinopathy found in the dog. Whether these diagnoses accurately reflect the true incidence of hypothyroidism in dogs is clouded by controversy concerning the best means of diagnosis and by the difficulties of early recognition of the disease, which are caused by the variety and subtleness of hypothyroidism's presenting signs. Even so, there is little doubt that hypothyroidism is a common endocrine disease of the dog.

In other companion animals, hypothyroidism is uncommonly recognized. Cats are known to develop hypothyroidism only as a result of bilateral thyroidectomy or ^{131}I therapy. Horses and caged birds with hypothyroidism have rarely been reported.

See also references 4, 11, 12, 14, 54, 66, and 77.

Incidence and Causes

Hypothyroidism is a disease most often affecting purebred mid-to large-size breeds of dogs, beginning during their middle years (4 to 6 years of age). There may be a higher incidence in female dogs. Breeds reported to have a greater-than-expected risk of hypothyroidism include spaniels, Doberman pinschers, Irish setters, Airedales, miniature schnauzers, Pomeranians, Shetland sheepdogs, dachshunds, and golden retrievers.[55] German shepherd dogs and mongrels have a lower-than-expected risk.[55] Hypothyroidism is unusual in most toy and miniature breeds.

Most cases of hypothyroidism in dogs are due to acquired primary destructive processes of the thyroid, especially idiopathic thyroidal atrophy and severe lymphocytic thyroiditis. Lymphocytic thyroiditis is generally regarded as an autoimmune disease that may or may not lead to primary hypothyroidism. Idiopathic thyroidal atrophy is most likely an "end-stage" immune-mediated process.

Rare causes of hypothyroidism in dogs include severe iodine deficiency from all meat or liver diets; congenital defects in thyroid development, hormonogenesis, or serum transport; neoplastic thyroidal destruction; and secondary causes (thyroid-stimulating hormone [TSH] deficiency) or tertiary causes (thyrotropin-releasing hormone [TRH] deficiency) caused by adenohypophyseal or hypothalamic disease. Hypothyroidism may also be iatrogenically caused by the administration of radioisotopes of iodine, goitrogens, or by surgical excision. Goitrogens include thioureas, iodides, lithium, sulfonylureas, and 6-mercaptopurine. More than 75% of both thyroid lobes must be nonfunctional before clinical hypothyroidism becomes apparent.

See references 5 and 13.

Clinical Signs

The clinical sign that seems to manifest first (and therefore occurs most often) depends on the clinician's interest, index of suspicion for hypothyroidism, and ability to do a thorough physical exam and conduct the necessary questioning of the animal's owners. Cardinal signs of hypothyroidism are shown in Figure 7–1. The most common finding suggestive of hypothyroidism is the development of alopecia, particularly of the dorsal proximal surface or distal aspect of the tail, in breeds with tails that are not docked (Fig. 7–2). Other early signs of hypothyroidism, affecting more than 90% of cases, are also related to the integument, including such signs as dry scaly skin, dull brittle hair, failure to regrow clipped hair, or bleaching of the normal hair color (Fig. 7–3). Less commonly (in 20% of subjects affected with hypothyroidism) an oily seborrhea, along with developing alopecia,

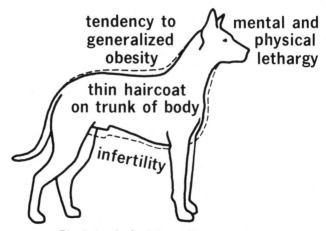

Fig. 7–1. Cardinal signs of hypothyroidism.

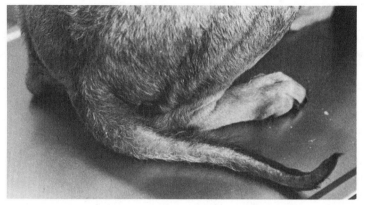

Fig. 7–2. Alopecia of the dorsum of the proximal portion of the tail is a common sign of hypothyroidism.

occurs. Skin changes, which are not usually associated with pruritus, may be pruritic, particularly if seborrhea and secondary infection are present. More subjective findings seen in the early stages of hypothyroidism include lethargy, exercise intolerance, mental torpor, and intolerance to a cold environment. When dogs who are to be used for breeding are affected, the admitting complaints may be abortion, infertility, a lack of libido, prolonged anestrus, or shortened estrus.

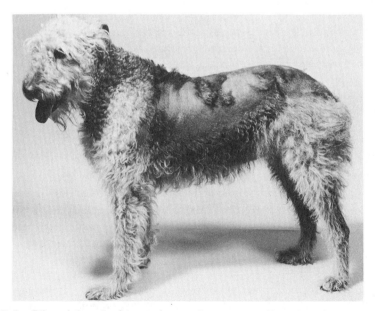

Fig. 7–3. Bilateral alopecia of the trunk occurs in most cases of hypothyroidism occurring in dogs. It may or may not be symmetrically distributed.

In severe hypothyroidism, not only are the earlier signs of illness more advanced, but additional signs also may be noted by the owner or clinician. Among these are hyperpigmentation of the skin, thickening of the skin from *myxedema* (a nonpitting swelling in the stroma of any organ), a gain in body weight (but rarely obesity), paresthesia of the limbs, paresis of the facial or vestibular nerves due to swelling of soft tissues around the external acoustic meatus, irritability and increased aggressiveness,[65] stiff locomotion, subnormal body temperature, delayed healing of wounds, constipation, sinus bradycardia with low electrocardiographic voltages,[60] and, in intact bitches, anestral galactorrhea. Myxedema is caused by an accumulation of acid and neutral mucopolysaccharides in the ground substance. The charged particles then attract and bind water.[42] The thickening of the dermis that results is most evident above the eyes and on the dorsum of the neck and shoulders.

Prepubertal and secondary or tertiary hypothyroidism are uncommon. Prepubertal hypothyroidism will cause disproportionate dwarfism with subnormal mentality. Secondary or tertiary hypothyroidism is usually concomitant with other signs of adenohypophyseal-hypothalamic dysfunction.

Secondary hyperlipidemia resulting from hypothyroidism may cause additional signs of disease. These signs particularly affect the eyes and include hypertensive retinopathy, lipemia retinalis, and annular lipid infiltration of the cornea and perilimbal sclera.[19, 44] Hypertension is presumably due to arteriosclerosis resulting from hyperlipidemia.[34, 49] Seizures, disorientation, and circling have been attributed to cerebrovascular atherosclerosis caused by hypothyroidism in the dog.[63]

Hypothyroidism in adult horses has been associated with poor work performance, thick crested necks, dull brittle hair coats, thickened scaly skin of the face and legs, and one possible case of alopecia.[45–47, 70, 76, 79]

Hypothyroidism in caged birds may be caused by iodine-deficient diets or idiopathic causes. Clinical findings reported with avian hypothyroidism have included dry skin, feather picking, obesity, lipomas, fatty liver, and hypercholesterolemia.[69]

See reference 26.

Laboratory Findings Suggestive of Hypothyroidism

Hypercholesterolemia occurs in two thirds of the canine cases of hypothyroidism. Hypercholesterolemia is a result of the greater decrease in the clearance of cholesterol compared with the lesser decrease in the synthesis of cholesterol. Although several other diseases may cause hypercholesterolemia (Table 7–1), severe fasting hypercholesterolemia (greater than 500 mg/dl) in a dog exhibiting clinical signs of advanced hypothyroidism only can be considered diagnostic of hypothyroidism until proved otherwise by definitive serum assays for thyroid function or by therapeutic failure. The next most probable cause for severe hypercholesterolemia is the nephrotic syndrome.

Table 7-1. Possible Causes for Hypercholesterolemia Other Than Hypothyroidism

Hyperadrenocorticism
Nephrotic syndrome
Various hepatic dysfunctions
Diabetes mellitus
Acute pancreatitis
Protein-losing enteropathies
Pregnancy

Less frequent laboratory findings that may alert the clinician to the possibility of hypothyroidism are a mild normochromic, normocytic nonregenerative anemia in 25% to 30% of cases and an increased serum creatinine phosphokinase (CPK) in less than 10% of cases. Mild elevations in serum levels of hepatic enzymes can occur in cases with hepatic lipidosis. Occasionally, serum triglycerides and uric acid levels are elevated. Platelet adhesiveness can decrease, thus aggravating bleeding in patients with von Willebrand's disease.[68]

Skin biopsy will not yield pathognomonic diagnostic data; however, finding epidermal thickness reduced to 1 to 2 cell layers, follicular hyperkeratosis, atrophy of the sebaceous glands, and no infiltration of cells of inflammation suggests a diagnosis of hypothyroidism (Fig. 7–4).[67,72] Myxedema can be confirmed by toluidine blue or Armed Forces Institute of

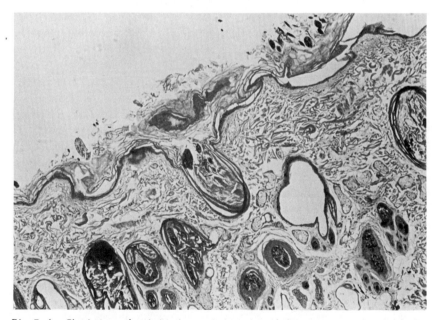

Fig. 7–4. Classic (nonseborrheic) changes in hypothyroid skin showing epidermal atrophy, follicular hyperkeratosis, and no cells of inflammation.

Pathology (AFIP) modification of Mowry's colloidal iron stains. Alcian blue, or periodic acid-Schiff reagent may be useful in some cases. Seborrheic hypothyroidism, which is less common, is characterized by follicular and epidermal acanthosis and mild infiltration of mixed cells associated with inflammation.[51] Evaluation of semen in hypothyroid male animals frequently shows oligospermia and, occasionally, azoospermia.

See reference 38.

Diagnostic Tests

Serum thyroxine (T_4) levels should be determined by radioimmunoassay (RIA). As sensitive as the RIA is for serum (or plasma) T_4, there is considerable (10% to 20%) overlapping of base-line serum T_4 between normal humans and humans with developing hypothyroidism. In dogs, because of breed differences, individual differences, serum protein binding, assay specificity, and other unknown reasons, overlapping may occur in up to 50% of hypothyroid cases.

Since the rate of thyroid metabolism (determined by the degree of negative adenohypophyseal-hypothalamic feedback) and the peripheral cellular effects are caused only by free (unbound) T_4, considerable change can occur in total serum T_4 in response to changes in protein binding while the quantity of free T_4 remains normal. Binding proteins can be increased by estrogens and pregnancy, and decreased by androgens, large doses of glucocorticoids, or hypoproteinemia when caused by the nephrotic syndrome, severe malnutrition, chronic hepatitis, hookworm disease, and protein-losing enteropathy. Protein-bound T_4 can be displaced by phenytoin, salicylates, chlorpropamide, aminoglutethimide, and tolbutamide, resulting in increased free T_4 leading to the decreased release of TSH and lowered total serum T_4 levels.

If baseline serum T_4 levels are in the low normal range, response to TSH (Dermathycin) should be evaluated (Table 7–2).[37] Horses double or nearly double their baseline serum T_4 levels 4 to 5 hours after receiving an intravenous dose of 5 U of TSH. Psittacine birds generally double their baseline T_4 levels 4 to 6 hours after receiving an intramuscular dose of 1 to 2 U of TSH. The purpose of T_4 stimulation with TSH is to assess the thyroids' reserve capacity to form and release T_4 while under maximum stimulation. Increases in serum T_3 concentrations following the administration of TSH are too variable to be of value.[6] Baseline T_4 levels can fluctuate for a few months before becoming consistently subnormal. During this period, the thyroid's reserve capacity to produce normal amounts of T_4 in response to TSH is decreased. This assessment is most meaningfully based on the maximum concentration of serum T_4 attained.

Regardless of the laboratory used, the minimum response recorded for serum T_4 after the administration of TSH should be twice that of the baseline serum T_4 and an increase of at least 1 μg/dl. Drugs that cause low serum T_4 levels because plasma proteins or their T_4-binding affinity has

Table 7–2. Recommended Thyroid-Stimulating Hormone
Response Tests

Daytime Method (Intramuscular or Intravenous TSH)
  1. 8:00 A.M.—Draw serum for baseline T_4, then give TSH intramuscu-
    larly or intravenously as follows:
      5 U for 1 to 5 kg body weight
      10 U for 5 kg body weight or more
  2. 5:00 P.M.—Draw serum for T_4 assay after stimulation with TSH.

Overnight Method (Subcutaneous TSH)
  1. 5:00 P.M.—Draw serum for baseline T_4, then give TSH (in same
    dose as above) subcutaneously.
  2. 9:00 A.M.—Draw serum for T_4 assay after stimulation with TSH.

TSH = thyroid-stimulating hormone; T_4 = thyroxine.

been decreased do not impair responsiveness to stimulation with TSH. Use
of the popular criterion that serum T_4 in dogs should double by 4 hours
after the intravenous administration of TSH ignores the knowledge that
serum T_4 does not reach peak concentrations until 8 hours (at least 6 hours)
after the intravenous administration of TSH (Fig. 7–5). The 4-hour, intra-

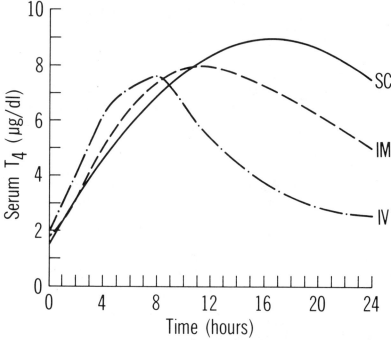

Fig. 7–5. Mean serum thyroxine concentrations after the injection of thyroid-stimulating
hormone in dog by intravenous, intramuscular, and subcutaneous routes showing different
times of peak response. T_4 = thyroxine; IV = intravenous; IM = intramuscular; SC = subcutaneous. (From Chastain, C.B.: Canine hypothyroidism. J. Am. Vet. Med. Assoc., *181*:349,
1982.)

venous TSH stimulation test also allows for the following possibilities: that a euthyroid dog with normal baseline T_4, sampled near peak natural production of T_4, might not have doubled levels of serum T_4 after receiving TSH; and that a hypothyroid dog's baseline T_4, sampled while serum T_4 concentration was low or subnormal, might double even though the animal's total reserve capacity was abnormally low.

Assessing normal thyroid function by measuring serum T_4 levels requires knowledge of normal values from the laboratory doing the assays. Normal serum T_4 values, as determined by the RIA, vary among laboratories, but if the technique is done correctly, differences are slight. The recommended interpretation of absolute serum T_4 levels, before and after the administration of TSH, may require minor changes depending on the values considered normal by the laboratory being used (Table 7–3). The same methodology and interpretation of testing may be used for cats.

Recent treatment with thyroid hormones will decrease but not negate the response to TSH. Repeated injections of TSH for 3 to 8 days will increase the magnitude of response if decreased baseline serum T_4 levels, or those measured after the administration of TSH, are caused by spontaneous or iatrogenic secondary hypothyroidism. If hypothyroidism is due to hypothalamic dysfunction, baseline T_4 levels will be abnormally low, but serum T_4 levels will often rise after an injection of either TSH or TRH.

If desired, adrenocorticotropic hormone (ACTH) stimulation tests for assessing adrenocortical function can be done on the same day as the TSH response tests, without affecting either serum cortisol or T_4 response levels[64]; however, if hypothyroidism is present, it can impair the response of the adrenal cortex to ACTH. Hypothyroidism can also impair the secretion of growth hormone (GH), but plasma prolactin levels may be elevated.

Table 7–3. Interpretation of Serum T_4 Levels by Radioimmunoassay Before and After the Administration of Thyroid-stimulating Hormone*

Baseline T_4	T_4 Values After the Administration of TSH†	Interpretation‡
<1.0	—	Hypothyroid
<2.0	≤4.0	Hypothyroid
<2.0	4–5.0	Probably hypothyroid— therapeutic trial or retest is recommended
1.0–4.0	≥5.0	Normal

* Dose: 5 U if animal is ≤ 5 kg body weight; 10 U if animal is > 5 kg body weight. T_4 = thyroxine; TSH = thyroid-stimulating hormone.

† Time necessary to wait before sampling T_4 levels after the administration of TSH, according to route of administration: intramuscular, 8 to 12 hours; subcutaneous, 14 to 18 hours; and intravenous, 8 hours.

‡ Normal serum T_4 levels measured by radioimmunoassay vary slightly among different laboratories.

Claims that 25% to 30% of all cases of hypothyroidism in dogs are caused by the failure of deiodinating T_4 to produce sufficient T_3 are unsubstantiated and unprecedented for any other species.[1,33] Low serum levels of T_3 alone do not justify a diagnosis of hypothyroidism unless they are accompanied by low serum T_4 levels before or after stimulation with TSH or by evidence of hypothyroidism shown by less common means of evaluating thyroid function such as radioiodine uptake[75]; therefore, serum T_3 levels have no true value in the diagnosis of hypothyroidism because the usefulness of measuring T_3 levels is superceded by the diagnostic value of measuring serum T_4 levels before and after the administration of TSH.

Empiric trials with thyroid hormones are rarely worthwhile. In a large dog the cost of treatment for 6 weeks exceeds the cost of the T_4 assay and TSH response test. Inappropriate treatment with levothyroxine also causes a delay in reaching a proper diagnosis and may cause detrimental catabolism. The clinical response to an empiric trial with thyroid hormone may be confusing. Due to the pharmacologic effects of thyroid hormones in synchronizing the hair growth cycle and stimulation of wakefulness, euthyroid patients with alopecia or depression may transiently improve. Such patients will not completely recover and usually relapse into more severe alopecia or depression than was present before treatment with thyroid hormones.

Three tests of thyroid function have recently been investigated in dogs and seem to have potential value in screening suspected dogs for hypothyroidism. The first is measurement of serum T_4 by enzyme-linked immunosorbent assay (ELISA). If the technique's precision and accuracy in the lower serum T_4 ranges are improved, measurement of T_4 by ELISA could provide an in-office assay method, eliminating the need for special instrumentation and licensing necessary for RIAs. The second test is the RIA for free T_4 measured by microdialysis. Direct assay of free T_4 eliminates the interpretative problems created by changes in T_4 binding protein levels and by bound T_4 displacement by drugs. In dogs, normal serum free T_4 levels determined by microdialysis are about 0.7 to 2.0 ng/dl.[56] The third test is a validated homologous RIA for canine TSH. In humans, using the RIA to measure TSH has proved the most sensitive diagnostic determination for hypothyroidism.

Treatment

Preparations of thyroid hormone are either of animal or synthetic origin. Products of animal origin, for example, dessicated thyroid, thyroglobulin, and soluble pork thyroid, have no advantage over synthetic products. They do have the disadvantage of having variable potency since they are usually standardized by iodine content.[8]

Synthetic forms of T_4 (levothyroxine), T_3 (liothyronine), and combinations of T_3 and T_4 are available. Synthetic T_3 and combination T_3-T_4 products have no established therapeutic advantage over synthetic T_4. Both the synthetic T_3 and T_3-T_4 combinations must be administered more frequently and are more expensive than synthetic T_4. Synthetic T_4 is readily deiodinated to T_3 as needed in all patients who are not ill or anorexic for other reasons.

Proof is lacking that primary spontaneous deiodination defects occur in dogs. For ease of administration and economic reasons, sodium levothyroxine should be used exclusively as replacement therapy for hypothyroidism. Sodium levothyroxine is available under several common trade names (Synthroid, Soloxine, Levothroid, Levoid, and Thyro-Tabs).

Sodium levothyroxine is effectively administered once daily to most hypothyroid dogs. Only about 15% of the orally administered dose is absorbed in the dog. The serum half-life of T_4 in the normal dog is about 12 hours, but metabolic effects are much longer. The duration of serum and tissue T_4 levels in hypothyroid dogs may be twice as long as the normal duration, as happens in hypothyroid persons. The duration of administered T_4 is also affected by dose. Since only 1% to 30% of the possible T_4 serum binding proteins are bound at normal concentrations of T_4, the longer effects of larger doses of T_4 are caused by the increase in circulating reserve T_4; however, iatrogenic thyrotoxicosis is uncommon unless recommended doses are exceeded by severalfold.

Treatment may usually be initiated at the full replacement dose. A more conservative approach, in which small doses are gradually increased to full replacement doses, is advisable if the patient has congestive heart failure, cardiac arrhythmias, or diabetes mellitus. Replacement of thyroid hormone should not be started before replacement of steroid hormone if the patient being treated also has hypoadrenocorticism.

The dose necessary for the replacement of thyroid hormone correlates better with the metabolic rate than with body weight. If the dosage is based on body weight (for example, a dose of 0.02 mg/kg body weight), it must be adjusted to a higher dose per kg for very small dogs and a lower dose per kg for very large dogs. Dosage is better determined by correlating it with body surface area (Table 7–4). If liothyronine is used, the recommended dosage is 5 μg/kg body weight three times daily. Overdosage can be very detrimental by depleting the muscle and liver of glycogen, causing exercise intolerance.[10] Other effects of overdosage are weight loss, undesirable changes in temperament, demineralization of the bones, polyuria, polydipsia, and failure to regrow hair. Thyroid hormone should never be used to treat obesity or aging changes in euthyroid dogs. Hypothyroidism in cats caused by thyroidectomy can be maintained with a daily dose of 0.1 mg of sodium levothyroxine.

The response to treatment should be unequivocally favorable 6 weeks after the initiation of replacement therapy. Apparent failure to respond to sodium levothyroxine at recommended doses within 6 weeks should be considered an error in diagnosis until proved otherwise by diagnostic reevaluation.

Determining a favorable response to treatment does not require serum

Table 7-4. Recommended Dosage Table of Sodium Levothyroxine Based on 0.5 mg per Square Meter of Body Surface

Kg Body Weight	Lb Body Weight	Mg/Day
0–1	0–2	0.05
2–3	3–7	0.1
4–5	8–11	0.15
6–8	12–18	0.2
9–11	19–24	0.25
12–15	25–32	0.3
16–19	33–40	0.35
20–23	41–50	0.4
24–27	51–60	0.45
28–31	61–70	0.5
32–36	71–80	0.55
37–41	81–90	0.6
42–47	91–103	0.65
48–53	104–115	0.7

T_4 or T_3 assays. Improved mental alertness, physical activity, regrowth of hair, cessation of seborrhea, or other regression of previous physical abnormalities plus the return to normal values recorded for hemoglobin, packed cell volume, serum cholesterol, and serum CPK denote a favorable response to treatment. The expense of post-treatment serum T_4 or T_3 testing is only justified if the following conditions are present: apparent failure to respond, suspected toxicity, possible drug interaction (anticonvulsants induce rapid biliary excretion of T_4), or chronic heart, gastrointestinal, or kidney disease. When necessary, post-treatment testing of serum T_4 and T_3 should be done 4 to 6 hours after oral administration and immediately before the next dose (24 hours after the first dose) is given to determine peak serum T_4 levels, T_4 duration, and the degree of T_4 deiodination.

Possible causes of failure to respond to the replacement of thyroid hormone are listed in Table 7-5 in decreasing order of probability.[8] Misdiagnosis is the most common cause. Various conditions associated with hypothyroidism in dogs, such as idiopathic alopecias, keratitis sicca, obesity, infertility, and others, have not been adequately corrected by replacement with thyroid hormone.[38,59] Conditions such as feline endocrine

Table 7-5. Possible Causes for Failures in Response to Thyroid Hormone Replacement in Decreasing Order of Probability

Inaccurate diagnosis
Failure to receive medication
Inadequate dose or frequency of administration
Inactive preparation
Poor absorption
Peripheral tissue resistance

alopecia that do not completely and permanently resolve when adequate serum levels of T_4 are achieved should not be considered the result of hypothyroidism.[73]

Horses with hypothyroidism have been reported to respond to iodinated casein in doses of 5 g/day. Because iodinated casein is not currently available, treatment of equine hypothyroidism would have to be empirically attempted with sodium levothyroxine.

See references 22 and 36.

Cautions

Since the first clinical use of thyroid hormone in 1891, replacement preparations of thyroid hormone have been used indiscriminately. The only indication for the therapeutic use of thyroid hormones in dogs is the confirmed diagnosis of hypothyroidism. The use of these products for obesity, convulsions, infertility, or other miscellaneous reasons without a laboratory evaluation of thyroid function is not recommended.

The greatest risk resulting from inappropriate therapy with thyroid hormones is the failure to find and correct the true cause of the patient's problem. Other risks include any of the signs of hyperthyroidism, such as weight loss, irritability, and muscle tremors.

Special Forms of Hypothyroidism

SECONDARY HYPOTHYROIDISM.   Secondary hypothyroidism is rare in the dog. It is not known how rare its existence is in dogs. In humans, about 4% of cases of hypothyroidism are caused by TSH deficiency. In neonates and juveniles, congenital hypopituitarism is the most common cause of secondary hypothyroidism. In adults, it is usually caused by adenohypophyseal adenomas. More than 20% of humans with adenohypophyseal adenomas develop secondary hypothyroidism.

Clinical signs suggestive of canine secondary hypothyroidism are indications of hypothyroidism concomitant with an excess or deficiency of ACTH, secondary hypogonadism, diabetes insipidus, or various dysfunctions of the central nervous system such as seizures, a change in temperament, amaurosis, or head pressing. The diagnosis can be confirmed by showing the lack of colloid vacuoles in biopsies of the thyroid, along with radiographic evidence of adenohypophyseal enlargement shown by cranial sinus venography or cranial tomography. Characteristically, baseline serum T_4 levels are low, and serum T_4 levels are normal or near normal after 3 to 8 days of injections of TSH. Images produced by thyroid scans will also increase in response to the administration of TSH for 3 days, if secondary or tertiary hypothyroidism is the cause of low baseline serum T_4 levels.

See references 17 and 20.

INAPPROPRIATE GALACTORRHEA AND INFERTILITY.   Hyperprolactinemia occurs in animals with severe hypothyroidism caused by an excess of TRH and deficient concentrations of hypothalamic dopamine. Hyperprolactinemia may cause inappropriate galactorrhea in some dogs if their mammae have been adequately primed for lactation (Fig. 7–6). This phenomenon occurs most often in intact bitches and must be differentiated from other possible causes of galactorrhea, particularly pregnancy, pseudocyesis, and mammary trauma. Hyperprolactinemia may also be at least partially responsible for infertility in dogs with severe hypothyroidism since prolactin may interfere with gonadotropin-releasing hormone (GnRH) or directly with gonadal production of steroids.

See also reference 18.

HYPOTHYROID MYOPATHY. Severe hypothyroidism can cause profound muscle weakness (Fig. 7–7). Some dogs exhibit slow, stiff locomotion or signs described by owners as muscle cramps. The weakness can be so severe that the condition has been mistaken for wobbler's syndrome or polyradiculoneuritis. Affected dogs have elevated serum CPK values and usually hypercholesterolemia. Other more characteristic signs of hypothyroidism are present, but may be overshadowed by the degree of muscular weakness. In affected dogs, there is a preferential metabolic dysfunction in Type II fibers leading to Type II fiber atrophy.[7] Muscles in affected humans are deficient in α-glucosidase.[39] Complete clinical recovery after replacement of thyroid hormone provides definitive proof of hypothyroid myopathy.

See reference 61.

MYXEDEMA COMA. The most dangerous possible sequelae of severe hypothyroidism is myxedema coma. Most recognized cases have involved Doberman pinschers. Associated mortalities are high. Suggestive clinical signs are hypothermia without shivering, stupor leading to coma, hypoven-

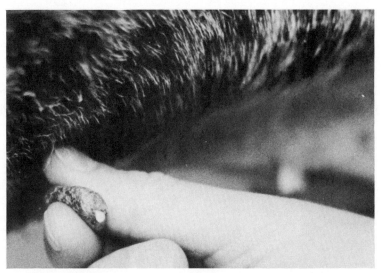

Fig. 7–6. Galactorrhea can occur in anestral, sexually intact female dogs who develop severe hypothyroidism. (From Chastain, C.B., and Schmidt, B.: Galactorrhea associated with hypothyroidism in intact bitches. J. Am. Anim. Hosp. Assoc., *16:*851, 1980.)

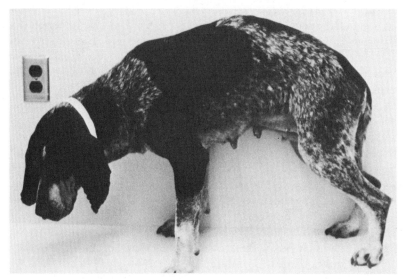

Fig. 7–7. Severe hypothyroidism can be present in animals with the primary complaint of muscle weakness and reluctance to move because of hypothyroid myopathy. (From Chastain, C.B., and Schmidt, B.: Galactorrhea associated with hypothyroidism in intact bitches. J. Am. Anim. Hosp. Assoc., *16:*851, 1980.)

tilation, hypotension, and bradycardia (Fig. 7–8). Laboratory findings may include hyponatremia, hypercarbia, hypoglycemia, hypocortisolemia, and hypoxemia. The protein and CPK levels of cerebrospinal fluid may be elevated. Serum levels of T_4 will be low, but myxedema coma is a medical emergency and must be treated as such.

Treatment must begin before the results of measuring T_4 levels are received. Treatment consists of an intravenous dose of sodium levothyroxine prepared for injection (Synthroid for Injection) or an oral dose of liothyronine given by gastric tube, mechanical respiratory support, intravenous administration of glucocorticoids, broad-spectrum antibiotics, and passive rewarming. Fluid administration, vasopressors, and active attempts to warm

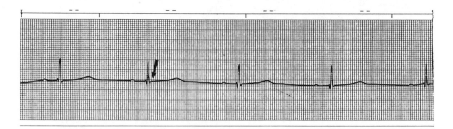

Fig. 7–8. Lead II electrocardiogram from a dog with myxedema coma showing bradycardia, first-degree atrioventricular blockade, prolongation of the QRS duration and QT interval, and equivocal J wave (*arrow*). (From Chastain, C.B., Graham, C.L., and Riley, M.G.: Myxedema coma in two dogs. Canine Pract., *9:*20, 1982.)

should be avoided, at least until T$_4$ has been administered and a response noted. Precipitating factors of myxedema coma are respiratory depressant drugs, infectious diseases (especially pneumonia), heart failure, or exposure to a cold environment.

See references 15, 43, and 62 for further information.

CONGENITAL HYPOTHYROIDISM. Most dogs and cats with congenital hypo-thyroidism probably die before weaning. The two most probable potential causes include thyroid dysgenesis (responsible for 80% to 90% of congeni-tal hypothyroidism in humans), and dyshormonogenesis (usually an inability to organify iodine, dyshormonogenesis is the second most common cause of congenital hypothyroidism). Other forms of dyshormonogenesis (defects in uptake, coupling, dehalogenase deficiencies, production of abnormal iodo-proteins, or proteolysis), serum transport abnormalities, congenital TSH deficiency, goitrogens, and severe iodine deficiency are also possible causes, but they are far less likely. If the condition is not severe or the puppy or kitten is reared by hand, it can survive.

Clinical signs may go unnoticed until the period after weaning, when impaired growth and maturation of skeletal and nervous systems become obvious. Severe congenital hypothyroidism causes disproportionate (short-legged) dwarfism and subnormal mentality. Other physical signs can include short-broad skull, shortened mandible, protruding tongue, lateral strabis-mus, exophthalmus, alopecia, hypothermia, bradycardia, muscular weak-ness, delayed dental eruption, and (depending on the cause) goiter (Fig. 7–9).

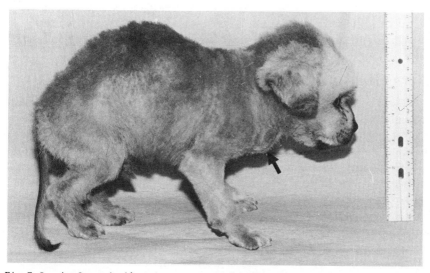

Fig. 7–9. An 8-month-old cretinous pup with kyphosis, goiter (*arrow*), disproportionate dwarfism, and hair loss. (From Chastain, C.B., et al.: Congenital hypothyroidism in a dog due to an iodide organification defect. Am. J. Vet. Res., *44:*1257, 1983.)

Suggestive laboratory findings can include hypercholesterolemia, nonregenerative anemia, elevated serum CPK levels, impaired secretion of GH, and hypoglycemia. Diagnosis is based on clinical signs and assays for baseline serum T_4 levels and T_4 levels after the administration of TSH. It should be noted that normal levels of serum T_4 in neonates is 10 to 20 times that of normal concentrations of serum T_4 in adults.

Thyroid dysgenesis is made evident by abnormal findings in a thyroid scan. A defect in organification is substantiated by abnormal findings in a perchlorate discharge test.

Some clinicians consider radiographic evidence of epiphyseal dysgenesis (ragged epiphyses with few foci of calcification) pathognomonic for congenital hypothyroidism (Fig. 7–10). Other radiographic findings include delayed epiphyseal closure, deformities of the open cranial sutures joints, kyphosis, and arthritis. Although administration of thyroid hormones can promote some physical growth after prolonged cretinism, treatment must be begun very early, even before 3 months of age in children, to preserve normal intelligence levels (Fig. 7–11).

Congenital hypothyroidism in foals has been reported to cause defective ossification of the central and third tarsal bones leading to their collapse. Delayed epiphyseal closure and delayed dental eruption have also occurred in hypothyroid foals.[40, 41, 74]

See also references 2, 9, 16, and 71.

SCHMIDT'S SYNDROME. People with hypothyroidism caused by lymphocytic thyroiditis can concurrently develop hypoadrenocorticism, hypoparathyroidism, primary hypogonadism, or diabetes mellitus. These concurrent endocrinopathies represent autoimmune (lymphocytic) destruction of multiple endocrine glands. Although concurrent endocrinopathies in dogs with hypothyroidism have been clinically recognized, well-substantiated reports of Schmidt's-like syndrome in dogs and other companion animals are lacking.[35]

THYROIDITIS

Inflammatory disorders of the thyroid may be acute or chronic, infectious or noninfectious. Acute or subacute thyroiditis is usually the result of an infective process such as cellulitis of the neck or septicemia. Acute or subacute thyroiditis is generally subclinical in companion animals.

Chronic thyroiditis is frequently seen in dogs, but in other companion animals, it seems to be rare to nonexistent. Chronic thyroiditis in dogs is characterized histologically as a multifocal interstitial infiltration of lymphocytes, plasma cells, and macrophages.[52] Destruction of thyroid follicles with antigen-antibody complexes on follicular basement membranes also occurs. Chronic thyroiditis in dogs is apparently immune-mediated.[29, 48, 57] Similar lesions have been produced experimentally by injections with thyroglobulin or thyroid antigens with adjuvants, intrathyroidal injection of autoantibodies, or intrathyroidal injection of allogeneic lymphocytes.[21, 27, 30, 31]

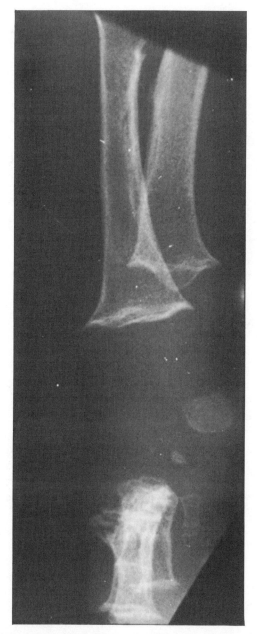

Fig. 7–10. Epiphyseal dysgenesis in an 8-month-old cretinous pup. The epiphyses of the distal radius and ulna are not ossified, the distal metaphyseal bone margin is flared, and most of the carpal bones have not ossified. (From Chastain, C.B., et al.: Congenital hypothyroidism in a dog due to an iodide organification defect. Am. J. Vet. Res., *44:*1257, 1983.)

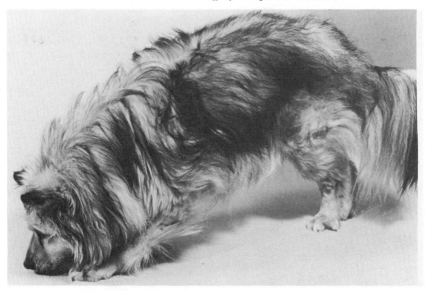

Fig. 7–11. The same cretinous dog seen in Figure 7–9 after 8 months of thyroid hormone replacement therapy. Mental retardation persisted. (From Chastain, C.B., et al.: Congenital hypothyroidism in a dog due to an iodide organification defect. Am. J. Vet. Res., *44:*1257, 1983.)

A familial chronic lymphocytic thyroiditis has been noted in some colonies of beagles used for research.[24, 25, 28, 50, 53, 58, 78] The incidence among young adult beagles in affected colonies is about 20%. Male and female dogs are affected with equal frequency. Most affected beagles do not develop clinical hypothyroidism. Gross enlargement of affected thyroids does not occur. Antibodies have been detected against thyroglobulin, microsomal antigen, and a second colloid antigen. Fluorescent examinations of antibodies are consistently positive. Precipitating antibodies are not detected, passive hemagglutinations are in low titers, and complement fixation titers vary. Some may form antinuclear antibodies (ANA) or antihepatic antibodies. Concomitant inflammatory lesions of testes and salivary glands have been noted in some dogs with lymphocytic thyroiditis.[23]

The experimentally produced thyroiditis lesion and familial thyroiditis of beagles are very similar to such phenomena seen in Hashimoto's thyroiditis in humans.[3] Hashimoto's thyroiditis is a Gell and Coombs Type II, immune-mediated destructive process affecting the thyroid. It is a genetically linked trait aggravated by biologic or emotional stress.

The ELISA method has determined that the incidence of antithyroglobulin antibodies in the general canine population is 13%. The incidence of thyroid lesions similar to those seen in beagles with lymphocytic thyroiditis is estimated to be 0.4%. In a survey of spontaneous hypothyroid dogs, about half the dogs had antithyroglobulin antibodies (in ratios of 1:20 or greater), a finding determined by chromic chloride passive hemagglutination and by the ELISA method. Antimicrosomal antibodies were found in 4%. Twenty percent of hypothyroid dogs were also tested as positive for circulating immune complexes.[32] In humans, antimicrosomal antibodies best correlate with developing hypothyroidism and with histologic findings of active thyroiditis. The presence of antithyroglobulin antibodies with hypothyroidism is suggestive of primary (not secondary or tertiary) hypothyroidism. Low antithyroglobulin titers have also been associated with acanthosis nigricans in some dogs.[32] The significance of this latter finding is unknown.

REFERENCES

1. Anderson, R.F.: Canine hypothyroidism. Compend. Contin. Ed., *1:*103, 1979.
2. Arnold, U., et al.: Goitrous hypothyroidism and dwarfism in a kitten. J. Am. Anim. Hosp. Assoc., *20:*753, 1984.
3. Beierwaltes, W.H., and Nishiyama, R.H.: Dog thyroiditis: occurrence and similarity to Hasimoto's struma. Endocrinology, *83:*501, 1968.
4. Belshaw, B.E.: Diagnosis and treatment of hypothyroidism in dogs. Proceedings of the 6th Kal Kan Symposium. Columbus, OH, 1982, p. 85.
5. Belshaw, B.E., and Becker, D.V.: Necrosis of follicular cells and discharge of thyroidal iodine induced by administering iodide to iodine-deficient dogs. J. Clin. Endocrinol. Metabol., *36:*466, 1971.
6. Belshaw, B.E., and Rijnberk, A.: Radioimmunoassay of plasma T_4 and T_3 in the diagnosis of primary hypothyroidism in dogs. J. Am. Anim. Hosp. Assoc., *15:*17, 1979.
7. Braund, K.G., et al.: Hypothyroid myopathy in two dogs. Vet. Pathol., *18:*589, 1981.
8. Brennan, M.D.: Thyroid hormones. Mayo Clin. Proc., *55:*33, 1980.
9. Brouwers, J.: Goitre et hérédité chez le chien. Ann. Méd. Vet., *94:*173, 1950.
10. Brzezinska, Z., and Kaciuba-Uscilko, H.: Low muscle and liver glycogen contents in dogs treated with thyroid hormones. Horm. Metab. Res., *11:*675, 1979.
11. Bush, B.M.: Thyroid disease in the dog. A review: Part I. J. Small Anim. Pract., *10:*95, 1969.
12. Bush, B.M.: Thyroid disease in the dog. A review: Part II. J. Small Anim. Pract., *10:*185, 1969.
13. Calvert, C.A., Chapman, W.L., and Toal, R.L.: Congestive cardiomyopathy in Doberman pinscher dogs. J. Am. Vet. Med. Assoc., *181:*598, 1982.
14. Chastain, C.B.: Canine hypothyroidism. J. Am. Vet. Med. Assoc., *181:*349, 1982.
15. Chastain, C.B., Graham, C.L., and Riley, M.G.: Myxedema coma in two dogs. Canine Pract., *9:*20, 1982.
16. Chastain, C.B., et al.: Congenital hypothyroidism in a dog due to an iodide organification defect. Am. J. Vet. Res., *44:*1257, 1983.
17. Chastain, C.B., Riedesel, D.H., and Graham, C.L.: Secondary hypothyroidism in a dog. Canine Pract., *6:*59, 1979.
18. Chastain, C.B., and Schmidt, B.: Galactorrhea associated with hypothyroidism in intact bitches. J. Am. Anim. Hosp. Assoc., *16:*851, 1980.
19. Crispin, S.M., and Barnett, K.C.: Arcus lipoides corneae secondary to hypothyroidism in the Alsatian. J. Small Anim. Pract., *19:*127, 1978.
20. Eigenmann, J.E.: Diagnosis and treatment of dwarfism in the German shepherd dog. J. Am. Anim. Hosp. Assoc., *17:*798, 1981.
21. Evans, T.C., Beierwaltes, W.H., and Nishiyama, R.H.: Experimental canine Hashimoto's thyroiditis. Endocrinology, *84:*641, 1969.
22. Evinger, J.V., and Nelson, R.W.: The clinical pharmacology of thyroid hormones in the dog. J. Am. Vet. Med. Assoc., *185:*314, 1984.
23. Fritz, T.C., et al.: Pathology and familial incidence of orchitis and its relation to thyroiditis in a closed beagle colony. Exp. Mol. Pathol., *24:*142, 1976.
24. Fritz, T.C., Norris, W.P., and Kretz, N.D.: Influence of lymphocytic thyroiditis on iodine metabolism in the beagle. Proc. Soc. Exp. Biol. Med., *134:*450, 1970.

25. Fritz, T.C., Zeman, R.C., and Zelle, M.R.: Pathology and familial incidence of thyroiditis in a closed beagle colony. Exp. Mol. Pathol., *12:*14, 1970.
26. Goldberg, R.C., and Chaikoff, I.L.: Myxedema in the radiothyroidectomized dog. Endocrinology, *50:*115, 1952.
27. Gosselin, S.J., et al.: Lymphocytic thyroiditis in dogs: induction with a local graft-versus-host reaction. Am. J. Vet. Res., *42:*1856, 1981.
28. Gosselin, S.J., Capen, C.C., and Martin, S.L.: Animal model of human disease: lymphocytic thyroiditis in the dog. Am J. Pathol., *90:*285, 1978.
29. Gosselin, S.J., Capen, C.C., and Martin, S.L.: Histologic and ultrastructural evaluation of thyroid lesions associated with hypothyroidism in dogs. Vet. Pathol., *18:*299, 1981.
30. Gosselin, S.J., et al.: Autoimmune lymphocytic thyroiditis in dogs. Vet. Immunol. Immunopathol., *3:*185, 1982.
31. Gosselin, S.J., et al.: Induced lymphocytic thyroiditis in dogs: effect of intrathyroidal injection of thyroid autoantibodies. Am. J. Vet. Res., *42:*1565, 1981.
32. Gosselin, S.J., et al: Biochemical and immunological investigations on hypothyroidism in dogs. Can. J. Comp. Med., *44:*158, 1980.
33. Greene, J.A., Knecht, C.D., and Roesel, O.F.: Hypothyroidism as a possible cause of canine intervertebral disk disease. J. Am. Anim. Hosp. Assoc., *15:*199, 1979.
34. Gwin, R.M., et al.: Hypertensive retinopathy associated with hypothyroidism, hypercholesterolemia, and renal failure in a dog. J. Am. Anim. Hosp. Assoc., *14:*200, 1978.
35. Hargis, A.M., et al.: Relationship of hypothyroidism to diabetes mellitus, renal amyloidosis, and thrombosis in purebred beagles. Am. J. Vet. Res., *42:*1077, 1981.
36. Hightower, D., Kyzar, J.R., and Chester, D.K.: Replacement therapy for induced hypothyroidism in dogs. J. Am. Vet. Med. Assoc., *163:*979, 1973.
37. Hoge, W.R., Lund, J.E., and Blakemore, J.C.: Response to thyrotropin as diagnostic aid for canine hypothyroidism. J. Am. Anim. Hosp. Assoc., *110:*167, 1974.
38. Hollander, C.S., et al.: Repair of the anemia and hyperlipidemia of the hypothyroid dog. Endocrinology, *81:*1007, 1967.
39. Hurwitz, L.J., McCormick, D., and Allen, I.V.: Reduced muscle alpha-glucosidase (acid maltase) activity in hypothyroid myopathy. Lancet, *1:*67, 1970.
40. Irvine, C.H.G.: Hypothyroidism in the foal. Equine Vet. J., *16:*302, 1984.
41. Irvine, C.H.G., and Evans, M.J.: Hypothyroidism in foals. N.Z. Vet. J., *24:*354, 1977.
42. Johnson, J.A., and Patternson, J.M.: Multifocal myxedema and mixed thyroid neoplasm in a dog. Vet. Pathol., *18:*13, 1981.
43. Kelly, M.J., and Hill, J.R.: Canine myxedema coma stupor and coma. Compend. Contin. Ed., *6:*1049, 1984.
44. Kern, T.J., and Riis, R.C.: Ocular manifestations of secondary hyperlipidemia associated with hypothyroidism and uveitis in a dog. J. Am. Anim. Hosp. Assoc., *16:*907, 1980.
45. Lowe, J.E., et al.: Semen characteristics in thyroidectomised stallions. J. Reprod. Fertil., *Suppl. 23:*81, 1975.
46. Lowe, J.E., et al.: Equine hypothyroidism: the long term effects of thyroidectomy on metabolism and growth in mares and stallions. Cornell Vet., *64:*276, 1974.
47. Lowe, J.E., and Kallfelz, F.A.: Thyroidectomy and the T_4 test to assess thyroid dysfunction in the horse and pony. Proc. Am. Assoc. Equine Pract., *16:*135, 1970.
48. Lucke, V.M., Gaskell, C.J., and Wotton, P.R.: Thyroid pathology in canine hypothyroidism. J. Comp. Pathol., *93:*415, 1983.
49. Manning, P.J.: Thyroid gland and arterial lesions of beagles with familial hypothyroidism and hyperlipoproteinemia. Am. J. Vet. Res., *40:*820, 1979.
50. Manning, P.J., Corwin, L.A., and Middleton, C.C.: Familial hyperlipoproteinemia and thyroid dysfunction of beagles. Exp. Mol. Pathol., *19:*378, 1973.
51. Martin, S.L., and Capen, C.C.: Hypothyroidism and the skin. Vet. Clin. North Am., Small Anim. Pract., *9:*29, 1979.
52. Mawdesley-Thomas, L.E.: Lymphocytic thyroiditis in the dog. J. Small Anim. Pract., *9:*539, 1968.
53. Mawdesley-Thomas, L.E., and Jolly, D.W.: Autoimmune disease in the beagle. Vet. Rec., *80:*553, 1967.
54. Meir, H., and Clark, S.T.: The clinico-pathologic aspect of thyroid disease in the dog and cat. II. Clinical features. Zentralbl. Veterinarmed., *5:*120, 1958.
55. Milne, K.L., and Haynes, H.M.: Epidemiologic features of canine hypothyroidism. Cornell Vet., *71:*3, 1981.

56. Mincey, E.K., and McTaggart, M.P.: Direct determination of free thyroxine in canine serum using single tube radioimmunoassay. Vet. Clin. Pathol., *10:*25, 1981.
57. Mizejewski, G.J., Baron, J., and Poissant, G.: Immunologic investigations of naturally occurring canine thyroiditis. J. Immunol., *107:*1152, 1971.
58. Musser, E., and Graha, W.R.: Familial occurrence of thyroiditis in purebred beagles. Lab. Anim. Care, *18:*58, 1968.
59. Nesbitt, G.H., et al.: Canine hypothyroidism: a retrospective study of 108 cases. J. Am. Vet. Med. Assoc., *177:*1117, 1980.
60. Nijhuis, A.H., et al.: ECG changes in dogs with hypothyroidism. Tijdschr. Diergeneeskd., *103:*736, 1978.
61. Norris, F.H., and Panner, B.J.: Hypothyroid myopathy clinical, electromyographical and ultrastructural observations. Arch. Neurol., *14:*574, 1966.
62. Noxon, J.O.: Accidental hypothermia associated with hypothyroidism. Canine Pract., *10:*17, 1983.
63. Patterson, J.S., Rusley, M.S., and Zachary, J.F.: Neurologic manifestations of cerebrovascular atherosclerosis associated with primary hypothyroidism in a dog. J. Am. Vet. Med. Assoc., *186:*499, 1985.
64. Reimers, T.J.: Radioimmunoassays and diagnostic tests for thyroid and adrenal disorders. Compend. Contin. Ed., *4:*65, 1982.
65. Reinhard, D.W.: Aggressive behavior associated with hypothyroidism. Canine Pract., *5:*69, 1978.
66. Rijnberk, A.: Iodine Metabolism and Thyroid Disease in the Dog. Doctoral thesis. Utrecht, The Netherlands, Drukkerij Elinkwijk, 1971.
67. Rojko, J.L., Hoover, E.A., and Martin, S.L.: Histological interpretation of cutaneous biopsies from dogs with dermatologic disorders. Vet. Pathol., *15:*579, 1978.
68. Romatowski, J.: Intercurrent hypothyroidism, autoimmune anemia, and a coagulation deficiency (von Willebrand's disease) in a dog. J. Am. Vet. Med. Assoc., *185:*309, 1984.
69. Rosskopf, W.J., and Woerpel, R.W.: Remission of lipomatous growths in a hypothyroid budgerigar in response to L-thyroxine therapy. Vet. Med. Small Anim. Clin., *78:*1415, 1983.
70. Schlotthauer, C.F.: The incidence and types of disease of the thyroid gland of adult horses. J. Am. Vet. Med. Assoc., *78:*211, 1931.
71. Schwalder, V.P.: Zwergwuchs beim Hund. Kleintier Prax, *23:*3, 1978.
72. Scott, D.W.: Histopathologic findings in endocrine skin disorders of the dog. J. Am. Anim. Hosp. Assoc., *18:*173, 1982.
73. Scott, D.W.: Thyroid function in feline endocrine alopecia. J. Am. Anim. Hosp. Assoc., *11:*798, 1975.
74. Shaver, J.R., et al.: Skeletal manifestations of suspected hypothyroidism in two foals. J. Equine Med. Surg., *3:*269, 1979.
75. Slade, E.A., et al.: Serum thyroxine and triiodothyronine concentrations in canine pyoderma. J. Am. Vet. Med. Assoc., *185:*216, 1984.
76. Stanley, O., and Hillidge, C.J.: Alopecia associated with hypothyroidism in a horse. Equine Vet. J., *14:*165, 1982.
77. Stogdale, L.: The diagnosis and treatment of canine hypothyroidism. J. S. Afr. Vet. Assoc., *51:*46, 1980.
78. Tucker, W.E., Jr.: Thyroiditis in a group of laboratory dogs. Am. J. Clin. Pathol., *38:*70, 1962.
79. Waldron-Mease, E.: Hypothyroidism and myopathy in racing thoroughbreds and standardbreds. J. Equine Med. Surg., *3:*269, 1979.

8

Goiters, Hyperthyroidism, and Hypercalcitoninism

Goiter is defined as any gross enlargement of the thyroid. Since normal thyroids are not palpable in the dog and cat, the term goiter infers that the thyroids are palpable.

Goiters may be categorized according to cause or functional state. Causes of goiter include neoplasms, hyperplasia, cysts, or inflammation. Several functional states may be associated with goiter: hypothyroidism, hyperthyroidism, or euthyroidism; or hypocalcitoninism, hypercalcitoninism, or eucalcitoninism.

NON-NEOPLASTIC GOITER: SIMPLE, ENDEMIC, NONTOXIC, DIFFUSE, AND COLLOID GOITERS

Non-neoplastic enlargements of the thyroid are the result of biochemical disorders in the synthesis or release of thyroid hormones, resulting in a partial or complete failure to suppress the release of TSH. Increased levels of TSH produce bilateral thyroid hypertrophy and hyperplasia.

See also references 3, 4, 11, 16, 18, 19, 40, 59, and 69.

Causes

Causes for non-neoplastic goiters are listed in Table 8–1. Since dogs and cats are carnivorous, goitrogenic plants are unlikely causes for goiters in these species. Ingestion of goitrogenic plants is a more common cause of goiter in horses and birds, particularly if the diet is low in iodine or if the enzymes necessary for the synthesis of thyroid hormone are deficient.

Non-neoplastic goiters, which were most often due to dietary iodine deficiency, are now rare in dogs and cats in the United States. Goiters resulting from iodine deficiency were once common in dogs from the iodine-deficient belt of the Great Lakes, as well as other areas of the world.[60, 64] Mountainous and other areas that ancient seas never covered, or areas where frequent rainfalls took place, washing iodine from the soil, were also places endemic in iodine-deficient goiters.

In dogs and cats, unsupplemented diets of meat or liver could cause goiter if used exclusively because meat and liver are deficient in iodine. Dietary iodine requirements in dogs are 34 μg/kg body weight/day in dogs and 100 μg/day in cats. These requirements are met by feeding the animals commercial pet foods supplemented with iodine, iodates used in bread making, and iodized table salt.

Table 8-1. Causes for Non-neoplastic Goiter

Dietary iodine deficiency
Dietary iodine excess
Dyshormonogenesis
Goitrogenic diet
    Turnips
    Cabbage
    Kale
    Soybeans
    Lentil
    Linseed
    Peas
    Peanuts

Goitrogenic drugs
    Aminosalicylic acid
    Sulfonylureas
    Sulfonamides
    Phenylbutazone
    Lithium
    Iodine-containing drugs
    Propylthiouracil
    Methimazole

Diets too high in iodine are uncommon. Kelp is high in iodine and can cause goiter in foals if fed to nursing mares.[20,41] Since the Wolff-Chaikoff effect is normally transient, up to 2 weeks long, goiters should not result from excessive dietary iodine unless there is concomitant deficiency of enzymes necessary for the synthesis of thyroid hormone.

Known familial defects in the synthesis of thyroid hormone (dyshormonogenesis) are rare. A few have been reported in dogs and, possibly, in one cat.[2] Five types of congenital goiter have been described in humans. These are: defective transport of iodine; thyroid peroxidase deficiency; impaired coupling; absence or deficiency of iodotyrosine deiodinase; and production of an abnormal iodoprotein. Congenital goiter caused by a deficiency in peroxidase (an organification defect) has been described in the dog.

Goitrogenic drugs are rarely administered in sufficient doses or for a duration sufficient to cause clinical goiter. Their effects may be potentiated if the diet is low in iodine or dyshormonogenesis is present. Youth and pregnancy potentiate the effects of all goitrogens since iodine requirements and the synthesis of thyroid hormone per kg body weight during growth and pregnancy are greater than the iodine requirements and rate of thyroid hormone synthesis in the average adult.

Clinical Signs

The clinical sign characteristic of non-neoplastic goiters, regardless of cause, is bilateral, palpable enlargements of the thyroids. Non-neoplastic goiters are movable and unattached to the skin or trachea. Marked enlargements may cause dysphagia, dysphonia, dyspnea, or vascular compression. Most non-neoplastic goiters are euthyroid, since the enlarged thyroids are often capable of compensating for the potential deficiency of circulating thyroid hormones. However, goiters resulting from dyshormonogenesis are likely to be incapable of compensation, and overt signs of hypothyroidism (cretinism) coexistent with palpable thyroids are usually noted.

Treatment

Treatment of non-neoplastic goiter depends on the cause. Dietary or drug-induced goiters may be corrected by dietary management or the drug's withdrawal. Congenital goiters can be reduced with the replacement of thyroid hormone, but complete regression to normal size is unlikely because of fibrosis.

THYROID NEOPLASIA

Thyroid neoplasms are infrequent, but not rare in dogs and cats. In fact, any tumor in the ventral cervical area should be considered a thyroid neoplasm until proved otherwise. Types are listed in Table 8–2. Most thyroid neoplasms in the cat and horse are difficult to palpate and are benign. Most neoplasms in the dog are easy to palpate and are malignant. Follicular carcinomas (adenocarcinomas) in dogs and adenomas or multinodular adenomatous hyperplasia in cats can produce excesses of triiodothyronine (T_3) or thyroxine (T_4), causing hyperthyroidism. In other cases, neoplastic destruction of functional thyroid tissue by thyroid carcinomas may cause hypothyroidism. Some are euthyroid. At least some thyroid medullary carcinomas in dogs produce calcitonin in excess. A few cases of hypercalcitoninism from thyroid medullary carcinomas have caused hypocalcemia. Possible clinical signs of neoplastic goiter, particularly thyroid carcinomas in dogs, are listed in Table 8–3.

The cause for neoplasia of the thyroid is rarely determined; however, low-dose external irradiation to the neck is an established cause for papillary cacinomas in humans. Diagnostic radiography and the use of radioisotopes for diagnostic or therapeutic purposes are not known causes of thyroid neoplasia. Chronic iodine deficiency can cause hyperplasia of follic-

Table 8–2.   Types of Thyroid Neoplasms

Adenoma
  Follicular
  Papillary

Carcinoma
  Follicular
  Papillary
  Mixed papillary-follicular
  Medullary
  Anaplastic

Table 8–3.   Possible Clinical Signs Associated with Canine
Neoplastic Goiters

Palpable mass in neck
Dyspnea (tracheal compression or invasion)
Dysphonia (tracheal or recurrent laryngeal nerve
    compression or invasion)
Dysphagia (invasion or compression of the esophagus)
Horner's syndrome (damage to the cervical sympathetic
    nerves)
Edema of the head and neck (venous occlusion)
Ophthalmoplegia (venous occlusion)
Hyperthyroidism (20% to 25% of follicular carcinomas)
Hypocalcemia (some medullary carcinomas)
Watery diarrhea (some medullary carcinomas)

---

ular cells, and this has been suspected to induce thyroid neoplasia in some
persons. Multinodular adenomatous changes have been proposed to result
from successive cycles of hypertrophy and involution of the thyroid's follicular cells. Medullary carcinomas in humans are often familial. Other medullary carcinomas are sporadic (idiopathic).

See also references 15, 24, 30, 33, 34, and 67.

Thyroid Neoplasms in Dogs

Thyroid neoplasia accounts for about 2% to 3% of all canine tumors.
Follicular carcinomas are the most common type. The average age of the
clinical occurrence of canine thyroid neoplasia is about 10 years. Beagles,
boxers, and golden retrievers are the breeds reported to have a predisposition for thyroid neoplasms, whereas for miniature and toy Poodles the risk
is lower than expected. There is no predisposition for sex.

Many thyroid adenomas in dogs are not clinically detected. About one
third of thyroid neoplasms in dogs discovered at necropsy are adenomas;
however, because most thyroid adenomas are less than 2 cm in diameter,
only 10% to 15% of thyroid neoplasms clinically detected are adenomas.

About 90% of thyroid neoplasms discovered ante mortem are thyroid
carcinomas greater than 7 cm in diameter. More than half are noticed by the
owners, whose primary complaint is finding a palpable mass in the ventral
neck area. The dyspnea in nearly half the affected dogs is caused by invasion
or compression of the larynx and trachea or metastasis to the lungs (Fig. 8–
1). Approximately 10% have a mediastinal mass. Five percent to ten
percent of canine tumors at the base of the heart are thyroid tumors.[44, 63, 68]

The thyroid, the site of 20% to 25% of all canine carcinomas, is second
only to the mammary gland in the frequency of carcinomas. Follicular carcinomas are bilateral in about one third of the cases. They may be locally
invasive and are usually firmly attached to the larynx, trachea, and other
surrounding structures. There is often considerable delay (1 month to over

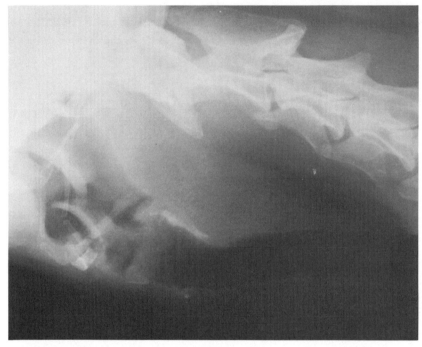

Fig. 8–1. A follicular carcinoma of the thyroids compressing the larynx and trachea in a dog. (Courtesy of Dr. Jimmy Lattimer, University of Missouri.)

6 months) in the time between the owner's discovery of a mass in the dog's neck and a definitive diagnosis of thyroid carcinoma.

Follicular carcinomas metastasize early to the lungs via the venous circulation. Metastasis to regional lymph nodes (retropharyngeal, cervical, and submandibular) can also occur. About 15% of primary tumors less than 20 ml in volume have already metastasized. If the tumor volume is 20 to 100 ml, about 75% of the primary tumors have metastasized, and virtually all follicular carcinomas greater than 100 ml in volume have metastasized. Overall, about one half of all follicular carcinomas presented for medical care have already metastasized. Metastasis to the bones is rare in the dog in comparison to metastasis in humans.[32] One third of dogs with thyroid neoplasia have another primary tumor.

Medullary (C-cell) carcinomas of the canine thyroid arise from the calcitonin-secreting parafollicular cells.[36, 48, 70] Medullary carcinomas have not been reported in the cat. Some medullary carcinomas of the canine thyroid have been associated with hypocalcemia caused by hypercalcitoninism. In humans, medullary carcinomas can also produce histaminase, adrenocorticotropic hormone (ACTH), serotonin, prostaglandins, or gastrointestinal hormones. In one survey of thyroid tumors, medullary carcinomas comprised only 2% to 3% of the carcinomas of the canine thyroid. Familial predisposition is known to occur in humans, but families of affected dogs have not been reported. Medullary carcinomas may metastasize to regional lymph nodes, the retropharyngeals. Medullary carcinomas in dogs may not contain amyloid as they do in humans. Definitive diagnosis is based on electron microscopy and antiperoxidase immunocytochemical tests for thyroglobulin and calcitonin.[42]

Multiple endocrine neoplasia, Type II (IIa), has been reported in a dog.[56] It is a triad of tumors derived from amine precursor uptake and decarboxylation cells (APUDomas) involving medullary carcinoma of the thyroid, pheochromocytoma, and parathyroid hyperplasia. *Multiple endocrine neoplasia, Type III (IIb)*, has not been reported in companion animals. In humans, it is a variable combination of medullary carcinoma, neuromas (ganglioneuromas of the lips and intestines), and pheochromocytoma.

Based on necropsy surveys, thyroid adenomas are common in dogs over 10 years of age. Many are subclinical, being neither toxic nor palpable in the dog. Nearly all canine thyroid adenomas are follicular adenomas. Papillary adenomas are very rare in dogs. About 15% are palpable. These are more freely movable than carcinomas. Thyroid adenomas may be solid (compact) or cystic. In dogs, thyroid adenomas are not likely to be associated with endocrine dysfunction as thyroid carcinomas are. Unfortunately, tumors of the thyroid may appear microscopically like adenomas, but clinically act like carcinomas. Adenomas may also convert by metaplasia into carcinomas; therefore, palpable thyroid adenomas, like thyroid carcinomas in dogs, should carry a guarded prognosis for 1 year after excision.

Fibrosarcomas, teratomas, and other miscellaneous primary thyroid tumors rarely occur in the dog and cat. Secondary tumors in the thyroid are usually subclinical, being overshadowed by the primary tumor.

Several diagnostic examinations may be considered if thyroid neoplasia is suspected. Fine needle biopsy of the mass can be done to confirm the mass as the thyroid.[65] Thyroid scans can be used to evaluate the possibility of ectopic or metastatic lesions and also to assess the tumor's ability to take up technetium (and presumably iodine).[8] Thoracic radiographs may detect ectopic thyroid neoplasms or lung metastasis. Echography can be used to determine if the tumor is cystic. Functional studies for hyperactivity such as the radioimmunoassay (RIA) for serum T_4, the RIA for T_3, the RIA for calcitonin, or radioactive iodine uptake should be considered in each case of thyroid neoplasia.

Thyroid scans show that three fourths of follicular carcinomas take up technetium, called a "hot" nodule or tumor. Papillary carcinomas, more common in humans than in dogs, do not take up technetium. Medullary carcinomas and anaplastic carcinomas also do not take up technetium. These are called "cold" nodules or tumors. Whether a thyroid tumor is "hot" or "cold" does not indicate its degree of malignancy; however, "hot" nodules should be evaluated further for thyrotoxicity. "Hot" nodules also indicate that radioactive iodine may be considered for treatment of the tumor.

Once a cervical mass is confirmed as a thyroid neoplasm, total excision is the preferred method of treatment. Care should be taken while a total thyroidectomy is being done to avoid the recurrent laryngeal nerves and preserve one cranial parathyroid. If all parathyroids are excised, supplements of oral doses of calcium gluconate (0.5 to 2 g/day) and vitamin D (0.01 mg/kg body weight/day of dihydrotachysterol) should be administered and the doses adjusted to need based on serum calcium levels. Severe postsurgical hypocalcemia must be treated more rapidly with a 10% intravenous solution of calcium gluconate (0.5 to 1.5 ml/kg body weight).

Ancillary therapy for a subtotal thyroidectomy can include the administration of thyroid hormone or radiotherapy. Therapy with thyroid hormone can be used for the replacement of hormones and to suppress the secretion of TSH, which might stimulate the growth of remaining neoplastic cells. Radiotherapy with ^{131}I, primarily a gamma emitter, is possible for "hot" tumors. Administration of ^{131}I is best delayed until 2 weeks after a partial thyroidectomy. The resulting increase in the endogenous secretion of TSH promotes the uptake of ^{131}I into the remaining thyroid tissue. Subtotal thyroidectomy also increases the efficiency of ^{131}I in its action on remaining tissue, while increasing the margin of safety at the same time by reducing the required dose. Intravenous doses for the dog are usually about 5 to 10 mCi of [131]I. Radioiodine therapy must be administered by specialists in veterinary radiology and the animal housed in special facilities for radioisotope therapy. All animals treated with radioiodine must be isolated for approximately 3 weeks, and all urine and feces collected for safe disposal.

If available and economically feasible, external irradiation (cobalt) can be considered after a subtotal thyroidectomy. A recommended therapeutic course for the dog is 400 rads, given three times per week for ten treatments for a total dose of 4000 rads.[40]

Doxorubicin (Adriamycin) has been useful in some dogs with thyroid carcinoma.[28] The drug is quite toxic and should be restricted for use in cases of inoperable carcinoma or dissemination. It is administered every third week in an intravenous dose of 30 mg/m² diluted in saline. Toxic reactions that may occur early in treatment include anxiety, urticaria, swelling of the face, acute cardiac arrhythmias, and hemorrhagic enterocolitis. Most dogs require concomitant treatment with cyclophosphamide (Cytoxan) in a dose of 100 mg/m² for 4 days, beginning the third day after treatment with doxorubicin, or require vincristine (Oncovin) in an intravenous dose of 0.025 mg/kg body weight on the same day doxorubicin is administered.

See also references 1, 6, 9, 10, 12, 13, 21, 22, 38, 40, 43, 57, 61, and 62.

Thyroid Neoplasms in Cats

The average age of cats detected with thyroid neoplasia is about 13 years. There is no known predisposition for sex or breed. More than 95% of thyroid neoplasms in the cat are adenomas. As many as 15% to 30% of older cats have subclinical multinodular adenomas, which are classified by some pathologists as hyperplasia. Medullary carcinomas have not been described in the cat.

Treatment of neoplastic goiter in the cat is similar to that in the dog. Surgical excision is preferable. Radiotherapy with ^{131}I has been successfully used in cats with "hot" nodules. The use of external irradiation or chemotherapy has not been reported in cats.

See also references 13, 18, 26, 29, 37, 46, and 47.

HYPERTHYROIDISM

Hyperthyroidism may be caused by "toxic" thyroid tumors, overdosage (iatrogenic administration), overstimulation by ectopic production of TSH, TSH-secreting adenohypophyseal adenomas, or hyperfunctional ectopic thyroid tissue such as that found in the ovary (struma ovarii). In dogs, the cause is usually a follicular carcinoma of the thyroid; in cats, hyperthyroidism is usually caused by a thyroid adenoma or multinodular adenomas.

The only known cause for spontaneous canine or feline hyperthyroidism is excessive production of thyroid hormones by a thyroid neoplasm. The most common cause for hyperthyroidism in humans is Grave's disease, which is usually associated with, and apparently caused by, an immunoglobulin G (thyroid-stimulating immunoglobulin [TSI] or long-acting thyroid stimulator [LATS]). TSI stimulates enlargement of the thyroid and excessive production of follicular hormones. Grave's disease is frequently accompanied by exophthalmos and pretibial myxedema. Grave's disease, hyperthyroid exophthalmos, pretibial myxedema, and TSI are not known to occur in the dog or cat, or any other companion animal.

Hyperthyroidism in Dogs

One half of follicular carcinomas in dogs secrete enough T_4, T_3, or both to cause atrophy of the contralateral lobe. One half of these (one fourth of the total) produce excesses of T_4, T_3, or both, sufficient to cause clinical signs of thyrotoxicity. Production must reach considerable excesses before causing clinical signs. For example, serum T_4 or T_3 usually must exceed 8 μg/dl and 400 ng/dl, respectively. Young healthy dogs can tolerate acute overdoses up to 25 times the usual replacement doses of thyroid hormones before clinical signs appear. The clinical signs of spontaneous (neoplastic) and iatrogenic hyperthyroidism are listed in Table 8–4.

Some clinical signs (polyuria, polydipsia, weight loss, increased appetite, and hyperthermia) are attributable to an increased metabolic rate; some (muscular tremors and increased heart rate) are due to increased sensitivity to catecholamines; and some can be caused by the tumor's local invasion of surrounding structures or metastasis (see Table 8–3). Increased catecholamine effects are the result of increased beta-adrenergic receptors, increased receptor sensitivity, and an increase in free catecholamine levels in the tissues. Thyrotoxicosis can cause increases in the cardiac rate and output. In addition, peripheral resistance can be lowered, leading to "high output" heart failure.

Laboratory findings that may occur in hyperthyroid dogs are polycythemia, hypocholesterolemia, hypercalcemia, and hypercalciuria. Liver function can be impaired by the chronic depletion of glycogen caused by hyperthyroidism.

The diagnostic examinations indicated for animals with possible hyperthyroidism are the same as those indicated for any animal with suspected thyroid neoplasm. Measuring serum T_4 and T_3 levels is also indicated in patients without a palpable tumor in the neck but showing signs of hyperthyroidism, such as polyuria and polydipsia, unexplained weight loss, and excessive appetite. Ectopic thyroid tissue, especially in the mediastinum, can cause hyperthyroidism without cervical goiter. Barium swallows or technetium scans of the chest may show intrathoracic thyroid neoplasia when plain thoracic radiography is inconclusive.

Serum T_3 levels should be determined when the animal is suspected to be hyperthyroid. In humans, thyrotoxic nodules may produce excesses of T_3 before those of T_4. Thyrotoxic carcinomas deprived of adequate iodide may preferentially produce excess T_3. About 4% of thyrotoxicity in humans is exclusively a T_3 excess. Exclusive T_3 excess has been reported in a dog, but the excess in T_3 was not sufficiently high to cause clinical signs of toxicosis.[14]

Functional thyroid neoplasms can be autonomous and produce near normal serum T_4 and T_3 levels. If measurement of baseline serum T_4 and T_3 levels is not conclusive for the diagnosis of an autonomous thyroid tumor, injections of TSH can be given for 3 or more days after the thyroid scan has been taken. Suppressed normal thyroid tissue should appear on scans done after stimulation with exogenous TSH. Conversely, T_4 or T_3 can be given for 1 week after a thyroid scan. Nodules appearing on scans immediately subsequent to suppression of T_4 or T_3 should be suspected to be autonomous.

Treatment of canine hyperthyroidism preferably consists of excision of the autonomous tumor. In most cases of follicular carcinoma, this is impossible. Subtotal thyroidectomy can be attempted after serum T_4 and T_3 levels

Table 8–4.   Clinical Signs of Hyperthyroidism in the Dog

Polyuria and polydipsia (most frequent sign)
Weight loss
Excessive appetite
Fine muscular tremors
Muscular weakness, wasting, and fatigue
Behavioral change, especially fearfulness
Pacing
Increased heart rate
Increased body temperature
Increased ECG amplitudes in all leads
Frequent defecation
Demineralization of bone

become normal. The thyroidectomy may then be followed by ^{131}I therapy, external irradiation, or treatment with doxorubicin. Elevated serum T_4 and T_3 levels can be reduced by the oral administration of five drops of saturated potassium iodide solution per day. The administration of iodide can temporarily block organification, inhibit proteolysis, and decrease thyroid vascularity, but eventually its effects lessen. Iodides can cause inflammation of the salivary glands, conjunctivitis, dermatitis, and, in some cases, aggravate hyperthyroidism. Thiocarbamides, derivatives of thiouracil, inhibit iodination of monoiodothyronine and block coupling. The most common thiocarbamides are propylthiouracil (PTU) and methimazole (Tapazole). PTU also inhibits the deiodination of T_4 to T_3. Thiocarbamides must be titrated to the needs of each patient. If T_4 levels are suppressed to below normal levels, the resulting increased secretion of TSH may cause enlargement of the thyroid neoplasm. PTU is the most often used of the thiocarbamides. The initial dose of PTU in dogs is 10 mg/kg body weight/day.

Cardiac complications resulting from increased sensitivity to catecholamines may be controlled by reserpine, phentolamine, guanethidine, or propranolol (Inderal). Propranolol, the drug of choice, is a beta-adrenergic blocker capable of reducing tachycardia and lowering serum T_3 levels. Serum T_4 levels can still be monitored for signs of improvement after the thyroidectomy or radiotherapy with ^{131}I. Serum T_4 levels should become euthyroid within 3 months of radiotherapy with ^{131}I; otherwise, the treatment should be repeated. If a thyroidectomy is planned, treatment with propranolol should begin at least 2 days before the surgery. If ^{131}I radiotherapy is to be used, propranolol should be administered 1 month before and 1 month after the administration of ^{131}I. Dogs are given 5 to 40 mg three times daily. The presence of congestive heart failure necessitates extreme care if propranolol is used. A history of bronchial spasms is a contraindication to the use of propranolol.

Thyroid storms have not been reported in thyrotoxic companion animals, but the possibility of its occurrence should not be forgotten. Thyroid storm is a very serious complication in some persons who have concurrent infections, are inadequately prepared for surgery, or are just recovering from a subtotal thyroidectomy or ^{131}I therapy. It is characterized by delirium, tachycardia, vomiting, diarrhea, and fever. The plasma T_4 and T_3 levels of persons with thyroid storm do not differ from those in patients who do not develop thyroid storm. Therapy consists of the administration of propranolol, treatment of the underlying disease, the use of glucocorticoids, and general supportive care.

See reference 58.

Hyperthyroidism in Cats

Recognized in cats more frequently than other companion animals, hyperthyroidism was virtually unknown until 1976. Now it is the first or second most commonly diagnosed endocrinopathy in the cat. Feline hyperthyroidism serves as a prime example of the occurrence of many more endocrine diseases in companion animals that go unrecognized or underestimated.

See references 25, 27, 31, 39, 45, 49, and 55.

Causes

Hyperthyroidism in cats is usually caused by a solitary adenoma (feline Plummer's disease) or multinodular adenomatous hyperplasia (feline Marine-Lenhart Syndrome). Thyroid carcinomas are rare in cats. Older cats (6 to 20 years old) are most often affected. There is no predisposition for breed or sex. Both thyroid lobes are involved in about 70% of cases; 30% are unilateral.

Clinical Signs and Laboratory Findings

Clinical signs are caused by an increased metabolic rate and increased sensitivity to catecholamines. Most (90%) are palpable near the larynx. The most frequently recognized clinical signs are listed in Table 8–5 and shown in Figure 8–2. Less common clinical signs include anorexia, apathy, mild fever, polypnea and dyspnea, muscle weakness and tremors, congestive heart failure, hair loss, and increased nail growth. In about 10% of affected cats, severe depression, anorexia, and weakness occur. This "apathetic hyperthyroidism" is usually associated with cardiac arrhythmias or congestive heart failure.

The reasons for some of the observed clinical signs are speculative. Polyuria and polydipsia may be caused by a decrease in the threshold of the thirst center, increased renal blood flow, or decreased renal medullary osmolality. Vomiting may be caused by thyroid hormone stimulation of the chemoreceptor trigger zone in the medulla. Diarrhea may result from increased ingested food volume, decreased pancreatic secretions, intestinal hypermotility, and malabsorption. Daily fecal fat excretion can be increased 2 to 15 times normal excretion in hyperthyroid cats. Normal fecal fat should not exceed 0.5 g/kg body weight/day or 3.5 g in 48 hours.

Cardiac complications can be life-threatening.[54] One half of thyrotoxic cats have cardiomegaly.[35] Some have pulmonary edema and pleural effu-

Table 8–5.   Common Clinical Signs of Hyperthyroidism in Cats in Decreasing Order of Appearance

Weight loss
Polyphagia
Hyperactivity
Tachycardia
Polyuria and polydipsia
Vomiting
Cardiac murmur
Diarrhea and increased fecal volume

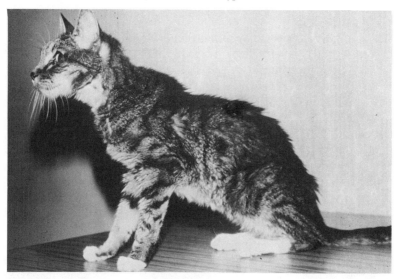

Fig. 8–2. Hyperthyroid cat showing weight loss and poor hair coat. (Courtesy of Dr. Mark Peterson, Animal Medical Center, New York, New York.)

sion. Two thirds have sinus tachycardia (heart rates exceeding 240 beats per minute) and tachyarrhythmias. One third have increased QRS voltages in lead II exceeding 0.9 mv. Many have second-degree atrioventricular blocks and left anterior fascicular blocks. Echocardiograms may show that the size of the left ventricle, aortic root, and left atrium has increased.[7] Changes in the ECG revert to normal in at least 80% of patients whose serum T_4 and T_3 levels are successfully lowered. No other form of hypertrophic cardiomyopathy can be so effectively corrected. All cases of feline cardiomyopathy should be screened by measuring serum T_4 and T_3 levels to rule out or substantiate hyperthyroidism as a cause.

Laboratory findings associated with feline hyperthyroidism include the stress leukogram, mild to moderate erythrocytosis, macrocytosis, increased serum inorganic phosphorus, increased fecal fat, hyperbilirubinemia, and elevated serum hepatic enzymes. Increased serum phosphorus may be caused by the release of calcium from the thyroid hormone's effects on bone, which in turn suppresses PTH release. The decreased release of PTH leads to the retention of phosphorus. Increased serum enzymes of hepatic origin occur in more than one-half the affected cats. These serum enzymes include alkaline phosphatase, lactic dehydrogenase, aspartate transaminase, and alanine transaminase. All older cats with weight loss and elevated serum liver enzymes should be screened for hyperthyroidism by measurement of serum T_4 and T_3 levels.

Histologic changes that occur in the liver are centrolobular fatty infiltration and mild hepatic necrosis. Adrenocortical hyperplasia occurs in one third of hyperthyroid cases as a compensatory change caused by the increased clearance of cortisol.

Diagnosis

The definitive diagnosis of feline hyperthyroidism is usually based on elevated serum T_4 levels (above 4 μg/dl) or T_3 levels (above 200 ng/dl). In nearly all cases both serum T_3 and T_4 levels are abnormally elevated. In a few cases, serum T_3 levels may remain within normal limits. This may be more common in cats with mild to moderate T_4 elevations who also have a concurrent illness impairing peripheral T_4 deiodination. Borderline elevations can be further differentiated by the TSH stimulation test, because autonomous thyroid tumors are not stimulated by the administration of TSH, or by administering liothyronine (T_3), because autonomous thyroid tumors do not cease producing T_4 when T_3 is supplemented.

Thyroid scans can yield useful information in hyperthyroid cats with and without palpable goiter.[51] Scans can detect aberrant "hot" thyroid nodules or metastasis (Fig. 8–3). Scans also indicate whether involvement is unilat-

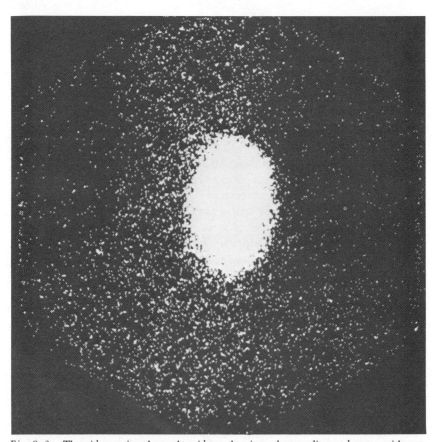

Fig. 8–3. Thyroid scan in a hyperthyroid cat showing a large solitary adenoma with atrophied (not visible) normal thyroid lobe. (From Peterson, M.E., et al.: Feline hyperthyroidism: pretreatment clinical and laboratory evaluation of 131 cases. J. Am. Vet. Med. Assoc., *183:*103, 1983.)

eral or bilateral (Fig. 8–4). When unilateral hyperthyroid neoplasia exists, the contralateral lobe should not be evident on a thyroid scan. If serum T_4 or T_3 levels are persistently high, any thyroid tissue visible on thyroid scans should be excised, if possible.

Radioiodine uptake is increased in hyperthyroid cats, but the procedure is difficult, expensive, and adds little, if any, additional information.

Treatment

Treatment of hyperthyroidism can be accomplished with antithyroid drugs, radioactive iodine, and surgery. The treatment of choice for feline hyperthyroidism is partial or complete thyroidectomy. The hypermetabolism and hypersensitivity to catecholamines should be controlled before surgery. PTU or methimazole (Tapazole) are used to suppress glandular

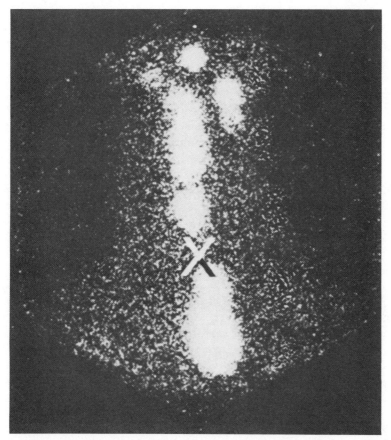

Fig. 8–4. Thyroid scan in a hyperthyroid cat showing multiple areas taking up technetium caused by a follicular carcinoma with extension into the thoracic cavity (*X* marks the thoracic inlet). (From Peterson, M.E., et al.: Feline hyperthyroidism: pretreatment clinical and laboratory evaluation of 131 cases. J. Am. Vet. Med. Assoc., *183:*103, 1983.)

hypersecretion.[50] Treatment with PTU is begun with a dose of 50 mg (if methimazole is used, the dose is 5 mg) every 8 hours and continued for 2 weeks before the thyroidectomy.

Since PTU and methimazole primarily block organification in the thyroid, stored hormone is continued to be released and must be allowed to dissipate before surgery. In the treatment of severe hyperthyroidism PTU is preferable to methimazole, because PTU also inhibits deiodination of T_4 to the more metabolically active T_3.[17] Serum T_4 levels begin to drop within 24 to 48 hours of treatment, but it should be confirmed that serum T_4 and T_3 levels are less than 4 μg/dl and 200 ng/dl, respectively, before surgery is done. If there is little decline in serum T_4 and T_3 levels after 2 weeks' treatment, PTU or methimazole can be increased to a dose of 200 to 300 mg/day or 20 to 30 mg/day, respectively.

Adverse effects develop in 5% to 10% of cats treated with PTU.[53] Common adverse effects of PTU in the first 2 weeks of treatment include anorexia, vomiting, and lethargy. These effects are often transient. After 2 weeks of treatment, drug allergy is more likely, manifesting as skin rash, facial swelling and pruritis, and hepatopathy. A drug-induced, lupus-like reaction may occur. Affected cats may develop weak antinuclear antibody titers, have a positive response to the Coombs' test with hemolysis, or have thrombocytopenia. Weekly hematocrit and platelet counts are advisable after the second week of treatment with PTU. Methimazole may cause fewer adverse effects, but its use has been associated with granulocytopenia. The adverse effects of PTU and methimazole resolve after treatment is discontinued. An oral dose of potassium iodide, or an intravenous dose of sodium iodide, 50 to 100 mg/day for 1 to 2 weeks, can be used as an alternative to treatment with PTU and methimazole. Iodides may cause hypersalivation and anorexia.

Propranolol (Inderal) should be considered if tachyarrhythmias or other excessive adrenergic effects are present, or if adverse reactions to PTU develop. The initial dosage of propranolol should be 2.5 to 5 mg three times per day for at least 2 days before the thyroidectomy is done. Propranolol should not be used alone, if at all, if congestive heart failure is evident.

Because of the risks of the surgical procedure and the poor risk inherent in doing surgery on debilitated aged cats, thyroidectomies should be done by experienced surgeons. Surgically related mortalities are 5% to 10%.[5] The use of atropine and halothane should be avoided because of their adverse effect on tachyarrhythmias. Acetylpromazine, glycopyrrolate, methoxyflurane, or fluothane are preferred. A cardiac monitor should be used throughout the procedure. If a unilateral thyroidectomy is done, the cranial parathyroid should be spared in case a relapse necessitates later removal of the remaining thyroid. If a bilateral thyroidectomy is done, at least one cranial parathyroid should be preserved. After the surgery, serum calcium levels should be monitored for signs of hypocalcemia for at least 2 days. Parathyroid function may be temporarily or permanently impaired by post-surgical trauma. Treatment for hypocalcemia is usually unnecessary, until serum calcium levels have fallen below 7 mg/dl. Severe hypocalcemia should be treated with an intravenous dose of calcium gluconate. Persistent hypocalcemia may be controlled with an oral dose of 0.2 mg of dihydrotachysterol per week.

After a unilateral thyroidectomy, serum T_4 levels should be monitored. Because the remaining thyroid will have been suppressed, serum T_4 levels will be low and may remain so for 2 to 3 months, but replacement therapy with thyroid hormone should not be administered unless marked lethargy occurs or low serum T_4 levels persist more than 3 months. Premature thyroid hormone replacement therapy could perpetuate the atrophy of remaining normal thyroid tissue. If a bilateral thyroidectomy is done, a dose of 0.05 to 0.1 mg of sodium levothyroxine should be given daily. When the patient has recovered from the thyroidectomy, the replacement dosage of thyroxine can be gradually reduced to allow any remaining normal ectopic thyroid tissue to hypertrophy and possibly to eliminate the need for replacement of thyroid hormone. Other possible postsurgical problems include Horner's syndrome or vocal cord paralysis.

Therapy with radioactive iodine can be safer than a thyroidectomy in some patients.[52, 66] Therapy with radioactive iodine is also a valuable salvage procedure when subtotal thyroidectomy is not curative. The disadvantages of ^{131}I therapy are the need for 3 to 4 weeks' isolation, difficulty in accurately titrating the dose so that the hyperthyroidism is corrected without causing hypothyroidism, and the necessity of specialists to administer the treatment and monitor the post-treatment isolation. An intravenous dose of 1 to 5 mCi of ^{131}I is administered to deliver approximately 20,000 rads to the "hot" nodules. Improvement should be noticeable within 1 month, and a euthyroid state should occur within 3 months. Repeat treatments are sometimes necessary. Until euthyroidism results, symptomatic control of clinical signs may be achieved with propranolol, phenobarbitol, a high caloric and protein diet, and supplementation with vitamins.

Regardless of whether a surgical excision is done or treatment with radioactive iodine is used, relapse may occur. Most relapses occur within 9 months of the initial treatment. Re-evaluation of serum T_4 and T_3 should be done 6 months and 12 months after treatment for hyperthyroidism in cats.

If for various reasons a thyroidectomy or therapy with radioactive iodine is not possible or undesirable, indefinite therapy using PTU may be tried as a last resort. After the initial suppression of elevated serum T_4 and T_3 levels to normal levels with a 50-mg dose of PTU three times daily, a 50-mg dose two times daily, or a single daily dose of 50 mg to 150 mg may be tried for maintenance. Alternately, methimazole may be used at one-tenth the dosage of PTU. Suppressing serum T_4 and T_3 levels allows the release of TSH. If thyroid nodules remain, increasing the response levels of TSH could result in accelerated growth of the nodules and a refractory response to the previous dosage of PTU. Toxic drug reactions may occur at any time; therefore, monthly determinations for serum T_4 and serum T_3 and complete blood cell counts are advised.

HYPERCALCITONINISM

Two forms of hypercalcitoninism have been described in the dog. *Primary hypercalcitoninism,* an autonomous secretion of calcitonin by a neoplasm, has been clinically associated with some medullary carcinomas of the thyroid in dogs, as in humans. *Secondary hypercalcitoninism,* hypersecretion of calcitonin dependent on hypercalcemia-promoting factors, has supposedly been produced by dietary imbalances in the dog. Plasma calcitonin can also be elevated by hypergastrinemia due to chronic renal failure and gastrinomas. Clinical hypocalcitonin disorders have not been recognized.

So little calcitonin is present in the feline thyroid that it has been reported undetectable by present methods. Medullary carcinomas and clinical disorders related to calcitonin are not known to occur in cats.

Primary Hypercalcitoninism in Dogs

Medullary carcinomas of the thyroid arise from the calcitonin-secreting parafollicular cells.[36,48,70] Increased amounts of calcitonin are often found in these tumors in dogs. Serotonin and 5-hydroxytryptophan have also been found in a canine medullary carcinoma. Instances of hypocalcemia associated with medullary carcinoma have been reported in the dog. In one case, serum calcium levels improved, returning toward near normal levels after the tumor's removal, and hypocalcemia developed again when the tumor recurred. Consequently, the parathyroids are unable to normalize serum calcium levels in some cases of canine medullary carcinoma. In other cases, hypocalcemia may result from the destruction of the parathyroids by the medullary carcinoma's expansion.

In addition to hypocalcemia, diarrhea can also result from medullary carcinomas of the thyroid. The cause of diarrhea is presumed to be an elaboration of serotonin, or prostaglandins, or both. Fasting plasma calcitonin levels produced by medullary carcinomas can attain unequivocally excessive levels (greater than 25 pg-eq/ml) compared to levels recorded in normal dogs. In cases in which fasting baseline levels are not diagnostic, provocative stimulation with an intravenous dose of calcium chloride or pentagastrin, followed by the determination of stimulated plasma calcitonin levels 2 to 5 minutes later, has proved diagnostically valuable in affected humans. Whenever a medullary carcinoma is diagnosed, the possibility of other endocrine neoplasms, especially pheochromocytoma, should be investigated.

Treatment of primary hypercalcitoninism consists of the surgical removal of the tumor. There is no known effective radiotherapy or chemotherapy for medullary carcinomas. If a pheochromocytoma is also present, the pheochromocytoma should be excised first.

Secondary Hypercalcitoninism in Dogs

An excessive production of calcitonin is the physiologic response to any hypercalcemia-promoting factor. In some instances, such as primary hyperparathyroidism, pseudohyperparathyroidism, or hypervitaminosis D, secondary hypercalcitoninism is insufficient to normalize serum calcium and prevent bone resorption. With mild to moderate hypercalcemia-promoting stimulation, the serum calcium concentration may remain within normal limits, but the remodeling of bone is inhibited.

In Great Danes experimentally fed excessive amounts of calcium (200% of National Research Council [NRC] requirements) and vitamin D (1500% of NRC requirements) for slightly more than 1 year after weaning, numerous skeletal problems developed, apparently from hypercalcitoninism and the resulting impaired bone remodeling. Skeletal problems included lateral deviation of the front legs, "cow-hocked" pelvic limbs, skeletal pain, ataxia, disinterest in play, pronounced enlargement of the metaphyseal areas of the long bones, overextension of the carpus and tarsus, early closure of the epiphyseal plates, osteochondrosis dissecans, bulging costochondral junctions, "Wobbler's syndrome," hip dysplasia, enostosis, coxa valga, and hypertrophic osteodystrophy. The results of this experiment did not conclusively establish that excessive dietary intake of calcium and vitamin D were totally responsible for the lesions produced. Assays of serum calcitonin were not done, and the diet also included excessive phosphorus (150% of NRC requirements), vitamin A (300% of NRC requirements), and magnesium (500% of NRC requirements), among others.

Treatment of secondary hypercalcitoninism of endogenous origin consists of the removal, destruction, or suppression of the tumor responsible for promoting elevation of serum calcium. The treatment of secondary hypercalcitoninism of dietary origin consists of a balanced diet without additional vitamin or mineral supplementation, especially calcium or vitamin D.

See also reference 23.

REFERENCES

1. Andersen, A.C., and Johnson, R.M.: Carcinoma of the thyroid in a beagle. Am. J. Vet. Res. *25:*861, 1964.
2. Arnold, U., et al.: Goitrous hypothyroidism and dwarfism in a kitten. J. Am. Anim. Hosp. Assoc., *20:*753, 1984.
3. Baker, J.R.: Case of equine goiter. Vet. Rec., *112:*407, 1983.
4. Baker, H.J., and Lindsey, J.R.: Equine goiter due to excess dietary iodide. J. Am. Vet. Med. Assoc., *153:*1618, 1968.
5. Birchard, S.J., Peterson, M.E., and Jacobson, A.: Surgical treatment of feline hyperthyroidism: results of 85 cases. J. Am. Anim. Hosp. Assoc., *20:*705, 1984.
6. Birchard, S.J., and Roesel, O.F.: Neoplasia of the thyroid gland in the dog: a retrospective study of 16 cases. J. Am. Anim. Hosp. Assoc., *17:*369, 1981.
7. Bond, B.R., Fox, P.R., and Peterson, M.E.: Echocardiographic evaluation of 30 cats with hyperthyroidism. New York, Proceedings of Am. Coll. Vet. Intern. Med. 1983, p. 39.
8. Branam, J.E., Leighton, R.L., and Hornof, W.J.: Radioisotope imaging for the evaluation of thyroid neoplasia and hypothyroidism in a dog. J. Am. Vet. Med. Assoc., *180:*1077, 1982.
9. Brodey, R.S., and Kelly, D.F.: Thyroid neoplasms in the dog. A clinicopathologic study of 57 cases. Cancer, *22:*406, 1968.
10. Buergelt, C.: Mixed thyroid tumors in two dogs. J. Am. Vet. Med. Assoc., *152:*1658, 1968.
11. Bush, B.M.: Thyroid disease in the dog—a review: Part I. J. Small Anim. Pract., *10:*95, 1969.
12. Bush, B.M.: Thyroid disease in the dog—a review: Part II. J. Small Anim. Pract., *10:*185, 1969.

13. Capen, C.C.: Tumors of the endocrine glands. *In* Tumors in Domestic Animals. Edited by J.E. Moulton. Berkeley, University of California Press, 1978, p. 372.
14. Chastain, C.B., Hill, B.L., and Nichols, C.E: Excess triiodothyronine production by a thyroid adenocarcinoma in a dog. J. Am. Vet. Med. Assoc., *177:*172, 1980.
15. Clark, S.T., and Meier, H.: A clinicopathological study of thyroid disease in the dog and cat. Part I. Thyroid pathology. Zentralbl. Veterinarmed., *5:*17, 1958.
16. Conway, D.A., and Cosgrove, J.S.: Equine goitre. Ir. Vet. J., *34:*29, 1980.
17. Cooper, D.S.: Antithyroid drugs. N. Engl. J. Med., *311:*1353, 1984.
18. Cowen, P.N., and Jackson, P.: Thyroid carcinoma in a cat. Vet. Rec., *114:*521, 1984.
19. Drew, B., Barber, W.P., and Williams, D.G.: The effect of excess dietary iodine on pregnant mares and foals. Vet. Rec., *97:*93, 1975.
20. Driscoll, J., Hintz, H.F., and Schryver, H.F.: Goiter in foals caused by excessive iodine. J. Am. Vet. Med. Assoc., *173:*858, 1978.
21. Harkema, J.R., King, R.R., and Hahn, F.F.: Carcinoma of thyroglossal duct cysts: a case report and review of the literature. J. Am. Anim. Hosp. Assoc., *20:*319, 1984.
22. Hayes, H.M., and Fraumeni, J.F.: Canine thyroid neoplasms: epidemiologic features. J. Nat. Cancer Inst., *55:*931, 1975.
23. Hedhammar, A., et al.: Overnutrition and skeletal disease. An experimental study in growing Great Dane dogs. Cornell Vet., *64*(Suppl. 5):1, 1974.
24. Hillidge, C.J., Sanecki, R.K., and Theodorakis, M.C.: Thyroid carcinoma in a horse. J. Am. Vet. Med. Assoc., *181:*711, 1982.
25. Hoenig, M., et al.: Toxic nodular goiter in the cat. J. Small Anim. Pract., *23:*1, 1982.
26. Holzworth, J., Husted, P., and Wind, A.: Arterial thrombosis and thyroid carcinoma in a cat. Cornell Vet., *45:*487, 1955.
27. Holzworth, J., et al.: Hyperthyroidism in the cat: ten cases. J. Am. Vet. Med. Assoc., *176:*345, 1981.
28. Jeglum, K.A., and Whereat, A.: Chemotherapy of canine thyroid carcinoma. Compend. Contin. Ed., *5:*96, 1983.
29. Johnson, K.H., and Osborne, C.A.: Adenocarcinoma of the thyroid gland in a cat. J. Am. Vet. Med. Assoc., *156:*906, 1970.
30. Joyce, J.R., Thompson, R.B., and Kyzar, J.R.: Thyroid carcinoma in a horse. J. Am. Vet. Med. Assoc., *168:*610, 1976.
31. Keene, B., and Peterson, M.E.: Electrocardiogram of a hyperthyroid cat. J. Am. Vet. Med. Assoc., *176:*712, 1980.
32. Krook, L., Olsson, S., and Rooney, J.R.: Thyroid carcinoma in the dog. A case of bone-metastasizing thyroid carcinoma stimulating hyperparathyroidism. Cornell Vet., *50:*106, 1960.
33. Leav, I., et al.: Adenomas and carcinomas of the canine and feline thyroid. Am. J. Pathol., *83:*61, 1976.
34. Lewis, G.T., et al.: Ophthalmoplegia caused by thyroid adenocarcinoma invasion of the cavernous sinuses in the dog. J. Am. Anim. Hosp. Assoc., *20:*805, 1984.
35. Liu, S-K, Peterson, M.E., and Fox, P.R.: Hypertrophic cardiomyopathy and hyperthyroidism in the cat. J. Am. Vet. Med. Assoc., *185:*52, 1984.
36. Long, G.G., Clemmon, R.H., and Heath, H.: Metastatic canine medullary thyroid carcinoma. Vet. Pathol., *17:*323, 1980.
37. Lucke, V.M.: An histological study of thyroid abnormalities in the domestic cat. J. Small Anim. Pract., *5:*351, 1964.
38. McClelland, R.B.: Carcinoma of the thyroid: a report of five cases in dogs. J. Am. Vet. Med. Assoc., *98:*38, 1941.
39. McMillian, F.D., and Sherding, R.G.: Feline hyperthyroidism. Feline Pract., *11*(5):25, 1981.
40. Mitchell, M., Hurov, L.I., and Troy, G.C.: Canine thyroid carcinomas: clinical occurrence staging by means of scintiscans, and therapy of 15 cases. Vet. Surg., *8:*112, 1979.
41. Miyazawa, K., Motoyoshi, S., and Usui, K.: Nodular goiters of three mares and their foals, induced by feeding excessive amount of seaweed. Jpn. J. Vet. Sci., *40:*749, 1978.
42. Moore, F.M., et al.: Thyroglobulin and calcitonin immunoreactivity in canine thyroid carcinomas. Vet. Pathol., *21:*168, 1984.
43. Neer, T.M.: Disseminated intravascular coagulation associated with metastatic thyroid carcinoma—a case report. J. Am. Anim. Hosp. Assoc., *18:*107, 1982.

44. Nilsson, T.: Heart-base tumours in the dog. Acta Pathol. Microbiol. Scand., *37:*385, 1955.
45. Noxon, J.O., et al.: An adenoma in ectopic thyroid tissue causing hyperthyroidism in a cat. J. Am. Anim. Hosp. Assoc., *19:*369, 1983.
46. O'Brien, S.E., Riley, J.H., and Hagemoser, W.A.: Unilateral thyroid neoplasm in a cat. Vet. Rec., *107:*199, 1980.
47. Patnaik, A.K., and Lieberman, P.H.: Feline anaplastic giant cell adenocarcinoma of the thyroid. Vet. Pathol., *16:*687, 1979.
48. Patnaik, A.K., et al.: Canine medullary carcinoma of the thyroid. Vet. Pathol., *15:*590, 1978.
49. Peterson, M.E.: Diagnosis and treatment of feline hyperthyroidism. Columbus, OH, proceedings of the 6th Kal Kan Symposium, 1982, p. 63.
50. Peterson, M.E.: Propylthiouracil in the treatment of feline hyperthyroidism. J. Am. Vet. Med. Assoc., *179:*485, 1981.
51. Peterson, M.E., and Becker, D.V.: Radionuclide thyroid imaging in 135 cats with hyperthyroidism. Vet. Radiol., *25:*23, 1984.
52. Peterson, M.E., et al.: Radioactive iodine (131-I) treatment of feline hyperthyroidism. New York, Proceedings of Am. Coll. Vet. Intern. Med., 1983, p. 40.
53. Peterson, M.E., et al.: Propylthiouracil-associated hemolytic anemia, thrombocytopenia, and antinuclear antibodies in cats with hyperthyroidism. J. Am. Vet. Med. Assoc., *184:*806, 1984.
54. Peterson, M.E., et al.: Electrocardiographic findings in 45 cats with hyperthyroidism. J. Am. Vet. Med. Assoc., *180:*934, 1982.
55. Peterson, M.E., et al.: Feline hyperthyroidism: pretreatment clinical and laboratory evaluation of 131 cases. J. Am. Vet. Med. Assoc., *183:*103, 1983.
56. Peterson, M.E., et al.: Multiple endocrine neoplasia in a dog. J. Am. Vet. Med. Assoc., *180:*1476, 1982.
57. Reid, C.F., et al.: Functioning adenocarcinoma of the thyroid gland in a dog with mitral insufficiency. J. Am. Vet. Radiol. Soc., *4:*36, 1963.
58. Rijnberk, A., and der Kingeren, P.J.: Toxic thyroid carcinoma in the dog. Acta Endocrinol., Suppl. *138:*177, 1969.
59. Rijnberk, A., and Van Der Horst, C.J.G.: Investigations on iodine metabolism of normal and goitrous dogs. Zentralbl. Veterinarmed., *16:*495, 1969.
60. Schlotthauer, C.F., McKenney, F.D., and Caylor, H.D.: The incidence of goiter and other lesions of the thyroid gland in dogs of southern Minnesota. J. Am. Vet. Med. Assoc., *76:*811, 1930.
61. Stephens, L.C., Saunders, W.J., and Jaenke, R.S.: Ectopic thyroid carcinoma with metastases in a beagle dog. Vet. Pathol., *19:*669, 1982.
62. Susaneck, S.J.: Thyroid tumors in the dog. Compend. Contin. Ed., *5:*35, 1983.
63. Thake, D.C., Cheville, N.F., and Sharp, R.F.: Ectopic thyroid adenomas at the base of the heart of the dog. Vet. Pathol., *8:*421, 1971.
64. Thompson, T.: Iodine-deficiency goitre in a bitch. N.Z. Vet. J., *27:*113, 1979.
65. Thompson, E.J., et al.: Fine needle aspiration cytology in the diagnosis of canine thyroid carcinoma. Can. Vet. J., *21:*186, 1980.
66. Turrell, J.M., et al.: Radioactive iodine therapy in cats with hyperthyroidism. J. Am. Vet. Med. Assoc., *184:*554, 1984.
67. Von Sandersleben, J., and Hanichen, T.: Tumours of the thyroid gland. Domestic Animals Bull. W.H.O., *50:*35, 1974.
68. Walsh, K.M., and Diters, R.W.: Carcinoma of ectopic thyroid in a dog. J. Am. Anim. Hosp. Assoc., *20:*665, 1984.
69. Wise, R.D.: Hyperplastic goiter in a budgerigar. Vet. Med. Small Anim. Pract., *75:*1013, 1980.
70. Zarrin, K.: Naturally occurring parafollicular cell carcinoma of the thyroid in dogs. Vet. Pathol., *14:*556, 1977.

Section IV

THE PARATHYROIDS

9

The Normal Parathyroids and Clinical Tests
of Their Function

The canine parathyroids usually consist of four small oval glands in the neck, whose entire weight is about 2 to 5 mg (Fig. 9–1). The two largest glands (2 to 5 mm in length) are generally found on the craniolateral pole of each thyroid gland. Two smaller glands are located within the fibrous capsule or parenchyma of the thyroids, on the medial aspect between the thyroids' middle and caudal third. The only known secretion of the parathyroids is *parathyroid hormone* (PTH) (Parathyrin), which interacts with calcitonin and vitamin D to maintain calcium homeostasis.

DEVELOPMENT OF THE PARATHYROIDS

The parathyroids originate from the endodermal lining of the third and fourth pharyngeal pouches. These are most often referred to as *parathyroids III and IV*. Parathyroid III develops as an evagination from the dorsocranial face of the third pharyngeal pouch in close association with the thymus (Fig. 9–2). Parathyroid III migrates to the craniolateral pole of the thyroids, where it is called the *cranial (external) parathyroid*. Parathyroid IV develops as an evagination of the fourth pharyngeal pouch. Parathyroid IV, trailing the movement of the thymus, migrates to the thyroid's medial surface or within the thyroid on the medial side near the middle to caudal third, where it is called the *caudal (internal) parathyroid*. In the horse, the caudal parathyroids are larger than the cranial parathyroids and are found at or near the level of the first rib.

ANOMALIES OF THE PARATHYROIDS

After the evagination of pharyngeal pouches III and IV, a duct communicating with the pharynx is temporarily present. Incomplete involution of this duct tends to produce cysts, which are usually associated with the development of the cranial parathyroids (III).

Accessory and aberrant parathyroid tissue are common. Fragments of parathyroid III or IV may be found in the thyroid. Because of parathyroid III's close association with the thymus, accessory tissue may be found around the larynx, in the carotid sheath, cranial mediastinum, or within the thymus.

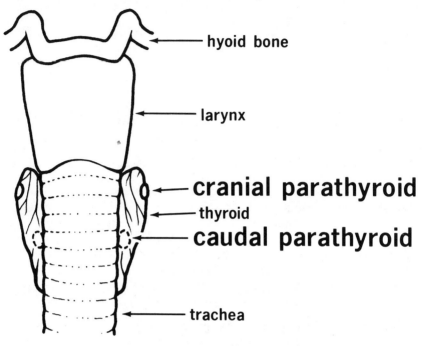

Fig. 9–1.   Normal canine parathyroids.

MICROSTRUCTURE AND FUNCTION OF THE PARATHYROIDS

The parathyroids consist of two types of cells: the *chief ("principal") cells* and the *oxyphil cells*. Chief cells have a clear cytoplasm and are the PTH-secreting cells. Oxyphil cells are apparently inactive. The numbers of oxyphil cells increase with aging and are generally more rare in dogs and

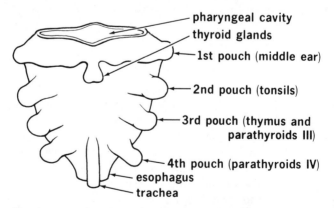

Fig. 9–2.   Development of the thyroids and parathyroids. (Adapted from Netter, F.H.: Endocrine system and selected metabolic diseases. *In* The CIBA Collection of Medical Illustrations. Vol 4. Summit, New Jersey, CIBA, 1965.)

cats than in horses. A variant of the chief cells that is much larger than chief cells is called the *"water clear" (Wasserhelle) cell*. The function of the "water clear" cell is unknown, but their numbers increase with the chronic stimulation of persistently low ionized serum calcium.

In the species studied, ribosomes of the chief cell produce a large polypeptide chain of 113 amino acids, *pre pro-PTH*, which first is reduced to *pro-PTH* (containing 90 amino acids), then to PTH, a straight polypeptide chain containing 84 amino acids. The PTH, with a molecular weight of 9500, is temporarily stored until the stimulus for release, primarily low levels of ionized calcium, is present in the serum. Normally, small quantities of PTH are almost continuously secreted, but if calcium levels drop as little as 1.5 mg/dl, serum levels of PTH increase fourfold. Low levels of serum magnesium also stimulate the release of PTH, but magnesium is not equipotent (one half to one third as strong on a molar basis) to ionized calcium. Beta-adrenergic stimuli, dopamine, secretin, prostaglandin E_1, glucocorticoids, and histamine also may cause the release of PTH.

Before its release into the circulation, some PTH is reduced to its *N-terminal (amino)* and *C-terminal (carboxyl) fragments*. More PTH is reduced to fragments by the liver and kidney. The N-terminal fragment containing the initial 34 amino acids is biologically active (Fig. 9–3). The C-terminal fragment comprises the bulk of the circulating PTH fragments, but is biologically inactive. The N-terminal fragment's structure differs among species studied, whereas the C-terminal fragment is identical whether it is human, bovine, or porcine.

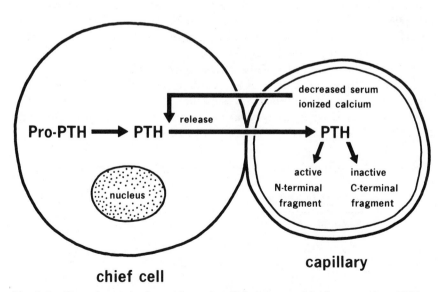

Fig. 9–3. Formation and release of parathyroid hormone and its fragmentation. PTH = parathyroid hormone.

The structure of PTH is unknown in the dog, horse, and cat, but it is assumed that the C-terminal fragment is the same in all companion animals. In humans, the plasma half-life of the C-terminal fragment of PTH is approximately 7 to 10 days. The half-life of the N-terminal fragment in plasma is less than 30 minutes. The onset of effects at the target cell may take 15 minutes or longer. With normocalcemia, plasma levels of PTH reported in normal dogs vary among laboratories: 10 to 82 μl Eq/ml, 65 to 213 μl Eq/ml, 255± 92 pg/ml, 322± 33 pg/ml, 30 to 100 μl Eq/ml, 600 to 885 ng/L, and 213 to 279 pg Eq/ml have been reported.[1, 5, 14] Plasma levels of PTH also fluctuate at 12-minute intervals in the dog.[8] In humans, PTH levels increase slightly with age and decreased degradation. Reported plasma PTH levels in cats are about 310 to 420 μl Eq/ml.[21] The effects of PTH are mediated through the adenyl cyclase-cyclic adenosine monophosphate (cAMP) system. The liver and kidney inactivate PTH.

Parathyroid hormone has several target tissues: bones, kidney, and perhaps the intestines. In the kidney, PTH promotes activation of vitamin D to its most active metabolite (1,25 dihydroxy D_3). PTH also promotes the distal tubular reabsorption of filtered calcium and, to a lesser extent, other ions. It decreases the proximal tubular reabsorption of phosphorus and other ions (Table 9–1). PTH indirectly causes the release of renin because of increased sodium excretion.

Parathyroid hormone increases the number and activity of osteoclasts and osteocytes, resulting in resorption of bone. The bones serve as a storehouse of calcium. Over a period of time, to maintain normal serum levels of calcium, bones can be depleted to the point of pathologic fracture. The action of PTH on bone requires the permissive presence of vitamin D and magnesium. Estrogens inhibit the action of PTH on bone. PTH directs the amount of bone remodeling. Mechanical stresses determine the location and direction of the remodeling process.

Intestinal absorption of calcium is also promoted by PTH, but not directly. It facilitates the activity of vitamin D in absorbing calcium from the intestines. This is accomplished, at least in part, by activating a weak metabolite of vitamin D by hydroxylation in the proximal convoluted tubule of the kidney.[20] The action of PTH is illustrated in Figure 9–4.

Table 9–1.   Renal Effects of Parathyroid Hormone

Promotes Retention of:	Promotes Excretion of:
Calcium	Phosphates
Magnesium	Potassium
Ammonia	Bicarbonate
H^+ ions	Sodium
	Amino acids
	cAMP*

* cAMP = cyclic adenosine monophosphate.

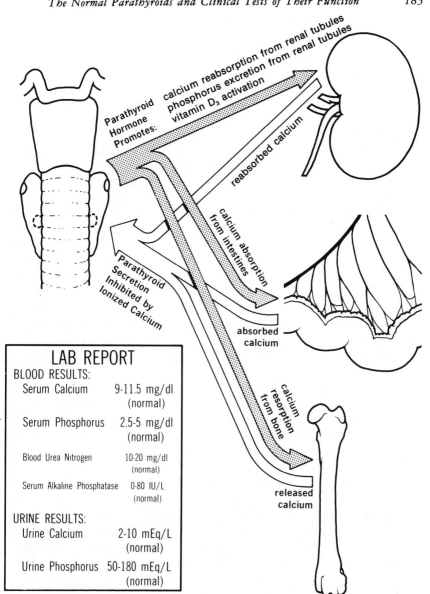

LAB REPORT

BLOOD RESULTS:

Serum Calcium 9-11.5 mg/dl
(normal)

Serum Phosphorus 2.5-5 mg/dl
(normal)

Blood Urea Nitrogen 10-20 mg/dl
(normal)

Serum Alkaline Phosphatase 0-80 IU/L
(normal)

URINE RESULTS:

Urine Calcium 2-10 mEq/L
(normal)

Urine Phosphorus 50-180 mEq/L
(normal)

Fig. 9–4. Parathyroid hormone and serum calcium in normal animals.

Parathyroid hormone from beef sources is available commercially (Parathyroid Hormone Injection), but its expense and antigenicity limit its use primarily to diagnostic tests. Parathormone, a trade name for a commercial preparation of PTH, should not be used as a synonym when referring to PTH.

See also references 3, 9, 13, 15, 18, 23, 25, and 26.

CALCIUM, PHOSPHORUS, AND MAGNESIUM HOMEOSTASIS

Calcium

Calcium is necessary for many vital and nonvital functions (Table 9–2). It is the fifth most abundant element in the body. Nearly 99% of calcium is found in the skeletal system, where it is essential for skeletal strength and serves as a storehouse to replenish serum deficits. Less than 1% of skeletal calcium is available for free exchange with extracellular fluid. The extraskeletal calcium is necessary for life, being essential for the normal contraction of cardiac and skeletal muscle, nerve function, and blood coagulation.

Dietary calcium requirements are affected by the stage of growth and by the intake of vitamin D and phosphorus. Dietary calcium requirements for the dog and cat are 120 to 260 mg/kg body weight/day and 200 to 400 mg/kg body weight/day, respectively. Younger dogs and cats who are growing need calcium in the upper range of these requirements. Calcium and phosphorus should exist in a ratio of 1.2 to 1.4:1 by weight (this is generally provided in commercial diets as 1.1% calcium and 0.9% phosphorus by weight). The dietary intake of vitamin D can increase the amount of absorbed calcium; normal requirements for the dog and cat are 11 to 22 IU/kg body weight/day and 50 to 100 IU/day, respectively. Of the total amount of calcium absorbed, most passes back into the intestines, some is excreted in the urine, and the remainder is retained by the skeletal system, depending on need and hormonal influences.

Serum calcium levels are very closely maintained, at approximately 10 mg/dl (5 mEq/L), in all domestic species by the action of vitamin D and PTH in order to raise serum calcium levels, and are counterbalanced by calcitonin, which serves to lower serum calcium levels. Other hormones, such as glucocorticoids, estrogens, glucagon, and growth hormone (GH), play minor regulatory roles.

Serum calcium exists in more than one form—about 50% is ionized. Ionized calcium is the only form that inhibits the secretion of parathyroid and is utilizable for the maintenance of neuromuscular excitability and blood coagulation. Approximately 10% to 15% of serum calcium is complexed to phosphate, citrate, or bicarbonate, and 40% is protein-bound to albumin or, to a much lesser extent, alpha- and beta-globulins. The complexed and protein-bound forms are circulating storage forms from

Table 9–2.   Functions in Which Calcium is Involved

Neuromuscular excitement
Membrane permeability
Muscular contraction
Enzyme activation
Hormone release
Blood coagulation
Bone formation

---

which ionized calcium can be readily released. Routine clinical determinations detect total serum calcium levels.

The ionized calcium portion of total serum calcium in the dog has been reported to be 4 to 5 mg/dl, but the determination of ionized serum calcium requires special instrumentation unavailable to most practices. Because about 40% of the total calcium is protein-bound, total calcium levels should be interpreted with plasma protein levels in mind. For example, hypoproteinemia will lower total levels of serum calcium, whereas ionized serum calcium levels may remain normal. Total serum calcium levels that meet or exceed 12 mg/dl or fall below 6.5 mg/dl are not likely to be caused by altered serum protein binding alone.

Calcium is absorbed from the brush border of the proximal small intestine by active transport and a carrier protein from the intestinal wall. Phosphorus is transported secondarily (passively) to calcium. Normally, about 20% to 30% of ingested calcium is absorbed. Intestinal absorption is increased by the administration of vitamin D, PTH (at least indirectly), acidification of the gastrointestinal tract, and, perhaps, lactose and some amino acids such as lysine. Intestinal absorption is decreased by dietary phytates, oxalates, cellulose, and phosphates. It is also decreased with steatorrhea, the nephrotic syndrome, glucocorticoid therapy, aging, and alkalinization of the gastrointestinal tract.

Serum calcium not bound to serum proteins passes the glomerulus, but most of the filtrated calcium is reabsorbed (70% in the proximal convoluted tubules, 20% in the loops of Henle, and 8% in the distal convoluted tubules). Daily urinary calcium losses normally are equal to absorbed dietary calcium. Although the reabsorption of calcium in the loops of Henle and distal convoluted tubules is calcium-specific, calcium's reabsorption in the proximal convoluted tubule is linked to the reabsorption of sodium. Urinary calcium excretion is enhanced by the excretion of sodium in the tubules and by certain tubular dysfunctions. It is decreased by the administration of thiazides, which enhance distal tubular reabsorption, and by conditions causing a reduced glomerular filtration rate.

Phosphorus

Eighty-five percent of the body's phosphorus is located in bone. Two thirds of the remaining phosphorus is found in organic compounds, most of it in the liver and skeletal muscle, and one third is inorganic phosphorus. Total plasma phosphorus (organic and inorganic) levels are approximately 12 mg/dl. In clinical situations, measurements of serum phosphorus assess concentrations of inorganic phosphorus. Normal concentrations of serum inorganic phosphorus for adult companion animals are approximately 2.5 to 5 mg/dl. Normal values for young growing animals are higher, up to 7 to 8 mg/dl. The entrance of phosphorus into cells is facilitated by insulin.

Phosphorus combines with calcium to form the mineral structure of bone. It is also an important component of nucleic acids, cellular and subcellular membranes, and aerobic and anaerobic metabolism.

Many foods are high in phosphorus, especially organ meats and grains. Ingested phosphorus is absorbed by active and passive processes in a direct relationship with the amount ingested. Factors such as vitamin D that increase calcium absorption from the gastrointestinal tract also facilitate phosphorus absorption. Aluminum hydroxide binds dietary phosphorus, thus preventing gastrointestinal absorption. On normal diets, about 70% of the ingested phosphorus is absorbed. Serum inorganic phosphorus is not protein bound, so it readily passes through the glomeruli. Usually 85% to 90% of phosphorus in the glomerular filtrate is reabsorbed in the proximal convoluted tubule. This renal reabsorption process is inhibited by PTH and, to a lesser extent, by expansion of extracellular fluid volume, increased intake of sodium, hypercalcemia, calcitonin, glucocorticoids, and growth hormone. Elevated serum phosphorus levels tend to inhibit indirectly the secretion of PTH by suppressing serum calcium levels.

Magnesium

Half of the body's magnesium is present in insoluble form in the skeletal system. Most (35%) of the remainder is intracellular, being necessary for the synthesis of some protein and DNA. It is also necessary for a wide variety of enzymes' activity in intracellular metabolism. Magnesium is the second most prevalent intracellular cation. About 1% is found in extracellular fluid. The effects of magnesium on the central and peripheral nervous system mimic those of calcium—that is, magnesium enhances excitation when deficiencies exist and depresses excitation when excesses occur. The synthesis, release, and target cell effects of PTH require magnesium, but excessive levels of serum magnesium also inhibit the secretion of PTH and possibly its peripheral action; therefore, the optimal secretion and action of PTH depend on normal serum magnesium levels.

The gastrointestinal absorption of ingested magnesium is amplified by vitamin D and inhibited by increased ingested calcium. Normal plasma magnesium concentrations are about 1.5 to 2.5 mEq/L. One fourth of plasma magnesium is protein-bound. Magnesium that is not protein-bound is able to pass through the glomerulus. Most filtrated magnesium is reabsorbed. The renal reabsorption process is increased by PTH. Serum magnesium concentrations decrease with acute PTH deficiency resulting from parathyroidectomy.

TESTS OF PARATHYROID FUNCTION

Routine Assessments

Most parathyroid disorders may be diagnosed correctly by correlating the baseline data listed in Table 9–3.

Serum tests needed to evaluate parathyroid function and calcium metabolism are listed in Table 9–4. Hypercalcemia and hypophosphatemia are indicative of hyperparathyroidism. The reverse—hypocalcemia and hyper-

Table 9–3. Baseline Data for Evaluating Parathyroid Function and Calcium Metabolism

Clinical signs and dietary history
Current physical findings
Plasma protein level
Acid-base balance
Serum analysis (see Table 9–4)
Urinalysis
Skeletal radiographs

phosphatemia—is consistent with hypoparathyroidism. Most secondary parathyroid disorders are fully compensated so that the serum calcium is within low normal range and kept that way by increased secretion of PTH. Decreased serum magnesium levels can stimulate the parathyroid's secretion, as can low serum calcium concentrations.

In the critical interpretation of total serum calcium values, it is important to know the patient's state of hydration, acid-base balance, and serum albumin level.[6, 16] Plasma protein-bound calcium levels fluctuate with changes in plasma proteins without necessarily affecting ionized calcium. A decrease in serum albumin of 1 g/dl decreases the serum calcium level of 0.8 mg/dl. Serum calcium levels can be corrected for hypoproteinemia by calculations (Table 9–5).[2, 16] Severe dehydration can cause increased concentration of serum calcium and mild hypercalcemia.

Another factor to consider in interpreting total serum calcium levels is the patient's acid-base balance. Calcium ionizes better in an acid environment; therefore, the total serum calcium can be very low without producing hypocalcemic dysfunctions if acidosis is present or if less plasma protein is available for binding. This is important for therapy because alkalinization of a patient with low total serum calcium carries the risk of precipitating hypocalcemic dysfunctions. For example, if the pH of blood increases by 0.1, ionized calcium will decrease 0.4 mg/dl. Total serum calcium levels can be determined most accurately by atomic absorption spectrophotometry, and ionized serum calcium can be specifically determined by calcium-sensitive electrodes.

Spurious hypercalcemia can be caused by prolonged venous occlusion and by hyperlipidemia. Venous occlusion for longer than 2 to 3 minutes can

Table 9–4. Minimum Serum Determinations Necessary to Evaluate Parathyroid Function and Calcium Metabolism*

Calcium
Phosphorus
Magnesium
Urea nitrogen (BUN)
Alkaline phosphatase (SAP)

* BUN = blood urea nitrogen; SAP = serum alkaline phosphatase.

Table 9–5.   Formulas for Correcting the Total Serum Calcium Level for Altered Serum Protein Levels

---

Corrected serum calcium (mg/dl) = Measured serum calcium (mg/dl) − serum albumin (g/dl) + 3.5

Corrected serum calcium (mg/dl) = Measured calcium (mg/dl) − [0.4 × total plasma protein (g/dl)] + 3.3

---

elevate serum calcium measurements as much as 0.8 mg/dl. Hyperlipidemia can falsely elevate measured serum calcium, phosphorus, and, to a lesser extent, alkaline phosphatase if measurements are done by routine spectrophotometry.[10]

The measurement of blood urea nitrogen (BUN) value is useful in assessing renal insufficiency, which may lead to secondary (compensatory) parathyroid changes, or renal damage, which may be caused by the unregulated (autonomous) secretion of PTH.

The determination of concentrations of urinary calcium and phosphorus can be helpful in assessing parathyroid function. They are best interpreted on the basis of 24-hour excretion. Normal urine values of calcium in dogs have been reported to be about 0.5 to 1 mg/kg body weight/24 hours. Urine phosphorus values are approximately 10 to 30 mg/kg body weight/24 hours.[4, 19] The concentration of urinary calcium in horses varies widely.[17] Increased urinary calcium occurs with hyperparathyroidism, hypervitaminosis D, hyperthyroidism, high sodium diets, hypercalcitoninism, and increased secretion of GH. Increased urinary phosphorus is expected with hyperparathyroidism, hypercalcitoninism, and hypervitaminosis D. Decreased urinary calcium and phosphorus may occur in patients with rickets (vitamin D deficiency) and hypoparathyroidism. Urinary phosphorus concentrations are quite variable and depend on the amount of dietary phosphorus ingested.

Serum alkaline phosphatase (SAP) originates from the liver, bone, placenta, kidney cortex, and intestines.[11, 22] In the dog, most of the SAP normally comes from the liver. The cat is able to clear the SAP rapidly from the blood.[12] As a result, the SAP level is of little diagnostic value in the cat with parathyroid disease. In the dog, unless the liver is concurrently affected, elevations of SAP do not usually occur until parathyroid-induced osteopenia is radiographically overt. Modest increases in SAP values are associated with osteoblastic activity. Normal values are higher in young, actively growing animals. In parathyroid disorders, increased SAP levels are indicative of attempted osseous repair rather than the degree of osteoclastic resorption.

Radiographs of the skeletal system may be used to assess crudely the extent of damage caused by autonomous or compensatory secretion of PTH. Demineralization is not radiographically evident until about one half of mineralization is depleted. In the case of compensatory secretion of PTH caused by renal disease, dietary imbalances, or intestinal malabsorption, radiographs of the bones may be the main initial diagnostic tool. Some skeletal areas show visible changes earlier than others. Osteopenia can be seen initially surrounding the tooth roots (dissolution of the laminae dura dentes), and other changes include osteomalacia of the body and dorsal processes of the vertebrae, and subperiosteal resorption in the phalanges. Thinning of the cortex of long bones and eventually pathologic (spontaneous) fractures may be evident in later stages.

Special Assessments

Special tests for solving diagnostic dilemmas involving parathyroid and calcium metabolic disorders are often expensive, difficult to interpret, or both.

PLASMA PTH ASSAY.   Potentially, the most informative is the plasma PTH assay; however, because of its expensiveness, species specificity, cross-reactions with other hormone fragments, short plasma half-life, and other reasons, the PTH assay has been attempted on a clinical basis on only a small number of dogs and even a smaller number of cats. Since the plasma half-life of the N-terminal fragment is so short, its diagnostic accuracy for hyper- and hyposecretion disorders is poor. Most commercial laboratories use a radioimmunoassay (RIA) for the C-terminal fragment because its half-life is much longer and better parallels the mean secretory rate.

Even though the C-terminal fragment is inactive, its increase in the plasma seems to correlate with increased secretory disorders of PTH. Fortunately, the C-terminal fragment structure is similar in several species, including presumably the human, dog, and cat. The appropriateness of the degree of PTH levels in the serum must be interpreted with the concomitant knowledge of serum calcium levels. For example, when serum calcium levels exceed 12 mg/dl virtually all stimulus for the secretion of PTH is nonexistent. Serum PTH and calcium levels are simultaneously elevated in primary hyperparathyroidism. Serum PTH levels are often much higher in cases of secondary hyperparathyroidism than in primary hyperparathyroidism. Simultaneous with elevated serum levels of PTH, serum calcium levels are low normal with secondary hyperparathyroidism.

Clinical investigators have reported normal canine values in different units: pg/ml, ng/L, pg Eq/ml, and μl Eq/ml. It is not always clear if these values represent PTH and all, or only some, of its fragments. Indications for PTH assay include persistent borderline calcium elevations, undiagnosed bone diseases, and recurrent urinary calcium stone formation. Serum for C-terminal PTH fragment assay does not need to be frozen to be shipped to laboratories doing the analysis.

URINARY CYCLIC ADENOSINE MONOPHOSPHATE.   Canine urinary concentrations of cyclic adenosine monophosphate (cAMP) have been reported to be approximately 5 to 7 μM/L and 1 to 4 μM/g creatinine.[24] Plasma cAMP levels in normal dogs are about 11 to 16 nM/L. Between 30% to 50% of urinary cAMP is of nephrogenous origin. Nephrogenous concentrations of cAMP should parallel the plasma concentrations of PTH (this concept is controversial in the dog).[7] Nephrogenous cAMP can be calculated by measuring urinary and plasma cAMP and urinary and plasma creatinine. Nephrogenous concentrations of cAMP increase with primary hyperparathyroidism. In normal subjects, nephrogenous cAMP should decrease if calcium is infused intravenously. Injections of PTH should increase nephrogenous cAMP if renal PTH receptors are normal.

URINARY HYDROXYPROLINE. The urinary concentration of hydroxyproline, a degradation product of collagen, has been suggested as an index of parathyroid destruction of bone. Bone is one-third osteoid, and osteoid is 97% collagen; however, an increase in urinary hydroxyproline is not specific for breakdown of bone collagen. As a result, the cause of increased urinary hydroxyproline must be based on case history, skeletal radiographs, or bone biopsies. Reported urinary concentrations of hydroxyproline in normal dogs is about 0.25 to 0.75 mg/kg body weight/24 hours.[19]

IONIZED SERUM CALCIUM. Ionized serum calcium can be measured by calcium ion-specific electrodes. This eliminates estimating the significance of plasma protein and acid-base alterations on ionized calcium from the total serum calcium determination. The practicality of determining ionized serum calcium is limited by the necessity of obtaining anaerobic venous samples with little or no occlusion of the vein and having the sample analyzed within minutes.

GLUCOCORTICOID SUPPRESSION OF SERUM CALCIUM. The administration of glucocorticoids has no clinically significant effect on normal levels of serum calcium or on hypercalcemia induced by autonomous parathyroid neoplasm or hyperplasia. Glucocorticoids suppress the hypercalcemia caused by lymphoreticular neoplasms, the most common known cause for pseudohyperparathyroidism in the dog and cat. If the administration of 0.5 to 1.0 mg/kg body weight/day of prednisone or prednisolone does not normalize or markedly decrease serum calcium elevations in 10 days, primary hyperparathyroidism should be suspected.

For further information on tests of parathyroid function, see references 6 and 11.

REFERENCES

1. Anderson, C., and Danylchuk, K.D.: Plasma levels of immunoreactive parathyroid hormone in dogs chronically exposed to low levels of calcium chloride. J. Environ. Pathol. Toxicol., *2:*1151, 1979.
2. Chew, D.J., and Meuten, D.J.: Disorders of calcium and phosphorus metabolism. Vet. Clin. North Am., *12:*411, 1982.
3. Cramer, C.F.: Participation of parathyroid glands in control of calcium absorption in dogs. Endocrinology, *72:*192, 1963.
4. DiBartola, S.P., Chew, D.J., and Jacobs, G.: Quantitative urinalysis including 24-hour protein excretion in the dog. J. Am. Anim. Hosp. Assoc., *16:*537, 1980.
5. Feldman, E.C., and Krutzik, S.: Parathyroid hormone levels in spontaneous canine parathyroid disorders. Proceedings of Am. Coll. Vet. Intern. Med., p. 102, 1979.
6. Finco, D.R.: Interpretations of serum calcium concentration in the dog. Compendium on Continuing Educ. for the Practicing Vet., *5:*778, 1983.

7. Fox, J., and Heath, H.: Parathyroid hormone does not increase nephrogenous cyclic AMP excretion by the dog. Endocrinology, *107:*2124, 1980.
8. Fox, J., Offord, K.P., and Heath, H.: Episodic secretion of parathyroid hormone in the dog. Am. J. Physiol., *241:*E171, 1981.
9. Grunbaum, D., et al.: Bioactive parathyroid hormone in canine progressive renal insufficiency. Am. J. Physiol., *247:*E442, 1984.
10. Handelman, C.T.: Laboratory data: read beyond the numbers. Compendium on Continuing Educ. for the Practicing Vet., *5:*687, 1983.
11. Hoffmann, W.E.: Diagnostic value of canine serum alkaline phosphatase and alkaline phosphatase isoenzymes. J. Am. Anim. Hosp. Assoc., *13:*237, 1977.
12. Hoffman, W.E., Renegar, W.E., and Dorner, J.L.: Serum half-life of intravenously injected intestinal and hepatic alkaline phosphatase isoenzymes in the cat. Am. J. Vet. Res., *38:*1637, 1977.
13. Hruska, K.A., et al.: Metabolism of immunoreactive parathyroid hormone in the dog. J. Clin. Invest., *56:*39, 1975.
14. Jorch, U.M., et al.: Concentrations of plasma C-terminal immunoreactive parathyroid hormone in the standardized research beagle. Am. J. Vet. Res., *43:*350, 1982.
15. Martin, K.J., et al.: The peripheral metabolism of parathyroid hormone. N. Engl. J. Med., *301:*1092, 1979.
16. Meuten, D.J., et al.: Relationship of serum total calcium to albumin and total protein in dogs. J. Am. Vet. Med. Assoc., *180:*63, 1982.
17. Morris, D.D., Divers, T.J., and Whitlock, R.H.: Renal clearance and fractional excretion of electrolytes over a 24-hour period in horses. Am. J. Vet. Res., *45:*2431, 1984.
18. Neuman, M.W., Newman, W.F., and Lane, K.: Formation and serum disappearance of fragments of parathyroid hormone in the infused dog. Calcif. Tissue Int., *28:*79, 1979.
19. Norrdin, R.W., et al.: Observations on calcium metabolism, [47]Ca absorption, and duodenal calcium-binding activity in chronic renal failure: Studies in beagles with radiation-induced nephropathy. Am. J. Vet. Res., *41:*510, 1980.
20. Oldham, S.B., Mitnick, S.A., and Coburn, J.W.: Intestinal and parathyroid calcium-binding proteins in the dog. J. Biol. Chem., *255:*5789, 1980.
21. Ross, L.A., Finco, D.R., and Corwell, W.A.: Effect of dietary phosphorus restriction on the kidneys of cats with reduced renal mass. Am. J. Vet. Res., *43:*1023, 1982.
22. Saini, P.K., and Saini, S.K.: Origin of serum alkaline phosphatase in the dog. Am. J. Vet. Res., *39:*1510, 1978.
23. Stevenson, R.W., and Parsons, J.A.: Effects of parathyroid hormone and the synthetic 1–34 amino-terminal fragment in rats and dogs. J. Endocrinol., *97:*21, 1983.
24. Weller, R.E., and Cowgill, L.D.: Urinary cyclic AMP levels in dogs as determined by radioimmunoassay. A preliminary investigation. 21st Annual Proceedings of Am. Assoc. Vet. Lab. Diagn., p. 481, 1978.
25. Wild, P.: Correlative light- and electron-microscopic study of parathyroid glands in dogs of different age groups. Acta Anat., *108:*340, 1980.
26. Wild, P., and Becker, M.: Response of dog parathyroid glands to short-term alterations of serum calcium. Acta Anat., *108:*361, 1980.

10

Hyperparathyroidism

Hyperparathyroidism can be primary, secondary, or tertiary. *Primary hyperparathyroidism* is an autonomous hypersecretion of parathyroid hormone (PTH) caused by a parathyroid neoplasm or spontaneous hyperplasia of parathyroid glands. *Secondary hyperparathyroidism* is a compensatory hypersecretion of PTH and hyperplasia-hypertrophy of the parathyroids induced by a variety of possible disorders tending to decrease serum ionized calcium levels. Occasionally, secondary hyperparathyroidism becomes autonomous after prolonged stimulation from low serum ionized calcium, a condition called *tertiary hyperparathyroidism.*

Some neoplasms of nonparathyroid origin may cause hypercalcemia and other changes that mimic those of primary hyperparathyroidism. This condition is called *pseudohyperparathyroidism.* Pseudohyperparathyroidism may or may not be caused by the ectopic production of PTH or PTH-like peptides.

PRIMARY HYPERPARATHYROIDISM

Pathogenesis

Primary hyperparathyroidism is caused by neoplasia or, occasionally, hyperplasia of the parathyroid, which secretes excessive amounts of PTH and is unresponsive to the suppressive effects of hypercalcemia (Fig. 10–1). Too few cases have been described in the dog to estimate the relative frequency of causes. Primary hyperparathyroidism has only rarely been diagnosed in the horse, and no cases have yet been reported in birds or cats. The relative frequency of causes for primary hyperparathyroidism in humans is reported as follows: single adenomas, 80%; hyperplasia of all four glands, 15%; single carcinomas, 4%; and multiple adenomas, about 1%. It is presumed that the relative frequency of causes is similar in companion animals. Affected parathyroid tissue may be found near the thyroid, in the thyroid, the neck, the pericardial sac, or the cranial mediastinum.

Parathyroid hyperplasia in humans is often familial. It may be concurrent with adenomatous changes in other organs such as the pituitary, pancreatic islets, and adrenal cortices. This constellation of signs is called multiple endocrine neoplasia, Type I (Werner's syndrome). Parathyroid hyperplasia may also be concurrent with neoplasia of the adrenal medulla and parafollicular cells of the thyroid, a condition called multiple endocrine neopla-

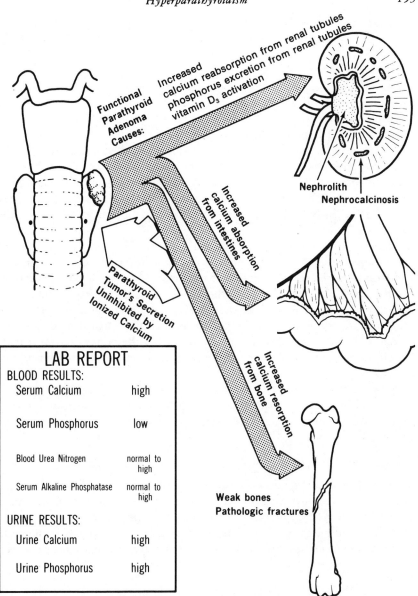

Functional Parathyroid Adenoma Causes:

Increased calcium reabsorption from renal tubules

phosphorus excretion from renal tubules

vitamin D₃ activation

Nephrolith
Nephrocalcinosis

Increased calcium absorption from intestines

Parathyroid Tumor's Secretion Uninhibited by Ionized Calcium

Increased calcium resorption from bone

Weak bones
Pathologic fractures

LAB REPORT
BLOOD RESULTS:
Serum Calcium — high
Serum Phosphorus — low
Blood Urea Nitrogen — normal to high
Serum Alkaline Phosphatase — normal to high
URINE RESULTS:
Urine Calcium — high
Urine Phosphorus — high

Fig. 10–1. Primary hyperparathyroidism.

sia, Type II. This second type of parathyroid hyperplasia has been reported in a dog.[58] Familial parathyroid hyperplasia has been reported in two female German shepherds, who were littermates; the condition was suspected to result from an autosomal recessive trait.[70]

Parathyroid neoplasms (or autonomous hyperplasia) may follow secondary hyperparathyroidism (hypocalcemia-dependent hyperplasia). Hyperparathyroidism resulting from parathyroid neoplasms and preceded by secondary hyperparathyroidism is called tertiary hyperparathyroidism.

Clinical Signs

The clinical signs of primary hyperparathyroidism ("bones, groans, and stones") are produced by hypercalcemia, bone resorption, and calcium nephropathy resulting from the excessive secretion of PTH. Effects and clinical signs of hypercalcemia are listed in Table 10–1.

Electrocardiographic effects of hypercalcemia include bradycardia, decreased QT interval (proportional to hypercalcemia), increased PR interval, elevated ST segment, and ventricular dysrhythmias. Other effects and clinical signs of excess PTH are also listed in Table 10–2. Some of these are associated with the uremic syndrome resulting from calcium nephropathy (Table 10–3).

Affected dogs are usually more than 8 years old. The incidence of primary hyperparathyroidism in dogs is rare, but undiagnosed cases may be common as, until recently, they were in humans. Primary hyperparathyroidism has not yet been described in the cat. One reason for its seemingly rare occurrence is that clinical signs and, rarely, hypercalcemia may be intermittent, making recognition of the condition difficult. Most canine cases are recognized only after considerable alterations in the bones or after urinary calculi have occurred. Except for the rare carcinomas, parathyroid tumors are not palpable.

Bony facial swelling (hyperostosis), loose teeth, and pliability of the mandible ("rubber jaw") are thought to result from demineralization, multiple infractions, hemorrhage, and replacement of bone by fibrous connective tissue and osteoid.

Radiographic Findings

Skeletal demineralization, osteopenia (osteomalacia), can be seen radiographically in patients with primary hyperparathyroidism[68]; however, mineralization must be depleted by more than 25% before it becomes evident on routine radiographs. In humans, less than 20% have skeletal demineralization evident radiographically at the time of diagnosis. The earliest detect-

Table 10–1.   Effects and Clinical Signs of Hypercalcemia

Anorexia (gastric atony)
Vomiting (gastric atony)
Constipation (intestinal atony)
Muscle weakness
Bradycardia and arrhythmias
Depression, coma, or seizures
Polyuria, compensatory polydipsia, and dehydration
Uremia (nephrocalcinosis and nephrolithiasis)
Gastric ulcer (hypergastrinemia)

Table 10-2. Other Possible Effects and Clinical Signs Caused by Excessive Parathyroid Hormone

Soft bones and spontaneous fractures
Facial hyperostosis
Loosening or loss of teeth
Painful mastication and malodorous breath
Weight loss
Bone pain, lameness, or neck pain
Acute pancreatitis

able changes usually are radiolucency of the sockets of the teeth (laminae dura dentes), the vertebral bodies, and the dorsal processes of the vertebrae. Eventually there is a general loss of bone density, but the overall size of the bones may increase with fibrous connective tissue and osteoid (*hyperostotic osteomalacia*). Subperiosteal cortical resorption and bone cysts (*osteitis fibrosa cystica*) may be visualized radiographically in long bones, especially the phalanges. Multiple pathologic fractures are rare but may occur in advanced cases. Neurologic impairment may occur if a fracture compresses or severs the spinal cord. Subclinical demineralization may be made evident by a technetium pyrophosphate bone scan. Demineralization of the skeleton can be reduced or delayed if dietary intake of calcium is high.

In primary hyperparathyroidism, the incidence of soft tissue metastatic mineralization outside the kidney is uncommon compared with secondary hyperparathyroidism or vitamin D intoxication. The risk of soft tissue mineralization is decreased by hypophosphatemia and hyperchloremic metabolic acidosis in animals with primary hyperparathyroidism. Other possible causes of metastatic mineralization of soft tissues are pseudohyperparathyroidism, vitamin D intoxication, chronic irritation resulting in metaplasia, secondary hyperparathyroidism of renal origin, and hyperadrenocorticism.[30]

Nephroliths and uroliths are found easily in radiographs, since they are composed of calcium phosphate or oxalate. Nephrocalcinosis is less distinct in radiographs, but may appear as diffuse mild radiopacity of the kidneys.

Table 10-3. Clinical Signs and Other Effects of the Uremic Syndrome

Depression
Vomiting
Diarrhea
Oral ulcerations and uremic breath
Anemia
Dehydration
Metabolic acidosis
Polyuria-polydipsia (eventually oliguria or anuria)
Mild hyperglycemia
Thrombocytopathy
Immunodepression

The uremic syndrome is another cause of metastatic mineralization, and would be accompanied by the signs listed in Table 10–3. Chondrocalcinosis and periarticular calcification may be noted in animals with primary or secondary hyperparathyroidism.

Contrast studies with selective arteriography and parathyroid scintigraphy with selenomethionine are generally of little value. Parathyroid adenomas can be best identified radiologically by thallium-201 and technetium-subtraction scans. This technique has not been described in dogs and would require several weeks of isolation. Thyroid scans with technetium to show thyroid compression by a parathyroid tumor are more practical but not as sensitive.

Laboratory Findings and Diagnosis

Persistent hypercalcemia is the best single diagnostic determinant of hyperparathyroidism. The hypercalcemia of primary hyperparathyroidism is usually of mild to moderate magnitude (12 to 14 mg/dl). Rarely, serum calcium levels may be normal or intermittently elevated. Other possible causes for hypercalcemia are listed in Table 10–4.[3, 18, 19, 38, 83] Repeated measurements (at least three) of serum calcium levels are recommended in patients with clinical signs and history suggestive of primary hyperparathyroidism. Although compensatory changes in calcium regulation (hypercalcitoninism) or concurrent diseases that cause hypoalbuminemia can cause normocalcemia in cases of primary hyperparathyroidism, these instances are rare. Ionized calcium levels are rarely necessary. Early in the development of primary hyperparathyroidism, hypercalcemia often is accompanied by

Table 10–4.   Possible Causes for Hypercalcemia Other Than Primary Hyperparathyroidism

Increased intestinal absorption of calcium (hypervitaminosis D)

Increased release of calcium from bone
  Non-parathyroid tumors producing PTH or PTH-like peptides
  Malignant tumors with bone metastasis
  Malignant hematolymphatic neoplasia
  Acute immobilization
  Hyperthyroidism
  Septic osteomyelitis
  Hypervitaminosis A

Increased renal tubular reabsorption of calcium
  Thiazide diuretics
  Severe hypoadrenocorticism

Spurious lab results (hyperlipidemia)

Decreased glomerular clearance and increased circulating
    complexed calcium
  Congenital renal diseases in dogs
  Chronic renal disease in horses

serum phosphorus levels below normal or in the low end of the normal range and by decreased plasma bicarbonate levels.

Frequently, the loss of bicarbonate and phosphorus in the urine leads to hyperchloremia and an increased serum chloride to bicarbonate ratio. Ratios of serum chloride (mEq/L) to phosphorus (mg/dl) that exceed 30:1 suggest the diagnosis of primary hyperparathyroidism. Ratios exceeding 33:1 are typical but not diagnostic of primary hyperparathyroidism.

If the clinician has confidence in a laboratory's procedures for a PTH assay, the use of a radioimmunoassay (RIA) for C-terminal PTH may be considered.[21] In any case, the RIA for PTH is expensive and should be reserved for those cases for which less expensive means cannot rule out the diagnosis of primary hyperparathyroidism as the cause of hypercalcemia (Table 10–5).

The condition that most closely mimics primary hyperparathyroidism is pseudohyperparathyroidism, a nonparathyroid tumor producing hypercalcemia. The differentiation of pseudohyperparathyroidism and primary hyperparathyroidism is summarized in Table 10–6. Normalization of serum calcium levels after the administration of large trial doses of glucocorticoids is diagnostic for pseudohyperparathyroidism. Unfortunately, the serum calcium levels are not affected in some cases of pseudohyperparathyroidism treated with glucocorticoids.

Hypercalcemia results in excess calcium in the urine in more than three fourths of reported persons with primary hyperparathyroidism. Concentrations of urinary phosphorus may also be increased as a direct effect of increased PTH in the renal tubules. Determination of urinary calcium and phosphorus is best based on excretion values for a 24-hour period. Normal total urinary excretion of calcium and phosphorus in the dog is approximately 0.5 to 1 mg and 10 to 30 mg/kg body weight/24 hours, respectively. Excessive calcium in the filtrate leads to impaired tubular reabsorption caused in part by decreased sodium reabsorption and decreased medullary tonicity. In addition, tubular calcification, tubular degeneration, and tubular necrosis can occur, especially if serum calcium levels exceed 14 mg/dl. Mineralization first becomes evident at the corticomedullary junction. The polyuria that results is not responsive to water deprivation or administration of antidiuretic hormone (ADH).

Nephrocalcinosis is often too advanced to be reversed once it is clinically evident; however, clinical nephrocalcinosis is not necessarily fatal. Measure-

Table 10–5. Basic Preliminary Criteria for a Diagnosis of Primary Hyperparathyroidism

---

Hypercalcemia (may be intermittent)
Hypophosphatemia (inconsistently present)
Hypercalciuria (inconsistently present)
Elimination of other causes of hypercalcemia

---

ments of excretory function (blood urinary nitrogen [BUN], serum creatinine, creatinine clearance) may or may not be abnormal, depending on the extent of renal damage. Functional renal impairment must be evaluated by the results of tests of excretory function, their change following diuresis, and urinalysis. All patients with calcium phosphate or oxalate nephroliths or uroliths should be suspected to have primary hyperparathyroidism. Clinicians need to be alert to the possibility that once calcium oxalate or calcium phosphate stones become infected they may be covered with magnesium ammonium phosphate and therefore not suspected to be associated with hyperparathyroidism.

Primary hyperparathyroidism increases the urinary excretion of nephrogenous cyclic adenosine monophosphate (cAMP) in humans, but controversy exists about whether this is true for the dog. The measurement of nephrogenous cAMP is an expensive test that has not been adequately evaluated in companion animals. Additional diagnostic tests may be considered, but have limited value.

Serum alkaline phosphatase (SAP) levels may be mildly elevated if overt bone disease is present, but have little diagnostic value for primary hyperparathyroidism. Only about 25% of human cases of primary hyperparathyroidism have elevated SAP levels. The meaningfulness of increased urinary hydroxyproline is also diagnostically nonspecific other than assessing the degree of current bone degradation of osteoid. Bone biopsy may be considered, but is rarely necessary. Undecalcified sections especially should show decalcified osteoid and increased numbers of osteoclasts and osteoblasts.

Treatment

Surgical removal of the parathyroid neoplasm (or three-and-one-half of the hyperplastic parathyroids) is necessary to treat primary hyperparathy-

Table 10–6. Comparison Between Clinical Findings Typical of Primary Hyperparathyroidism and Those of Pseudohyperparathyroidism

Clinical Finding	Primary Hyperparathyroidism	Pseudohyperparathyroidism
Onset of clinical signs	Insidious	Sudden
Primary clinical signs	Lameness and urinary calculi	Weight loss and anemia
Skeletal radiographs	Subperiosteal resorption	Normal
Serum chemistries		
Calcium	11–14 mg/dl	More than 14 mg/dl
Chloride (Cl)	Increased	Normal
Phosphorus (P)	Normal to low	Normal
Alkaline phosphatase	Normal to mild increase	Often elevated
Cl/P ratio	More than 30:1	Less than 30:1
Plasma PTH level	Elevated	Rarely elevated
Corticosteroid response	Little to no decrease in serum calcium	Serum calcium often becomes normal or decreases markedly

roidism. Chemotherapy and radiation therapy do not hold much promise at present. Before surgery, the patient should be evaluated for the extent of functional renal impairment. Thoracic radiographs are also indicated to search for metastasis of parathyroid carcinomas or for cranial mediastinal ectopic parathyroid neoplasms.[55]

During surgery all parathyroids should be examined and their sizes compared to each other. Enlarged glands should be removed, with the exception that if all are enlarged, then one half of one cranial parathyroid should be left. Strict hemostasis must be practiced to avoid discoloration of the muscles while searching for ectopic hyperplastic or neoplastic parathyroid tissue. A second operation should be avoided, because after the first operation scar tissue virtually eliminates the chance of finding a parathyroid adenoma. Multiple, minute, white foci seen in the thyroids are hyperplastic parafollicular cells. The hypercalcemia of hyperparathyroidism induces secondary hypercalcitoninism.

Transient but serious hypocalcemia may develop in 12 to 96 hours after the operation because the source of excess PTH has been removed with unaccommodated parathyroid tissue remaining and because of rapid calcium uptake by mineral-starved bone ("recalcification tetany"). By adjusting oral doses of calcium gluconate and vitamin D to maintain serum calcium levels between 7.5 to 9.0 mg/dl, the production of PTH from the remaining parathyroid tissue will normalize without the risk of acute hypocalcemia. Possible signs and effects of acute hypocalcemia are listed in Table 10–7.

If postoperative serum calcium levels are lower than 7.5 mg/dl, and no hypocalcemic signs are noted, oral calcium gluconate should be given in divided doses of 50 to 75 mg/kg body weight/day. Vitamin D or an isomer (dihydrotachysterol) should also be given. Dihydrotachysterol's action is more rapid in onset than other forms of vitamin D, and its elimination is also more rapid. The initial dose of 0.125 to 0.2 mg/day should be reduced after 3 to 4 days. Benefits from vitamin D and its isomers are slow in onset (taking several days), and the effects are cumulative; toxicosis resulting from excessive levels of vitamin D can occur if one overdoses from impatience. Supplementation with vitamin D and calcium may be necessary for only a few days to as long as 3 months.

Postoperative hypocalcemia with tetany or seizures is an emergency situation. An intravenous solution of 10% calcium gluconate should be slowly

Table 10–7.   Possible Signs and Effects of Acute Hypocalcemia

Muscle fasciculation and tremors of facial muscles and forelegs
Nervousness and restlessness
Prolonged QT on ECG
Tetanic convulsions
Death from laryngeal spasm

administered in a dose of 1 ml/kg body weight, up to a total of 10 ml. The heart rate and ECG should be monitored for bradycardias and dysrhythmias. Prolonged administration at a slow drip with 5% dextrose may be continued. Preparations of calcium precipitate when added to fluids containing bicarbonate. This should be avoided. Parathyroid extract is commercially available, but the administration of calcium is more practical, as commercial parathyroid extracts are antigenic, expensive, short-lived, and require parenteral administration.

Hypomagnesemia (levels of magnesium <1 mEq/L) and hyperkalemia (levels of potassium >5.5 mEq/L) potentiate the effects of hypocalcemia. Postoperative hyperkalemia is uncommon and responds adequately to correction of hypocalcemia. Serum magnesium levels, however, should be monitored with serum calcium levels after parathyroid surgery. Hypomagnesemia may be corrected by 2 mEq/kg body weight of magnesium sulfate given intravenously over a 4-hour period.

The production of parathyroid hormone by the remaining parathyroid tissue should normalize in 1 to 3 weeks. Skeletal recovery after successful surgery should be nearly complete in 2 months. If serum calcium remains elevated after surgery, additional ectopic tissue in the neck or cranial mediastinum should be sought, or the diagnosis of primary hyperparathyroidism re-evaluated. Medical management of inoperable parathyroid tumors is not a desirable situation. Attempts to control the hypercalcemia can include low dietary intake of calcium and administration of oral phosphates. Mineralization of soft tissue is likely to become worse.

For further information on primary hyperparathyroidism, see references 12, 14, 19, 20, 35, 36, 39, 56, 69, and 79.

PSEUDOHYPERPARATHYROIDISM (Hypercalcemia of Malignancy)

Pseudohyperparathyroidism is more common than primary hyperparathyroidism. In comparison to primary hyperparathyroidism, pseudohyperparathyroidism is usually characterized by a more rapid onset, weight loss, lack of overt bone demineralization, and hypercalcemia of greater magnitude. Other differentiating criteria are listed in Table 10–6.

See also references 9, 10, 16, 43, 51–54, 60, 74, and 75.

Causes

The term *pseudohyperparathyroidism* is used here to describe any hypercalcemia resulting from malignancy not caused by metastasis to bone. Only a minority of these cases cause hypercalcemia by producing PTH or a PTH-like peptide. Some lymphosarcomas in dogs can apparently produce PTH.[81] In humans, malignant tumors most likely to produce PTH or similar peptides are carcinomas of the lung or kidney. Other pathologic mechanisms that cause hypercalcemia include production of epidermal growth factor, transforming growth factor, prostaglandin E_2, osteoclast-activating factor, vitamin-D-like sterols, activators of 1α-hydroxylase, or production of increased serum calcium-binding globulins.[52, 76]

Hypercalcemia resulting from malignancy is most frequently associated with lymphosarcoma in dogs.[28, 29, 67, 71, 80] Lymphosarcoma comprises about 4.5% of all canine neoplasia, and 10% to 40% of dogs with lymphosarcoma develop hypercalcemia. A much lower percentage of cats with lymphosarcoma seem affected with hypercalcemia.[15] Hypercalcemia associated with lymphosarcoma and with gastric carcinoma[48, 49] has also been noted in the horse.[6] Canine breeds considered at a greater-than-expected risk for lymphosarcoma include boxers, basset hounds, St. Bernards, Scottish terriers, and various hunting breeds. The second most common cause of hypercalcemia in dogs is apocrine gland adenocarcinomas of the anal sacs.[24, 27, 46, 47, 61] Reported causes of pseudohyperparathyroidism in dogs are listed in Table 10–8.[1, 17, 26, 33, 41, 44, 45, 78, 82]

Although lymphosarcoma in dogs may produce PTH or PTH-like peptides,[81] most cases of lymphosarcoma in dogs associated with hypercalcemia seem to cause hypercalcemia by producing a lymphokine, osteoclast-activity factor. Multicentric and thymic (cranial mediastinal) forms of lymphosarcoma are most commonly associated with hypercalcemia. About 10% of dogs with multicentric lymphosarcoma and 50% of dogs with thymic forms develop hypercalcemia. Over 80% of dogs with hypercalcemia from lymphosarcoma have a cranial mediastinal mass. About 70% have bone marrow involvement. There is no evidence that prostaglandin E_2 (PGE_2) or vitamin D-like sterols are involved in the hypercalcemia caused by lymphosarcoma.

In humans, PGE_2-induced hypercalcemia is generally caused by carcinomas of the lung or kidney, and vitamin D-like sterols are usually produced by carcinomas of the breast. Multiple myeloma, like lymphosarcoma, can cause hypercalcemia by producing osteoclast-activating factor in humans. In addition, multiple myeloma can produce abnormal serum globulins that bind calcium.[4, 19]

Table 10–8. Reported Causes of Canine Pseudohyperparathyroidism

Lymphosarcoma (malignant lymphoma)
Apocrine gland adenocarcinoma of the anal sacs
Mammary gland adenocarcinomas
Fibrosarcoma
Pancreatic adenocarcinoma
Multiple myeloma
Lymphatic leukemia
Primary epidermoid carcinoma of the lungs
Interstitial cell tumor of the testis
Perianal squamous cell carcinoma
Nasal adenocarcinoma
Undifferentiated adenocarcinoma

Apocrine gland adenocarcinomas of the anal sacs in dogs are presumed to cause hypercalcemia by producing a stimulating factor for 1α-hydroxylase. 1α-Hydroxylase is a renal enzyme necessary for hydroxylation of vitamin D (25, hydroxy-D_3) to form the more potent 1,25 dihydroxy-D_3. More than 90% of dogs affected with apocrine gland adenocarcinoma of the anal sacs are female dogs with an average age of 10 years. About 80% of the apocrine gland adenocarcinomas are unilateral, and despite the relative lack of anaplastic appearances, more than 90% have metastasized to the iliac or sublumbar lymph nodes by the time of diagnosis. This tumor usually, but not invariably, causes hypercalcemia. It is often occult, not being discovered until a digital examination of the anus and rectum is done.[46]

There is no known successful treatment for apocrine gland adenocarcinoma of the anal sacs. Excision followed by therapy with cyclophosphamide and 5-fluorouracil has been suggested. The average length of survival after diagnosis is approximately 9 months. Apocrine gland adenocarcinomas of the anal sacs should not be confused with the more common perianal gland adenomas. Perianal gland adenomas (hepatoid tumors) occur in older sexually intact male dogs. Perianal gland adenomas, usually benign, are easily seen as lobulated tumors elevated from the surface of the skin. They are usually found near the anus but can occur elsewhere on the skin. Pseudohyperparathyroidism is rarely, if ever, caused by perianal gland adenomas.

Clinical Signs and Laboratory Findings

Many of the clinical signs of pseudohyperparathyroidism are attributable to hypercalcemia and are identical to those seen in animals with primary hyperparathyroidism (see Table 10–1). Additional clinical signs may be produced by the nonparathyroid tumor itself, including such signs as enlarged lymph nodes, perianal tumors, mammary tumors, cough from lung metastasis, and others. The osteomalacia seen in subjects with primary hyperparathyroidism is not evident radiographically in subjects with pseudohyperparathyroidism. This is presumably because the nonparathyroid neoplasm causes earlier debilitation resulting from nonhormonal effects and more severe hypercalcemia, whereas parathyroid adenomas or hyperplasia more gradually affect the animal's health by means of the hormone's excess and mild hypercalcemia.

Other possible reasons for the absence of osteomalacia in association with pseudohyperparathyroidism include production of local osteolytic factors or vitamin-D-like sterols that do not cause generalized osteomalacia. Serum alkaline phosphatase elevations are more likely associated with metastasis of the nonparathyroid neoplasm into the liver than with overt bone disease in pseudohyperparathyroidism. Elevated serum alkaline phosphatase levels occur more often, and to a greater magnitude, in animals with pseudohypoparathyroidism than in animals with primary hyperparathyroidism.

Calcium nephropathy is present in most cases of pseudohyperparathyroidism. Urinalysis usually shows isosthenuria or hyposthenuria, no casts, and an occasional red or white blood cell in the sediment. Crystals of calcium phosphate or oxalate may be found. Retention of BUN, creatinine, organic acids, and other metabolic waste products depends on the severity of renal failure at the time of examination. Mineralization of soft tissue outside the kidneys is rare in animals with pseudohyperparathyroidism.

Diagnosis

The clinical diagnosis of pseudohyperparathyroidism is based on correction of the elevated serum calcium levels after the removal, destruction, or suppression of the nonparathyroid neoplasm suspected to be producing hypercalcemia-promoting substances. A minimal data base, necessary to arrive at a tentative diagnosis of pseudohyperparathyroidism, requires a thorough and accurate history. Physical examination should include palpation of the skeleton, all superficial lymph nodes, anal sacs, deep abdominal structures, and an ophthalmologic examination. Radiologic examination of the bones for subperiosteal resorption should include the dental arcade and metacarpals-phalanges. Films of the thorax and abdomen are also recommended. Thyroid or bone scans may be useful in selected cases.

Recommended laboratory data useful in differentiating pseudohyperparathyroidism from primary hyperparathyroidism include a complete hemogram, serum chemistries (urea nitrogen [UN], alanine aminotransferase [ALT], alkaline phosphatase, creatinine, total protein, albumin, calcium, phosphorus, and magnesium), urinalysis, bone marrow biopsy, and an aspirate biopsy of the lymph nodes. Since some tumors responsible for pseudohyperparathyroidism are occult but are suppressed by glucocorticoids, normalization of serum calcium after the administration of glucocorticoid (3 to 10 days of 0.5 to 1 mg/kg body weight/day of prednisone) is tentatively diagnostic for pseudohyperparathyroidism when a nonparathyroid neoplasm is not readily found. Primary hyperparathyroidism is little affected by glucocorticoids, but some reduction of serum calcium is theoretically possible, resulting from reduced urinary calcium excretion, decreased intestinal calcium absorption, and other minor effects on calcium metabolism by glucocorticoids.

Treatment

Ideally, the nonparathyroid tumor responsible for pseudohyperparathyroidism should be excised or totally destroyed by radiation or immunotherapy. Within 2 days of excision, the hypercalcemia should be resolved. Regrettably, total elimination is rarely possible. Most frequently, suppression by chemotherapy is the only alternative to euthanasia. The chemotherapy indicated varies with the neoplasm, and suggested regimens are constantly changing. The degree of functional renal disability should be determined before undertaking any form of therapy. Nephropathologic changes caused by calcium may not be reversible.

Hypercalcemic crisis resulting from serum calcium levels in excess of 14 mg/dl occurs more often with pseudohyperparathyroidism than with primary hyperparathyroidism. Clinical signs of hypercalcemic crisis can include constipation, muscle tremors, and mental depression. Serum calcium levels that exceed 18 mg/dl can result in renal failure and shock, rapidly leading to death.

It is advisable to attempt to reduce the serum calcium levels with an intravenous solution of sterile isotonic saline with added potassium chloride, 10 mEq/L, and furosemide, 1 mg/kg body weight, every 2 hours. In addition to the dilutional effects of an intravenous saline solution, sodium loading with saline and treatment with furosemide inhibit calcium's reabsorption in the renal tubules. Thiazide diuretics can aggravate hypercalcemia and should be avoided.

Prednisone, 2 mg/kg body weight/day, may be beneficial if the hypercalcemia is being caused by lymphosarcoma, malignant myeloma, some other malignant tumors, or vitamin D intoxication. One-half to 2 g daily of oral phosphate (Neutra-Phos) in divided doses and a low-calcium diet may be of benefit in reducing or managing hypercalcemia. Because oral phosphates can cause a laxative effect, the dosage should be reduced if bowel movements are excessively soft. Nonsteroidal, anti-inflammatory drugs that inhibit prostaglandin synthetase (ibuprofen [Motrin]) are not recommended because PGE_2-mediated hypercalcemia has not been reported in hypocalcemic companion animals, and because ibuprofen and most similar drugs are not eliminated or tolerated as well in companion animals as in humans.

Other means of reducing hypercalcemia can be considered after conservative attempts with the intravenous administration of saline, furosemide, and glucocorticoids have failed. Mithramycin (Mithracin) is an antibiotic anticancer agent that decreases DNA-directed RNA synthesis and decreases osteoclastic activity. An intravenous dose of 10 to 25 mg/kg body weight once or twice per week effectively reduces hypercalcemia without risking the mineralization of soft tissue. Potential adverse effects include thrombocytopenia, hepatic and renal necrosis, and hypocalcemia. Calcitonin (Calcimar-Solution) is effective, but has a short duration and is expensive. The intravenous administration of disodium or monopotassium phosphate or sodium sulfate decahydrate is more hazardous than any of the other suggested means to reduce hypercalcemia. Phosphate and sulfate solutions lower serum calcium levels by promoting soft tissue mineralization. Both are contraindicated if renal failure is present. Peritoneal dialysis is indicated if serum calcium levels exceed 18 mg/dl, and conservative therapy or treatment with mithramycin has been unsuccessful.

SECONDARY HYPERPARATHYROIDISM

Secondary hyperparathyroidism is associated with excessive production of PTH, leading to demineralization of the bones. Unlike primary hyperparathyroidism or pseudohyperparathyroidism, the serum calcium levels are in the low normal range or, occasionally, the abnormally low range. Secondary hyperparathyroidism is an appropriate response to nonparathyroid disorders promoting a decrease in serum calcium or magnesium levels.

The most important disorders that lead to secondary hyperparathyroidism are chronic renal disease, intestinal malabsorption, and dietary imbalances of calcium, phosphorus, or vitamin D. Other diseases that can cause secondary hyperparathyroidism as a more minor portion of their spectrum of pathology are calcitonin-secreting medullary carcinomas of the thyroid and hyperadrenocorticism.

Secondary hyperparathyroidism causes defective mineralization of the osteoid of bone, particularly bones of the appendicular skeleton. Defective mineralization results in softening of the bones, called *osteomalacia.* During growth, the epiphyses of long bones and endochondral growth of bones are also affected, a condition called *rickets.*

Secondary Hyperparathyroidism of Renal Origin

This ramification of chronic renal failure is usually overshadowed by the severe clinical syndrome associated with the final stages of renal failure. Actually, secondary hyperparathyroidism and osteopenia begin to occur early in renal failure, but the changes are subclinical until late in the course of disease.

Decreased glomerular filtration accompanying renal failure promotes potential hypocalcemia in two major ways. One is the potential fall in serum calcium levels as serum phosphorus levels increase, which results from decreased glomerular filtration. This inverse relationship has been called the "mass-law equation." In vivo, serum calcium usually does not become abnormally low because of the compensatory increase in PTH. The other process leading to lower serum calcium levels is the impaired activation of vitamin D, a phenomenon associated with many renal diseases. The deficiency of renal-activated vitamin D (1,25-dihydroxy D_3) leads to poor gastrointestinal absorption of calcium. The slow onset of chronic renal failure allows the compensatory secretion of PTH to maintain normal or near-normal serum calcium concentrations. Concomitant hypoproteinemia or acidosis may reduce total serum calcium levels, but is not necessarily associated with decreased levels of ionized calcium.

When the cause of renal failure is acquired, it usually occurs in dogs older than the age of 5 years; if it is congenital and inherited, it usually occurs before the age of 5 years. Some types of acquired and congenital renal disease that can cause secondary hyperparathyroidism are listed in Table 10–9.[34] Congenital and inherited renal disease, "renal dysplasia," has been reported in Norwegian elkhounds, cocker spaniels, Lhasa apsos, shih tsus, beagles, German shepherd dogs, dachshunds, miniature schnauzers, samoyeds, and Alaskan malamutes.

Osteomalacia (rickets) occurring from congenital or inherited renal disease is more severe than that occurring from acquired renal disease. In growing animals, the osteomalacia is likely to be followed by excessive fibrous connective tissue repair, leading to excess volume of bone (especially involving the maxilla and the other bones of the skull). Isostotic

Table 10–9.   Causes for Secondary Hyperparathyroidism of Renal Origin

Acquired disease
  Chronic interstitial nephritis
  Glomerulonephritis
  Nephrosclerosis
  Renal amyloidosis

Congenital or hereditary abnormalities
  Congenital renal cortical hypoplasia
  Polycystic kidneys
  Bilateral hydronephrosis

osteomalacia is more common than hyperostotic osteomalacia in secondary hyperparathyroidism whose origin is from acquired renal disease. The bones of the maxilla may become soft enough to permit excessive movement of the canine teeth if upper canines are pressed toward each other. The mandible may become unusually pliable, a condition referred to as "rubber jaw." Subperiosteal resorption of long bones and elevation of tendinous attachments may be noted on radiographs. In addition to PTH-induced osteomalacia, PTH is considered a major toxin of the uremic syndrome, being responsible in part for behavioral abnormalities and anemia resulting from uremia; therefore, secondary hyperparathyroidism of renal origin is most often seen in an animal with renal failure, exhibiting signs of the uremic syndrome (see Table 10–3) and excessive levels of PTH (see Table 10–2).

Laboratory findings generally include isosthenuric urine, increased blood urea nitrogen, low normal serum calcium, increased serum phosphorus, and possibly increased serum alkaline phosphatase (Fig. 10–2). Whenever the serum calcium X phosphorus product exceeds 70, mineralization of soft tissues occurs. Calcium nephropathy and urinary calculi are unlikely with secondary hyperparathyroidism of renal origin, but mineralization in other soft tissues is common (Table 10–10).

The treatment of secondary hyperparathyroidism of renal origin in companion animals initially consists of improving renal filtration by diuresis or peritoneal dialysis. Additional measures that may be taken to correct the serum calcium and phosphorus concentrations are dietary supplementation with calcium, a diet low in phosphorus,[64] and oral administration of phosphorus binders—aluminum hydroxide gel or aluminum carbonate gel. Aluminum hydroxide gel (Amphojel) can be given at 1 ml/kg body weight three times daily to affected dogs. Calcium lactate (0.5 to 2 g/day), calcium gluconate (1 to 3 g/day), or calcium carbonate (0.25 to 1 g/day) are often used to supplement the diet with calcium.

Aluminum gels to bind dietary phosphorus should be used cautiously. Aluminum may be absorbed in excess from the gastrointestinal tract and has been implicated as a cause of dementia, microcytic anemia, and osteomalacia with a poor response to vitamin D in humans.

Once the product resulting from the multiplication of calcium and phosphorus is less than 70, vitamin D may be administered to facilitate the

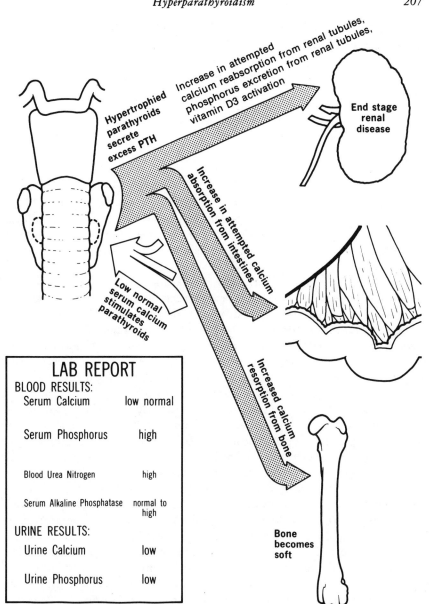

Labels within figure:
Hypertrophied parathyroids secrete excess PTH

Increase in attempted calcium reabsorption from renal tubules, phosphorus excretion from renal tubules, vitamin D3 activation

End stage renal disease

Increase in attempted calcium absorption from intestines

Low normal serum calcium stimulates parathyroids

Increased calcium resorption from bone

Bone becomes soft

LAB REPORT

BLOOD RESULTS:

Serum Calcium	low normal
Serum Phosphorus	high
Blood Urea Nitrogen	high
Serum Alkaline Phosphatase	normal to high

URINE RESULTS:

Urine Calcium	low
Urine Phosphorus	low

Fig. 10–2. Renal secondary hyperparathyroidism. PTH = parathyroid hormone.

intestinal absorption of calcium. Dihydrotachysterol, an isomer of vitamin D, is preferred because renal activation is not necessary. The dose for dogs is approximately 0.125 to 0.2 mg every 1 to 7 days. Serum calcium levels should be closely monitored, and the treatment interrupted for a few weeks if hypercalcemia is discovered. The rate of dihydrotachysterol excretion is slow, but after 1 to 2 weeks of withdrawal, it may be reinstituted at a lower dose. Cimetidine (Tagamet), an H_2-receptor antagonist, decreases plasma

Table 10–10. Common Sites of Soft Tissue Mineralization Produced by Secondary Hyperparathyroidism

Gastric mucosa
Subcutis
Periarticular tissue
Pleura
Endocardium and myocardium
Arterial walls
Lung

PTH levels in chronic renal disease, possibly by blocking histamine receptors in the parathyroid or accelerating the degradation of PTH.[32] A dosage commonly used in the dog to block H_2 receptors is 5 mg/kg body weight of cimetidine given twice daily. Subtotal parathyroidectomy may be beneficial in selected cases.

Renal tubular anomalies causing hypercalcinuria are rare causes for secondary hyperparathyroidism and osteomalacia. Idiopathic canine Fanconi's (De Toni-Fanconi-Debre's) syndrome in basenjis and other breeds, and acquired Fanconi's syndrome of the proximal convoluted tubules caused by ingestion of outdated tetracycline or heavy metal poisoning, can cause hypercalciuria, secondary hyperparathyroidism, and osteomalacia. Classic renal tubular acidosis of the distal tubules is characterized by hypercalciuria, secondary hyperparathyroidism, osteomalacia, and nephrocalcinosis.

About 5% of dogs with chronic renal disease develop hypercalcemia rather than low-normal or low serum calcium levels characteristic of secondary hyperparathyroidism. Most are young dogs with congenital renal anomalies. Several possible reasons have been proposed for hypercalcemia associated with some cases of chronic renal disease. Among these are autonomous hyperplasia or adenomas of the parathyroids induced by the prior existence of compensatory parathyroid hyperplasia caused by chronic renal disease (tertiary hyperparathyroidism), decreased degradation of PTH, decreased renal ability to excrete calcium, increased citrates causing increased levels of complexed calcium, and the rebound of serum calcium resulting from decreasing serum phosphorus and other events subsequent to therapy for secondary hyperparathyroidism.[22, 73] In horses, paradoxical hypercalcemia is usually co-existent with chronic renal disease.[6, 7] The cause is unknown.

See also references 2, 8, 11, 42, and 77.

Secondary Hyperparathyroidism of Intestinal Origin (Malabsorption-Maldigestion)

Again, secondary hyperparathyroidism is overshadowed by the primary disease. Maldigestion and intestinal malabsorption may produce secondary hyperparathyroidism as sequelae to the impaired absorption of vitamin D, calcium, and phosphorus (Fig. 10–3). Treatment consists of correcting or

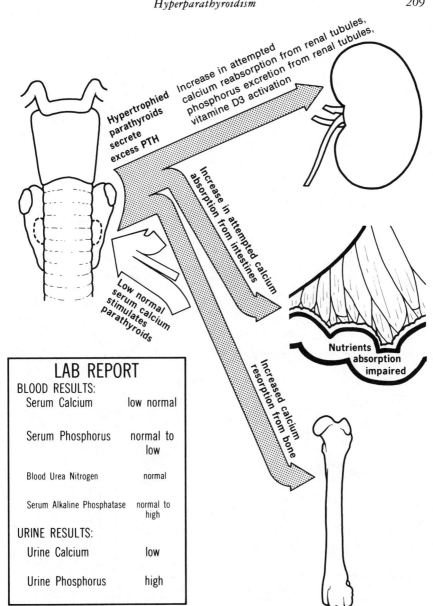

Fig. 10–3. Malabsorption secondary hyperparathyroidism. PTH = parathyroid hormone.

controlling the cause of maldigestion or malabsorption and the parenteral administration of vitamin D.

Secondary Hyperparathyroidism of Dietary Origin: Osteogenesis Imperfecta, Juvenile Osteoporosis, Paper Bone Disease

Secondary hyperparathyroidism of dietary origin differs from the other causes of secondary hyperparathyroidism in that the presenting complaints are

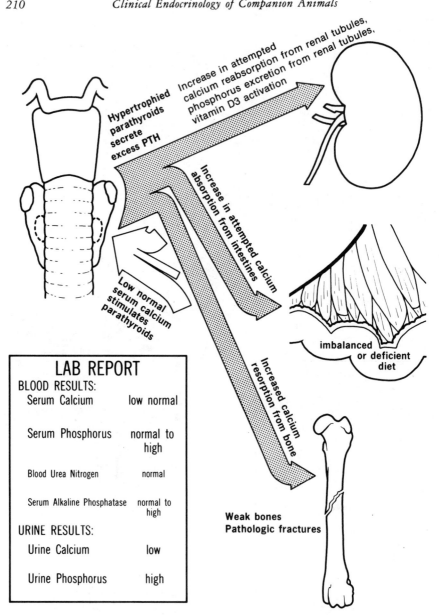

Fig. 10–4.   Nutritional secondary hyperparathyroidism. PTH = parathyroid hormone.

directly associated with the osteomalacia (Fig. 10–4). The osteomalacia is not overshadowed by uremia or diarrhea. In many cases, the affected animal seems in good health, has a lustrous haircoat, and may even be obese.

Dietary imbalances or deficiencies that may lead to secondary hyperparathyroidism include a high dietary intake of phosphorus with deficient or adequate intake of calcium (examples listed in Table 10–11), low dietary

Table 10–11.   Example Calcium:Phosphorus Ratios in Various Foods*

Meat	1:22
Potatoes	1:7.6
Bananas	1:3.3
Boiled eggs	1:3.8
Liver	1:50
Bread	1:3
Rice	1:6
Corn meal	1:10

* The ideal ratio is 1.2:1.

intake of calcium, or low dietary intake of vitamin D coupled with little or no exposure to ultraviolet light. In 1983, almost one fourth of the commercial cat foods surveyed were imbalanced, containing more phosphorus than calcium.[40] Growing puppies require about 550 mg of calcium and 450 mg of phosphorus/kg body weight/day. Kittens require 200 to 400 mg

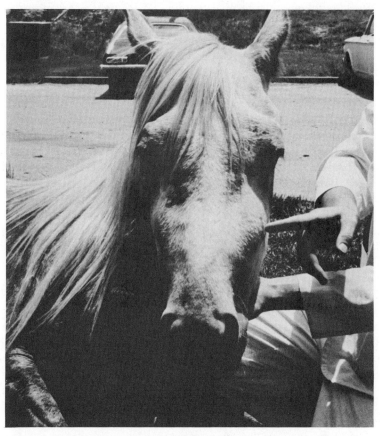

Fig. 10–5. "Big head." Swelling of the maxilla in a horse with nutritional secondary hyperparathyroidism. (Courtesy of Dr. Lou Tritschler.)

Table 10–12.   Clinical Signs and Effects of Secondary
Hyperparathyroidism of Dietary Origin in Quadrupeds

Posterior lameness of "shifting leg lameness"
Uncoordinated gait
Reluctance to move and play
Medial deviation of paws
Sternal recumbency
Pain in mastication
Swollen maxilla or other skull bones (in the young)
Loose teeth
Enlargement of costochondral junctions
Impaired growth
Bowing of the legs
Persistent extrusion of claw in felidae
Lordosis of the lumbar vertebrae

calcium/day. The per kg body weight requirements of adult dogs and cats are approximately one-half those of puppies and kittens. Certain species of New World monkeys must receive vitamin D_3 because they are incapable of utilizing vitamin D_2.

Dietary imbalances are often the result of an owner's pampering his pet by feeding the animal excessive quantities of meat, liver, rice, potatoes, bread, or eggs, to the exclusion of balanced commercial pet foods.[23, 25, 50, 57, 59, 66, 72] This practice, which is most often noted in cats, is called "Siamese cat disease," and is disastrous in the young.[62, 63] A diet of beef hearts or liver causes lameness in kittens within 4 to 8 weeks. All seed diets in budgerigars have a calcium to phosphorus ratio of 1:37 and can rapidly cause secondary hyperparathyroidism, which is first recognized by soft distorted beaks and pathologic fractures. Grain diets with little or no legumes or diets high in oxalate that bind dietary calcium can lead to secondary hyperparathyroidism in horses. For example, wheat bran has a calcium to phosphorus ratio of 1:11. Alfalfa (a legume) hay has a calcium to phosphorus ratio of 6:1. Affected horses develop an enlarged mandible and maxilla, loose teeth, and dysphagia, a condition called "big head" (bran disease, Millers' disease) (Fig. 10–5). Focal periosteal avulsion, torn or detached ligaments and tendons, and enlarged carpi, fetlocks, and hocks may also occur.

Animals are usually capable of producing sufficient vitamin D if their skin is exposed to enough ultraviolet light without supplementation of their diet with vitamin D; however, if the animal is deprived of adequate exposure to ultraviolet light, severe liver or kidney disease can eventually lead to vitamin D deficiency even if dietary sources are of normally sufficient amounts. This is because liver or kidney disease results in the animal's inability to store or activate (hydroxylate) natural vitamin D. Among their other antivitamin D effects, anticonvulsant drugs (primidone, phenobarbital, and phenytoin) also impair the activation of vitamin D.

Clinical signs of secondary hyperparathyroidism of dietary origin are listed in Table 10–12. Radiographic findings are similar to those of secondary hyperparathyroidism of renal origin (Figs. 10–6 and 10–7). In young animals on a severely deficient or imbalanced diet, bone resorption may exceed bone repair. When this happens, the volume of bone may be less than normal resulting in hypostotic osteomalacia. Epiphyses may appear wide and "moth eaten." Clinical signs of rickets, such as enlargement of costochondral junctions ("rachitic rosary"), precede radiographic changes in young affected animals.

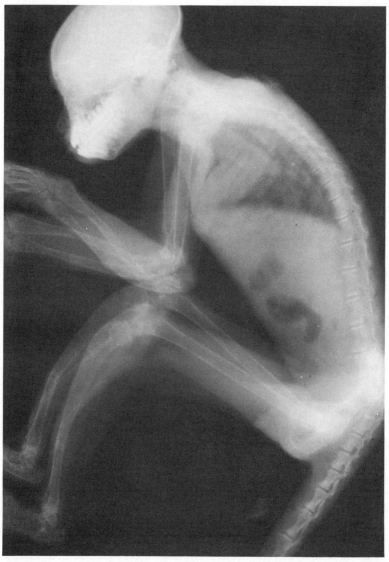

Fig. 10–6. Osteomalacia from nutritional secondary hyperparathyroidism in a monkey. Note the decreased bone density in comparison to the teeth and the pathologic fractures of the legs and arms.

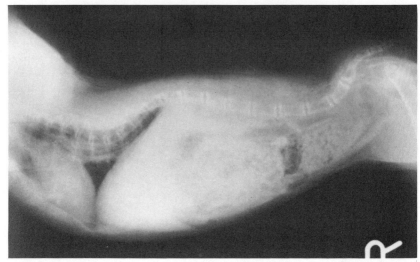

Fig. 10–7. Nutritional secondary hyperparathyroidism in a young cat showing osteomalacia and lordosis. (Courtesy of Dr. Jimmy Lattimer.)

Laboratory findings include low-normal serum levels of calcium, normal or increased serum levels of phosphorus, decreased levels of urinary calcium, and increased or normal levels of urinary phosphorus. Increased serum levels of alkaline phosphatase may occur in the presence of overt bone disease. Aminoaciduria may be caused by the increased secretion of PTH. A focal necrotic myopathy may develop, and serum creatinine phosphokinase may be elevated.

Treatment of secondary hyperparathyroidism of dietary origin is most safely done by simply restricting the diet to a reputable commercial pet food. Since the specific content of calcium and phosphorus is not required on labels of pet food, the clinician must rely on the company's good reputation. Homemade diets have been described, but they are troublesome and potentially hazardous, depending on the stage of bone recovery. Once the animal is on an adequate diet, clinical improvement may be noted in as soon as 5 days.[57] Skeletal recovery requires 2 to 3 months.[37] Since the patient's attitude improves more rapidly than skeletal strength, solitary cage confinement to eliminate jumping and rough-housing is advisable for 4 to 8 weeks. Cuttlebone, mineral blocks, crushed oyster or egg shells, green vegetables, and alfalfa pellets are adequate calcium supplements for budgerigars.

Virtually complete skeletal recovery is to be expected if fractures have been minor; however, spinal compression from vertebral fractures or neurologic deficits from severed peripheral nerves can occur. Also, dystocia, constipation, or obstipation may occur due to pelvic fractures narrowing the pelvic canal.

See also references 5, 13, 31, 62, 63, and 65.

REFERENCES

1. Beebe, M.A.: Pseudohyperparathyroidism associated with adenocarcinoma in three dogs. Mod. Vet. Pract., *61:*582, 1980.
2. Bergdahl, L., and Boquist, L.: Hyperparathyroidism in transient experimental renal failure in dogs. Pathol. Eur., *8:*89, 1973.
3. Blank, R.E.: Differential diagnosis of hypercalcemia in dogs. Compendium on Continuing Educ. for the Practicing Vet., *1:*220, 1979.
4. Braund, K.G., et al.: Neurologic complications of IgA multiple myeloma associated with cryoglobulinemia in a dog. J. Am. Vet. Med. Assoc., *174:*1321, 1979.
5. Bray, N.C.: Nutritional secondary hyperparathyroidism in a kitten. Feline Pract., *14:*31, 1984.
6. Brewer, B.D.: Disorders of equine calcium metabolism. Compendium on Continuing Educ. for the Practicing Vet., *4:*244, 1982.
7. Brobst, D.F., Lee, H.A., and Spencer, G.R.: Hypercalcemia and hypophosphatemia in a mare with renal insufficiency. J. Am. Vet. Med. Assoc., *173:*1370, 1978.
8. Brodey, R.S., Medway, W., and Marshak, R.R.: Renal osteodystrophy in the dog. J. Am. Vet. Med. Assoc., *139:*329, 1961.
9. Brown, N.O.: Paraneoplastic syndromes of humans, dogs and cats. J. Am. Anim. Hosp. Assoc., *17:*911, 1981.
10. Brown, S.R., and Walsh, M.B.: Pseudohyperparathyroidism in a dog. Vet. Med. Small Anim. Clin., *75:*61, 1980.
11. Burk, R.L., and Barton, C.L.: Renal failure and hyperparathyroidism in an Alaskan malamute pup. J. Am. Vet. Med. Assoc., *172:*69, 1978.
12. Capen, C.C.: Diagnosis and management of parathyroid diseases in animals. Proceedings of the 6th Kal Kan Symposium, p. 67, 1982.
13. Capen, C.C., and Rowland, G.N.: Ultrastructural evaluation of the parathyroid glands of young cats with experimental hyperparathyroidism. Z. Zellforsch., *90:*495, 1968.
14. Carrillo, J.M., Burk, R.L., and Bode, C.: Primary hyperparathyroidism in a dog. J. Am. Vet. Med. Assoc., *174:*67, 1979.
15. Chew, D.J., et al.: Pseudohyperparathyroidism in a cat. J. Am. Anim. Hosp. Assoc., *11:*46, 1975.
16. Cohen, S.J.: Pseudohyperparathyroidism in a dog. Canine Pract., *4:*57, 1977.
17. DeSchepper, J., Van Der Stock, J., and DeRick, A.: Hypercalcemia and hypoglycaemia in a case of lymphatic leukaemia in the dog. Vet. Rec., *94:*602, 1974.
18. Drazner, F.H.: Hypercalcemia in the dog and cat. J. Am. Vet. Med. Assoc., *178:*1252, 1981.
19. Dust, A., Norris, A.M., and Valli, V.E.O.: Cutaneous lymphosarcoma with IgG monoclonal gammopathy, serum hyperviscosity and hypercalcemia in a cat. Can. Vet. J. *23:*235, 1982.
20. Fasnacht, D.W., and Maksic, D.: Primary hyperparathyroidism in a dog. Mod. Vet. Pract., *43:*38, 1982.
21. Feldman, E.C., and Krutzik, S.: Case reports of parathyroid levels in spontaneous canine parathyroid disorders. J. Am. Anim. Hosp. Assoc., *17:*393, 1981.
22. Finco, D.R., and Rowland, G.N.: Hypercalcemia secondary to chronic renal failure in the dog: a report of four cases. J. Am. Vet. Med. Assoc., *173:*990, 1978.
23. Goddard, K.M., et al.: A comparison of all-meat, semi-moist, and dry-type dog foods as diets for growing beagles. J. Am. Vet. Med. Assoc., *157:*1233, 1970.
24. Goldschmidt, M.H., and Zoltowski, C.: Anal sac gland adenocarcinoma in the dog: 14 cases. J. Small Anim. Pract., *22:*119, 1981.
25. Gorham, J.R., Peckham, J.C., and Alexander, J.: Rickets and osteodystrophia fibrosa in foxes fed a high horsemeat ration. J. Am. Vet. Med. Assoc., *156:*1331, 1970.
26. Grain, E., and Walder, E.J.: Hypercalcemia associated with squamous cell carcinoma in a dog. J. Am. Vet. Med. Assoc., *181:*165, 1982.
27. Hause, W.R., et al.: Pseudohyperparathyroidism associated with adenocarcinomas of anal sac origin in four dogs. J. Am. Anim. Hosp. Assoc., *17:*373, 1981.
28. Heath, H., Weller, R.E., and Mundy, G.R.: Canine lymphosarcoma: a model for study of the hypercalcemia of cancer. Calcif. Tissue Int., *30:*127, 1980.
29. Hirsch, V.M., McLaughlin, B.G., and Parent, J.: Lymphosarcoma with hypercalcemia and osteolysis in a dog. Can. Vet. J., *24:*301, 1983.

30. Howerth, E.W.: Fatal soft tissue calcification in suckling puppies. J. S. Afr. Vet. Assoc., 54:21, 1983.
31. Hubbard, G.B., et al.: Effects of hyperparathyroidism and dietary calcium supplementation on bone healing. Am. J. Vet. Res., 40:288, 1979.
32. Jacob, A.I., et al.: Reversal of secondary hyperparathyroidism by cimetidine in chronically uremic dogs. J. Clin. Invest., 67:1753, 1981.
33. Johnson, J.T.: Pseudohyperparathyroidism associated with metastatic adenocarcinoma of undetermined origin in the dog. J. Am. Vet. Med. Assoc., 173:82, 1978.
34. Kaufman, C.F., Soirez, R.F., and Tasker, J.P.: Renal cortical hypoplasia with secondary hyperparathyroidism in the dog. J. Am. Vet. Med. Assoc., 155:1679, 1969.
35. Klopper, P.J., and Moe, R.E.: Demonstration of the parathyroids during surgery in dogs, with preliminary report of results in some clinical cases. Surgery, 59:1101, 1966.
36. Krook, L.: Spontaneous hyperparathyroidism in the dog. A pathologic-anatomical study. Acta Pathol. Microbiol. Scand., 41:1, 1957.
37. Krook, L., et al.: Reversibility of nutritional osteoporosis: physicochemical data on bones from an experimental study in dogs. J. Nutr., 101:233, 1971.
38. Krook, L., Olsson, S.E., and Rooney, J.R.: Thyroid carcinoma in the dog. A case of bone metastasizing thyroid carcinoma simulating hyperparathyroidism. Cornell Vet., 50:106, 1960.
39. Legendre, A.M., Merkley, D.F., and Carrig, C.B.: Primary hyperparathyroidism in a dog. J. Am. Vet. Med. Assoc., 168:694, 1976.
40. Lewis, L.D., and Morris, M.L.: Feline urologic syndrome: causes and clinical management. Vet. Med. Small Anim. Clin., 79:323, 1984.
41. Nafe, L.A., Patnaik, A.K., and Lyman, R.: Hypercalcemia associated with epidermal carcinoma in a dog. J. Am. Vet. Med. Assoc., 176:1253, 1980.
42. Norrdin, R.W., et al.: Observations on calcium metabolism, [47]CA absorption, and duodenal calcium-binding activity in chronic renal failure: studies in beagles with radiation-induced nephropathy. Am. J. Vet. Res., 41:510, 1980.
43. Norrdin, R.W., and Powers, B.E.: Bone changes in hypercalcemia of malignancy in dogs. J. Am. Vet. Med. Assoc., 183:441, 1983.
44. MacEwen, E.G., and Siegel, S.D.: Hypercalcemia. A paraneoplastic disease. Vet. Clin. North Am., 7:187, 1977.
45. Meuten, D.J., et al.: Hypercalcemia associated with malignancy in dogs. Proceedings of the 6th Kal Kan Symposium, p. 95, 1982.
46. Meuten, D.J., et al.: Hypercalcemia of malignancy: hypercalcemia associated with an adenocarcinoma of the apocrine glands of the anal sac. Am. J. Pathol., 108:366, 1982.
47. Meuten, D.J., et al.: Hypercalcemia associated with an adenocarcinoma derived from the apocrine glands of the anal sac. Vet. Pathol., 18:454, 1981.
48. Meuten, D.J., et al.: Gastric carcinoma with pseudohyperparathyroidism in a horse. Cornell Vet., 68:179, 1978.
49. Miller, S.: Squamous cell carcinoma in the stomach of a pony with hypercalcemia. Vet. Med. Small Anim. Clin., 78:1891, 1983.
50. Morris, M.L., Teeter, S.M., and Collins, D.R.: The effects of the exclusive feeding of an all-meat dog food. J. Am. Vet. Med. Assoc., 158:477, 1971.
51. Morrison, W.B.: Paraneoplastic syndromes of the dog. J. Am. Vet. Med. Assoc., 175:559, 1979.
52. Mundy, G.R., et al.: The hypercalcemia of cancer: clinical implications and pathogenic mechanisms. N. Engl. J. Med., 310:1718, 1984.
53. Osborne, C.A., et al.: Renal lymphoma in the dog and cat. J. Am. Vet. Med. Assoc., 158:2058, 1971.
54. Osborne, C.A., and Stevens, J.B.: Pseudohyperparathyroidism in the dog. J. Am. Vet. Med. Assoc., 162:125, 1973.
55. Patnaik, A.K., et al.: Mediastinal parathyroid adenocarcinoma in a dog. Vet. Pathol., 15:55, 1978.
56. Pearson, P.T., et al.: Primary hyperparathyroidism in a beagle. J. Am. Vet. Med. Assoc., 147:1201, 1965.
57. Pedersen, N.C.: Nutritional secondary hyperparathyroidism in a cattery associated with the feeding of a fad diet containing horsemeat. Feline Pract., 13:19, 1983.
58. Peterson, M.E., et al.: Multiple endocrine neoplasia in a dog. J. Am. Vet. Med. Assoc., 180:1476, 1982.

59. Price, D.A.: Dogs need more than meat. J. Am. Vet. Med. Assoc., *156:*681, 1970.
60. Rijnberk, A.: Pseudohyperparathyroidism in the dog. Tijdschr. Diergenesskd., *95:*575, 1970.
61. Rijnberk, A., et al.: Pseudohyperparathyroidism associated with perirectal adenocarcinomas in elderly female dogs. Tijdschr. Diergenesskd., *103:*1069, 1978.
62. Riser, W.H., Brodey, R.S., and Shirer, J.F.: Osteodystrophy in mature cats: a nutritional disease. J. Am. Vet. Rad. Soc., *9:*37, 1968.
63. Rowland, G.N., Capen, C.C., and Nagode, L.A.: Experimental hyperparathyroidism in young cats. Pathol. Vet., *5:*605, 1968.
64. Rutherford, W.E., et al.: Phosphate control and 25-hydroxycholecalciferol administration in preventing experimental renal osteodystrophy in the dog. J. Clin. Invest., *60:*332, 1977.
65. Saville, P.D., et al.: Nutritional secondary hyperparathyroidism in a dog. Morphologic and radioisotope studies with treatment. Cornell Vet., *59:*155, 1969.
66. Scott, P.P., Greaves, J.P., and Scott, M.G.: Nutrition of the cat. 4. Calcium and iodine deficiency on a meat diet. Br. J. Nutr., *15:*35, 1961.
67. Siegel, E.T., Larsen, A.S., and Galvin, C.: Clinicopathologic conference. Lymphosarcoma stimulating hyperparathyroidism. J. Am. Vet. Med. Assoc., *158:*244, 1971.
68. Siemering, B.: Metabolic bone diseases of the dog and cat. Compendium on Continuing Educ. for the Practicing Vet., *1:*544, 1979.
69. Starron, D.: Beitrag zum Hyperparathyroidismus des Hundes. Dtsch. Tierarztl. Wchnschr., *75:*117, 1968.
70. Thompson, K.G., et al.: Primary hyperparathyroidism in German shepherd dogs: a disorder of probable genetic origin. Vet. Pathol., *21:*370, 1984.
71. Turnwald, G.H.: Pseudohyperparathyroidism in a dog caused by lymphosarcoma: a case report. Southwest Vet., *31:*115, 1978.
72. Wallach, J.D.: Nutritional diseases of exotic animals. J. Am. Vet. Med. Assoc., *157:*583, 1970.
73. Watson, A.D.J., and Canfield, P.J.: Renal failure, hyperparathyroidism and hypercalcemia in a dog. Aust. Vet. J., *55:*177, 1979.
74. Weller, R.E.: Paraneoplastic disorders in companion animals. Compendium on Continuing Educ. for the Practicing Vet., *4:*423, 1982.
75. Weller, R.E.: Cancer-associated hypercalcemia in companion animals. Compendium on Continuing Educ. for the Practicing Vet., *6:*639, 1984.
76. Weller, R., Heath, H., and Mundy, G.R.: Etiopathogenesis of malignant hypercalcemia in dogs with lymphosarcoma. New York, Proceedings of Am. Coll. Vet. Intern. Med., p. 111, 1979.
77. Werner, L.L.: Renal secondary hyperparathyroidism, fibrous osteodystrophy, and hypocalcemia in a young dog with end-stage kidney disease. Compendium on Continuing Educ. for the Practicing Vet., *5:*195, 1983.
78. Wilson, J.W., et al.: Primary hyperparathyroidism in a dog. J. Am. Vet. Med. Assoc., *164:*942, 1974.
79. Wilson, R.B., and Branstad, D.C.: Hypercalcemia associated with nasal adenocarcinoma in a dog. J. Am. Vet. Med. Assoc., *182:*1246, 1983.
80. Yarrington, J.T., Hoffman, W., and Macy, D.: Pseudohyperparathyroidism. An animal model of hypercalcemia associated with lymphosarcoma in dogs. Am. J. Pathol., *89:*531, 1977.
81. Yarrington, J.T., et al.: Morphologic characteristics of the parathyroid and thyroid glands and serum immunoreactive parathyroid hormone in dogs with pseudohyperparathyroidism. Am. J. Vet. Res., *42:*271, 1981.
82. Zenoble, R.D., Crowell, W.A., and Rowland, G.N.: Adenocarcinoma and hypercalcemia in a dog. Vet. Pathol., *16:*122, 1979.
83. Zenoble, R.D., and Rowland, G.N.: Hypercalcemia and proliferative, myelosclerotic bone reaction associated with feline leukovirus infection in a cat. J. Am. Vet. Med. Assoc., *175:*591, 1979.

11

Hypoparathyroidism

Hypoparathyroidism is an endocrine disorder characterized by hypocalcemia and, frequently, hyperphosphatemia. Hypocalcemia leads to presenting complaints of muscular spasms and convulsions. The degree of hypocalcemia can be life-threatening. Hypoparathyroidism may be caused by a deficiency of parathyroid hormone (PTH), target cell resistance, or ineffective circulating PTH.

HYPOPARATHYROIDISM ASSOCIATED WITH DEFICIENCY OF PARATHYROID HORMONE

Pathogenesis

Partial or complete deficiency of PTH may be transient or permanent. Possible causes for PTH deficiency are listed in Table 11–1. The most commonly reported spontaneous cause in the dog is *lymphocytic parathyroiditis* (idiopathic hypoparathyroidism), which is presumed to be an autoimmune disease. Identical histologic lesions in the parathyroids have been experimentally produced in dogs by repeated injections of homologous parathyroid tissue. A similar hypoparathyroidism in humans is familial, sex-linked to male patients, and often associated with hypoadrenocorticism, hypogonadism, diabetes mellitus, hypothyroidism, and moniliasis. Familial hypoparathyroidism or hypoparathyroid-associated endocrinopathies have not been reported in the dog.

Small breeds, such as toy poodles, miniature schnauzers, and various small terriers, have the greatest incidence of canine hypoparathyroidism. It is most common in 2-to-8 (average, 5.5)-year-old female dogs.

Agenesis of the parathyroids has been reported in puppies. In humans, agenesis of the parathyroids is often associated with agenesis of the thymus, a condition called DiGeorge's syndrome. If this occurs in companion animals, they would likely die early in neonatal life. Death would result from either infections or hypocalcemia.

The only reported cause for hypoparathyroidism in cats is iatrogenic destruction of the parathyroid glands associated with surgery of the neck. Unintentional postsurgical hypoparathyroidism can be temporary or permanent, depending on the extent of parathyroid damage.

Table 11–1. Possible Causes for Parathyroid Hormone Deficiency

Iatrogenic (radiation or surgical) destruction of parathyroids
Parathyroid agenesis or hypoplasia (dysembryogenesis)
Lymphocytic parathyroiditis
Magnesium deficiency
Nonfunctional parathyroid neoplasia
Parathyroid atrophy from prolonged calcium or vitamin D therapy
Viral-induced (canine distemper)

Clinical Signs

Most clinical signs of hypoparathyroidism are directly related to the resulting hypocalcemia (Table 11–2). Some signs of hypocalcemia (tetanic convulsions, muscle fasciculations, spasms, weakness, and pain) can resemble those of idiopathic epilepsy or cervical disk disease (Fig. 11–1). These, plus nervousness, restlessness, and abdominal pain, can temporarily subside after treatment with anticonvulsants, muscle relaxants, or analgesics. Temporary satisfactory response to these medications can reinforce an erroneous diagnosis of epilepsy or disk disease. Because of the hair coat in animals, muscle fasciculations affecting the tongue can be seen most easily.

Behavioral changes reported in hypoparathyroid dogs have included groaning, circling, disorientation, hyperexcitability, startle reactions, and aggressiveness. Electroencephalographic changes may occur with hypoparathyroidism, but these are not necessarily corrected by normalizing the serum calcium concentration. Numbness and paresthesia of the face and extremities have occurred in affected humans. Paresthesia of the face has been suspected in affected dogs preoccupied with face rubbing.

Two classic clinical tests for latent hypocalcemic tetany in humans have not been well evaluated in companion animals. One is Chvostek's sign, a spasm of the facial muscles induced by gentle tapping on the facial nerve. The other, the Trousseau sign, is a spasm in an extremity to which a tourniquet has been applied.

Table 11–2. Signs and Effects of Hypocalcemia Noted in Companion Animals

Focal or generalized muscle fasciculations
Muscle spasms leading to hyperthermia, weakness, and pain
Cataracts
Nervousness and restlessness, confusion, irrational behavior, or depression
Abdominal pain
Anorexia, vomiting, and constipation
Tachycardia
Prolonged QT on ECG (corrected for heart rate)
Diaphragmatic contractions synchronous with the heart beat
Tetanic convulsions
Laryngeal stridor and death from laryngeal spasm

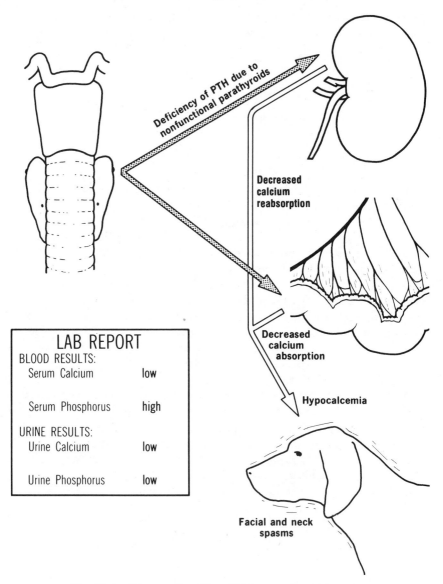

LAB REPORT

BLOOD RESULTS:

Serum Calcium	low
Serum Phosphorus	high

URINE RESULTS:

Urine Calcium	low
Urine Phosphorus	low

Deficiency of PTH due to nonfunctional parathyroids

Decreased calcium reabsorption

Decreased calcium absorption

Hypocalcemia

Facial and neck spasms

Fig. 11–1.   Hypoparathyroidism. PTH = parathyroid hormone.

Clinical signs of hypocalcemia are usually absent until the total serum calcium level goes below 7 mg/dl. Even then, the ionized calcium level, which is not generally clinically determined, more directly parallels the onset and degree of clinical signs. For instance, alkalosis deionizes serum calcium levels. In association with respiratory alkalosis from hyperventilation, or the administration of alkalinizing agents such as sodium bicarbonate, clinical signs of hypocalcemia can occur when the serum calcium levels are above 7 mg/dl. Additionally, hyperkalemia potentiates hypocalcemic tetany and can cause signs of hypocalcemia at total serum calcium levels that exceed 7 mg/dl. Conversely, total serum levels of calcium can be abnormally low with normal levels of ionized serum calcium if the low levels of total serum calcium are caused by low levels of serum albumin.

Cataracts have occurred in hypoparathyroid dogs with histories of prolonged hypocalcemia. The cataracts appear as small, white, punctate, and linear opacities in the anterior and posterior subcapsular areas. Once formed, the cataracts do not resolve with normalized serum calcium levels.

An uncommon clinical manifestation of hypocalcemia is diaphragmatic contractions synchronous with the heart beats. Other factors leading to its occurrence are hypokalemia, hypochloremia, alkalosis, or phrenic nerve trauma. Urinary calcium loss, hypokalemia, hypochloremia, and alkalosis are effects of calcium-depleting diuretics such as furosemide. The administration of furosemide to a patient with yet undiagnosed hypoparathyroidism is likely to result in signs of hypocalcemic tetany, including diaphragmatic contractions synchronous with the heart beats.

Some clinical signs of hypoparathyroid humans have not been noted in companion animals. Among these are defects of the dental enamel; alopecia; brittle nails; scaly skin; soft tissue mineralization of the skin, muscle, and basal ganglia; and papilledema with increased intracranial pressure.

See also reference 6 and 9.

Laboratory Findings and Diagnosis

The hallmark of hypoparathyroidism is hypocalcemia (less than 8.5 mg/dl) and hyperphosphatemia (more than 5 mg/dl in adults). When interpreting the upper limit of serum phosphorus levels, one should remember that the normal range in pups and kittens (less than 18 months of age) is as high as 9 mg/dl and that phosphorus is retained in renal diseases associated with a decreased glomerular filtration rate. Causes for hypocalcemia other than hypoparathyroidism are listed in Table 11-3.[1, 2, 5, 7, 17 19, 21]

Table 11-3. Possible Causes for Hypocalcemia Other than Hypoparathyroidism

Hypoalbuminemia
Acute necrotizing pancreatitis
Chronic renal disease
Puerperal tetany in dogs and cats
Hypercalcitoninism
Ethylene glycol or oxalate toxicity
Intravenous phosphate infusion or phosphate enemas
Lactation tetany in mares
Blister beetle toxicosis in horses
Vitamin D deficiency
Mithramycin

Hypoalbuminemia is the most common cause for abnormally low serum calcium levels. It does not affect ionized calcium levels. If hypoalbuminemia is the sole cause for hypocalcemia in a patient, it is not associated with hypocalcemic tetany. Common causes for hypoalbuminemia are intestinal malabsorption, especially lymphangiectasia; hepatic cirrhosis; glomerulonephritis; and hookworm infection. Acute necrotizing pancreatitis can cause hypocalcemia by saponification of peripancreatic fat, hypomagnesemia, and secondarily induced hypercalcitoninism. Chronic renal disease leads to hypocalcemia by decreased activation of vitamin D and hyperphosphatemia-induced hypocalcemia. Hyperphosphatemia-induced hypocalcemia can also result from intravenous infusions of phosphate or phosphate enemas. Puerperal tetany in dogs and cats and lactation tetany in mares are caused, at least in part, by maternal depletion of calcium through losses in the production of milk.[1, 2, 5, 21]

Hypercalcitoninism from medullary carcinomas of the thyroid can produce hypocalcemia by facilitating urinary loss of calcium and inhibition of osteolysis. Ingestion of ethylene glycol (antifreeze) or oxalate-containing vegetation can form a complex with serum calcium and cause hypocalcemia in small companion animals and horses, respectively. Blister beetles (Epicauta) contain a hypocalcemia-producing toxin, cantharidin. The beetles are found in grasshopper-infested hay, where they eat the grasshopper eggs. Horses that eat blister beetles with their hay can develop hypocalcemia. Vitamin D deficiency is an unlikely cause of hypocalcemia unless multiple causes occur concurrently. Such combinations of causes can include dietary deficiency, intestinal malabsorption, seclusion from sunlight, and impaired activation of vitamin D caused by glucocorticoids, phenobarbital, phenytoin, severe liver disease, or severe kidney disease. Mithramycin can cause hypocalcemia by inhibition of osteolysis.

After eliminating other possible causes of hypocalcemia by review of the patient's history and gathering an initial laboratory data base (Table 11–4), confirmation of hypoparathyroidism should be sought. Hypoparathyroidism is characterized by an inappropriately low plasma PTH level in relation to the simultaneously low serum calcium level (Table 11–5). After treatment for the hypocalcemia, exploration of the parathyroid and biopsy may be considered to aid in the diagnosis of PTH-deficient hypoparathyroidism.

See also references 3, 4, 7, 8, 10, 11, 15, 16, 18, and 20.

Table 11–4.   Laboratory Tests for Suspected Hypoparathyroidism

Serum calcium, phosphorus, and magnesium
Urine calcium and phosphorus
Routine urinalysis
Plasma protein determination
BUN (blood urea nitrogen)

Table 11–5. Differential Laboratory Tests and Results for Hypocalcemia

Causes for Hypocalcemia	Serum Calcium	Serum Phosphorus	Plasma PTH*	Serum Alkaline Phosphatase
Hypoparathyroidism	Decreased	Increased	Decreased	Normal or decreased
Secondary hyperparathyroidism				
Intestinal malabsorption	Decreased or normal	Decreased	Normal or increased	Increased
Nutritional deficiencies	Decreased or normal	Decreased	Normal or increased	Increased
Chronic renal failure	Decreased or normal	Increased or normal	Increased	Increased
Acute pancreatitis	Decreased	Normal	Increased or normal	Normal
Hypomagnesemia	Decreased	Increased	Decreased or normal	Normal

*PTH = parathyroid hormone.

HYPOPARATHYROIDISM ASSOCIATED WITH EXCESSIVE LEVELS OF PARATHYROID HORMONE
(Pseudohypoparathyroidism)

Circulating levels of PTH may be normal or in excess but without biologic effect. This may occur because the target cells are unresponsive or because the PTH is ineffective. Neither condition has been documented in companion animals.

In humans, the unresponsive state of target cell receptors may be due to deficiencies of action or number of the cell receptors *Pseudohypoparathyroidism Type I)*, or to abnormal intracellular response *(Pseudohypoparathyroidism Type II)*. Also, abnormal PTH formation has been reported. Although abnormal PTH molecules may be detected by PTH assays, they are not biologically active. Caution should be exercised in making the diagnosis of pseudohyperparathyroidism because magnesium deficiency, vitamin D deficiency, hypercalcitoninism, excess glucocorticoids, and mithramycin each may impair the action of PTH by various means, leading to relative hypoparathyroidism.

Pseudohypoparathyroidism in humans is an inherited disorder, X-linked dominant with incomplete penetrance. Mental retardation and characteristic somatic features accompany the lack of PTH responsiveness. These features include a round face, short neck, short fourth and fifth metacarpals, and subcutaneous calcification. In pseudo-pseudohypoparathyroidism, the somatic features of pseudohypoparathyroidism are not accompanied by hypocalcemia because of an intermittent PTH refractory state, probably as a result of incomplete expression of pseudohypoparathyroidism I. Although pseudohypoparathyroidism and pseudo-pseudohypoparathyroidism have not yet been reported in companion animals, their possibility should be considered if developmental defects display somatic features similar to those features seen in affected humans.

If the determination of plasma PTH levels or exploration and biopsy of the parathyroids do not confirm that the hypoparathyroidism is caused by a deficiency in PTH, nor that the parathyroids are atrophied, hypomagnesemia or pseudohypoparathyroidism should be considered. If serum magnesium levels are normal, pseudohypoparathyroidism should be confirmed by evaluating the patient's and a normal control animal's responsiveness to PTH injections (the Ellsworth-Howard test). Both animals should remain on a similar diet with equal amounts of phosphorus for several days before the test.

After collecting three random urine samples to measure phosphorus levels, PTH (Parathyroid Injection USP) should be given in an intravenous dose of 200 U every 6 hours for 24 hours. Empty the urinary bladder before the last injection. Collect hourly urine samples 3 to 5 times to determine phosphorus levels after the last injection of PTH. The normal control animal's urinary phosphorus concentration should increase more than two- to threefold. If the patient's urinary phosphorus concentration is less than double its baseline levels, its PTH target cells are refractory. If the patient's urinary phosphorus concentration increases to a much greater extent than does that of the normal control animal, perhaps ten times its baseline level, it is likely that the endogenous PTH is an ineffective molecule. Similar evaluations using urinary cyclic adenosine monophosphate (cAMP) in place of urinary phosphorus concentrations might also be useful.

TREATMENT OF HYPOPARATHYROIDISM

Parathyroid hormone is available commercially, but its use is limited to diagnostic purposes and treatment of acute hypocalcemia. This is because of its poor availability, cost, short duration of action, and immunogenicity. Because of these problems, intravenous preparations of calcium are generally used for the treatment of acute hypocalcemia and the emergency treatment of severe hypocalcemia. Pharmacologic doses of vitamin D and oral doses of calcium are generally used to maintain normal levels of serum calcium in subjects with chronic hypoparathyroidism. If hypoparathyroidism is caused by trauma or surgery, asymptomatic hypocalcemia should be monitored for several weeks before treatment is initiated. Since accessory parathyroid tissue is common, premature treatment with calcium and vitamin D may impair or prevent compensatory hypertrophy of remaining parathyroid tissues.

See also references 7, 8, 12, 13, and 18.

Acute or Severe Hypocalcemia

Numerous parenteral preparations of calcium for intravenous use are commercially available for emergency treatment of hypocalcemia (Table 11–6). Because of their potentially hazardous effects on the cardiovascular system and because of their differences in available calcium (per ml), caution is advised. The treatment of choice for initial management of hypocalcemic seizures or tetany is 10% calcium gluconate, given in doses of

Table 11–6. Common Calcium Preparations for Parenteral and Oral Therapy

Parenteral preparations	Approximate mg calcium/ml
10% Calcium gluconate	9
10% Calcium levulinate	14
23% Calcium gluceptate	18
10% Calcium chloride	27
Oral preparations	Approximate mg calcium/g
Calcium gluconate	90
Calcium levulinate	130
Calcium lactate	130
Calcium chloride	270
Calcium carbonate	400

approximately 1 ml/kg body weight, up to a total of 10 ml. The administration should be a slow intravenous infusion over 15 to 30 minutes. The heart rate should be monitored during the infusion, preferably by ECG. If bradycardia, an elevated ST segment in lead II, or a prolonged QT interval occurs, the infusion should be temporarily discontinued. Rapid infusion, of calcium chloride especially, can also cause vasodilation through inducing metabolic acidosis and serious hypotension. After completing the injection and monitoring the patient's response, the serum calcium levels should be determined.

A single injection of intravenous calcium usually lasts only a few hours before symptoms reappear in hypoparathyroid patients; therefore, continued intravenous infusion is generally necessary at a slower rate with 20 to 30 ml of 10% calcium gluconate/L of 5% dextrose. The rate should be adjusted to maintain normal or near-normal serum calcium levels or detectable calcium in the urine by the Sulkowitch test. Oral calcium and a preparation of vitamin D for maintenance should be begun as soon as the patient can safely be administered oral medication.

Some situations that require calcium infusion warrant special considerations. Calcium binds more easily to protein, phosphates, citrate, or bicarbonate in an alkaline environment. Alkalinizing solutions should never be mixed with calcium because of the formation and precipitation of calcium bicarbonate. Treatment of hypocalcemic patients with alkalinizing solutions should be withheld until the hypocalcemia is corrected.

Calcium potentiates the effects of cardiac glycosides. Extreme caution should be exercised when administering intravenous calcium to digitalized patients.

Chronic Hypocalcemia

The treatment of chronic hypocalcemia from hypoparathyroidism involves the oral administration of pharmacologic doses of a preparation of vitamin D and supplementation of ingested calcium. Oral calcium supplements vary in the concentration of calcium per gram (Table 11–6). Calcium carbonate has the advantage that the ingestion of less than one fourth of a gram is equivalent to the same supplement of elemental calcium as 1 g of calcium gluconate. Usually 50 to 75 mg of elemental calcium/kg body weight/day is adequate for supplementation. For a 10-kg dog, this would be 1.25 to 1.88 g of calcium carbonate or 5.6 to 8.3 g of calcium gluconate per day. Daily doses should be divided into three to four administrations per day.

In the absence of PTH, vitamin D can facilitate sufficient intestinal absorption of calcium to raise serum calcium levels to acceptable levels near 9 mg/dl. But because PTH is necessary for normal hydroxylation of vitamin D_2, the vitamin D_2 must be initially administered in megadoses (250 to 500 times normal dietary requirements) to correct hypocalcemia resulting from hypoparathyroidism. Vitamin D_2-ergocalciferol (Calciferol, Disdol, and

Deltalin), is usually administered orally to hypoparathyroid dogs in daily doses of 25,000 to 50,000 U (0.625 to 1.25 mg)/day until serum levels of calcium are 9 mg/dl. Then the dose is reduced by 50% and administered two to three times per week or as necessary to maintain a serum calcium near 9 mg/dl.

Dihydrotachysterol (DHT and Hytakerol) is not as dependent on PTH as is vitamin D_2 for adequate hydroxylation. Dihydrotachysterol is generally three times more effective per mg than vitamin D_2. In hypoparathyroidism, it may even be more than three times more effective than vitamin D_2. Dihydrotachysterol's biologic activity is considered to be intermediate between 25, hydroxy D_3 and 1,25 dihydroxy D_3. Recommended dosage for dihydrotachysterol is 0.03 mg/kg body weight/day for 2 days, then 0.02 mg/kg body weight for 2 days, then 0.01/kg body weight/day, adjusted as necessary to maintain the serum calcium level near 9 mg/dl. Daily administration is not usually necessary after desirable serum calcium levels are attained. Administration once or twice per week may be sufficient. The oral solution of dihydrotachysterol permits more convenient adjustment of the dose in small companion animals than is possible with tablets and capsules.

Calcifediol (Calderol) is synthesized 25, hydroxy-D_3. It requires the presence of PTH for hydroxylation to 1,25 dihydroxy D_3. It is less effective per mg and less safe than dihydrotachysterol. It is more expensive than vitamin D_2 or dihydrotachysterol.

Calcitriol (Rocaltrol) is synthesized 1,25 dihydroxy D_3, the most potent form of vitamin D. Its efficacy in the treatment of hypoparathyroidism is presumably identical to that seen during treatment with vitamin D_2 and dihydrotachysterol. Calcitriol's safety is greater than that of vitamin D_2 and dihydrotachysterol because of its short serum half-life, but its expense is much greater than the alternative therapeutics.

Regardless of the form of vitamin D used to treat hypoparathyroidism, all forms of vitamin D can cause hypercalcemia and mineralization of soft tissues if overdosed. The risk of soft tissue mineralization is thought to parallel the calculated value of the product of serum calcium times serum phosphorus. When this product reaches 70, soft tissue mineralization and hypercalcemic nephropathy are likely. Unfortunately, therapy with vitamin D raises levels of both serum calcium and phosphorus.

The goals of treatment are to prevent hypocalcemic seizures and tetany while avoiding hypercalcemia and soft tissue mineralization. To achieve these goals the serum calcium should be maintained between 8 to 10 mg/dl, and the product of calcium times phosphorus should be maintained at less than 70 if possible. The approximate times required to stabilize the serum calcium with various vitamin D products and the time required to relieve toxicity in humans are listed in Table 11–7. Owners should be instructed to watch for signs of polyuria, which would suggest developing hypercalcemic nephropathy. Since estrogens augment the activity of 1 α-hydroxylase, fluctuating serum estrogen levels could alter the response to vitamin D; there-

Table 11–7. Approximate Times Required With Vitamin D Therapy to Stabilize the Serum Calcium in Hypoparathyroidism and to Relieve Toxicity in Humans

Product	Treatment Time Required to Stabilize Serum Calcium	Withdrawal Time Required to Relieve Hypercalcemia
Vitamin D_2	4 weeks	6 weeks
Dihydrotachysterol	10 days	2 weeks
Calcifediol	3 weeks	4 weeks
Calcitriol	4 days	1 week

fore, ovariectomy (ovariohysterectomy) is advisable for affected sexually intact female dogs.

In addition to supplementation with calcium and the administration of a preparation of vitamin D, other means of managing chronic hypoparathyroidism include avoidance of foods high in phosphorus such as milk and cheese. A nutritionally balanced, low phosphorus diet for dogs and cats is commercially available (Prescription Diet k/d). Furosemide and other less common calcium-depleting diuretics should be avoided. Aluminum hydroxide gels to bind dietary phosphorus may be useful if serum calcium is less than 12 mg/dl and phosphorus levels are elevated.

Thiazides decrease calcium excretion in urine and increase serum calcium. Thiazides are most often used as diuretics because they inhibit sodium reabsorption in the renal tubules. If a thiazide is administered and dietary sodium intake is decreased, the retention of sodium and calcium in serum is enhanced. This can cause iatrogenic hypercalcemia in normal patients or hypoparathyroid patients already being treated with pharmacologic doses of vitamin D.

This hypercalcemic effect of thiazides has been used to treat hypocalcemia without using pharmacologic doses of vitamin D. Administration of a thiazide-like sulfonamide diuretic (chlorthalidone) and a low-sodium diet has been successful in normalizing the serum calcium of hypoparathyroid persons without some of the side effects, such as the nephroliths that may result from pharmacologic doses of vitamin D.[14] The effectiveness of chlorthalidone and therapy using the low dietary intake of sodium has not yet been evaluated in companion animals.

Iatrogenic Hypercalcemia

Overzealous administration of vitamin D or its isomers can lead to metastatic calcification of soft tissues, renal damage, acute pancreatitis, or even fatal cardiac dysrhythmia. Treatment of iatrogenic hypercalcemia consists of withdrawing treatment using calcium and vitamin D and placing the patient on a low-calcium diet. Acute or life-threatening hypercalcemia should be treated with furosemide and normal saline diuresis to promote calcium excretion in the urine, and glucocorticoids to inhibit hydroxylation of vitamin D. Thiazide diuretics should be strictly avoided since they promote the reabsorption of renal calcium.

REFERENCES

1. Austad, R., and Bjerkas, E.: Eclampsia in the bitch. J. Small Anim. Pract., *17:*793, 1976.
2. Bjerkas, E.: Eclampsia in the cat. J. Small Anim. Pract., *15:*411, 1974.
3. Bovee, K.C., Crabtree, B.J., and Steinberg, S.: Idiopathic hormone-deficient hypoparathyroidism in dogs. Proceedings of Am. Coll. Vet. Intern. Med., p. 110, 1980.
4. Burk, R.L., and Schaubhut, C.W.: Spontaneous primary hypoparathyroidism in a dog. J. Am. Anim. Hosp. Assoc., *11:*784, 1975.
5. Edney, A.T.B.: Lactation tetany in the cat. J. Small Anim. Pract., *10:*231, 1969.
6. Kirk, G.R., Breazile, J.E., and Kenny, A.D.: Pathogenesis of hypocalcemic tetany in the thyroparathyroidectomized dog. Am. J. Vet. Res., *35:*407, 1974.
7. Kornegay, J.N.: Hypocalcemia in dogs. Compendium on Continuing Educ. for the Practicing Vet., *4:*103, 1982.
8. Kornegay, J.N., et al.: Idiopathic hypocalcemia in four dogs. J Am. Anim. Hosp. Assoc., *18:*723, 1980.
9. Kunze, R., and Wingfield, W.E.: ECG of the month. Hypocalcemia. J. Am. Vet. Med. Assoc., *174:*1080, 1979.
10. McKelvey, D., and Post, K.: Hypocalcemia in a dog. Can. Vet. J., *24:*214, 1983.
11. Meyer, D.J., and Terell, T.G.: Idiopathic hypoparathyroidism in a dog. J. Am. Vet. Med. Assoc., *168:*858, 1976.
12. Neuman, N.B.: Acute pancreatic hemorrhage associated with iatrogenic hypercalcemia in a dog. J. Am. Vet. Med. Assoc., *166:*381, 1975.
13. Peterson, M.E.: Treatment of canine and feline hypoparathyroidism. J. Am. Vet. Med. Assoc., *181:*1434, 1982.
14. Porter, R.H., et al.: Treatment of hypoparathyroid patients with chlorthalidone. N. Engl. J. Med., *298:*577, 1978.
15. Prieur, W.D.: Hypocalcemic tetany in the dog due to parathyroid disorders. Kleintier Prax, *11:*173, 1966.
16. Resnick, S.: Hypocalcemia and tetany in the dog. Vet. Med. Small Anim. Clin., *67:*637, 1972.
17. Schaer, M., et al.: Iatrogenic hyperphosphatemia, hypocalcemia, and hypernatremia in a cat. J. Am. Anim. Hosp. Assoc., *13:*39, 1977.
18. Sherding, R.G., et al.: Primary hypoparathyroidism in the dog. J. Am. Vet. Med. Assoc., *176:*439, 1980.
19. Thrall, M.A., Grauer, G.F., and Mero, K.N.: Clinicopathologic findings in dogs and cats with ethylene glycol intoxication. J. Am. Vet. Med. Assoc., *184:*37, 1984.
20. Weisbrode, S.E., and Krakowka, S.: Canine distemper virus-associated hypocalcemia. Am. J. Vet. Res., *40:*147, 1979.
21. Wolfersteig, D., Schaer, M., and Kirby, R.: Hypocalcemia, hyperkalemia, and renal failure in a bitch at term pregnancy. J. Am. Anim. Hosp. Assoc., *16:*845, 1980.

12

Vitamin D and Its Hormone Metabolites

Vitamins occur in various foods in small quantities and are necessary for normal intermediary metabolism. Ergosterol and 7-dehydrocholesterol occur in plant and animal food sources, respectively. They are best described as provitamins, being transformed in the body into the metabolites: *vitamins D_2 (ergocalciferol)* and D_3 *(cholecalciferol)*. Vitamin D_1, a substance once thought to be another vitamin D, was found to be a product of vitamin D_2. Vitamins D_2 and D_3 may be taken into the body directly from the diet. They can also be produced in the body by ultraviolet (290 to 320 μ wave length) irradiation of ergosterol or 7-dehydrocholesterol in the skin. Endogenously produced vitamins D_2 and D_3 are released from the skin into the bloodstream and modulate target cell functions, especially after hydroxylation in the liver and the kidney; therefore, D vitamins may be considered vitamins and their hydroxylated metabolites may be considered hormones.

Vitamin D is one of several factors necessary for calcium homeostasis. It and its metabolites increase calcium and phosphorus gastrointestinal absorption and are necessary for normal parathyroid hormone (PTH) action. Excess levels of vitamin D cause metastatic mineralization in soft tissues. A deficiency in D vitamins results in secondary hyperparathyroidism and, eventually, rickets or osteomalacia.

SOURCES, ACTIVATION, AND ACTIONS OF VITAMIN D

Natural dietary sources of vitamin D for the dog and cat come primarily from animal sources (in the form of D_3) such as fish liver oil, animal skin, liver, and eggs. Commercial vitamin D_2 produced by irradiating ergosterol from yeast is added to many foods prepared for animals. Vitamins D_2 and D_3 are absorbed with fat into the lacteals of the intestine and transported to the liver bound to α-globulins. Although the serum half-lives of vitamins D_2 and D_3 are only about 1 day, the D vitamins can be stored for months in the liver or skin.

Endogenously produced vitamin D_2 and D_3 are also transported to the liver by α-globulins. The liver then hydroxylates D_2 and D_3 from either exogenous or endogenous sources to *25, hydroxy D_2 (25, OH-D_2)* and *25, hydroxy D_3 (25, OH-D_3)*. The serum half-life of 25, OH-D_2 and 25, OH-D_3 is more than 2 weeks. Serum concentrations are about 10 to 50 ng/ml, depending on dietary intake and exposure to sunlight. Twenty-five hydroxylated vitamin D metabolites are the most abundant form of vitamin D in the circulation. Serum concentrations of 25, OH-D$_3$ are about 1000 times those of its more potent metabolite 1,25(OH)$_2$-D$_3$.

Further hydroxylation of 25, OH-D$_3$ by *1-α hydroxylase* to the more active *1,25(OH)$_2$-D$_3$* occurs in the kidney. 1 α-Hydroxylase activity is primarily stimulated by low serum levels of phosphorus or high serum levels of PTH. To a lesser degree, prolactin, estradiol, placental lactogen, and growth hormone (GH) also enhance 1 α-hydroxylase activity. These latter stimuli result in higher serum 1,25(OH)$_2$-D$_3$ levels during pregnancy and lactation, which aid in providing calcium sufficient for gestation and the production of milk. When serum calcium is elevated and serum PTH is low, the secretion of 1,25(OH)$_2$-D$_3$ is inhibited and hydroxylation of 25, OH-D$_3$ to relatively inactive metabolites (24,25(OH)$_2$-D$_3$; 25,26(OH)$_2$-D$_3$; and 1,24,25(OH)$_3$-D$_3$) is favored. Normal serum levels of 1,25(OH)$_2$-D$_3$ in dogs are approximately 15 to 35 pg/ml. Factors affecting serum levels of 1,25(OH)$_2$-D$_3$ are listed in Table 12–1.

The most important sites of action of D vitamins are the gastrointestinal tract and the bones. Calcium absorption from the intestines is an active process requiring a calcium-binding protein. Vitamin D induces the secretion of calcium-binding protein from goblet cells and enhances calcium movement across the intestinal wall in both directions. Most calcium absorption occurs in the proximal small intestine. Some of the phosphorus's absorption is dependent on the absorption of calcium, so vitamin D indirectly governs some of the absorption of phosphorus. Most absorption of phosphorus occurs in the distal small intestine.

The effects of vitamin D on bone are not well understood. In small amounts, vitamin D$_2$ promotes the formation of bone. In higher amounts, vitamin D$_2$ increases bone resorption synergistically with parathyroid hormone (PTH) by stimulating osteoclasts and recruiting new osteoclasts. In large amounts, vitamin D$_2$ may have a direct action on bone resorption independent of PTH. The hydroxylated metabolite of vitamin D$_3$, calci-

Table 12–1. Conditions Affecting Serum 1,25(OH)$_2$-D$_3$ Levels

Conditions That May Increase Serum 1,25(OH)$_2$-D$_3$ Levels	Conditions That May Decrease Serum 1,25(OH)$_2$-D$_3$ Levels
Primary hyperparathyroidism	Secondary hyperparathyroidism
Hypothyroidism	Hyperthyroidism
Hypervitaminosis D	Hypoparathyroidism
Pregnancy	Metabolic acidosis
	Glucocorticoid excess
	Calcitonin excess
	Lead intoxication
	Type I vitamin-D-dependent rickets
	Insulin deficiency

triol, when administered in pharmacologic doses, inhibits bone resorption from disuse, presumably by inhibiting the secretion of PTH.[-2]

Although the kidney has renal receptors for vitamin D, vitamin D's promotion of the reabsorption of calcium is a minor aspect of vitamin D's metabolic action. Renal reabsorption of calcium is enhanced by vitamin D_2 in the proximal convoluted tubule. Small doses of vitamin D_2 promote phosphorus reabsorption from the renal tubules, but large doses increase the excretion of phosphorus in the urine. The metabolism and actions of vitamin D are summarized in illustrative form in Fig. 12–1.

Vitamin D_2 and D_3 metabolites are not equipotent. The effects of the same metabolite in different species of animals also can differ. For example,

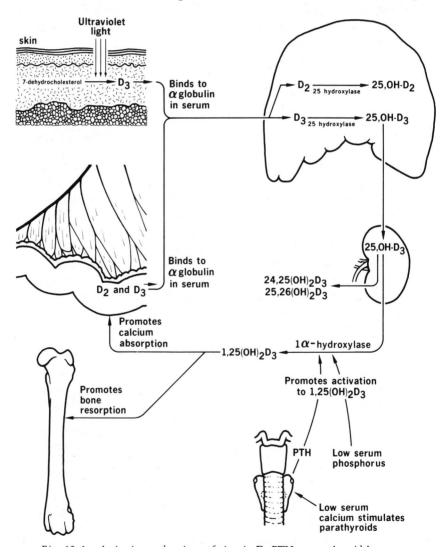

Fig. 12–1. Activation and actions of vitamin D. PTH = parathyroid hormone.

compared to vitamin D_3, vitamin D_2 is relatively inactive in birds and certain New World monkeys.[10, 13] Also, in humans and horses, vitamin D_3 has a greater potential for toxicity than does vitamin D_2, even though vitamin D_2 is generally considered equal on a weight basis in effects to vitamin D_3.[5, 6] The hydroxylated metabolite, 25, OH-D_3, is about 12 times more active than D_3 in stimulating the intestinal absorption of calcium. 1,25(OH)$_2$-D_3 is 100 times more effective than 25, OH-D_3 in promoting the absorption of calcium from the intestines.

See also references 4, 7, 8, 11, and 15.

HYPOVITAMINOSIS D (Rickets)

Minimum dietary requirements for vitamin D in companion animals are low in comparison to what is normally available in their diets. Adult dogs require 11 IU/kg body weight/day; puppies, 22 IU/kg body weight/day; cats, 50 IU/kg body weight/day; and horses, 6.6 IU/kg body weight/day. Most of the requirements for D vitamins are met by ultraviolet irradiation of 7-dehydrocholesterol in the skin, especially between March and October in North America. Storage of vitamin D in the liver and skin has a duration of months. Even circulating intermediate metabolites (25, OH-D_3) persist for weeks. Unless dietary deficiencies are prolonged, occur during growth periods, and are accompanied by confinement without exposure to sunlight, vitamin D deficiency is unlikely in otherwise normal companion animals.

Some disease states and the administration of certain drugs predispose to, and can even directly cause, hypovitaminosis D. Renal diseases can prevent final hydroxylation of 25, OH-D_3 to 1,25(OH)$_2$-D_3, thus contributing to secondary hyperparathyroidism of renal origin.[14] In humans, 50% to 80% of the patients with chronic renal disease are reported to have osteodystrophy. Intestinal malabsorption can prevent the absorption of vitamin D as well as calcium, leading to secondary hyperparathyroidism. But it should be remembered that liver diseases do not present with the signs of secondary hyperparathyroidism, despite impaired hydroxylation of D_3 to 25, OH-D_3, because little 25, OH-D_3 is necessary to serve as a precursor to 1,25(OH)$_2$-D_3 and because of the seriousness of the loss of other important liver functions. Anticonvulsants, especially phenytoin and phenobarbital, reduce the synthesis and enhance the degradation of 25, OH-D_3. Impaired gastrointestinal absorption of calcium and gastrointestinal response to 1,25(OH)$_2$-D_3 have also been implicated as causes of the bone resorption that can develop from anticonvulsant therapy.

Glucocorticoids inhibit 25, OH-D_3 hydroxylation to 1,25(OH)$_2$-D_3, an action that can be useful in treating hypervitaminosis D. One form of vitamin-D-dependent rickets (Type I) occurring in humans is caused by defective 1 α-hydroxylase. It is an autosomal, recessive inherited trait that has not yet been recognized in companion animals.

Regardless of the cause of hypovitaminosis, the pathogenesis of bone disease is the same. The resulting hypocalcemia from hypovitaminosis D stimulates excessive secretion of PTH, a secondary hyperparathyroidism, in an effort to maintain a normal concentration of serum calcium. Secondary hyperparathyroidism can lead to bowing of the legs, enlargement of costochondral junctions, and loosening of the teeth.

See also references 3 and 12.

HYPERVITAMINOSIS D (Vitamin D Intoxication)

Excess ingestion of D vitamins in companion animals is often iatrogenically caused or produced by the owner. The results of oversupplementation can be lethal. Day-blooming jessamine (*Cestrus diurnum*), a house plant that contains vitamin D, could cause hypervitaminosis D in house pets if eaten. Wild jessamine is also a source of hypervitaminosis D in horses in the southern United States.

Hypervitaminosis D produces hypercalcemia and hyperphosphatemia.[5,6] When the product of the calcium and phosphorus levels exceeds 70, metastatic calcification of soft tissues may occur. Most affected are the lungs, heart, wall of large blood vessels, kidneys, and stomach. Clinical signs and laboratory findings of hypervitaminosis D are listed in Tables 12–2 and 12–3. Many are caused by the uremic syndrome associated with hypercalcemic nephropathy.

In women, some carcinomas of the breast have been shown to produce a vitamin-D-like tachysterol, resulting in a pseudohyperparathyroidism hypercalcemic syndrome. The endogenous overproduction of D vitamins or similarly acting sterols has not been recognized in dogs or cats, but some apocrine gland adenocarcinomas of the anal sacs in dogs are thought to stimulate excessive hydroxylation of $25, OH-D_3$ to $1,25(OH)_2-D_3$ by increasing the activity of $1\ \alpha$-hydroxylase.

Treatment of exogenous hypervitaminosis D consists of providing a diet low in vitamin D and ceasing supplementation of vitamin D. Diuresis with sterile saline and furosemide aid in producing calciuria. Glucocorticoids inhibit further hydroxylation of $25, OH-D_3$. Intoxication may last more than 1 month. Unfortunately, most cases are recognized in postmortem examination.

See also references 9 and 16.

Table 12–2. Clinical Signs Associated With Hypervitaminosis D

Vomiting
Diarrhea, sometimes bloody
Limb stiffness
Excess lacrimation
Weight loss
Rapid respiration
Muscular weakness
Anorexia
Cessation of growth
Polyuria-polydipsia
Urinary calculi

Table 12–3.   Laboratory Findings of Hypervitaminosis D

Inconsistent hypercalcemia and persistent hyperphosphatemia
Depressed serum alkaline phosphatase
Isosthenuric urine
Azotemia
Glucosuria

THERAPEUTIC USES OF VITAMIN D

Several oral and parenteral preparations of vitamin D are commercially available for the treatment of hypovitaminosis D and hypoparathyroidism (Table 12–4). Provided there is no problem with the intestinal absorption of fat, the oral route is preferred. Intramuscular injections of vitamin D in oil are poorly absorbed in patients whose intramuscular circulation is impaired by immobility, or hypothermia, or both. Intramuscular injections also preclude critical adjustment of vitamin D dosages when hypercalcemia or other signs of toxicity develop. Vitamin D may need to be administered intramuscularly in severe cases of liver failure or intestinal malabsorption.

Fish oil products, vitamin D_2, and vitamin D_3 are generally considered equipotent. One international unit (IU) or USP unit is equal to 25 ng of crystalline vitamin D (1 μg = 40 units). Dihydrotachysterol USP, an isomer of vitamin D, is three times more potent per mg than vitamin D_2 or D_3. It is more rapid in onset of action and rate of metabolism than vitamin D_2 or vitamin D_3. Dihydrotachysterol is hydroxylated to $25,(OH)_2$-tachysterol in the liver and does not require renal hydroxylation.

Therapy with vitamin D is potentially dangerous. The possibility of inducing hypercalcemia and metastatic calcification is always present. Dosages must be individualized by titration. Titration is complicated by vitamin D's cumulative action and by a lag period of usually 3 to 4 days before absorption, hydroxylation, and target cell metabolic modifications produce a maximum response.

Table 12–4.   Vitamin D Preparations, Relative Potency, and Relative Rates of Maximum Effect

Preparation	Form of Vitamin D	Relative Potency Per Mg	Approximate Days Until Maximum Effect
Fish liver oil	D_3	1	30
Ergocalciferol (Califerol, Drisdol)	D_2	1	30
Cholecalciferol	D_3	1	30
Dihydrotachysterol (DHT)	Dihydrotachysterol	3	15
Calcifediol (Calderol)	25, OH-D_3	15	15
Calcitriol (Rocaltrol)	$1,25(OH)_2$-D_3	2,000	3

Effective doses of vitamin D depend on the condition to be treated. Vitamin-D-deficient rickets caused by an insufficient diet and lack of exposure to sunlight or intestinal malabsorption requires a dosage that is similar to normal daily requirements. However, dosages required to successfully treat hypoparathyroidism are often 100 to 200 times normal daily requirements. For example, a young 10-kg dog with vitamin-D-deficient rickets would require about 200 IU vitamin D_2/day, but a 10-kg dog with hypoparathyroidism would require approximately 20,000 to 40,000 IU/day of vitamin D_2. Although yet unreported in companion animals, the (so-called) vitamin-D-dependency rickets resulting from defective 1 α-hydroxylase (Type I) or target cell resistance to $1,25(OH)_2$-D_3 (Type II) that occurs in humans would require even greater doses of vitamin D_2 than hypoparathyroidism for successful treatment.[1] If calcitriol, synthetic $1,25(OH)_2$-D_3, is used for Type I dependency rickets, only small doses would be necessary. Therapy with vitamin D is also recommended during the initial treatment of osteomalacia or rickets due to renal tubular acidosis. After bone healing is accomplished, vitamin D therapy is not necessary for long-term maintenance, although continued treatment with alkali would be required.

REFERENCES

1. Brooks, M.H., et al.: Vitamin-D dependent rickets type II. Resistance of target organs to 1,25-dihydroxy-vitamin D. N. Engl. J. Med., *298:*996, 1978.
2. Caywood, D.D., et al.: Effects of 1,25-dihydroxycholecalciferol on disuse osteoporosis in the dog: a histomorphometric study. Am. J. Vet. Res., *40:*89, 1979.
3. Gallagher, J.C., and Riggs, B.L.: Current concepts in nutrition. Nutrition and bone disease. N. Engl. J. Med., *298:*193, 1978.
4. Goormaghtigh, N., and Handovsky, H.: Effect of vitamin D (Calciferol) on the dog. Arch. Pathol., *26:*1144, 1938.
5. Harrington, D.D.: Acute vitamin D_2 (ergocalciferol) toxicosis in horses: case report and experimental studies. J. Am. Vet. Med. Assoc., *180:*867, 1982.
6. Harrington, D.D., and Page, E.H.: Acute vitamin D_3 toxicosis in horses: case reports and experimental studies of the comparative toxicity of vitamins D_2 and D_3. J. Am. Vet. Med. Assoc., *182:*1358, 1983.
7. Haussler, M.R., and McCain, T.A.: Basic and clinical concepts related to vitamin D metabolism and action. Part I. N. Engl. J. Med., *297:*974, 1977.
8. Haussler, M.R., and McCain, T.A.: Basic and clinical concepts related to vitamin D metabolism and action. Part II. N. Engl. J. Med., *297:*1041, 1977.
9. Howerth, E.W.: Fatal soft tissue calcification in suckling puppies. J. S. Afr. Assoc., *54:*21, 1983.
10. Hunt, R.D., Garcia, F.G., and Hegsted, D.M.: A comparison of vitamin D_2 and D_3 in New World primates. I. Production and regression of osteodystrophia fibrosa. Lab. Anim. Care, *17:*222, 1967.
11. Juan, D.: Vitamin D metabolism. Update for the clinician. Postgrad. Med., *68:*210, 1980.
12. Krook, L., and Barrett, R.B.: Simian bone disease—a secondary hyperparathyroidism. Cornell Vet., *52:*459, 1962.
13. Lehner, N.D.M., et al.: Biological activities of vitamin D_2 and D_3 for growing squirrel monkeys. Lab. Anim. Care, *17:*483, 1967.
14. Norman, A.W., and Henry, H.: The role of the kidney and vitamin D metabolism in health and disease. Clin. Orthop. Rel. Res., *98:*258, 1974a.
15. Scriver, C.R., et al.: Serum 1,25-dihydroxy-vitamin D levels in normal subjects and in patients with hereditary rickets or bone disease. N. Engl. J. Med., *299:*976, 1978.
16. Spangler, W.L., Gribble, D.H., and Lee, T.C.: Vitamin D intoxication and the pathogenesis of vitamin D nephropathy in the dog. Am. J. Vet. Res., *40:*73, 1979.

Section V

The Pancreatic Islets and Gastrointestinal Hormones

13

The Normal Pancreatic Islets and Tests of Their Function

The pancreatic islets were first described by Paul Langerhans in 1869 as islands of cells within the pancreas. They produce at least four peptide hormones in adult animals: insulin, glucagon, somatostatin, and pancreatic polypeptide (PP). Insulin promotes the storage of glycogen, fatty acids, and amino acids, whereas glucagon promotes their mobilization. Insulin lowers the blood glucose level, and glucagon raises it. Somatostatin inhibits the secretion of insulin and glucagon. The function of PP is unknown. The most commonly known endocrine dysfunctions of the pancreas are hyposecretion of insulin (diabetes mellitus) and hypersecretion of insulin (insulin-secreting islet cell tumors, "insulinomas").

REGIONAL ANATOMY

The normal canine and feline pancreas is a "V"-shaped organ in the frontal plane that lies dorsomedial to the descending duodenum and ventrocranial to the transverse colon (Fig. 13–1). It is composed of a thin right (duodenal) lobe and a thicker, wider left (splenic) lobe, which is two thirds as long but 50% wider than the right lobe. Lobes are also called limbs. The angle formed by the two lobes is about 45°. In the 15-kg dog, it is about 20 cm long and weighs approximately 30 g, or 0.23% of the total body weight.

DEVELOPMENT OF THE ISLETS

Islet cells are thought to be derived from the neural crest. After migrating to the duodenal entoderm, the islet cells mature from buds from the pancreatic ducts of the dorsal and ventral pancreatic lobes. Buds from the dorsal pancreatic lobe contain more A cells than F cells, and buds from the ventral pancreatic lobe have more F cells than A cells. During development the terminal connections to the exocrine duct system disappear, leaving the islet cells isolated and separated from the exocrine tissue by reticular fibers. Consequently, the islets are clusters of roughly oval vascular islands of cells in the pancreas without ducts of their own. Islets comprise about 2% of the normal pancreas by weight. Venous drainage is into the portal vein.

See also reference 1.

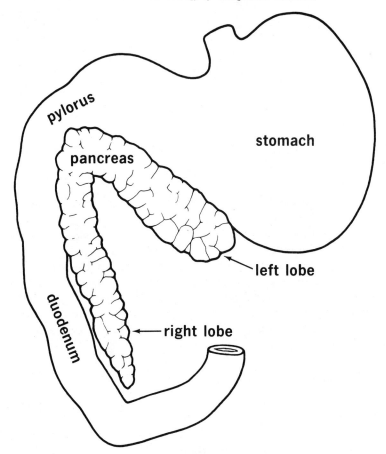

Fig. 13–1. The normal canine pancreas.

ANOMALIES OF THE ISLETS

Accessory pancreatic tissue has occasionally been seen in dogs in the wall of the gallbladder, wall of the small intestines, stomach wall, spleen, omentum, and mesentery. The frequency of accessory pancreatic tissue in dogs and cats has not been reported. Selective islet cell aplasia has been rarely reported in dogs.

STRUCTURE AND FUNCTION OF THE ISLETS

The pancreatic islets in mammals (Fig. 13–2) are composed of several cell types that are tabulated with their secretory products and relative concentrations (Table 13–1). Generally, B cells comprise most of the islets' medulla. A cells form the outer rim, and D cells are concentrated between A and B cells.[11, 13] It is thought that paracrine (local) intercommunications occur between islet cells. For example, insulin inhibits the secretion of

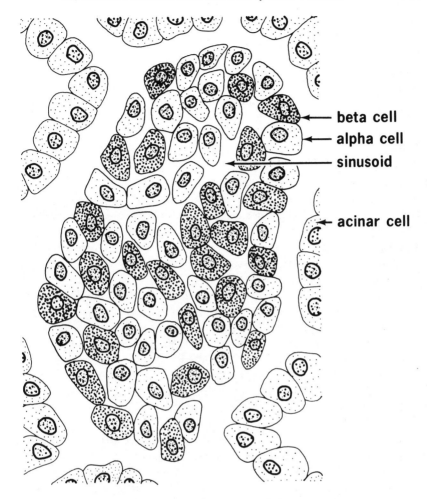

beta cell

alpha cell

sinusoid

acinar cell

Fig. 13–2. Normal islets of Langerhans.

glucagon, which stimulates the secretion of insulin and somatostatin. Somatostatin inhibits the secretion of insulin, glucagon, and pancreatic polypeptides. The right (duodenal) lobe of the pancreas in the dog has relatively few islets and is deficient in A cells, but has some B and F cells. The uncinate ("hooked") process of the human pancreas, an analogue to the canine or feline right pancreatic lobe, is also deficient in A cells. An uncinate process does not exist in the pancreas of dogs or cats. Birds' islets contain more A cells than do mammalian pancreatic islets.

Insulin

Insulin has a special place in the history of endocrine treatments. After its discovery in 1921 by a surgeon (F.G. Banting) and a biochemistry student (C.H. Best), it was the first hormone to have its structure characterized, to

Table 13–1.   Islet Cells in Mammals

Cell Type	Product	Percent
B (β)	Insulin	40–60
A (α)	Glucagon	20–30
D (Δ)	Somatostatin (and gastrin?)	5–15
F (PP)	Pancreatic polypeptide	5–10

be synthesized chemically, and to be measured by radioimmunoassay.[40] Insulin is a polypeptide with a molecular weight of 5733 and is composed of two chains of amino acids linked by disulfide bridges. There are minor structural differences in insulin among most domestic species. Insulin from cattle and pigs is biologically effective in companion animals, but is also immunologically different and weakly antigenic. The structure of insulin in the pig and dog is identical. The structure in cats is presumed similar to that in the dog.

Insulin is first synthesized as *preproinsulin* in the endoplasmic reticulum of the B cell. A fragment consisting of 23 amino acids is removed from the C-terminal, after which the molecule folds to form *proinsulin* (with a molecular weight of 9000), and then the A chain with 21 amino acids and B chain with 30 amino acids are linked by sulfide bridges. Proinsulin is transported to the Golgi complex, where it gains a membrane. Inside the secretory granule the connection between the A and B chain, which has 31 amino acids and is called the C (connecting)-peptide, is removed (Fig. 13–3).

There are considerable differences among C-peptide structures of different species as opposed to the relative lack of differences in the A and B chains of species.[27] At the cell membrane, the secretory granule is expelled by exocytosis. Insulin and C-peptide are released in equimolar amounts. Although the C-peptide is not active, it has a longer half-life, so it exceeds the concentration of insulin in the blood. Normal fasting C-peptide levels in canine serum are about 0.15 to 0.25 pM/ml. Measurements of C-peptide have been used to assess the endogenous secretion of insulin in human patients receiving insulin therapy.

Some proinsulin is also normally secreted. Its activity is about 10% to 15% that of insulin. Functional islet cell tumors may secrete an excess ratio of proinsulin to insulin.

The secretion of insulin is mediated through the cyclic adenosine monophosphate (cAMP) system and requires the presence of calcium, magnesium, and potassium. The secretion of insulin has two phases. The first phase peaks 4 to 5 minutes after the onset of secretion and represents stored insulin ready for release. The second phase peaks in 30 to 60 minutes because it represents the migration of packets and the new synthesis of insulin.

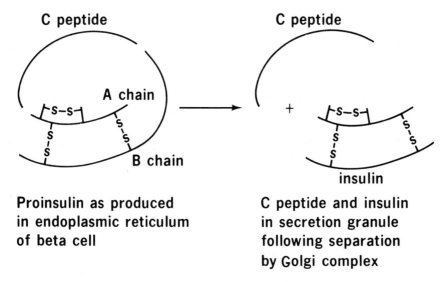

C peptide

A chain

B chain

**Proinsulin as produced
in endoplasmic reticulum
of beta cell**

C peptide

insulin

**C peptide and insulin
in secretion granule
following separation
by Golgi complex**

Fig. 13–3. Formation of insulin.

Insulin-like activity in the blood consists of about 7% immunoreactive insulin (IRI) and of 93% nonspecific insulin-like activity (NSILA). Almost all (95%) of NSILA consists of nonsuppressible, insulin-like protein of unknown origin. About 5% of NSILA is insulin-like growth factors (IGFs), including IGF-I, IGF-II, somatomedin A, and multiplication-stimulating activity. Normal fasting IRI in the peripheral serum of dogs is about 0.078 to 1.0 ng/ml or 5 to 30 μU/ml. Postprandial serum IRI is about 50 to 150 μU/ml. Portal vein IRI is four to eight times as concentrated as peripheral blood IRI. Insulin circulates unbound to plasma proteins and has a half-life of 5 minutes. About 50% of secreted insulin is bound by the liver during the first pass.

Insulin secretion is stimulated by rising or high levels of plasma glucose, which diffuses into B cells of the islets without facilitation by insulin. B cells act as their own glucostats. Less important stimuli for secretion of insulin include several gastrointestinal hormones such as gastric inhibitory polypeptide (GIP), gastrin, secretin, cholecystokinin (CCK), and glicentin; sugars—other than glucose—such as mannose and fructose; other hormones such as progesterone, estrogens, growth hormone, pancreatic glucagon, thyroxine, adrenocorticotropic hormone (ACTH), and cortisol; potassium; right vagal stimulation; ketoacids; amino acids such as leucine and arginine; and several drugs such as theophylline, isoproterenol, phentolamine, and sulfonylureas. GIP is considered the principal postprandial stimulus of gastrointestinal origin for the secretion of insulin. Small surges of insulin secretion normally occur in fasting dogs because of growth hormone (GH)-induced bursts of secretion and spontaneous neural discharges.

The secretion of insulin is decreased by falling or low levels of plasma glucose. Less important inhibitors include somatostatin, epinephrine, norepinephrine, serotonin, angiotensin II, hypothermia, hypokalemia, hypocalcemia, and some drugs such as propranolol, phenformin, diazoxide, thiazide diuretics, and phenytoin. Principal insulin antagonists that protect against hypoglycemia are epinephrine and glucagon. GH and cortisol provide more sustained protection from hypoglycemia.

The actions of insulin include facilitation of the entry of glucose into most cells. Exceptions are red blood cells, brain (except part of the hypothalamus), liver, kidney tubules, intestinal mucosa, and B cells of pancreatic islets. Insulin is not a requirement for glucose to enter cells and the glycolytic cycle, but it facilitates glucose's entry and phosphorylation as much as threefold.

Exercise, probably because of decreased O_2, and inhibitors of oxidative phosphorylation such as the biguanides also facilitate the entry of glucose into cells without the aid of insulin. Insulin especially favors glucose's movement across muscle and fat cell membranes. It induces the synthesis of the rate-limiting glycolytic enzymes glucokinase, phosphofructokinase, and pyruvic kinase. It suppresses the synthesis of four key gluconeogenic enzymes: pyruvic carboxylase, PEP carboxykinase, fructose diphosphatase, and glucose-6-phosphatase. Insulin favors the storage of energy-rich phosphates. It facilitates the storage of fat and glycogen and the anabolism of body proteins (Fig. 13–4). The actions of insulin on its three principal target tissues (fat, skeletal muscle, and liver) are listed in Tables 13–2, 13–3, and 13–4).

The principal insulin antagonists in the endocrine system include GH, cortisol, epinephrine, glucagon, thyroxine, estrogens, and progestins. They are frequently involved in clinical syndromes involving disorders of the homeostasis of blood glucose.

GH decreases glucose uptake by fat and skeletal muscle. It also enhances the B cell's response to glucose and glucose output by the liver. A deficiency in GH, which normally mobilizes free fatty acids from peripheral fat and decreases insulin receptor numbers and their affinity for insulin, causes insulin sensitivity (exaggerated hypoglycemic reactions to insulin). An excess of GH causes resistance to insulin's actions. Overt diabetes mellitus develops in about 25% of humans with acromegaly. Repeated injections of GH are diabetogenic in dogs and cats.

Cortisol enhances the availability of glucose precursors, increases the activity of hepatic gluconeogenic enzymes, and decreases peripheral utilization of glucose. Most animals on pharmacologic glucocorticoid therapy, or those with spontaneous hyperadrenocorticism with hypercortisolism, have diabetic glucose tolerance curves. Some develop overt diabetes mellitus.

Epinephrine activates hepatic and muscle glycogenolytic enzymes, decreases insulin secretion by B cells, and decreases the uptake of glucose by peripheral tissues. Functional pheochromocytomas can cause hyperglyce-

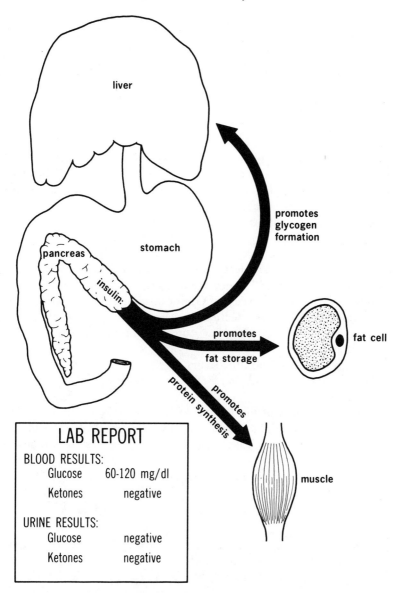

liver

promotes
glycogen
formation

stomach

pancreas

insulin

promotes
fat storage

fat cell

promotes
protein synthesis

muscle

LAB REPORT

BLOOD RESULTS:
    Glucose   60-120 mg/dl
    Ketones   negative

URINE RESULTS:
    Glucose   negative
    Ketones   negative

Fig. 13–4. Principal actions of insulin.

mia or abnormal results in the glucose tolerance test.

Thyroxine increases intestinal absorption of glucose, increases glucose output by the liver, enhances gluconeogenesis, and may increase the degradation of insulin. Required insulin dosage in diabetic patients may increase after the administration of thyroxine. Severe hypothyroidism can cause hypoglycemia.

Table 13–2. Actions of Insulin on Adipose Tissue

Increases entry of glucose, potassium, and phosphate
Increases synthesis of fatty acids
Increases synthesis of glycerol phosphate
Increases storage of triglycerides
Activates lipoprotein lipase
Inhibits hormone-sensitive lipase

Estrogens and progestogens are considered insulin antagonists, but their mechanisms of action have not been described. Estrus in diabetic dogs markedly increases insulin requirements. Megesterol acetate, a progestin, has induced temporary diabetes mellitus in some, as well as permanent diabetes mellitus in other cats treated with the drug.

At least some of the antagonism to insulin action caused by various factors is the result of effects on insulin receptors. Insulin receptors are constantly being formed and lost under normal conditions. The half-life of human insulin receptors is 7 hours. Among the factors producing a net loss of insulin receptors are an excess of GH or insulin, obesity,[23] and glucocorticoids. Glucocorticoids also decrease receptor affinity for insulin, as does acidosis. Factors that produce a net gain in receptors are exercise,[29] GH deficiency, and fasting.

Some degradation of insulin occurs in nearly all tissues, but 80% is degraded in the kidneys and liver.[41] The enzymes involved are collectively called *insulinases.*

Several preparations of insulin are commercially available. Most are of bovine or porcine origin, but human insulin is now available. This insulin is being produced by genetically engineered bacteria or by amino acid substitution.

See also references 2, 6, 10, 17, 30, and 36.

Glucagon

Glucagon is a straight-chained polypeptide from the A cells composed of 29 amino acids. It has a molecular weight of 3485, and its structure is similar to that of secretin. Glucagon's half-life in the circulation is about 5 to 10 minutes. Meaningful assays of circulating glucagon were initially hampered by two glucagon-like immunoreactive factors from the gastric and intestinal

Table 13–3. Actions of Insulin on Skeletal Muscle

Increases entry of glucose, potassium, and phosphate
Increases synthesis of glycogen
Increases uptake of branched chain amino acids and synthesis of protein
Increases uptake of ketoacids

Table 13–4.   Actions of Insulin on the Liver

Decreases cyclic adenosine monophosphate (cAMP)
Decreases ketogenesis and gluconeogenesis
Increases synthesis of proteins and lipids
Increases synthesis of glycogen and decreases production of glucose
Increases entry of potassium and phosphate

mucosa. One, from the stomach and duodenal A cells, is identical to pancreatic glucagon. The other, *glicentin* (glucagon-like immunoreactive [GLI] factor, enteroglucagon), is structurally different from glucagon. Its molecular weight is 11,000. It has the same N-terminal fragment as glucagon, and it possesses some of the same actions as glucagon. Small amounts of glicentin are also found in pancreatic A cells. Glucagon and glicentin are also present in the hypothalamus and brainstem, but their function in the central nervous system is unknown. Normal fasting serum levels of glucagon in the dog are reported to be approximately 225 to 275 pg/ml.

Glucagon is stimulated by amino acids, specifically alanine, arginine, serine, glycine, cysteine, and threonine; gastrointestinal hormones (CCK and gastrin); glucocorticoids; GH; exercise; β-adrenergic stimulators; theophylline; infections; and various stresses such as abdominal trauma. It is inhibited by high plasma glucose, secretin, somatostatin, phenytoin, free fatty acids, ketones, insulin, and α-adrenergic stimulators. Glucagon's major physiologic role may be to prevent hypoglycemia during protein stimulation of the secretion of insulin and during fasting. With diabetes mellitus, the suppression of glucagon's secretion by high blood glucose may be lost, resulting in its augmentation of hyperglycemia and ketogenesis.

The actions of glucagon are hyperglycemic and catabolic. Glucagon mobilizes glucose from the liver by activating hepatic phosphorylase, as well as by promoting gluconeogenesis and lipolysis. It also stimulates the oxidation of free fatty acids to ketones. Glucagon does not activate muscle phosphorylase. Glicentin has no effect on muscle or hepatic phosphorylase. Glucagon stimulates GH, insulin, pancreatic somatostatin, and the release of calcitonin. Hyperglucagonemia may contribute to or cause the hypocalcemia occasionally seen in acute attacks of pancreatitis.

Hyperglucagonemia has been associated with mild diabetes mellitus produced by functional pheochromocytomas or rare islet cell tumors called glucagonomas. Its role in the more common forms of diabetes mellitus is still being debated.

Hypoglucagonemia has been reported in some children with neonatal hypoglycemia. Although glucagonomas and hypoglucagonemic neonatal hypoglycemia have not been reported in dogs and cats, veterinary clinicians should be mindful of their possibility.

Glucagon is inactivated rapidly by the liver and by many other tissues but to lesser degrees. Glucagon (Glucagon for Injection Ampoules) is available commercially. Its clinical uses include diagnostic response tests for hyperadrenocorticism, glycogen storage disorders, insulinomas, and functional pheochromocytomas. It is also used to evaluate hepatic regeneration after the ligation of portosystemic shunts, and as therapy for acute hypoglycemia from insulin overdosage.

See also references 10, 12, 34, and 35.

Somatostatin

A 14-amino-acid polypeptide with a molecular weight of 1639, somatostatin is produced in the wall of the stomach, small intestines, pancreatic islets, central nervous system (in and out of the hypothalamus), peripheral ganglia, and perhaps, the thyroid gland. The half-life in the circulation is about 1 minute. Somatostatin inhibits secretion of GH, thyroid-stimulating hormone (TSH), ACTH, insulin, CCK, glucagon, gastric inhibitory polypeptide, pancreatic polypeptide, vasoactive intestinal peptide, gastrin, glicentin, secretin, renin, and motilin. It also inhibits the secretion of gastric acid, gastric motility, contraction of the gallbladder, and pancreatic exocrine secretions. Stimuli for the secretion of somatostatin are glucose, amino acids (arginine and leucine), and CCK.

Analogues have been investigated as a possible medical treatment for control of diabetic catabolism and ketonemia induced by hyperglucagonemia. Its diverse actions and short half-life currently preclude its possible clinical applications at this time. Somatostatinomas, tumors secreting excess somatostatin, are a rare cause for mild diabetes mellitus. Deficiency of somatostatin is not recognized as the cause of disease. Somatostatin is neither commercially available nor used clinically.

Pancreatic Polypeptide

A linear peptide with a molecular weight of 4328, pancreatic polypeptide (PP) consists of 36 amino acids produced by islet F (PP) cells. Its function is unknown. Plasma PP levels are increased by the ingestion of protein, fasting, exercise, or hypoglycemia. The secretion of PP is inhibited by hyperglycemia and somatostatin. More than half of all pancreatic islet tumors secrete excessive amounts of PP. It may be useful as a tumor marker (indicator).

Other Islet Cell Products

Little is known of the physiologic importance and actions of vasoactive intestinal peptide (VIP) and pancreatic serotonin. VIP has been recognized, however, as one cause for the pancreatic cholera (Verner-Morrison's) syndrome in humans associated with some islet cell tumors of the pancreas.

TESTS OF ISLET CELL FUNCTION

Most islet cell dysfunctions can be clinically assessed by measuring the fasting blood glucose level before and, occasionally, after challenge administrations of glucose, amino acids, glucagon, glucocorticoids, or tolbutamide. Glycosylated hemoglobin and plasma proteins provide retrospective assessments of blood glucose levels. Sometimes serum insulin or gastrin assays are necessary to evaluate islet cell function.

Fasting Blood and Urine Glucose

Normal fasting blood glucose values for dogs, cats, and horses are generally in the range of 60 to 120 mg/dl. Birds normally have blood glucose levels between 200 to 550 mg/dl. Plasma or serum values are about 15% higher than whole blood glucose values. Values from the same animal (or patient) may vary considerably due to the time the sample was taken in relation to the last meal, the psyche of the animal, the influence of concomitant drugs, and the degree of stress the patient is subjected to in obtaining the sample. Immaturity, especially the first 5 days of life, is often associated with erratic blood glucose levels. Repeated tests are necessary for meaningful interpretations. Glucose is not normally found in the urine until the renal threshold is exceeded. The renal threshold varies considerably among patients, and there are species differences as well. The mean blood glucose level above which glucose appears in the urine is about 180 mg/dl in dogs and about 300 mg/dl in cats.[16]

Blood cells consume glucose at a rate of about 20 mg/dl/hr at room temperature; therefore, it is necessary to do one of three things between obtaining the sample and performing the test: run the test within 30 minutes of collecting the sample; collect the blood in sodium fluoride (gray-top tubes), which inhibits glycolysis; or separate the serum or plasma from the packed cells and refrigerate as soon as possible.

Most methods of determining blood and urine glucose are now specific for glucose. Many of the older methods measured total reducing substances, not just glucose. One quantitative test for reducing substances (Clintest tablets) is still in general use. Clinicians should be aware of possible false-positive tests caused by reducing drugs, especially salicylates and ascorbic acid.

Glucose oxidase or o-toluidine methods are more specific. Glucose oxidase-impregnated paper strips are specific and sensitive to as little as 0.1% glucose, but they must be used with caution since they deteriorate with age and exposure to air. Only fresh strips from in-date bottles recently opened and properly stored less than 4 months should be relied on. Reflectance colorimeters are available to quantify the color change in many enzyme-impregnated paper strips.

Sodium fluoride inhibits the reaction between glucose and glucose oxidase. Only fresh blood or blood collected in heparin or EDTA tubes should be used with glucose oxidase-impregnated paper strips.

Glucose in the urine represents any hyperglycemia exceeding the patient's renal threshold since the last voiding of urine. As a screening test for hyperglycemia, urine glucose may be convenient, but it should not be relied on when monitoring changes in blood glucose in dogs or cats. Glucose may be detected in the urine even though blood glucose levels are normal, such as in the case of renal tubular dysfunction associated with ethylene glycol poisoning[32] or canine Fanconi-like syndrome.[9, 39] In addition, a "pseudoglucose" occurs in the urine of cats affected with feline urethritis syndrome, causing false-positive responses with the glucose oxidase method of determination. Only previous determinations of an individual's renal glucose threshold and collections of "double-voided" urine samples meaningfully reflect blood glucose values. Double-voided samples in dogs and cats can be obtained only by urinary catheterization and aspiration followed by collection of urine formed in the next 2 hours to be used for the determination of urine glucose. Fasting blood glucose infers no ingestion of food for 8 hours or more before the sample is taken.

See also reference 14.

Glucose Tolerance Test

In clinical veterinary medicine, glucose tolerance tests (GTTs) are rarely indicated. The indication for GTTs is only to determine the quantity and timing of the release of insulin in response to glucose challenge. There are three types of GTTs: oral, intravenous, and high dose. Clinical deficiencies or excesses of insulin in dogs or cats are rarely obscure enough to require GTTs.

More physiologic in their stimulus, oral GTTs are generally preferred over intravenous GTTs, except in the presence of concurrent malabsorption. In many cases, an intravenous GTT is more practical because of the difficulty in administering hypertonic glucose orally and because of the smaller possibility of vomiting. Oral GTTs are done on a patient in a fasted state by gastric intubation and administration of 2.2 g of dextrose/kg body weight (5 ml of 20% dextrose/lb). Greater dosages are not recommended because of the risk of vomiting and because gastric emptying will be delayed.

The stomach empties a specific number of calories per minute under the control of osmoreceptors in the duodenum.[18] A normal response to an oral GTT is shown in Figure 13–5. Intravenous GTTs are usually given in an intravenous dose of 0.5 g of dextrose/kg body weight over a period of 3 to 5 minutes (Fig. 13–6), but a high-dose, intravenous GTT (1.1 g/kg body weight) is sometimes recommended. A screening oral GTT can be done effectively by taking three blood glucose samples: a sample done before the test, a sample 1 hour after the test, and a sample 2 hours after the test. By 2 hours the blood levels should be normal. The 1-hour sample ensures the adequate absorption of the glucose challenge. If the results of the 2-hour postprandial oral GTT are questionable (more than 140 mg/dl), a 3-hour test should be done with blood glucose samples taken every 30 minutes. Acceptable results for the oral GTT are as follows: baseline blood glucose values of less than 120 mg/dl; 1 hour after the GTT, less than 200 mg/dl; and 2 hours after the GTT, less than 140 mg/dl. Blood glucose levels

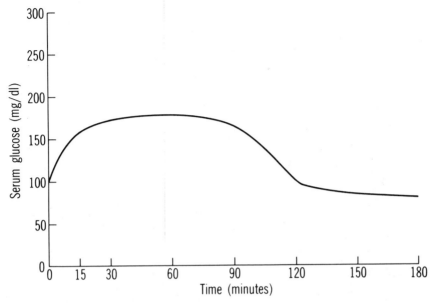

Fig. 13–5. An example of normal oral glucose tolerance in dogs (2.2 g/kg body weight).

should be less than 140 mg/dl within 1 hour if the intravenous GTT is used. If reactive hypoglycemia is suspected, a 5-hour oral GTT is indicated. Standard conditions to minimize stress on the patient, a fast lasting 8 hours at the minimum, a diet containing carbohydrates for at least 3 days before the test, and normal serum potassium levels are prerequisites to be attempted in each case.

A formula for interpreting the glucose tolerance curve has been described: $K = 69.3/T_2 - T_1$ (the percentage decrease of glucose per minute: normal values, $K > 2$; subclinical diabetes, K of 1–2; and overt diabetes, $K < 1$). However, blood glucose K formulas, cortisone-primed oral GTTs, and insulin asays taken during GTTs are research tools rarely required in clinical small animal endocrinology to assess islet cell function.

Possible endogenous and drug-related causes for an elevated GTT curve are listed in Tables 13–5 and 13–6.[5, 15, 24, 33]

See also references 7 and 26.

Glucagon Tolerance Test

Glucagon is capable of causing hyperglycemia if glycogen is present in the liver and the necessary glycogenolytic enzymes are present. The glucagon tolerance test has value in classifying causes for hypoglycemia. The test is done after a 12-hour fast by administering an intravenous dose of 0.03 mg/kg body weight of glucagon (Glucagon for Injection). Blood glucose is determined by samples taken before the test, and 1, 3, 5, 15, 30, 45, 60, 90,

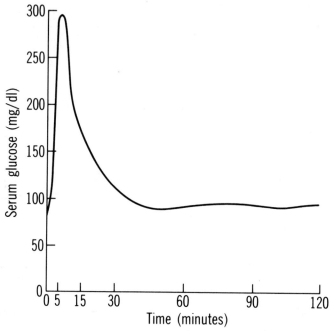

Fig. 13–6. An example of normal intravenous glucose tolerance in dogs (0.5 g/kg body weight).

and 120 minutes after the test. Multiple insulin assays taken after a glucagon challenge have been recommended by some, but their clinical usefulness does not outweigh the expense. An example of a normal blood glucose curve after an injection of glucagon is illustrated in Figure 13–7. Curves failing to rise indicate that the glucagon is inactive or that there is an absence of glycogen or glycogenolytic enzymes in the liver. Curves that rise but drop sharply to even subnormal levels suggest hyperinsulinemia.

See also reference 3.

Insulin (Immunoreactive Insulin) Assay

The immunoreactive insulin (IRI) assay is commercially available at many laboratories. Quantities of IRI are usually reported in μU/ml. Normal fasting values in the dog and cat are about 5 to 30 μU/ml.

Collection of samples requires more care than that necessary for the collection of thyroid or steroid hormones. Because IRI is a polypeptide hormone and some insulinases are present in the serum, insulin must be separated from the packed cells as soon as possible, and the IRI serum sample must be frozen before shipment. Shipment of samples should be done in dry ice. The time of sampling is critical, since IRI levels can increase fivefold in postprandial states.

More diagnostic than the absolute IRI level is its relative value in relation to the blood glucose. Normal insulin to blood glucose ratios are about 0.10

Table 13–5. Endogenous Causes for Elevated Glucose Tolerance
Test Curves

Diabetes mellitus
Hyperadrenocorticism
Functional pheochromocytoma
Oversecretion of growth hormone
Thyrotoxicosis
Chronic renal disease
Chronic liver disease

to 0.30 (also expressed as 10 to 30 $\mu U/mg \times 100$). Another means of assessing the insulin to blood glucose ratio is by the "amended insulin-glucose" ratio (IRI $\times$ 100/blood glucose $-$ 30). Normal amended ratios are less than 30. Although obesity can moderately raise the amended ratio, an amended ratio above 50 is diagnostic for hyperinsulinemia.

See also references 4, 25, 31, and 37.

Glycohemoglobin (Fast Hb, Glycosylated Hb, HbA₁c, GHb) and Glycosylated Plasma Proteins

Small amounts of glucose nonenzymatically and relatively irreversibly bind with a form of hemoglobin. This binding occurs slowly throughout the life of the red blood cell. By measuring the combination, called glycohemoglobin (GHb), an indirect assessment of the mean blood glucose can be determined for the preceding 3 to 8 weeks. This test has proved valuable in assessing control of diabetes in dogs and humans.

Table 13–6. Drug-Induced Causes for Elevated Glucose Tolerance
Test Curves

Hormones
  Corticosteroids
  Estrogens
  Progestins
  Thyroid hormones
  Sympathomimetics
Nicotinic acid
Phenytoin
Thiazides
Calcium-channel blocking agents
Isoniazid
Tranquilizers and anesthetics
  Phenothiazine-derivatives
  Thiopental
  Ketamine
  Xylazine
  Morphine

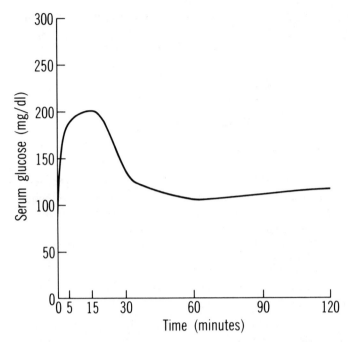

Fig. 13–7. An example of normal intravenous glucagon tolerance in dogs (0.03 mg/kg body weight).

GHb is a tissue glucose rather than a serum or plasma glucose. Values are altered if the concentration of red blood cells is abnormal or if recent red blood cell regeneration from anemia has occurred.

Glycohemoglobin may be measured by chromatographic or direct chemical means. The chromatographic method can be affected by other substances such as azotemia, salicylates, and some antibodies. Direct chemical determinations are less affected by interfering substances. The chromatographic method is not valid for feline GHb. Normal values in dogs are about 6% to 8% depending on the method used and the laboratory. Uncontrolled diabetes can have values as high as 15% to 20%.

Other blood proteins are also glycosylated like hemoglobin. By determining their glycosylated concentration and considering their half-life, a better estimate of the duration of hyperglycemia can be made. The concentration of glycosylated plasma proteins is normally about 9% to 12% in the dog. Normal concentrations of glycosylated albumin in the dog are about 8% to 14%. Canine glycosylated albumin concentration reflects the mean blood glucose exposure of the previous 7 to 10 days.

See also references 8, 19–22, 28, and 38.

Insulin-Tolerance Test

The insulin response test is rarely used to supplement the GTT when insulin resistance is suspected. Causes for an elevated GTT are the same causes for insulin resistance and an abnormal insulin response test. The greatest value of the insulin response test is in indirectly establishing the possible oversecretion of GH by showing insulin resistance and elimination of other causes.

The procedure requires a fast of 8 or more hours, followed by an intravenous injection of 0.4 U/kg body weight of regular (crystalline) insulin. A blood glucose curve is determined by samples taken before the test and 15, 30, 45, 60, and 90 minutes after the test. A normal response is exemplified by a decrease in blood glucose to 50% to 70% of baseline (pretest) values in 20 to 40 minutes with a rebound to normal values in 60 to 90 minutes.

Tests of Questionable Value

Tolbutamide is a sulfonylurea that stimulates the islet B cells to secrete insulin. Intravenous tolbutamide tests have been advocated to assess the ability of the islets to produce insulin in suspected insulin-deficient states or states of excessive secretion of insulin. It has not been proved that the diagnostic benefits outweigh the potentially lethal hazards of the diagnostic use of this drug in clinical patients.

Leucine is one of the amino acids that stimulates the secretion of insulin. Recommended as a challenge test in the diagnosis of hyperinsulinemia, it has never fallen into common use.

REFERENCES

1. Acosta, J.M., et al.: Distribution and volume of the islets of Langerhans in the canine pancreas. Acta. Physiol. Lat. Am., *19:*175, 1969.
2. Adesanya, T., Grillo, I., and Cunningham, J.G.: Serum insulin in totally pancreatectomized pregnant dogs. J. Endocrinol., *39:*307, 1967.
3. Atkins, C.E., and Chin, H.P.: Insulin kinetics in juvenile canine diabetics after glucose loading. Am. J. Vet. Res., *44:*596, 1983.
4. Belinger, R.E., and Siegel, E.T.: Double antibody radioimmunoassay in canine serum. Am. J. Vet. Res., *33:*2149, 1972.
5. Benson, G.J., et al.: Effect of xylazine hydrochloride upon plasma glucose and serum insulin concentrations in adult pointer dogs. J. Am. Anim. Hosp. Assoc., *20:*791, 1984.
6. Campbell, J., and Rastogi, K.S.: Effects of glucagon and epinephrine on serum insulin and insulin secretion in dogs. Endocrinology, *79:*830, 1966.
7. Church, D.B.: A comparison of intravenous and oral glucose tolerance tests in the dog. Res. Vet. Sci., *29:*353, 1980.
8. Delack, J.B., and Stogdale, L.: Glycosylated hemoglobin measurement in dogs and cats: implications for its utility in diabetic monitoring. Can. Vet. J., *24:*308, 1983.
9. Easley, J.R., and Breitschwerdt, D.B.: Glucosuria associated with renal tubular dysfunction in three basenji dogs. J. Am. Vet. Med. Assoc., *168:*938, 1976.
10. Eigler, N., Sacca, L., and Sherman, R.S.: Synergistic interactions of physiologic increments of glucagon, epinephrine, and cortisol in the dog. J. Clin. Invest., *63:*114, 1979.
11. Gingerich, R.L., et al.: Regional pancreatic concentration and in-vitro secretion of canine pancreatic polypeptide, insulin, and glucagon. Diabetes, *2:*96, 1978.
12. Goschke, H., et al.: Glucagon, insulin, cortisol and growth hormone levels following major surgery: their relationship to glucose and free fatty acid elevations. Horm. Metab. Res., *10:*465, 1978.
13. Hellman, B., Wallgren, A., and Hellerstrom, C.: Two types of islet cells in different parts of the pancreas of the dog. Nature, *194:*1201, 1962.
14. Hendriks, H.J., et al.: Studies on glucose and insulin levels in the blood of normal and diabetic dogs. Zentralbl. Veterinarmed., *23:*206, 1976.

15. Hsu, W.H., and Hembrough, F.B.: Intravenous glucose tolerance test in cats: influenced by acetylpromazine, ketamine, morphine, thiopental, and xylazine. Am. J. Vet. Res., 43:2060, 1982.
16. Kruth, S.A., and Cowgill, L.D.: Renal glucose transport in the cat. Proceedings of Am. Coll. Vet. Intern. Med., p. 78, 1978.
17. Kuzuya, T., Kajinuma, H., and Ide, T.: Effect of intrapancreatic injection of potassium and calcium on insulin and glucagon secretion in dogs. Diabetes, 23:55, 1974.
18. Leib, M.S., et al.: Canine gastric emptying of glucose. Proceedings of Am. Coll. Vet. Intern. Med., p. 50, 1984.
19. Mahaffey, E.A.: Glycosylated hemoglobulin measurement (Letter). Canad. Vet. J., 25:226, 1985.
20. Mahaffey, E.A., and Cornelius, L.M.: Evaluation of a commercial kit for measurement of glycosylated hemoglobulin in canine blood. Vet. Clin. Pathol., 10:21, 1981.
21. Mahaffey, E.A., and Cornelius, L.M.: Glycosylated hemoglobin in diabetic and nondiabetic dogs. J. Am. Vet. Med. Assoc., 180:635, 1982.
22. Mahaffey, E.A., Buonanno, A.M., and Cornelius, L.M.: Glycosylated albumin and serum protein in diabetic dogs. Am. J. Vet. Res., 45:2126, 1984.
23. Mattheeuws, D., et al.: Glucose tolerance and insulin response in obese dogs. J. Am. Anim. Hosp. Assoc., 20:287, 1984.
24. Mattheeuws, D., et al.: Effects of pentobarbitone anaesthesia and atropine on the intravenous glucose tolerance test in normal dogs. J. Small Anim. Pract., 22:779, 1981.
25. Reimers, T.J., et al.: Validation of a rapid solid-phase radioimmunoassay for canine, bovine, and equine insulin. Am. J. Vet. Res., 43:1274, 1982.
26. Rottiers, R., et al.: Glucose uptake and insulin secretory responses to intravenous glucose loads in the dog. Am. J. Vet. Res., 42:155, 1981.
27. Smith, L.F.: Species variation in the amino acid sequence of insulin. Am. J. Med., 40:662, 1966.
28. Smith, J.E., Wood, P.A., and Moore, K.: Evaluation of a colorimetric method for canine glycosylated hemoglobin. Am. J. Vet. Res., 43:700, 1982.
29. Soman, V.R., et al.: Increased insulin sensitivity and insulin binding to monocytes after physical training. N. Engl. J. Med., 301:1200, 1979.
30. Stevenson, R.W., Parsons, J.A., and Alberti, K.G.M.M.: Insulin infusion into the portal and peripheral circulations of unanaesthetized dogs. Clin. Endocrinol., 8:335, 1978.
31. Stockham, S.L., Nachreiner, R.F., and Krehbiel, J.D.: Canine immunoreactive insulin quantitation using five commercial radioimmunoassay kits. Am. J. Vet. Res., 44:2179, 1983.
32. Thrall, M.A., Grauer, G.F., and Mero, K.N.: Clinicopathologic findings in dogs and cats with ethylene glycol intoxication. J. Am. Vet. Med. Assoc., 184:37, 1984.
33. Tranquilli, W.J., et al.: Hyperglycemia and hypoinsulinemia during xylazine-ketamine anesthesia in thoroughbred horses. Am. J. Vet. Res., 45:11, 1984.
34. Unger, R.H., and Orchi, L.: Glucagon and the A cell. I. N. Engl. J. Med., 304:1518, 1981.
35. Unger, R.H., and Orci, L.: Glucagon and the A cell. II. N. Engl. J. Med., 304:1575, 1981.
36. Vanhelder, W.P., et al.: Diurnal episodic pattern of insulin secretion in the dog. Diabetes 29:326, 1980.
37. Wilson, R.B., and Martin, J.M.: Radioimmunoassay of plasma insulin in dogs and monkeys: application of the dextran coated charcoal separation method. Can. J. Comp. Med., 33:264, 1969.
38. Wood, P.A., and Smith, J.E.: Glycosylated hemoglobin and canine diabetes mellitus. J. Am. Vet. Med. Asoc., 176:1267, 1980.
39. Wright, R.P., and Wright, H.J.: Paradoxic glucosuria (canine Fanconi syndrome) in two basenji dogs. Vet. Med. Small Anim. Clin., 79:199, 1984.
40. Yalow, R.S., and Berson, S.A.: Immunoassay of endogenous plasma insulin in man. J. Clin. Invest., 39:1157, 1960.
41. Zaharko, D.S., Beck, L.V., and Blankenbaker, R.: Role of the kidney in the disposal of radioiodinated and nonradioiodinated insulin in dogs. Diabetes, 15:680, 1966.

14

Diabetes Mellitus

Diabetes mellitus (meaning "sweet diuresis") results from an absolute or relative deficiency of insulin. It is probably the first most commonly recognized endocrine disease in the cat (affecting about 1 in 800) and the second in the dog (affecting about 1 in 200). Diabetes is rare in horses[5, 6, 14, 54, 64, 122] and birds.[2, 3, 107] The incidence of diabetes mellitus in humans, 2% to 10% of the American population, is higher than that in companion animals. Diabetes mellitus has a variety of manifestations and heterogenic causes. Carbohydrate intolerance resulting from an insufficiency or deficiency of insulin is the hallmark of diabetes mellitus.

Without sufficient insulin, glucose cannot easily enter most of the cells of the body. Hyperglycemia and an intracellular deficiency of energy result. In addition to facilitating the entry of glucose into cells, insulin suppresses the mobilization of peripheral fat and protein stores and suppresses gluconeogenesis from fat and protein. With diabetes, muscles are catabolized and fat depots atrophy because of unsuppressed mobilization and gluconeogenesis resulting from insufficient insulin. The condition is augmented by increased levels of serum cortisol and glucagon.

The liver is capable of converting mobilized fat into an alternative energy source, ketones; however, the liver cannot regulate the need for ketones, most of which are acid. When excessive ketoacids are produced, they are buffered by circulating buffers in the plasma, excreted in the urine, and expired in the breath. Diabetic ketoacidosis occurs whenever the production of ketones exceeds the body's need for them as an energy source and exceeds the body's buffering capacity (Fig. 14–1).

Diabetics are affected, at least initially, with excessive thirst, urination, and recent weight loss, although many are still obese at the time of their diagnosis. Underlying these signs is hyperglycemia—that is, blood glucose values frequently or consistently in excess of 140 mg/dl.

The term "diabetes" is used synonymously, in clinics and by the public, with diabetes mellitus. The condition resulting from deficiencies in the action of antidiuretic hormone (ADH), diabetes insipidus, should never be referred to simply as "diabetes."

CAUSES AND CLASSIFICATION OF DIABETES MELLITUS

In 1979, the National Diabetes Data Group proposed a simplified classification of human diabetes mellitus. This classification, applicable to com-

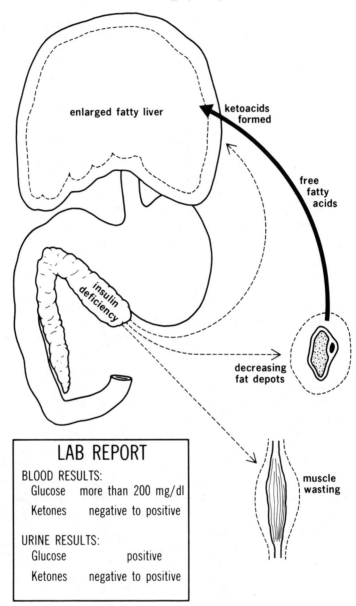

enlarged fatty liver

ketoacids
formed

free
fatty
acids

insulin
deficiency

decreasing
fat depots

muscle
wasting

LAB REPORT

BLOOD RESULTS:
  Glucose   more than 200 mg/dl

  Ketones   negative to positive

URINE RESULTS:
  Glucose   positive

  Ketones   negative to positive

Fig. 14–1.   Diabetes mellitus.

panion animals, eliminates less-well-defined descriptive terms such as latent, subclinical, chemical, prediabetes, maturity-onset, adult-onset, and juvenile-onset diabetes (Table 14–1).

See also references 26, 29, 30, 40, 43, 44, 50, 69, 77, 80, 105, 123, and 131.

Table 14–1. National Diabetes Data Group's Classification of Diabetes Mellitus

---

Spontaneous
   Type I (Insulin-dependent)
   Type II (Insulin-independent)
Secondary
   Generalized pancreatic disease or injury
   Excesses of antagonistic hormones
   Drug-induced
   Insulin-receptor abnormalities
   Genetic abnormalities causing multiple anomalies
Impaired glucose tolerance
Gestational

Spontaneous Types

Type I (insulin-dependent) and *Type II (insulin-independent)* diabetes mellitus are, in part, inherited in humans. The concordance rate in human twins, an indication of inheritability, is greater in twins with Type II than those with Type I diabetes. The risk of Type I is associated with the presence of certain human leukocyte antigens (HLAs). Determining whether HLAs are present can give some indication of the risk of diabetes in humans. Even though some breeds of dogs are predisposed to diabetes, it is difficult to assess the extent of familial occurrence in dogs and other companion animals. Accurate medical histories of the ancestors and siblings of affected animals are rarely available, except when the age of onset is less than 1 year of age. Other possible causes for diabetes are listed in Table 14–2.

Table 14–2. Possible Causes for Diabetes Mellitus

Genetic
Pancreatic injury by:
   Trauma
   Neoplasia
   Infection
   Autoantibodies
   Inflammation

Hormone-induced B cell exhaustion
   Growth hormone
   Thyroid hormones
   Glucocorticoids
   Catecholamines
   Estrogens
   Progestins

Target tissue insensitivity
   Decreased number of receptors
   Defective receptors
   Defect in post-receptor effects

Dyshormonogenesis of insulin

In humans and companion animals, diabetes mellitus is most common in late middle age. Type I diabetes is more common in companion animals; Type II is more common in humans. The typical diabetic human is diagnosed at approximately 50 years old, is overweight, has mild to moderate hyperglycemia, and is not ketonemic. Most diabetic dogs and cats are diagnosed at 8 to 10 years of age, are overweight, have moderate to severe hyperglycemia, and are ketonemic. Diabetes in humans can frequently be controlled by loss of excessive weight, exercise, and dietary control. Some patients are given drugs orally to increase the endogenous secretion of insulin and the sensitivity to insulin. Diabetic dogs and cats can rarely be controlled by such measures. Injections of insulin are virtually always necessary to control diabetes in companion animals.

About 15% of human diabetics are insulin-dependent (Type I diabetes mellitus). In most patients the onset of disease occurs before the age of 20 years. Less than 2% of dogs have juvenile-onset diabetes (onset of illness before the animal has reached 1 year of age). Canine juvenile diabetics are also insulin-dependent.

For several years a number of viruses, such as mumps, rubella, cytomegalovirus, and coxsackie B_4, have been suspected to play a role in the development of Type I diabetes in humans. Further evidence has shown that viruses induce diabetes in susceptible strains of mice. In 1979, a coxsackie B_4 virus was recovered from a person with Type I diabetes with a rapid onset following flu-like symptoms.[136] A histologic examination of the islets showed the lymphocytic infiltration of the islets. This case substantiated previous theories that genetic predisposition, when aided by viral stimulation, triggers the autoimmune destruction of the B cells.

In persons with Type I diabetes, 75% have recently formed anti-islet antibodies, and 70% have lymphocytic infiltration of the islets. Its incidence closely follows the occurrence of certain viral diseases. An association between viral disease, particularly canine parvovirus, and the onset of juvenile diabetes in dogs has been suspected. Autoantibodies to insulin or cytoplasmic antigens have been shown in more than 70% of dogs with diabetes.[47] Full expression of Type I diabetes requires a relative or absolute deficiency of insulin concomitant with a relative or absolute excess of glucagon.

Spontaneous diabetes mellitus has been described in cats and birds, but not in the horse. Diabetes in horses has been secondary to acinar pancreatitis, hyperadrenocorticism, or pheochromocytomas.[5, 6]

Secondary Causes

The most common cause of diabetes mellitus in the dog was once reported to be islet cell destruction secondary to the damage of acute and relapsing acinar necrotizing pancreatitis. The extension of damage from acinar pancreatitis is undoubtedly the most frequent known cause of diabetes in the dog, but this still represents a small percentage of cases. The cause of most cases of canine diabetes mellitus is still unknown. Microscopic islet lesions most commonly associated with canine diabetes mellitus include decreased or absent islet cells, hydropic degeneration or hyalinization of B cells, and selective amyloid infiltration. The B cells of diabetics are often described as "burned out." The pancreatic islets are the only endocrine cells that undergo atrophy from exhaustion. About 10% of human diabetics have islet cells that appear normal under light microscopy. Diabetes does not result from juvenile pancreatic atrophy of dogs; rather the exocrine function only is affected.[48, 121]

Pancreatic lesions in cats with diabetes mellitus are most often a selective deposition of amyloid in the islets.[57, 132–135] It is not generally associated with amyloidosis elsewhere in the body, and it is apparently not secondary to chronic suppurative processes. Although about half the older cats without diabetes have islet amyloid, the amount present in islets is less than in diabetic cats.[133] Both the amyloid present and the incidence of islet amyloid increase with diabetes in cats.

Sixty-five percent of diabetic cats have islet amyloidosis.[132] Selective islet amyloid differs from secondary systemic amyloid. Secondary systemic amyloid does not stain positive with Congo red stain after incubation with potassium permanganate; selective islet amyloid is stained by Congo red stain after incubation with potassium permanganate. It is thought that the increase of selective islet amyloidosis in diabetic cats is a result rather than a cause of diabetes. In comparison to dogs, even fewer diabetic cats develop diabetes as a result of generalized pancreatitis. Islet lesions other than amyloidosis that may be seen in diabetic cats include hydropic degeneration, decreased islet numbers, lymphocytic infiltration, nodular hyperplasia, neoplastic destruction, and extension of exocrine pancreatitis.[36]

Excesses of insulin-antagonistic hormones can lead to B-cell exhaustion. These excesses may be endogenous in origin or result from administration. Examples include an excess of glucocorticoids caused by iatrogenic or spontaneous hyperadrenocorticism,[16, 39, 63, 91, 97, 127] an excess of catecholamines resulting from functional pheochromocytoma, an excess of growth hormone (GH) resulting from the administration of GH or spontaneous acromegaly,[15, 31, 98] an excess of glucagon caused by glucagonomas or bacterial infections, and excessive thyroid hormone resulting from iatrogenic or spontaneous thyrotoxicosis, or the excessive administration of estrogen or progestin,[98, 119] or excessive estrogens or progesterone resulting from spontaneous or neoplastic secretion.[124]

Nonhormonal drug-induced causes of diabetes include the impaired release of insulin caused by tranquilizers, anesthetics, thiazides, and phenytoin. Permanent overt diabetes mellitus is more probable with chemical injury to B cells. The rodenticide, Vacor, and N-nitroso compounds in cured mutton have been linked to B-cell damage. Vacor was voluntarily withdrawn from the American market in May 1979. Streptozotocin is an antibiotic cytotoxic to B cells used to treat malignant tumors of B cells. Vacor and streptozotocin have a similar structure.

See also references 1 and 28.

Two types of insulin-receptor abnormalities have been identified in humans. The Type A abnormality is an idiopathic loss of receptors in young women. The Type B abnormality is caused by antireceptor antibodies in older humans. Neither type has been recognized in companion animals.

A possible genetic abnormality resulting in polyglandular failure has been reported in two German shorthaired pointer littermates who developed diabetes and hypothyroidism at the age of 7 years.[32] Several polyglandular failure syndromes have been described in humans. The underlying cause for these syndromes is apparently the autoimmune destruction of various combinations of endocrine organs. Other genetic abnormalities associated with diabetes such as leprechaunism, Klinefelter's syndrome, and Prader-Willi syndrome have been reported in humans.

Unlike humans, animals with impaired glucose tolerance are uncommonly identified. This is because there are no special facilities such as screening clinics to seek them out. Such attempts have not been warranted since companion animals are relatively free of the severe vascular and neurologic complications of diabetes that can occur in diabetic humans. Humans with diabetes are 25 times more likely to develop blindness and 17 times more likely to have heart disease than the general population. Transient overt diabetes, which is seen in companion animals under stress from infections such as osteomyelitis or treated with insulin-antagonistic drugs such as megestrol acetate or glucocorticoids, probably occurs only in animals with insufficient insulin and abnormal glucose tolerance before the stress or drug exposure occurs.

Gestational diabetes is the result of high plasma estrogens, cortisol, and the antagonism of progesterone to peripheral insulin action, along with the accelerated degradation of insulin, which is caused by placental insulinases. Overt diabetes generally does not result because of sufficient compensatory secretion of insulin. Female animals who become overtly diabetic during gestation are more susceptible to eventually developing permanent diabetes than is the general population.

INCIDENCE

Canine diabetes most frequently occurs in small breeds, especially the dachshund (standard, miniature, longhaired, and wirehaired) and poodle (toy, miniature, and standard), but all breeds are affected. German shepherd dogs, cocker spaniels, collies, and boxers are at significantly decreased risk. The age of onset is usually 8 to 9 years. Affected intact and neutered female dogs outnumber affected male dogs by two- to fourfold.

The diabetogenic effects of progesterone or progesterone-induced hypersecretion of GH during the metestrus of bitches have been proposed as a cause for the greater incidence of diabetes in female dogs. Although this may well be a contributing factor, it should be noted that sexually neutered female dogs still have a greater risk for diabetes than do male dogs.

Factors predisposing female dogs to diabetes have not yet been completely identified. The association between diabetes mellitus and benign mammary tumors in dogs is more frequent than would be expected by chance—there may be a common endocrine link between the two. The onset of diabetes may be more common in dogs during winter months.

Juvenile diabetes mellitus has been reported in the keeshond, golden retriever, Westhighland terrier, Alaskan malamute, poodle, old English sheepdog, Doberman pinscher, miniature schnauzer, miniature pinscher, shipperke, German shepherd dog, Labrador retriever, Finnish spitz, Manchester terrier, English springer spaniel, whippet, and mongrel.[66, 67, 72] It is usually recognized by the time the animal reaches 2 to 6 months of age. Male and female animals are affected with equal frequency. Keeshonds with juvenile diabetes have been best studied; it was found that they inherit B-cell atrophy as an autosomal recessive trait with incomplete penetrance. Islet A cells and acinar cells are unaffected. The pancreatic lesion reported in most other breeds with juvenile diabetes mellitus is atrophy of B cells and acinar cells.

Feline diabetes mellitus is slightly more common in male cats. Most of the affected cats are sexually altered (as is the usual feline hospital population). Domestic shorthairs are the most frequently affected breed, but again the incidence may not be in excess of the incidence of the general hospital population at risk. The usual age of onset, being more than 9 years, is slightly later than in dogs. The occurrence in cats seems more common in spring and summer.

See also references 4, 11, 41, 81, and 82.

CLINICAL SIGNS

The clinical signs of diabetes mellitus depend on the type of insulin insufficiency, the degree of insulin insufficiency, and the conditions preceding the onset of insulin insufficiency. Clinical forms of diabetes are categorized as nonketotic, ketoacidotic, and nonketotic hyperosmolar syndrome.

See also references 20, 23, 74, 85, 106, 108, and 111.

Nonketoacidotic (Uncomplicated) Diabetes Mellitus

Approximately 25% to 50% of dogs and cats with diabetes are seen for examination in a nonketotic state. Patients with uncomplicated diabetes mellitus are usually afebrile and are mentally alert. They also have nocturia, polyuria, and polydipsia with mild dehydration and are losing weight although the appetite is excessive (Fig. 14–2). Clinical signs have a duration of about 1 week to 1 month before presentation.

Polyuria, nocturia, and compensatory polydipsia with mild dehydration are the most frequent presenting signs. In each case, the conditions result from hyperglycemia, which induces an osmotic diuresis with glucosuria. Most patients are obese but have recently been losing weight because of the uninhibited gluconeogenesis. Polyphagia is the apparent result of failure to stimulate the hypothalamic satiety center with the entry of glucose. This allows the lateral hypothalamic appetite center to act without opposition. Hepatomegaly may be palpable in 10% to 20% of the patients and is the

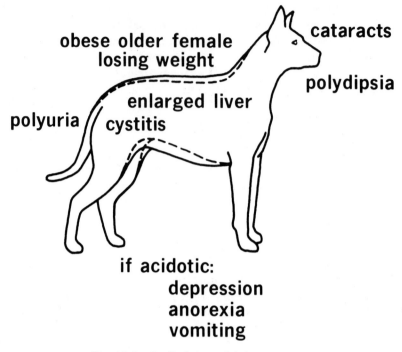

Fig. 14–2.   Cardinal signs of diabetes mellitus.

result of lipidosis caused by uninhibited hormone-sensitive lipase and peripheral fat mobilization.

Female companion animals, owing to their short, wide urethras, are especially predisposed to ascending urinary tract infections when glucose is present in the urine. Approximately one fourth to one half of female canine diabetics have bacterial cystitis at initial presentation. The cystitis may cause the clinical signs of dysuria and pollakiuria (increased frequency of urination). Rarely, proliferation of gas-forming bacteria (*Esherichia coli, Aerobacter aerogenes,* or *Clostridium* spp.) or yeast may cause emphysematous cystitis or cholecystitis to be visible radiographically.[75, 104] Emphysematous cystitis is not pathognomonic for diabetes.[84, 116]

Cataracts are found in about half of all canine diabetes patients at presentation. In many cases, stellate cataracts are the major presenting complaint. The development typically occurs over a period of a few days to 2 weeks. Diabetic cataracts are caused by sorbitol and fructose trapped in the lens. The osmotic influx of water separates the lenticular fibers.

Normally, the lens contains 10% of the concentration of glucose in the blood and aqueous humor. When insulin is deficient, the action of hexokinase permits glucose to undergo anaerobic glycolysis, but when hexokinase becomes saturated with glucose, aldose reductase irreversibly forms sorbitol from the excess glucose in the lens. Sorbitol may be con-

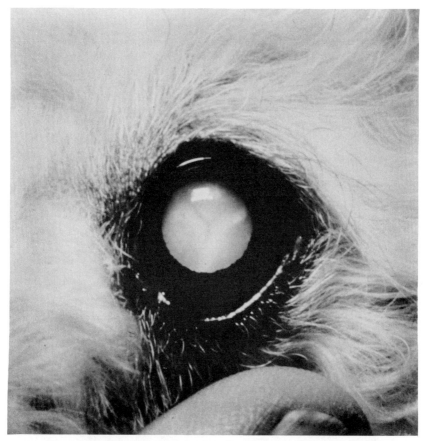

Fig. 14–3. Diabetic cataract in a poodle. (Courtesy of Dr. Dan Betts.)

verted to fructose by sorbitol dehydrogenase. Diabetic cataracts begin as vacuoles in the subepithelial equatorial cortex and progress to complete opacity with clefts in the lens' Y sutures (Fig. 14–3). Diabetic cataracts inexplicably do not occur in cats.

Mobilization of fat may be evident to the owner as atrophic fat depots. Hyperlipidemia, even during fasting, may be apparent on gross observation of blood taken for laboratory analyses (Fig. 14–4). Fundoscopic examination may also show that the blood in retinal vessels has a creamy appearance. This condition is called "lipemia retinalis." Elevated serum triglycerides and cholesterol occasionally lead to eruptive xanthomatosis of the skin and tendinous xanthomatosis, respectively.[18, 45, 70]

Xanthomas appear like papules, pustules, and nodules surrounded by bright red erythema (Fig. 14–5). They are most common in areas of friction or movement, like the ventral abdomen and legs. Pustules are bacteriologically sterile. Microscopically, the purulent exudate contains lipid-laden macrophages, called "foam cells."

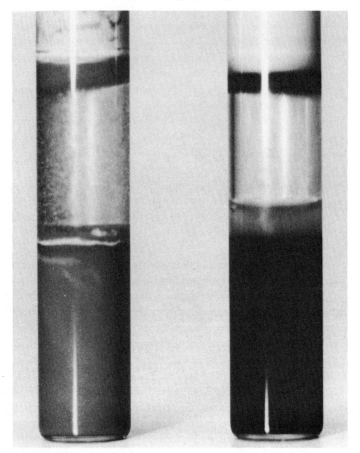

Fig. 14–4.　Left, hyperlipemic blood from a diabetic dog before treatment with insulin. *Right,* blood from the same diabetic dog after therapy with insulin.

Ketoacidotic Diabetes Mellitus

Ketoacidosis is present in most dogs and cats who initially present with diabetes mellitus. It represents the uncompensated stage of the body's attempts to buffer the ketoacids formed as an alternate energy source during severe or prolonged insulin deficiency. Ketonemia in companion animals is rare in nondiabetic conditions, but occasionally occurs if starvation is superimposed on late pregnancy, heavy lactation, or neonatal life. All the clinical signs of ketoacidotic diabetes mellitus may be explained by the greater insulin deficiency, longer duration of deficiency, metabolic derangements caused by the acidosis, and the serum hyperosmolarity resulting from hyperglycemia.

Ketoacidotic diabetes mellitus is characterized by laboratory findings of persistent fasting hyperglycemia in excess of 200 mg/dl, ketonemia, and metabolic acidosis. The clinician may note compensatory respiratory efforts in

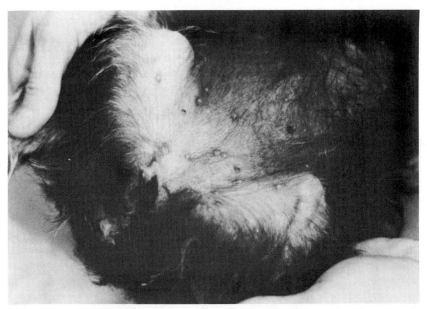

Fig. 14–5. Xanthomatic pustules on the ventral abdomen of a diabetic dog. (From Chastain, C.B., and Graham, C.L.: Xanthomatosis secondary to diabetes mellitus in a dog. J. Am. Vet. Med. Assoc., *172:*1209, 1978.)

the form of labored (Kussmaul's) breathing to blow off carbon dioxide and correct the metabolic acidosis. The plasma is often hyperosmolar. In addition to a history consistent with previous uncomplicated diabetes mellitus, affected patients may be febrile, have moderate to severe dehydration, be anorexic and mentally depressed, be vomiting or have diarrhea, and have oliguria or anuria.

Common initiating factors that cause diabetic patients to produce more ketones than they can buffer and excrete include infections, acute pancreatitis, administration of diabetogenic drugs such as glucocorticoids or megestrol acetate, spontaneous hyperadrenocorticism, dehydration, and anorexia.

Nonketotic Hyperosmolar Diabetic Coma

A rare form of diabetes mellitus reported in dogs, cats, and humans, nonketotic hyperosmolar diabetic coma is a condition in which the blood glucose level exceeds 600 mg/dl, serum sodium is often more than 145 mg/dl, and the plasma osmolality exceeds 340 mOsm. Each time blood glucose levels increase by 100 mg/dl, the plasma osmolality increases 5.6 mOsm/kg body weight. Ketonemia is not present. Patients with nonketotic hyperosmolar diabetic coma present with, or soon develop, stupor or coma caused by the plasma's hyperosmolality. It is believed that concurrent disease (for example, cardiac or renal disease) that impairs the body's ability to

Table 14–3. Common Abnormal Laboratory Findings in Diabetes Mellitus Before Treatment

	Nonketoacidotic	Ketoacidotic	Nonketotic-Hyperosmolar
Hemogram			
Total RBC and Hb	Normal	High to normal	High
Total WBC	Normal	Normal to high	Normal
Plasma or Serum			
Urea nitrogen	Normal	Normal to high	High
Ketones	Absent	Present	Absent
Glucose	>150 mg/dl	>250 mg/dl	>800 mg/dl
Cholesterol	Normal	High	Normal
Triglycerides	Normal to high	High	Normal to high
Alanine amino-transferase	Normal to high	High	Normal to high
Alkaline phos-phatase	Normal to high	High	Normal to high
Sodium	Normal	Normal to low	Low
Potassium	Normal	Normal to low	Normal to low
Calcium	Normal	Normal to low	Normal to low
Phosphorus	Normal	Normal to high	Normal to high
Bicarbonate	Normal	Low	Normal to low
Total CO_2	Normal	Low	Normal to low
pH	Normal	Low	Normal to low
Osmolality	280–310 mOsm/L	>310 mOsm/L	>340 mOsm/L
Urinalysis			
Glucose	Present	Present	Present
Ketones	Absent	Present	Absent

RBC = red blood cell; Hb = hemoglobin; WBC = white blood cell.

retain water and excrete sodium leads to nonketotic hyperosmolar coma in affected diabetics. Renal excretion should prevent blood glucose from exceeding 500 mg/dl if the glomerular filtration rate is normal.

See also references 110 and 114.

LABORATORY FINDINGS

Common abnormal laboratory findings in patients with nonketotic diabetes mellitus, ketoacidotic diabetes mellitus, and nonketotic hyperosmolar syndrome are summarized in Table 14–3. The total red blood cell count and hemoglobin rise with the dehydration that accompanies ketoacidosis or the hyperosmolar syndrome.

The stress of ketoacidosis (which often includes infections) elicits a leukocytosis with a left shift or a leukemoid reaction. Elevations of the blood or serum urea nitrogen and creatinine occur as the result of diabetic glomerulopathy, muscle catabolism, dehydration, or unrelated concurrent renal diseases. Serum amylase and lipase elevations are often unreliable as indicators of pancreatitis since they can also be elevated by decreased glomerular filtration.

Ketonemia is the result of free fatty acid mobilization with excess formation of acetyl CoA and acetoacetyl CoA. Acetoacetyl CoA is converted to acetoacetic acid, which may form acetone and β-hydroxybutyric acid.

Persistent fasting hyperglycemia, when glucose levels are greater than 140 mg/dl, is the hallmark of diabetes mellitus. It is the result of gluconeogenesis, glycogenolysis, and impaired entry of glucose into most cells of the body.

Uninhibited hormone-sensitive lipase mobilizes peripheral fat stores for energy. This leads to fatty infiltration of the liver. Mobilization of peripheral fat and the development of hepatic lipidosis are at least partially responsible for the tendency toward elevated serum enzymes (alanine amino transferase and alkaline phosphatase) from the liver. Uninhibited hormone-sensitive lipase is also responsible for serum elevations of cholesterol and triglyceride.

Some serum electrolyte concentrations tend to decrease with increasing blood glucose levels. Serum sodium and potassium levels are lowered by the osmotic diuretic action of glucosuria and ketonuria when organic anions cannot be adequately provided by hydrogen or ammonium ions. Ionized serum calcium usually remains normal despite low total levels of serum calcium because metabolic acidosis is frequently found in patients with diabetes mellitus.

The production of metabolic acidosis by ketoacids and by lactic acid depresses serum pH and bicarbonate. The pCO_2 should also become decreased if compensatory hyperventilation, Kussmaul's "air hunger," occurs as an attempt to correct the metabolic acidosis.

The probability of occurrence and degree of hyperosmolality are directly proportional to the elevation of blood glucose. Central nervous system dysfunction is not likely until the serum osmolality exceeds 340 mOsm/L. This is usually when levels of blood glucose approach 800 mg/dl.

Glucosuria—"sweet diuresis"—may occur in patients with diabetes mellitus, although it is not always present. Conversely, diabetes mellitus is not the only cause of glucosuria. The assumption that glucosuria is always present in patients with diabetes mellitus and reflects a certain degree of simultaneous hyperglycemia has created confusion in the diagnosis and control of diabetes mellitus. Other causes for glucosuria include ethylene glycol poisoning and a renal tubular disorder, canine Fanconi-like syndrome.[27] Fanconi-like syndrome has been reported in the basenji, Norwegian elkhound, Shetland sheepdog, and whippet. It is characterized by amino aciduria and hyperphosphaturia in addition to glucosuria. About 5% of glucosurias in humans are renal tubular dysfunctions not caused by diabetes. Because of dehydration and the concentration of urine, the urine ketones are more easily detected in the urine than in the plasma.

See also references 7, 34, 74, and 76.

DIAGNOSIS

The first step in the rational control of diabetes mellitus is arriving at a correct definitive diagnosis. Overt diabetes mellitus may be diagnosed if repeated fasting blood glucose values exceed 140 mg/dl or if fasting or postprandial-blood glucose values exceed 200 mg/dl. Occasionally, fasting blood glucose values may only periodically or transiently be in excess of 140 mg/dl, which may be caused by a mild to moderate impairment in patients who have glucose tolerance or a stress-related hyperglycemia. For example, 80% to 90% of dogs with acute pancreatitis have hyperglycemia, but less than 30% develop permanent secondary diabetes.[109] Stress hyperglycemia commonly occurs in cats with a variety of other illnesses, and treatment for diabetes mellitus is usually not required. Rarely in the dog or cat can a diagnosis of diabetes be based only on a glucose tolerance test. Glucose tolerance testing is affected by the patient's anxiety and chemical restraint; therefore, results are often not reproducible in the dog or cat. Glucosuria, classic clinical signs (polyuria, polydipsia, and weight loss), rapid onset of stellate cataracts in middle-aged or older dogs, or glucose detected in the tears can provide a presumptive diagnosis signaling the necessity for measuring blood glucose levels. These signals should never be used to make a definitive diagnosis of diabetes mellitus.

See also references 60 and 61.

GENERAL ASPECTS OF TREATMENT

Diabetes mellitus cannot yet be cured. In fact, current means of control are still crude and far less than satisfactory. Only replacement of a B cell capable of monitoring blood glucose and secreting a short-acting insulin into the portal circulation could completely correct diabetes mellitus—this is not meant to discourage veterinarians or their clients from attempting to control diabetes mellitus in a diabetic pet; it is hoped that all concerned will be encouraged to strive for the best possible control in each patient within the limits of reasonable expectations.

Before initiating therapy for diabetes mellitus, the owner and the veterinary clinician should have a realistic attitude toward the goals of therapy, its expense, surgeries possibly required in the future, and the burden of owner responsibility. In routine practice, approximately 30% of cases diagnosed as diabetic are given euthanasia by the owner's request in the first 7 days. At least 50% of those animals who are treated live more than 1 year without serious complications. Many animals have remained valuable pets while treated for 5 years or more. The decision whether to treat a patient should be made by the owners after they are made aware of the estimated expense and cautioned that therapy is a daily responsibility that must meet a schedule. Care for diabetic pets still must be done on schedule, including times when the owner wants to sleep late, go on vacation, or happens to get sick.

The possibility of cataracts, neuropathy, acute pancreatitis, and other complications should also be described to the owner, but not in a discouraging manner. When an owner elects to accept the responsibilities for a diabetic animal after being made aware of their ramifications, the probability of success is greatly improved. Successful management is dependent on owner cooperation.

Appropriate initial therapy is different in each presenting type of diabetes mellitus. Initial therapy of uncomplicated diabetes mellitus involves the use of insulins of intermediate duration, whereas therapy of ketoacidotic diabetes mellitus and nonketotic hyperosmolar coma involve the use of short-acting insulin. Fluid therapy of diabetic ketoacidosis and nonketotic hyperosmolar coma differ. Alkalinizing agents are contraindicated in nonketotic hyperosmolar coma, but they may be of benefit in ketoacidotic coma.

See references 19 and 38.

Goals of Therapy

Initially, the goals of therapy are to normalize the hyperglycemia and alterations in fluid balance, electrolyte balance, and plasma osmolality as carefully as possible. It is critical to begin therapy as soon as the diagnosis and classification are determined, but the speed at which corrections are made should be prudently controlled. Sudden alterations in blood glucose, fluid balance, serum electrolytes, or plasma osmolality can be as lethal as the original imbalance.

Once the patient's condition is stabilized, the long-term goals of therapy should be to maintain sufficient control of the blood glucose to permit maintenance of an ideal body weight for the patient's age, sex, and breed; normal growth in young patients; and maintenance of an alert attitude, normal physical activity, normal water consumption, and normal urine output.

These goals do not mean, nor should it be expected, that the blood glucose should be within ideal limits (60 to 150 mg/dl) each day. Because of the variance in delivering an exact amount of small doses (1 to 10 U) of insulin in small dogs and cats, variance in absorption from various injection sites, and variance in daily diets and exercise, achieving ideal limits each day is impossible with current techniques. Change in the administration of insulin should therefore be based on recurring effects, not on the effects produced in a single day.

Hyperglycemia, if it is moderate and does not change rapidly, is of little consequence in itself; however, even short-lived hypoglycemia can temporarily or permanently alter brain function and can be lethal. Hypoglycemia should be avoided by all means.

Recurrent hyperglycemia and insulin insufficiency are undesirable in animals, because, like their appearance in humans, they seem related to the incidence or severity of secondary infections, myopathy, retinopathy, glomerulopathy, neuropathy, hyperlipidemia, and cataracts in diabetic dogs. Diabetic neuropathy, glomerulopathy, and hyperlipidemia can also affect cats with recurrent hyperglycemia and insulin insufficiency. Recurrent hyperglycemia should be prevented as much as is practical without risking hypoglycemia.

Dietary Control and Oral Hypoglycemics

Oral hypoglycemics are subclassified as two types of drugs, sulfonylureas and biguanides. Biguanides are no longer available in the United States; however, several sulfonylureas are available in the United States, including acetohexamide, chlorpropamide, tolbutamide, tolazamide, glipizide, and glyburide. Sulfonylureas increase the endogenous secretion of insulin and number of insulin receptors. The use of sulfonylureas is usually restricted to human diabetics whose fasting blood glucose levels do not exceed 200 mg/dl and who have not become ketonemic. Based on these criteria, few canine or feline diabetics qualify as candidates for sulfonylureas. Most, but not all, studies on canine and feline diabetics have reported that more than 75% are insulin-deficient or prone to ketosis. Potential adverse reactions to sulfonylureas include hypoglycemia, skin reactions, visual disturbances, thyroid dysfunction, water intoxication, gastrointestinal disorders, hepatic disorders, and blood dyscrasias.

Sulfonylureas are not approved for veterinary use. Little is known of their toxicities in diabetic dogs and cats; however, it is known that tolbutamide can be hepatotoxic in dogs. Insufficient data on the efficacy and safety of sulfonylureas in dogs and cats prevent sulfonylureas from being advocated even for animals who may fulfill the criteria for this treatment.

See also references 24, 59, 73, 117, 118, and 129.

Insulins

Administration of exogenous insulin has been used as the mainstay of insulin-deficient diabetes mellitus for more than 60 years. Before 1921, the only form of therapy was Allen's treatment, a starvation diet. Despite many refinements in insulin and its administration, the successes are still not as great as desired.

After insulin was isolated and found to lower blood glucose levels, it was realized that multiple injections per day were required to maintain a lowered blood glucose concentration. In the 1930s, a Danish diabetologist, H.C. Hagedorn, found a solution to the problem of insulin's short duration of action. By combining zinc and a small protein from trout sperm, called "protamine," with insulin, the frequency of insulin injections could be reduced from several per day to one per day. The protamine insulin that is most often used today is isophane (meaning equal appearance or pure) insulin, which is also called NPH (neutral, protamine, Hagedorn) insulin. Protamine zinc insulin, like ultralente, is long-acting. Protamine insulins are buffered to neutral pH in phosphate buffer. No other insulin should be mixed with protamine zinc insulin, and NPH insulin should not be mixed with lente insulins.

Lente insulins are insulin suspensions of varying concentrations of zinc and crystal size in an acetate buffer. All are administered by subcutaneous injection. They do not contain any proteins other than insulin, and they may be mixed in any combination with each other. They were developed in the 1950s in an attempt to provide a better means of individualizing insulin dosages and durations.

There are now three types of insulin based on the duration of their effect: short-, intermediate-, and long-acting. At present there are 46 different formulations of insulin available. Primary categories of insulins, which are based on their reported onset and duration of action, are listed in Table 14–4. NPH insulin, an intermediate-acting insulin, is the most commonly used treatment, but should not be confused with "regular" (crystalline) insulin, which is short-acting. It may be that protamine zinc insulin will soon be discontinued because of its declining usage.

Most commercial insulins today are beef-pork combinations (in a 70:30 ratio), but insulin from either beef or pork only is available. It takes about 10,000 kg of raw pancreas to produce 1 kg of insulin. If an insulin preparation contains less than 25 ppm proinsulin, it is called "improved"; less than 10 ppm proinsulin is called "purified." Single peak insulin is 99% pure. Single component is more than 99% pure. Human insulin, or humulin, produced by genetically engineered bacteria, has become available. Another preparation of insulin designed to be identical with human insulin has been produced by enzymatically replacing alanine in pork insulin with threonine. All categories of insulin are currently available in concentrations of

Table 14–4. Type and Duration of Activities of Insulins

Type	Activity in Hours		
	Onset	Peak	Duration*
Short-acting			
Insulin injection USP (regular, crystalline)	$\frac{1}{4}$–$\frac{1}{2}$	2–4	5–7
Prompt insulin zinc suspension USP (semi-lente)	$\frac{1}{2}$–1	2–8	12–16
Intermediate-acting			
Isophane insulin suspension USP (NPH)	1–2	6–12	24–28
Insulin zinc suspension USP (lente)	1–2	6–12	24–28
Long-acting			
Protamine zinc insulin suspension USP	4–6	14–24	32–36
Insulin zinc suspension extended USP (ultra-lente)	4–6	18–24	32–36

* Duration is increased with increased dosages.

Note: Onset, peak effect, and duration of insulin are presumed to be similar among different species. The data provided in this table are standard guidelines for expected effects in humans. The actual onset, peak, and duration of effects should be determined on an individual basis for the type of insulin and dosage of insulin used in each patient.

40 and 100 U/ml. There is a 500 U/ml, short-acting pork insulin available for treatment of insulin resistance. Insulin is fairly stable at room temperature but is adversely affected by heat or freezing. Insulin is provided in multiple-dose vials, which should be refrigerated to prevent extremes in temperature.

Units were based on the amount necessary to decrease the blood glucose of a fasting, 2-kg rabbit from 120 to 45 mg/dl. Due to purification processes, units are now based on absolute weight of a recrystallized composite sample. One milligram of insulin is now equal to 24 U.

See also references 20, 88, and 112.

TREATMENT OF UNCOMPLICATED DIABETES MELLITUS

Initial Laboratory Assessments

The presence of diabetes can be ascertained quickly in many cases by placing a fresh strip of glucose oxidase-impregnated paper (TES-Tape) in the conjunctival sac. Any greenish tint evident in 60 seconds confirms the existence of hyperglycemia. Hyperglycemia also can be more accurately detected, directly or indirectly, by a variety of other glucose-determination techniques on blood or urine.

Selection of Patients

After establishing the diagnosis of diabetes, patients should be characterized in stages as having uncomplicated, ketoacidotic, or nonketotic hyperosmolar syndrome. Patients who are alert, with little or no dehydration and little or no ketonuria, and who are also willing and able to eat without vomiting, can be treated as having uncomplicated diabetes.

Basic Program of Therapy

Treatment of uncomplicated diabetes mellitus with insulin may begin with the subcutaneous administration of an intermediate-acting insulin, NPH or lente, at 0.5 U/kg body weight 30 minutes before the morning meal. Insulin is more efficient if it is present in adequate amounts while glucose is being absorbed from the intestines, rather than afterward. The response to intermediate insulin should be evaluated 8 to 12 hours after the injection, and the insulin dose should be appropriately modified by 1- to 2-U increments to attain a blood glucose value between 100 and 150 mg/dl in the evening. Morning blood glucose levels should also be measured and should not exceed 200 mg/dl. Crystalline insulin may be given in the evening if evening blood glucose levels exceed 250 mg/dl during the period of morning dosage adjustment. Exercise and caloric intake should remain as static as possible. Any nutritionally balanced diet with protein of high biologic value, such as Prescription Diet p/d, may be used. It is best to determine caloric requirements based on ideal body weight rather than on the present body weight. Reduction in body fat is beneficial because obesity reduces insulin receptors. Most 10- to 15-kg house dogs are estimated to require 40 to 60 kcal/kg body weight/day. Canned dog food is estimated to contain 500 to 600 kcal/lb. One fourth of the total daily requirements are given in the morning and three quarters are given 8 to 12 hours after the morning injection of insulin. An initial management checklist for uncomplicated diabetes is provided in Table 14–5.

Management of diabetes has been recommended in avians with intramuscular injections of intermediate-acting insulin at a dosage of about 0.002 U/30 g. Diabetes in the horse has been controlled with an intramuscular dose of approximately 0.5 U/kg body weight of protamine zinc insulin twice a day.

For further information on the treatment of uncomplicated diabetes mellitus, see also references 58 and 125.

TREATMENT OF DIABETES COMPLICATED BY KETOACIDOSIS AND HYPEROSMOLALITY

Diabetic ketoacidosis is a medical emergency requiring an aggressive approach; however, overly aggressive treatment, especially if the patient is not carefully monitored, can become the immediate cause of death. Proper intensive care of diabetic ketoacidosis, therefore, involves the prompt but judicious application of insulin and fluid therapy.

There is no magic formula for the successful treatment of diabetic ketoacidosis. Successful treatment depends on an accurate assessment of the patient's initial status, frequent reassessment of the patient's change in status during treatment, and appropriate therapeutic modifications during treatment.

See also reference 17.

Table 14–5. Initial Management Checklist of Uncomplicated Diabetes Mellitus*

---

1. Confine the animal to a cage and limit owner's visitations to keep exercise and excitement constant.
2. Calculate dietary requirements to maintain a thin ideal weight.
3. Feed one fourth of calculated diet at 7:00 to 8:00 A.M. 30 minutes after injecting intermediate-duration (NPH or lente) insulin subcutaneously at 0.5 U/kg body weight.
4. Collect blood sample for glucose determinations at 4:00 to 5:00 P.M. and feed three fourths of calculated diet.
5. Increase or decrease the next morning's insulin injection by no more than 1 to 2 U to attain an afternoon blood glucose value of 100 to 150 mg/dl.
6. Once the afternoon's blood glucose values have reached levels of 100 to 150 mg/dl, check one to two morning's blood glucose values (if >250 mg/dl, a long-lasting insulin or an insulin injection in the evening will also be necessary).

---

* Patient should have a good appetite and should not be vomiting.

Initial Laboratory Assessments

Ketones are easily measured in the blood or urine by nitroprusside reagents impregnated in paper strips (Ketostix) or by nitroprusside tablets (Acetest). Usually ketones are in greater concentration in the urine than in the blood because dehydration causes a greater concentration in the urine.

Unfortunately, the use of nitroprusside to detect ketones cannot by itself accurately assess ketoacidosis. For instance, ketones can be present with little or no change in blood pH if they are being adequately buffered and excreted. Conversely, ketoacidosis can be severe even though only a few ketones are detectable in the blood or urine. This is so because ketonemia results from mobilization of fat with the excessive formation of acetoacetic acid, which in turn may form acetone and β-hydroxybutyric acid, all of which are called ketones. Nitroprusside reacts well with acetoacetic acid, poorly with acetone, and not at all with β-hydroxybutyric acid. The normal β-hydroxybutyric acid to acetoacetic acid ratio is about 3:1, but in altered redox states, such as hypovolemia and cellular anoxia, the ratio of β-hydroxybutyric acid to acetoacetic acid may shift to values as great as 15:1; therefore, ketoacidosis may become more severe with hypotension, but detectable ketonemia or ketonuria may change little.

Other concomitant problems, such as lactic acidosis and azotemia, can cause severe acidosis with mild ketonemia or ketonuria in diabetic patients. Normal plasma lactate levels should not exceed 15 mg/dl in dogs, but direct measurements are frequently unavailable on a clinical basis. If serum sodium, potassium, chloride, and bicarbonate can be readily measured, the anionic gap (undetermined plasma anions) can be calculated by formula (Na + K − Cl − HCO_3 = normal anion gap [12 to 16 mEq/L]). An increased anionic gap in diabetic patients with little or no detectable ketones can usually be explained by the presence of β-hydroxybutyric acid, increased lactic acid, or retained organic acids of uremia.

Lactic acidosis is a sequela to impaired cardiopulmonary or hepatic function. Lactic acid is a product of anaerobic metabolism. Tissue hypoxia or deficient hepatic removal of lactic acid results in its accumulation in the blood. Treatment is directed at general attempts to improve cardiopulmonary or hepatic function and tissue oxygenation. Bicarbonate therapy is not particularly effective. Dichloroacetate is an anion that stimulates pyruvate dehydrogenase, an enzyme that catalyzes oxidation of lactate and pyruvate.[94] The clinical usefulness of dichloroacetate for the treatment of diabetic ketoacidosis is still under investigation.

The initial assessment of a diabetic patient with ketonemia or ketonuria and the selection of the most appropriate form of treatment obviously require more than quantitation of hyperglycemia and detection of ketones in the blood and urine. For the laboratory examination of the urine of a diabetic patient suspected of having ketoacidosis, a sample should be collected by cystocentesis to preclude contamination of the bladder. Venous blood samples, coagulated and anticoagulated (EDTA-treated), should be collected (Table 14–6).

Table 14–6. Blood and Urinary Values Needed for Management of Ketoacidotic Diabetes Mellitus

---

Blood
    Complete blood cell count
    Blood glucose
    Blood ketones
    Blood urea nitrogen (BUN)
    Serum sodium and potassium
    Blood pH
    Total CO_2 (complete blood gas analysis on arterial blood is preferred)
    Effective plasma osmolality [2 (Na) + blood glucose/20]
Urine
    Results of routine urinalysis, including cytologic examination of sediment
    Results of aerobic bacterial culture

Anticoagulated (heparinized) arterial blood is preferred for complete blood gas analysis. Samples for complete blood gas analysis must be collected in such a way that air bubbles are not left in the syringe with the blood sample, and samples must be placed in an ice water bath immediately after collection. Analysis of blood gas must be done within 3.5 hours of collection.

Frequent monitoring of the initial response to insulin is essential for the successful management of diabetic ketoacidosis. The variable rate of urine production, admixtures of urine collecting in the bladder from different times, individual variations in renal threshold, semiquantitative methods of determination, and risks of infection from indwelling urinary catheters make urine glucose determinations more difficult than serial blood glucose determinations. The blood glucose is generally determined each hour until the blood glucose level is less than 250 mg/dl. This can be done in a little over 1 minute with a few drops of whole blood using glucose oxidase impregnated strips (Dextrostix, Glucoscan Test Strips, and Stat-Tek Glucose Strips) and a reflectance colorimeter (Glucometer II, Glucoscan II, Glucochek II, Accu-check bG and Stat-Tek Meter).[22] Figure 14–6 shows a reflectance colorimeter being used. Alternately, two-color block strips impregnated with glucose oxidase (Chemstrip bG, Visidex and Visidex II) may be visually interpreted.

Qualitative estimates of the changes in serum potassium and serum bicarbonate in response to treatment for diabetes are sufficient for clinical purposes. Changes in concentrations of serum potassium and transmembrane potassium gradients can be monitored by electrocardiography. Total serum CO_2 can be determined by a CO_2 laboratory kit on as little as 100 μl of serum. Since 95% or more of total serum CO_2 consists of serum bicarbonate, total serum CO_2 can be substituted for serum bicarbonate for clinical purposes. Blood pH can be measured by an expanded pH meter.

Assessment of serum osmolality also should be included in the initial evaluation of diabetic patients. The serum of diabetic patients can become

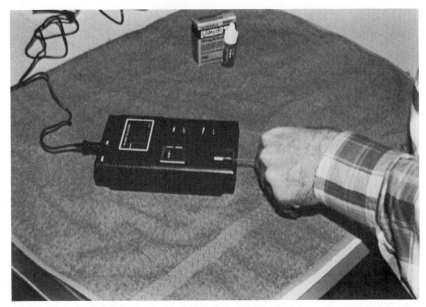

Fig. 14–6. A reflectance colorimeter quickly manages blood glucose levels with a few drops of whole blood. (From Chastain, C.B., and Nichols, C.E.: Current concepts on the control of diabetes mellitus. Vet. Clin. North Am., *14:*859, 1984.)

severely hyperosmolar with or without ketoacidosis. If the patient is clinically ill, as shown by such signs as depression, anorexia, weakness, and vomiting, serum hyperosmolality is possible. Direct determination on the serum by an osmometer measures all osmoles, but some—like urea—are freely permeable to cells. Tonicity or "effective osmolality" can be calculated in diabetics by the formula: $mOsm/L = 2 (Na) + glucose/20$. If the serum sodium is not available, low-normal serum sodium (140 mEq/L) can be used in the formula to calculate the serum osmolality for the purposes of selecting the most appropriate fluid therapy. Normal plasma effective osmolality in the dog and cat is about 280 to 310 mOsm/L. Serum osmolality above 340 mOsm/L can be dangerous in diabetic patients.

Once the existence of ketoacidosis has been determined by the laboratory, its clinical significance can be confirmed by the presence of mental depression, weakness, anorexia, or vomiting. An active, mentally alert patient who will eat and does not vomit does not have ketoacidosis to a degree sufficient to require intensive care.

Reassessments

The initial values to be reassessed during intensive care should be recorded on a flow sheet. The patient's clinical condition should be monitored hourly by appropriate examinations and tests during the initial treatment of diabetic ketoacidosis (Table 14–7). The initial blood pH and total serum CO_2 should be recorded. The frequency of later blood pH and total CO_2

Table 14-7. Clinical Conditions That Should Be Monitored
Hourly During Treatment of Diabetic Ketoacidosis

Blood glucose
Electrocardiographic QT interval (serum potassium determinations may be
   preferable)
Skin turgor
Urinary bladder size measured by palpation or the amount of urine voided
Pulse
Respiratory sounds by auscultation
Respiratory rate
Rectal temperature

reassessments depends on the initial value and on the apparent changes in
the patient's respiratory rate and depth, mental alertness, and color of the
mucous membranes. Hourly blood pH and total CO_2 determinations are
not necessary on a routine basis. Central venous pressure may be of value if
the patient is morbid. Most patients are ambulatory, so repeated measurements of central venous pressure often are impractical.

The measurement of urinary glucose concentrations is not a good means
of assessing the response to treatment. As previously mentioned, indwelling urethral catheterization is inadvisable unless the patient is comatose,
markedly azotemic, or apparently oliguric or anuric (the presence of oliguria or anuria is based on the lack of voided urine and urinary bladder
palpations). Indwelling urethral catheters introduce or aggravate bacterial
cystitis and bacteremias. Even transient urethral catheterization in healthy
dogs under conditions of carefully applied asepsis can contaminate female
urinary bladders. The incidence of iatrogenic infection is presumably
greater in debilitated females. Most diabetic dogs are female, and diabetic
patients have a higher-than-average risk of becoming infected due to impaired microcirculation and microbicidal functions.

Another reason urinary glucose concentrations should not be used to
monitor response to treatment is that the concentration of urinary glucose
does not correlate well with concentrations of plasma glucose. The concentration of urinary glucose varies with differences in the individual patient's
urinary glucose thresholds, volume output, and concentrating ability. For
example, urinary glucose thresholds in diabetic children may range from 45
to 270 mg/dl. Collection of a few drops of whole blood using a 23-gauge
needle for use in a reflectance colorimeter is a more accurate method of
assessing response to treatment and can be repeated numerous times without difficulty. It also is less hazardous and better tolerated by the patient
than indwelling urethral catheterization.

Fluid Therapy

Appropriate use of fluid therapy is the most important aspect of treatment for diabetic ketoacidosis. Invariably, patients with ketoacidosis of a
significant degree are moderately to severely dehydrated and hypotensive.

Hypotension is particularly likely if hyperosmolality is present, inasmuch as the resulting cellular dehydration of the myocardium weakens myocardial strength of contraction.[99] Proper administration of fluids should improve cardiac output, decrease serum osmolality, reduce hyperglycemia, reduce ketonemia, buffer ketoacids, maintain urinary excretion, and correct electrolyte imbalances.

See also reference 115.

ROUTES AND RATES OF ADMINISTRATION.   The basic guidelines of fluid therapy are to be followed. Owing to the immediacy of the need for fluid replacement, the intravenous route of administration should be used in all cases of clinically significant ketoacidosis. If the clinical significance of ketoacidosis is equivocal—that is, if the blood pH, serum osmolality, cardiac output, urine production, and serum potassium are all near normal— the subcutaneous route can be effectively used. The rate of the intravenous administration of fluids should not exceed 90 ml/kg body weight/hr. Slower rates are especially advisable if insufficiencies of cardiac or renal function are suspected or detected by thoracic auscultation or by monitoring urinary output.

In most cases, a rate of intravenous administration of 20 to 40 ml/kg body weight/hr is adequate until rehydration is complete, and then a slower rate is used to maintain urinary output. If possible, urinary output should be quantitated by using a metabolic cage that pools all voided urine. If a metabolic cage is not available, urinary output should be estimated by palpation of the urinary bladder and inspection of the cage and bedding for voided urine.

It is necessary to continue parenteral fluid therapy until the patient is willing to eat and does not vomit. Since several days of continuous fluid administration are frequently required, an indwelling intravenous catheter (Venocath) should be carefully and securely placed in a jugular vein. After taping the jugular catheter in place, a gauze-and-tape harness is placed around the thorax, to which extension tubing (Extension Set) from the intravenous catheter to the fluids' administration tubing is taped (Fig. 14–7). Tension on the tubing will not displace the jugular catheter. A strip of elastic banding can be attached from the top of the cage to the administration tubing to pull the tubing out of the patient's way, so that the patient is free to move about the cage at will without affecting the fluids' flow rate. Aseptically placed catheters can be left 2 to 3 days before being replaced.

SELECTION OF FLUIDS.   The selection of fluids is based on the patient's serum osmolality and blood pH (Table 14–8). Lactated Ringer's solution, half-strength normal saline solution (0.45% NaCl), and 5% dextrose are the most useful fluids in the treatment of diabetic ketoacidosis. Lactated Ringer's solution is a balanced isotonic polyionic electrolyte solution that, while replacing fluid volume, prevents dilution deficiencies in the concentration of electrolytes. It is used whenever the blood pH and serum osmolality are near normal. At half-strength, normal saline solution reduces

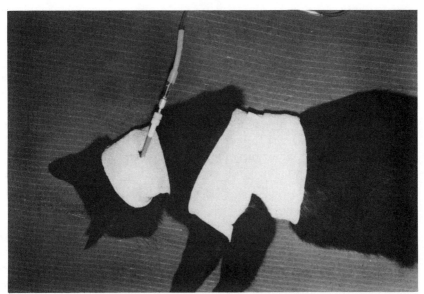

Fig. 14–7. The administration of intravenous fluids to a ketoacidotic patient is facilitated by a jugular catheter and a gauze-and-tape harness or saddle placed around the thorax to absorb tension caused by the patient's movements in the cage. (From Chastain, C.B.: Intensive care of dogs and cats with diabetic ketoacidosis. J. Am. Vet. Med. Assoc., *179:*972, 1981.)

serum hyperosmolality caused by profound hyperglycemia and dilutes the hyperosmolality of administered bicarbonate. One milliliter of 8.4% sodium bicarbonate contains 2,000 mOsm. Eight milliliters (mEq) of 8.4% sodium bicarbonate diluted in 1 L of fluids raise the osmolality by 160 mOsm/L. If added to isotonic fluids in such amounts, the dilution becomes undesirably hyperosmolar. Dextrose (5%) is reserved for whenever the administration of fluid and insulin lowers plasma glucose concentrations to less than 250 mg/dl.

SPECIAL FLUID THERAPY ADDITIVES. The need for fluid additives, such as potassium phosphate (Potassium Phosphate) and sodium bicarbonate, is determined by the blood pH and serum potassium concentration. If the concentration of serum potassium cannot be repeatedly determined directly, electrocardiography can be helpful in estimating serum potassium concentrations, especially if a baseline ECG and measurement of the concentration of serum potassium concentration were done at the initiation of treatment. Although electrocardiographic changes may not directly correlate with absolute concentrations of serum potassium, the ECG is a reliable monitor of changes in serum potassium concentrations and transmembrane potassium gradients. Prolongation of the QT interval (>0.22 seconds in the dog; >0.16 seconds in the cat) occurring in a patient with ketoacidosis should be interpreted as hypokalemia. Hypokalemia can also cause bradycardia and small biphasic T waves. Insulin facilitates the intracellular entry of phosphate as well as potassium. Resulting hypophosphatemia decreases the transfer of oxygen from hemoglobin to the tissues; therefore, potassium phosphate is preferred over potassium chloride as a potassium supplement in the treatment of ketoacidosis.

Although the excessive production of ketones leads to metabolic acidosis and insulin therapy can cause hypokalemia-hypophosphatemia, caution must be taken to avoid the injudicious administration of sodium bicarbonate or potassium phosphate. Rapidly, inappropriately, or excessively administered potassium phosphate can cause bradycardia, heart blocks, atrial standstill, and cardiac arrest. Bicarbonate should be administered when serum bicarbonate (or total CO_2) levels are less than 50% of normal (≤ 12 mEq/L), or when the blood pH is ≤ 7.1. Bicarbonate requirements are calculated by the following formula: base deficit (25 mEq/L − total CO_2 × 0.4 [the fluid space in which bicarbonate deficit is replaced in the first 3 to 4 hours]) × kg body weight. Only one half of the calculated bicarbonate deficit is replaced in the first 3 to 4 hours; then the patient's acid-base balance is reassessed.

Normal concentrations of serum potassium are about 3.5 to 5.5 mEq/L. Since fluid infusion is through an indwelling catheter with the tip in or near the cranial vena cava or right atrium, it is best not to infuse concentrations of potassium that exceed fourfold normal concentrations of serum potassium (20 mEq/L). Otherwise, the myocardium could be adversely affected by high concentrations of potassium. The administration of potassium should never exceed 0.5 mEq/kg body weight/hr.

Serum potassium levels are a poor index of potassium deficits. Approximately 60% of the body's water is intracellular, and normal intracellular

Table 14–8. Guidelines for the Selection of Fluid Therapy for Diabetic Ketoacidosis

Blood pH	Serum Osmolality (mOsm/L)	Serum Potassium (mEq/L)	ECG QT Interval	Recommended Fluids
>7.1	<340	>3.0	Normal	Lactated Ringer's solution.
>7.1	<340	≤3.0	Prolonged*	Lactated Ringer's solution plus 10–20 mEq/L of potassium phosphate.
>7.1	≥340	>3.0	Normal	0.45% saline solution plus 5–10 mEq/L of potassium phosphate.
>7.1	≥340	≤3.0	Prolonged*	0.45% saline solution plus 10–20 mEq/L of potassium phosphate.
≤7.1	>300	>3.0	Normal	0.45% saline solution plus 50% of calculated† bicarbonate deficit as sodium bicarbonate, given as 80 mEq/L or less; plus 5–10 mEq/L of potassium phosphate.
≤7.1	>300	≤3.0	Prolonged*	0.45% saline solution plus 50% of calculated† bicarbonate deficit as sodium bicarbonate, given as 80 mEq/L or less; plus 10–20 mEq/L of potassium phosphate.

* More than 0.22 seconds in the dog; more than 0.16 seconds in the cat.
† Serum or plasma bicarbonate deficit (mEq/L) × 0.4 × kg body weight = total bicarbonate deficit.

concentrations of potassium are 120 to 160 mEq/L; therefore, 98% of potassium is normally intracellular. If hypokalemia develops in a diabetic capable of taking oral doses of potassium, the oral supplementation of potassium (Micro-K Extencaps, Slow-K) at about 1.0 mEq/kg body weight/day should be given in divided doses, if possible, after meals. Urine potassium levels, as well as serum potassium levels, can be monitored to verify adequate supplementation.

Insulin Therapy

METHODS AND DOSES OF THE INITIAL ADMINISTRATION OF INSULIN.   After the patient's status has been assessed, a flow sheet of conditions to be re-assessed has been initiated, and fluid therapy has commenced, insulin ther-apy should begin. Regular (crystalline) or semilente insulin can be used in one of three administration programs. The insulin administration pro-grams include the conventional (bolus) method, the continuous low-dose intravenous method, and the low-dose intramuscular method.

The most frequent causes of death during treatment for diabetic ketoaci-dosis are cerebral edema, caused by a rapid decline in blood glucose con-centration or by the injudicious use of hypotonic fluids; hypokalemia, caused by the administration of insulin and bicarbonate plus fluid dilution and fluid-induced diuresis; and iatrogenic hypoglycemia or insulin shock. Low-dose administration of insulin permits a controllable, gradual decline in hyperglycemia, thereby reducing the risk of hypoglycemia and cerebral edema. The maximal effects of insulin are quantitative, with inhibition of ketogenesis and facilitation of glucose entry into cells in an amount less than that required to facilitate potassium entry into cells (Fig. 14–8). Because of this, the low-dose administration of insulin can also reduce the risks of insulin-induced hypokalemia. Mortality in dogs being treated with the con-ventional method of insulin administration for diabetic ketoacidosis ranges from 5% to 40%. Mortality in dogs treated with low-dose methods is much lower than with the conventional method. The conventional method of administering boluses of regular insulin for diabetic ketoacidosis has no advantages over low-dose methods that have been substantiated by clinical trials. Moreover, conventional insulin therapy has been associated with severe hypokalemia, hyperlactacidemia, late hypoglycemia, and decreased concentrations of serum phosphate and magnesium.

Intravenous low-dose administration of insulin is the preferred treatment if the patient is severely hypotensive or hypothermic, and if adequate super-vision is available to prevent malpositioning of catheters and to assure a regular rate of administration. If infusion pumps are not available, an intra-venous set ensuring the precise volume of insulin (Soluset) should be used. All tubing should be flushed with the insulin-containing fluids to saturate binding sites on the plastic. Recommended intravenous low-dose therapy is 0.1 U/kg body weight, followed by a dose of 0.1 U/kg body weight/hr of crystalline insulin diluted in replacement fluids, such as lactated Ringer's,

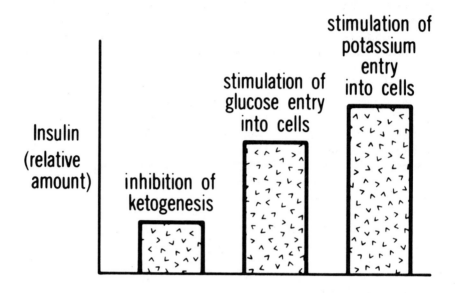

Fig. 14–8. Maximal effects on ketogenesis, glucose entry into cells, and stimulation of potassium entry into cells occur at different concentrations of insulin in the blood. (Modified from Alberti, K.G.M.M., and Nattrass, M.: Severe diabetic ketoacidosis. Med. Clin. North Am., 62:799, 1978.)

and administered by slow drip. With intravenous low-dose treatment there are potential problems in achieving proper dilution of insulin in the fluids and in knowing how much insulin is actually being administered, because insulin binds to glass and fluid administration equipment made of polyvinyl-chloride.

The low-dose, intramuscular administration of insulin permits more accurate measurement of administered insulin and requires a minimum of equipment and supervision. The low-dose, intramuscular method of administering regular insulin simply consists of giving a small initial priming dose, followed by hourly injections of even smaller doses of insulin, until the blood glucose has been reduced to less than 250 mg/dl. The priming dose binds unbound insulin-binding plasma proteins and sensitizes the target cells to the smaller doses that will follow.

The initial dose is 2 U of regular insulin, administered in the thigh muscles for cats and for small dogs weighing less than 10 kg. Very small dogs and cats under 3 kg should be treated initially with only 1 U of crystalline insulin followed by 1 U each hour. For dogs weighing more than 10 kg, the initial dose is 0.25 U/kg body weight. Treatment continues each hour thereafter until blood glucose levels are less than 250 mg/dl: for cats and small dogs, 1 U is administered; for dogs weighing more than 10 kg, 0.1

U/kg body weight is administered. Syringes measuring 1 U (Lo-Dose Insulin Syringes; 40–80 U Monoject Insulin Syringe) or a fresh dilution of regular insulin in sterile saline solution may be used.

After the blood glucose has been reduced to a concentration ranging between 250 and 150 mg/dl, the administration of intramuscularly administered insulin is discontinued. The mean time required is about 4 hours. Fluids are changed to 5% dextrose with 4 to 8 mEq/L of potassium phosphate added to prevent dilutional hypokalemia. Intravenously administered dextrose (5%) further reduces the risk of iatrogenic hypoglycemia and provides a source of energy to inhibit ketogenesis until the patient is willing to eat and does not vomit. If the blood glucose is less than 150 mg/dl, a solution of 5% dextrose with potassium phosphate is administered alone. Insulin is not given. If the blood glucose ranges between 150 and 250 mg/dl, the intravenous administration of 5% dextrose with potassium phosphate is given, and 0.5 U/kg body weight of regular insulin is administered subcutaneously every 6 to 8 hours. Doses are then changed by 1 to 2 U to maintain blood glucose concentrations between 100 and 200 mg/dl at 4 hours after the last injection. When the patient is able to eat without vomiting, fluids and regular administration of insulin can be discontinued. Therapy with NPH or lente insulin can then begin in a conventional manner.

Nonketotic hyperosmolar coma should also be treated with regular insulin. Because the coma is due to hyperosmolality, the reduction in hyperglycemia should be gradual to minimize the risk for iatrogenic cerebral edema. Patients affected with nonketotic hyperosmolar coma are not insulin-resistant. Low-dose administration is appropriate and preferred for the treatment of nonketotic hyperosmolar coma, as well as diabetic ketoacidosis. Once diabetics with ketoacidosis or nonketotic hyperosmolar coma are stabilized, willing, and capable of eating without vomiting, they can be treated as an uncomplicated diabetic.

See also references 17 and 42.

MAINTENANCE INSULIN THERAPY. If the patient's appetite, attitude, physical activity, consumption of water, and output of urine are within normal limits, and if the evening blood glucose is consistently between 100 and 150 mg/dl and the morning blood glucose does not exceed 200 mg/dl, the patient can be discharged and treated with a once daily injection of intermediate-acting insulin. In many cases, such conditions cannot be achieved, or control soon deteriorates.

Possible responses to insulin as described by Hallas-Moller are illustrated in Figure 14–9. Type "A" reactions may be caused by the *Somogyi effect,* an exaggerated response to insulin-induced hypoglycemia, or by a transient effect of intermediate-acting insulin, presumably from excessive insulinase activity, called the *"dawn phenomenon."* In our experience, transient insulin activity is more common in dogs and cats than is the Somogyi effect. Type "B" reactions are the desired response. Type "C" reactions result from the

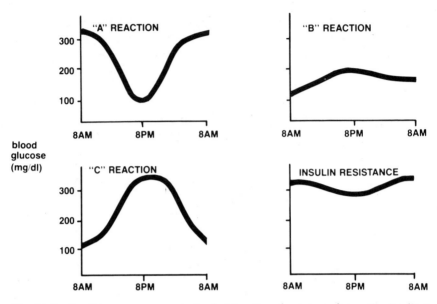

Fig. 14–9. Possible responses to a single administration of an intermediate-acting insulin at 8 A.M. (Modified from *Diabetes Mellitus.* 8th Ed. Indianapolis, Eli Lilly and Co., 1980.)

delayed action of insulin, which is caused by poor absorption from the injection site or binding with serum proteins.

Insulin resistance is arbitrarily defined as the failure to reduce blood glucose to normal levels with the administration of less than 2 U/kg body weight. Insulin resistance may be caused by decreased receptor affinity for insulin, the induction or administration of insulin-antagonistic hormones, insulin-antagonistic endocrinopathies, inactivation of insulin at the site of injection, anti-insulin antibodies, or postreceptor defects in insulin's action.

The inability to achieve or maintain adequate control of diabetes in dogs and cats occurs in more than one half of insulin-treated cases if they are closely monitored and re-evaluated. Several possible causes may be considered (Table 14–9). A rational progression of investigation to determine the cause for poor diabetic control is listed in Table 14–10.

Once the cause for poor control is known, the appropriate corrective measures are obvious. In the case of Type "A" reactions caused by the Somogyi effect, reducing the insulin dose will correct the hypoglycemic episodes and subsequent early morning hyperglycemia. Type "C" reactions may be corrected by changing insulins or injection sites or by giving more than one insulin injection per day. Insulin resistance may be corrected by successful management of the concurrent infectious disease, pancreatitis, obesity, pregnancy, estrus, uremia, or insulin-antagonistic endocrinopathy, or by the discontinuation of the administration of insulin-antagonistic drugs. Hormones antagonistic to insulin actions are epinephrine, glucagon, GH, glucocorticoids, progesterone, and thyroid hormones. Insulin resist-

Table 14–9. Possible Causes for Failure of Diabetic Control With Once-Daily Doses of Intermediate-acting Insulin

Storage or administration problems
  Improper storage of insulin
  Failure to agitate vial
  Improper injection technique

Decreased receptor affinity for insulin
  Obesity
  Insulin-antagonistic endocrinopathies
  Anti-insulin receptor antibodies

Induction of increased insulinase activity
Induction or administration of insulin-antagonistic hormones
  Infections
  Surgery
  Estrus
  Pregnancy
  Somogyi effect

Anti-insulin antibodies
Post-receptor defects in insulin action

ance caused by anti-insulin antibodies is probably rare because of the purity of insulins made since 1979.

If high titers to insulin or the elimination of other possibilities suggests the possibility of an insulin allergy, the administration of pork insulin should correct the resistance in dogs. The structure of pork insulin is identical to that of canine insulin. The structure of bovine insulin is different from pork and canine insulin, so it is more antigenic to dogs than is pork insulin. Most insulin preparations are pork and beef mixtures. The structure of feline insulin is not known, but it is thought that beef would also be more antigenic than pork in the cat. Inactivation of insulin by subcutaneous proteases has been reported in humans with apparent insulin resistance. This should be suspected if intravenous insulin is more effective than subcutaneous insulin in treatment. In theory, postreceptor defects in insulin's action may be responsible for insulin resistance. Unfortunately, such a possibility can only be suspected after all other possibilities have been eliminated.

Type "A" reactions, resulting from the transient effect of intermediate-acting insulin, are quite common in diabetic dogs and cats. One solution to this problem may be the use of a long-acting insulin. After a long-acting insulin injection (with the same number of units as had previously been given with the intermediate-acting insulin), measurements of blood glucose should be made every 2 hours. Unfortunately, protamine zinc insulin may have an undesirably long delay in its onset of action.

If the response to long-acting insulin does not produce a Type "B" response, twice daily NPH or lente insulin injections are often corrective. If further refinement is necessary or desired, "split and mixed" multiple daily injections should be tried. The best compromise between the insulin's ef-

Table 14–10. Algorithm for Investigating the Cause of Poor Diabetic Control or Apparent Failure to Respond to Insulin at More than 2 U/Kg Body Weight/Day

---

Review the history.
    Is the insulin being stored and administered correctly?
    Are the diet and allowed exercise proper?
    Are insulin-antagonistic drugs being administered?
    Has surgical stress recently occurred?
    Is the patient in estrus or pregnant?

If the cause of the lack of control is not apparent, continue routine feeding practices and insulin administration and measure blood glucose levels every 2 hours.

Type "A" reaction		Type "C" reaction Insulin is transiently sequestered by injection site or serum proteins.	Insulin resistance:
A period of hypoglycemia occurs before hyperglycemia (Somogyi effect).	Blood glucose is only transiently in normal range. Insufficient duration of effects.		Infectious processes Hyperadrenocorticism Functional pheochromocytoma Estrus Ovarian imbalance I Pregnancy Acromegaly Hyperthyroidism Uremia Obesity Anti-insulin antibodies Subcutaneous protease inactivation of insulin Post-receptor defects in insulin action.

---

fect and the effort to produce a desired effect is to give a mixture of intermediate-acting insulin and short-acting insulin twice daily 30 to 60 minutes before the morning and evening meal. A mixture composed of one third of short-acting and two thirds of intermediate-acting insulin is prepared. Mixtures are best prepared at the time of injection. Morning and evening meals should each be one half of the calculated daily requirements. Initially, the morning dose should be two thirds of the total daily requirements, and the evening dose should be one third of the total daily requirements. Using a greater insulin dose in the morning reduces the risk of night-time hypoglycemia. Morning and evening dosages are adjusted in 1- to 2-U increments in response to the blood glucose values produced. Many other split-dose regimens are possible. Some of these have been reported useful in dogs and cats.

Low-dose syringes and insulin diluent (Sterile Diluting Fluid for NPH Insulin and Sterile Diluting Fluid for Neutral Regular Insulin Injection) are recommended for cats and small dogs. Since sterile saline or bacterio-static water will alter the insulin pH, resulting in altered absorption of intermediate- and long-acting insulins, these diluents should not be used.[128] Needles and syringes from different manufacturers vary in their dead space and accuracy of dosage. The type of needles, syringes, and (of course) insulin should not vary.

See also references 19–21, 35, 37, 46, 52, 78, 86, 87, 89, and 113.

HOME MANAGEMENT

When the patient is regulated well enough to be sent home, an appointment with the owner should be made by the attending clinician. Sufficient time should be allotted to teach the owners how to care for their diabetic pet, quiet their apprehensions, and answer their questions.

Before bringing the pet into the conference room, the clinician should review written instructions for home care of the pet with owners. Emphasis should be placed on the scheduled diet and its amounts, as well as the timing and amount of insulin used in injections. The owners should be advised how to store the insulin when not in use. They should be shown how to agitate the suspension without causing foaming before it is aspirated into the syringe, how to aspirate aseptically the liquid from the vial into a syringe, how to remove the air bubbles, and how to tell precisely the amount of insulin they will be giving their pet. After telling and showing how to accomplish these tasks, the clinician should require the owners to demonstrate with sterile saline exactly how they plan to prepare for making the injections.

Once most of the discussion and questions have ended, have the animal brought into the room. Before this point, the animal would have been an unnecessary distraction for the owner. Finally, the clinician should indicate how to give the injections, showing the technique by giving the animal an injection in the same way the insulin should be given at home.

When the owners feel confident about caring for their pet at home, the patient can be discharged with insulin, syringes, and needles. The first recheck is requested in 2 weeks. All recommended subsequent rechecks should take place every 3 months, provided the patient is well regulated by the treatment.

MONITORING DIABETICS AT HOME AND DURING OUTPATIENT RECHECK EXAMINATIONS

At Home

Good control of diabetes mellitus cannot be assured by testing random urine samples for glucose each day. Besides being an inconvenience and an added expense to the owner, it is often misleading. The parameters best indicating the control of diabetes mellitus include the average highest value of blood glucose attained and the average range of variation in the blood glucose. Measurement of urine glucose cannot be assumed to reflect blood glucose values unless the renal threshold is established for patients on an individual basis, and urine voiding is monitored closely enough to know the length of the interval during which the urine tested was collected in the bladder. In dogs, the normal renal threshold for glucose is 175 to 220 mg/dl; in cats, it is 270 to 310 mg/dl.[68] If the urine glucose is undetectable, the blood glucose may be undesirably low.

There are two methods of testing for urine glucose. One is by glucose oxidase-impregnated strips (Tes-Tape and Clinistix), which may give false-negative results from inhibitory substances such as salicylates. The other method of testing for urine glucose is the copper reduction technique, which uses tablets (Clinitest Tablets) that may give false-positive results in the presence of other reducing substances such as ascorbic acid.

Even when control seems poor, the measurement of urine glucose levels is only an indication of the circumstances involving the last insulin injection, the last meal, recent exercise, and other recent unknown factors. Concern and changes in insulin dosage should be based on repeated abnormal findings involving more than one insulin injection, meal, period of exercise, and other events.

With this in mind, it seems more desirable to assess control at home by a variety of more practical means. The owner should keep a log of the parameters (listed in Table 14–11) to be reviewed by the veterinarian at times of apparent poor control and at routine re-examinations. Diabetic dogs or cats should be examined by a veterinarian if abnormalities are detected by monitoring at home for 2 or more days in a row or whenever ketones are detected in the urine. If urine glucose is used to supplement the means of monitoring listed in Table 14–11, the renal threshold should be established for each individual patient. In addition, for the urine glucose to be meaning-

Table 14–11. Recommended Means of Monitoring the Control of Diabetes Mellitus at Home

Evaluation	Assess and Record
Attitude	Daily
Appetite	Daily
Physical activity	Daily
Water consumption* (in ounces/24 hours)	Daily
Urinary continence	Daily
Body weight	Weekly
Urine ketones	As necessary†

* Daily water consumption should not exceed 60 ml/kg (1 oz/lb) body weight.
† Measurement of urine ketones should be done if there is concern about whether other assessments are normal.

ful as an indication of the proper control of diabetes, the time during which voiding is tested and the time of the last voiding of urine before the test should be recorded.

Outpatient Recheck Examinations

Diabetics should be physically re-examined, their home-monitoring log reviewed, and blood examinations repeated every 3 months. Recommended components of an outpatient recheck examination are listed in Table 14–12.

Glycohemoglobin is glycosylated hemoglobin A, which forms progressively and almost irreversibly throughout the lifespan of the red blood cells. Measuring the amount of glycohemoglobin in the dog is an excellent means of quantitatively assessing the average blood glucose in diabetics over several weeks. It is an assessment of the adequacy or inadequacy of home care, as opposed to the measurement of blood or urine glucose, which is only an indication of a part of the day the samples were collected. Diabetic animals often become excited when returning to the veterinary hospital, perhaps out of fear of being separated from the family, among other probable reasons; therefore, the in-office measurement of blood and urine glucose is much less reliable in assessing control of diabetes than are the monitoring log, physical examination, and glycohemoglobin value. Normal glycohemoglobin values in dogs are about 4% to 8%, depending on the laboratory and method of determination. Poorly controlled diabetic animals have values of 10% to 18%. This test is not valid in the cat.

POSSIBLE FUTURE CONTROL METHODS FOR DIABETES MELLITUS

Several methods of treating diabetes mellitus are being investigated and may become clinically useful in companion animal medicine. Some of these include "open-loop" portable insulin pumps, nasal administration of insulin-bile salt mixtures,[51] islet cell transplants, and immunotherapy to minimize

Table 14–12. Recommended Components of a Routine Outpatient Re-examination of Diabetics

1. Review owners' observations and home monitoring log.
2. Record body weight and results of complete routine physical examination.
3. Collect urine for urinalysis (if possible, without catheterization).
4. Collect blood for the following studies:
   Hemogram
   Blood glucose
   Serum urea nitrogen
   Cholesterol
   Serum alanine aminotransferase
   Serum alkaline phosphatase
   Glycohemoglobin (omit if a feline)

immune-mediated damage to the islets. Transplants of islet cells are the optimal form of therapy. A modified method of harvesting B cells by digesting pancreatic tissue with collagenase, followed by tissue culture and transplant into the spleen, has been successful in correcting experimentally induced diabetes in dogs.

SPECIFIC PROBLEMS

Infections

Ketoacidotic diabetic patients should be carefully examined for infections. Diabetes reduces resistance to infections by increasing extracellular glucose, impairing phagocytosis, causing cellular malnutrition, and impairing microcirculation. The most common precipitating cause for ketoacidosis in diabetics is infection, in some cases seemingly trivial infections. Infections induce the increased secretion of cortisol, glucagon, and possibly epinephrine, which antagonize the action of insulin and cause anorexia, a condition augmenting ketogenesis in excess of the body's ability to use or buffer ketoacids.

Common clinical signs of infection are not reliable indicators of infection in ketoacidosis. Ketoacidosis causes vasodilation, which tends to cause hypothermia, which then may counteract pyrexia from infection. Leukocytosis is caused by ketoacidosis with or without associated infection. Because trivial infections may precipitate ketoacidosis, because leukocytosis in ketoacidotic diabetic patients does not necessarily indicate infection, and because pyrexia may be absent with infections, diabetes-related infections may be easily overlooked.

Urinary tract infections in diabetic patients are common. Between 25% and 50% of diabetic dogs with ketoacidosis have urinary tract infections. Concentrations of leukocytes and protein in urine may be misleadingly low because of osmotic diuresis caused by glucosuria. As previously mentioned, samples for urinary culture should be collected aseptically as part of the initial assessment of every diabetic patient with ketoacidosis. Urethral catheters should be avoided except in morbid patients or in those otherwise suspected of having oliguria or anuria. Even if an infection cannot be found, broad-spectrum antimicrobial therapy should be used empirically in some cases. This is particularly true if the animal is resistant to insulin.

See also references 71 and 79.

Pancreatitis

The most commonly recognized cause of diabetes in the dog is acinar pancreatitis; however, pancreatitis is not necessarily the most common cause of diabetes in dogs (the most common cause is not known). In a recent retrospective study of diabetic ketoacidosis in dogs, 21% of the survivors were diagnosed as having concurrent acute pancreatitis; 5% had exocrine insufficiency. Of the nonsurvivors, 65% had acute pancreatitis;

15% had chronic pancreatitis. Acute pancreatitis is rare in the cat, with or without diabetes mellitus.

Acute pancreatitis should be suspected whenever vomiting continues after the blood glucose has decreased to less than 250 mg/dl. Other signs of acute pancreatitis associated with diabetes mellitus are pain in the cranial part of the abdomen and markedly elevated levels of serum amylase, serum lipase, serum alkaline phosphatase, serum bilirubin, or plasma fibrinogen. When the animal has acute pancreatitis, abdominal radiography may show duodenal ileus and local peritonitis in the area of the pancreas, and peritoneal lavage may yield fluid high in amylase and cells suggestive of aseptic peritonitis.

In the treatment of acute pancreatitis, patients should not be given food and water by mouth until serum amylase values are near normal. Fluids then are administered in the dosage described for the treatment of diabetic ketoacidosis. Calcium gluconate or gluceptate (200 mg of calcium/L) in 5% dextrose should be given intravenously in quantities sufficient to correct hypocalcemia in patients with hypocalcemia resulting from necrotizing acute pancreatitis (the dosage cannot be calculated beforehand). The subcutaneous administration of meperidine hydrochloride, in a dose of 10 mg/kg body weight, may be given to relieve pain. Antiemetics, corticosteroids, anticholinergics, and antibiotics have equivocal value in the treatment of acute pancreatitis. With concomitant diabetes mellitus, corticosteroids are contraindicated. Heroic attempts such as peritoneal lavage, abdominal drains, or pancreatectomy must be considered in cases that are unresponsive to conservative medical treatment.

See also references 2, 12, and 43.

Concurrent Endocrinopathies

The actions of insulin are best countered by GH, cortisol, glucagon, epinephrine, estrogens, and progesterone. In dogs, the most likely causes of endocrine-induced resistance to insulin not created by infection are hyperadrenocorticism, estrus,[124] and presumably the excessive production of glucagon caused by acute pancreatitis. In cats, endocrine-induced resistance to insulin usually is caused by the administration of glucocorticoids or megestrol acetate.[98]

Hyperadrenocorticism may be spontaneous or iatrogenic. The administration of corticosteroids, with few exceptions, is absolutely contraindicated in diabetic patients.

Estrus can be suppressed gradually with mibolerone (Cheque). Mibolerone is an anabolic steroid without effects on blood glucose values. The administration of mibolerone is advisable in all intact bitches with diabetes mellitus as soon as medication can be given orally without emesis. Megestrol acetate (Ovaban), another oral contraceptive hormone commonly used for behavioral modification and dermatoses in cats, is diabetogenic. It should not be given to diabetic patients.

Neuropathies

A diabetic polyneuropathy analogous to diabetic neuropathy of humans has been described in some diabetic dogs and cats. There are components of segmented demyelination and distal axonal degeneration leading to neurogenic myopathy. Atrophy of type II skeletal muscle fibers develops, but clinical signs have not been noted in dogs. Affected cats have had plantigrade stance, hind leg weakness, depressed patellar reflexes, and poor postural reactions (Fig. 14–10). Electromyopathy may show increased insertional activity, fibrillation potentials, positive sharp waves, and high frequency myotonic discharges. Nerve conduction velocities are decreased. Autonomic diabetic neuropathy has not been reported in companion animals. In humans, autonomic diabetic neuropathy is associated with gastroparesis, diarrhea, urinary and rectal incontinence, and impotence.

Diabetic polyneuropathy seems to be the result of the accumulation of sorbitol and fructose in the myelin of peripheral nerves. Dysfunction occurs from osmotic swelling. Mononeuropathies, not reported in companion animals, also occur in diabetic humans as an apparent result of ischemia caused by atherosclerotic changes or by an infarct of the vasa nervosum.

See also references 13, 56, 62, 65, 100, and 120.

Cataracts and Retinopathy

Cataracts develop in most diabetic dogs. Cataracts in juvenile diabetic dogs do not progress if insulin therapy is begun within 3 weeks of the onset

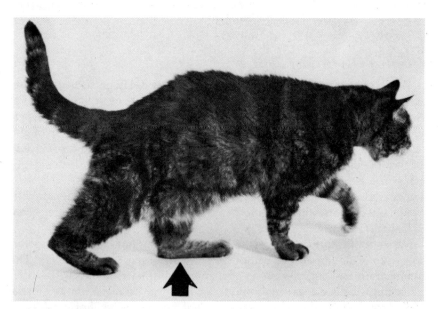

Fig. 14–10. Plantigrade stance (*arrow*) in a cat with diabetic neuropathy of the tibial nerve. (From Randolph, J.F., and Jorgensen, L.S.: Selected feline endocrinopathies. Vet. Clin. North Am., *14:*1261, 1984.)

of diabetes. It is thought the rapidity of onset and the severity of diabetic cataracts are inversely related to degree of control over hyperglycemia. Diabetic cataracts are not necessarily debilitating. In some cases the cataract opacity is not severe enough to result in blindness. Many dogs that are blinded adapt well as long as their daily routine is kept consistent and furniture is not moved. Surgical excision of the cataracts by an experienced veterinary ophthalmologist restores functional vision in 85% to 90% of affected dogs.

Retinopathies often occur in diabetic humans several years after the disease first occurred. Less than 10% have retinopathy in the first 10 years. After 15 years of having diabetes, about 60% of patients have retinopathy. Dogs rarely develop retinopathy, possibly because of their short life span and the insufficient time for retinopathy to develop. Occasionally, dogs do develop retinal capillary microaneurysms, hemorrhages, and shunts consistent with background (simple, benign, exudative) retinopathy of humans. Vision is not perceptibly affected. Humans, however, also can develop proliferative (neovascular, malignant) retinopathy that, if untreated, results in blindness. Dogs and other companion animals do not develop proliferative retinopathy. Postpubertal thickness of capillary basement membrane is positively related to the level and duration of hyperglycemia in humans. Basement membrane changes may be due to glycosylation similar to glycosylation of hemoglobin.

See also references 9, 10, 33, 49, 93, 95, 96, 101, and 126.

Renal Disease

Diabetic glomerulopathy is not as common or as severe in diabetic dogs and cats as it is in humans. The glomerular lesions in diabetic dogs and cats (thickening of the mesangial stalk and hypertrophy of the wall of the afferent arteriole) are not identical to signs of nodular glomerulosclerosis in diabetic humans. Still, 5% to 10% of diabetic dogs who survive have impaired renal function. More than 30% of those dogs who do not survive or who receive euthanasia early in the course of the disease have impaired renal function. Renal insufficiency causes insulin resistance by a number of mechanisms, including hyperglucagonemia and inhibition of insulin receptor synthesis. Peritoneal dialysis may be tried in uremic, anuric, or oliguric patients failing to respond to intravenous fluid therapy, but the prognosis is grave.

See also references 8, 12, 24, 52, 53, 55, and 130.

Cerebral Edema

Cerebral edema is a potential hazard resulting from the rapid reduction of hyperglycemia caused by the overzealous use of insulin or hypotonic fluid therapy to treat diabetes. The brain can adapt to hyperosmolality of hyperglycemia by slowly generating idiogenic osmols intracellularly. The dissipation of idiogenic osmols is also a slow process. If the osmolality of the blood drops rapidly, the brain's state will be hyperosmolar in comparison to that of the blood, and water will be drawn into brain cells. The ideal rate of reduction of hyperglycemia is 75 to 100 mg/dl/hr during the initial treatment of diabetes. If the brain is thought to be edematous, the intravenous administration of mannitol may be useful, but prevention is preferable to treatment.

Hyperlipidemia

Complications of secondary hyperlipidemia resulting from diabetes are infrequent. Possible complications include xanthomatosis, atherosclerosis, acute pancreatitis, and lipemia retinalis.[103] Xanthomatosis of the skin is easily mistaken for a superficial pyoderma.[18, 70] Xanthomata can be distinguished from pustules on the basis of repeated sterile cultures, a bright red hyperemia around the lesions, and remission after elevated levels of serum triglycerides have been reduced. Histologically, the xanthomata contain neutrophils and lipid-laden macrophages called "foam cells."

Miniature schnauzers are predisposed to a familial hyperlipidemia that can precipitate acute pancreatitis and precede diabetes mellitus.[102] Fasting hyperlipidemia in miniature schnauzers can usually be reduced by a low-fat (Prescription Diet i/d) with or without lipid-reducing agents (Choloxin).

See also references 83 and 92.

Insulin Allergy

After 2 months or less of insulin therapy, insulin antibodies are produced in all human diabetics. Very rarely, sufficient antibodies are produced to block the action of the injected insulin. The same seems true in the dog. If this were to occur, the problems that would be expected include any of the following: transient localized urticarial lesions, atrophy or hypertrophy of subcutaneous fat at the injection sites, injection site fibrosis, angioneurotic edema, anaphylaxis, and insulin resistance, without any reduction in blood glucose until large dosages (>3 U/kg body weight) are used. If insulin antibodies are suspected, the least antigenic commercially available insulin would be pure pork lente. Measurement of circulating anti-insulin antibodies is commercially available. In humans, titers of 1:64 or greater are considered significant, but titers of 1:512 may not cause insulin resistance. Hyposensitization kits for insulins are available. Corticosteroid immunosuppression has been used successfully in humans.

See also reference 90.

Insulin Shock

Insulin overdosage, called "insulin shock," should be carefully guarded against. Low-dose initial management programs are effective in minimizing the risk of iatrogenic hypoglycemia. The body's first defenses against hypoglycemia are glucagon and epinephrine. If the patient is receiving β-adrenergic-blocking drugs, the risk of severe hypoglycemia from insulin is greatly

Table 14–13. Management Checklist for Surgery on Diabetics

1. Attempt at least 2 weeks of good control on insulin before the procedure, if possible.
2. Give one-half the usual dose of intermediate-acting insulin at least 1 hour before anesthesia. Withhold the morning meal.
3. Reduce dose of preanesthetic narcotics. *Avoid nausea and vomiting.*
4. Infuse 5% to 10% dextrose intravenously during anesthesia, during surgery, and after surgery until the patient eats without vomiting. Check the blood glucose every 30 minutes during surgery. *Avoid hypoglycemia!*
5. Monitor cardiopulmonary function closely. *Avoid acidosis!*
6. Check the blood glucose every 6 hours and maintain blood glucose at 150 to 250 mg/dl. Administer regular insulin subcutaneously as necessary.
7. Continue subcutaneous administration of regular insulin three to four times daily and intravenous administration of dextrose until patient eats voluntarily without vomiting, then return to regular schedule. *Anticipate some insulin resistance* at least 3 days after surgery. Be careful of insulin overdosage after this time.

---

increased. Signs of hypoglycemia vary with the rate of the decline of blood glucose, the extent of cerebral hydration, and the degree of neural adaptation to previous cerebrospinal fluid glucose levels. Common signs of hypoglycemia are tremors of the hind legs when standing, confusion and apathy ("blank staring"), an unsteady gait, increased hunger, sleepiness, nervousness, fainting, and convulsions. Treatment for insulin shock should be initiated as soon as it is recognized. A sugar solution such as 50% dextrose, pancake syrup, or 40% dextrose in packets (Monojel) can be given orally, followed by additional food after normal mental function returns. If necessary, 10% to 50% dextrose should be given intravenously in sufficient quantities to effect a favorable response in the patient. A useful initial dose is the rapid intravenous infusion of approximately 2 ml/kg body weight of 50% dextrose. Alternately, an intramuscular injection of 1 mg of glucagon (Glucagon for Injection Ampoules) can be given.

Nonelective Surgery

Elective surgery should be avoided in diabetics. If surgery becomes necessary, it is mandatory to avoid nausea, vomiting, hypoglycemia, and acidosis. Many approaches to successful surgical management are possible. One method is suggested in Table 14–13.

REFERENCES

1. Altman, R.B., and Kirkmayer, A.H.: Diabetes mellitus in the avian species. J. Am. Anim. Hosp. Assoc., *12:*531, 1976.
2. Anderson, N.V., and Strafuss, A.C.: Pancreatic disease in dogs and cats. J. Am. Vet. Med. Assoc., *159:*885, 1971.
3. Appleby, R.C.: Diabetes mellitus in a budgerigar (Melopsittacus undulatus). Vet. Rec., *115:*652, 1984.
4. Atkins, C.E.: Disorders of glucose homeostasis in neonatal and juvenile dogs: hyperglycemia. Compendium on Continuing Educ. for the Practicing Vet. *5:*851, 1983.
5. Baker, J.R., and Ritchie, H.E.: Diabetes mellitus in the horse: a case report and a review of the literature. Equine Vet. J., *6:*7, 1974.

6. Baker, R.H.: Acute necrotizing pancreatitis in a horse. J. Am. Vet. Med. Assoc., *172:*268, 1978.
7. Bass, V.D., Hoffman, W.E., and Dorner, J.L.: Normal canine lipid profiles and effects of experimentally induced pancreatitis and hepatic necrosis on lipids. Am. J. Vet. Res., *37:*1355, 1976.
8. Bloodworth, J.M.B., Jr.: Experimental diabetic glomerulosclerosis. II. The dog. Arch. Pathol., *79:*113, 1965.
9. Bloodworth, J.M.B., Jr., and Engerman, R.L.: Diabetic microangiopathy in the experimentally diabetic dog and its prevention by careful control with insulin. Diabetes, *22:*290, 1973.
10. Bloodworth, J.M.B., Jr., and Molitor, D.L.: Ultrastructural aspects of human and canine diabetic retinopathy. Invest. Ophthal., *4:*1037, 1965.
11. Bloom, F.: Diabetes mellitus in a cat. N. Engl. J. Med., *217:*395, 1937.
12. Braca, G., and Pellegrin, N.: Pancreatic and renal lesions in dogs with diabetes mellitus. Atti. Soc. Ital. Sci. Vet., *23:*735, 1970.
13. Braund, K.G., and Steiss, J.E.: Distal neuropathy in spontaneous diabetes mellitus in the dog. Acta Neuropathol., *57:*263, 1982.
14. Bulgin, M.S., and Anderson, B.C.: Verminous arteritis and pancreatic necrosis with diabetes mellitus in a pony. Compendium on Continuing Educ. for the Practicing Vet., *5:*482, 1983.
15. Campbell, J., and Rastogi, K.W.: Growth hormone-induced diabetes and high levels of serum insulin in dogs. Diabetes, *15:*30, 1966.
16. Campbell, K.L., and Lattimer, K.S.: Transient diabetes mellitus associated with prednisone therapy in a dog. J. Am. Vet. Med. Assoc., *185:*299, 1984.
17. Chastain, C.B.: Intensive care of dogs and cats with diabetic ketoacidosis. J. Am. Vet. Med. Assoc., *179:*972, 1981.
18. Chastain, C.B., and Graham, C.L.: Xanthomatosis secondary to diabetes mellitus in a dog. J. Am. Vet. Med. Assoc., *172:*1209, 1978.
19. Chastain, C.B., and Nichols, C.E.: Low-dose intramuscular insulin therapy for diabetic ketoacidosis in dogs. J. Am. Vet. Med. Assoc., *178:*561, 1981.
20. Chastain, C.B., and Nichols, C.E.: Current concepts on the control of diabetes mellitus. Vet. Clin. North Am. [Small Anim. Pract.], *14:*859, 1984.
21. Church, D.B.: The blood glucose response to three prolonged duration insulins in canine diabetes mellitus. J. Small Anim. Pract., *22:*301, 1981.
22. Church, D.B., and Watson, A.D.J.: Whole blood glucose determinations in dogs using dextrostix and Eyetone reflectance colorimeter. J. Small Anim. Pract., *20:*163, 1979.
23. Cotton, R.L., Cornelius, L.M., and Theran, P.: Diabetes mellitus in the dog: a clinicopathologic study. J. Am. Vet. Med. Assoc., *159:*863, 1971.
24. Crowell, W.A., and Leininger, J.R.: Feline glomeruli: morphologic comparisons in normal, autolytic, and diseased kidneys. Am. J. Vet. Res., *27:*1075, 1976.
25. Davidson, J.L., Haas, K.B., and Conner, N.D.: Animal studies with tolbutamide, orally effective anti-diabetic agent. Vet. Med., *52:*497, 1957.
26. Drash, A.L.: The etiology of diabetes mellitus. N. Engl. J. Med., *300:*1211, 1979.
27. Easley, J.R., and Breitschwerdt, E.B.: Glucosuria associated with renal tubular dysfunction in three basenji dogs. J. Am. Vet. Med. Assoc., *168:*938, 1976.
28. Edwards, D.F.: Transient diabetes mellitus and ketoacidosis in a dog. J. Am. Vet. Med. Assoc., *180:*68, 1982.
29. Eigenmann, J.E.: Diabetes mellitus in dogs and cats. Proceedings of the 6th Kal Kan Symposium, p. 51, 1982.
30. Eigenmann, J.E.: Diabetes mellitus in elderly female dogs: recent findings on pathogenesis and clinical implications. J. Am. Anim. Hosp. Assoc., *17:*805, 1981.
31. Eigenmann, J.E., and Peterson, M.E.: Diabetes mellitus associated with other endocrine disorders. Vet. Clin. North Am., *14:*837, 1984.
32. Eigenmann, J.E., van der Haage, M.H., and Rijnberk, A.: Polyendocrinopathy in two canine litter mates: simultaneous occurrence of carbohydrate intolerance and hypothyroidism. J. Am. Anim. Hosp. Assoc., *20:*143, 1984.
33. Engerman, R.L., and Bloodworth, J.M.B., Jr.: Experimental diabetic retinopathy in dogs. Arch. Ophthalmol., *73:*204, 1965.
34. Feldman, E.C.: Diabetic ketoacidosis in dogs. Compendium on Continuing Educ. for the Practicing Vet., *2:*456, 1980.

35. Feldman, E.C., and Nelson, R.W.: Insulin-induced hyperglycemia in diabetic dogs. J. Am. Vet. Med. Assoc., *180:*1432, 1982.
36. Finn, J.P., Martin, C.L., and Manns, J.G.: Feline pancreatic islet cell hyalinosis associated with diabetes mellitus and lowered serum insulin concentrations. J. Small Anim. Pract., *11:*607, 1970.
37. Fischer, U., et al.: Insulin and insulin effect in a she-dog with spontaneous diabetes. J. Metab. Res., *2:*251, 1970.
38. Foster, S.J.: Diabetes mellitus: a study of the disease in the dog and cat in Kent. J. Small Anim. Pract., *16:*295, 1975.
39. Fox, J.G., and Beatty, J.O.: A case report of complicated diabetes mellitus in a cat. J. Am. Anim. Hosp. Assoc., *11:*129, 1975.
40. Gartner, K., and Melani, F.: Tendency of the bitch to develop diabetes mellitus. 1. Influence of the sexual cycle on glucose tolerance and the glucose space. 2. Insulin content of serum after glucose loading. Zentralbl. Veterinarmed. [A], *15:*517, 1968.
41. Gershwin, L.J.: Familial canine diabetes mellitus. J. Am. Vet. Med. Assoc., *167:*479, 1975.
42. Goriya, Y., et al.: Validation of I.V. small-dose insulin infusion therapy in diabetic ketoacidosis of depancreatized dogs. Acta. Diabetol. Lat., *15:*236, 1978.
43. Greve, T., Dayton, A.D., and Anderson, N.V.: Acute pancreatitis with coexistent diabetes mellitus: an experimental study in the dog. Am. J. Vet. Res., *34:*939, 1973.
44. Grillo, T.A.I., and Cunningham, J.G.: Serum insulin in totally pancreatectomized pregnant dogs. J. Endocrinol., *39:*307, 1967.
45. Gumbrell, R.C.: A case of multiple xanthomatosis and diabetes mellitus in a dog. N. Z. Vet. J., *20:*240, 1972.
46. Hallas-Moller, K.: The lente insulins. Diabetes, *5:*7, 1956.
47. Haines, D.M., and Penhale, W.J.: Autoantibodies to pancreatic islet cells in canine diabetes mellitus. Vet. Immunol. Immunopathol., *8:*149, 1985.
48. Hashimoto, A., et al.: Juvenile acinar atrophy of the pancreas of a dog. Vet. Pathol., *16:*74, 1979.
49. Hausler, H.R., Sibay, R.M., and Campbell, J.: Retinopathy in a dog following diabetes induced by growth hormone. Diabetes, *13:*122, 1964.
50. Hendriks, J.H., et al.: Studies on glucose and insulin levels in the blood of normal and diabetic dogs. Zentralbl. Veterinarmed. [A], *23:*206, 1976.
51. Hirai, S., Ikenaga, T., and Matsuzawa, T.: Nasal absorption of insulin in dogs. Diabetes, *27:*296, 1978.
52. Hommel, H., Fischer, U., and Kansy, H.: Insulin in the pancreatic blood and insulin half-life in a Alsatian bitch with spontaneous diabetes. Horm. Metab. Res., *3:*213, 1971.
53. Janle-Swain, E., et al.: Case study of a diabetic dog with chronic membranous glomerulopathy treated with continuous intraperitoneal insulin infusion. Am. J. Vet. Res., *43:*2044, 1982.
54. Jeffrey, J.R.: Diabetes mellitus secondary to chronic pancreatitis in a pony. J. Am. Vet. Med. Assoc., *153:*1168, 1968.
55. Jeraj, K., et al.: Immunofluorescence studies of renal basement membranes in dogs with spontaneous diabetes. Am. J. Vet. Res., *45:*1162, 1984.
56. Johnson, C.A., Kittleson, M.D., and Indrieri, R.J.: Peripheral neuropathy and hypotension in a diabetic dog. J. Am. Vet. Med. Assoc., *183:*1007, 1983.
57. Johnson, K.H., Osborne, C.A., and Barnes, D.M.: Intracellular substance with some amyloid staining affinities in pancreatic acinar cells of a cat with amyloidosis. Pathol. Vet., *7:*153, 1970.
58. Jost, H.: Treatment of diabetes mellitus in the dog. Schweiz. Arch. Terheilkd., *113:*517, 1971.
59. Kahil, M.E., et al.: Alcohol and the tolbutamide response in the dog. J. Lab. Clin. Med., *64:*808, 1964.
60. Kaneko, J.J., et al.: Glucose tolerance and insulin response in diabetes mellitus of dogs. J. Small Anim. Pract., *18:*85, 1977.
61. Kaneko, J.J., et al.: Renal clearance, insulin secretion and glucose tolerance in spontaneous diabetes mellitus of dogs. Cornell Vet., *69:*375, 1979.
62. Katherman, A.E., and Braund, K.G.: Polyneuropathy associated with diabetes mellitus in a dog. J. Am. Vet. Med. Assoc., *182:*522, 1983.
63. Katherman, A.E., et al.: Hyperadrenocorticism and diabetes mellitus in the dog. J. Am. Anim. Hosp. Assoc., *16:*705, 1980.

64. King, J.M., Kavanaugh, J.F., and Bentinck-Smith, J.: Diabetes mellitus with pituitary neoplasms in a horse and a dog. Cornell Vet., *52:*133, 1962.
65. Kramek, B.A., et al.: Neuropathy associated with diabetes mellitus in the cat. J. Am. Vet. Med. Assoc., *184:*42, 1984.
66. Kramer, J.W., and Evermann, J.F.: Early-onset genetic and familial diabetes mellitus in dogs. Proceedings of the 6th Kal Kan Symposium, p. 59, 1982.
67. Kramer, J.W., et al.: Inherited, early onset, insulin-requiring diabetes mellitus of Keeshound dogs. Diabetes, *29:*558, 1980.
68. Kruth, S.A., and Cowgill, L.D.: Renal glucose transport in the cat. Proceedings of the Am. Coll. Vet. Intern. Med., p. 78, 1978.
69. Kruth, S.A., Feldman, E.C., and Kaneko, J.J.: Serum immunoreactive insulin levels in normal dogs, dogs with functional B-cell tumors, and dogs with spontaneous diabetes mellitus. Proceedings of the Am. Coll. Vet. Intern. Med., p. 20, 1980.
70. Kwochka, K.W., and Short, B.G.: Cutaneous xanthomatosis and diabetes mellitus following long-term therapy with megestrol acetate in a cat. Compendium on Continuing Educ. for the Practicing Vet., *6:*185, 1984.
71. Lattimer, K.S., and Maffey, E.A.: Neutrophil adherence and movement in poorly and well-controlled diabetic dogs. Am. J. Vet. Res., *45:*1498, 1984.
72. Lettow, V.E., et al.: Juveniler Diabetes mellitus bei einem Hund. Kleintier Praxis, *28:*119, 1983.
73. Lewis, D.G.: A preliminary communication on the oral treatment of two cases of hyperglycemia in the dog presumed to be due to diabetes mellitus. J. Small Anim. Pract., *1:*201, 1960.
74. Ling, G.V., et al.: Diabetes mellitus in dogs: a review of initial evaluation, immediate, and long-term management, and outcome. J. Am. Vet. Med. Assoc., *170:*521, 1977.
75. Lord, P.F., and Wilkins, R.J.: Emphysema of the gallbladder in a diabetic dog. J. Am. Vet. Radiol. Soc., *13:*49, 1972.
76. Lorenz, M.D., and Cornelius, L.M.: Laboratory diagnosis of endocrinological disease. Vet. Clin. North Am., *6:*687, 1976.
77. Lukens, F.D.W., and Dohan, F.C.: Pituitary diabetes in the cat: recovery following insulin or dietary treatment. Endocrinology, *30:*175, 1942.
78. Maddison, J.E., Davis, A.C., and Johnson, R.P.: Stabilization of diabetic dogs (Letter). J. Am. Vet. Med. Assoc., *181:*756, 1982.
79. Mahaffey, M.B., and Anderson, N.V.: Effect of staphylococcal alpha toxin pancreatitis on glucose tolerance in the dog. Am. J. Vet. Res., *37:*947, 1976.
80. Manns, J.G., and Martin, D.L.: Plasma insulin, glucagon, and nonesterified fatty-acids in dogs with diabetes mellitus. Am. J. Vet. Res., *33:*981, 1972.
81. Marmor, M., et al.: Epidemiologic patterns of canine diabetes mellitus. Am. J. Epidemiol., *112:*436, 1980.
82. Marmor, M., et al.: Epizootiologic patterns of diabetes mellitus in dogs. Am. J. Vet. Res., *43:*465, 1982.
83. McCullagh, K.G.: Plasma lipoproteins in animal health and disease. Vet. Annual, *18:*41, 1978.
84. Middleton, D.J., and Lomas G.R.: Emphysematous cystitis due to Clostridium perfringens in a non-diabetic dog. J. Small Anim. Pract., *20:*433, 1979.
85. Milks, H.J.: Some cases of diabetes in dogs. J. Am. Vet. Med. Assoc., *81:*620, 1932.
86. Moise, N.S., and Reimers, T.J.: Insulin therapy in cats with diabetes mellitus. J. Am. Vet. Med. Assoc., *182:*158, 1983.
87. Mulnix, J.A.: Insulin dosage in canine diabetes. Mod. Vet. Pract., *54:*45, 1973.
88. Nelson, R.W.: Use of insulin in small animal medicine. J. Am. Vet. Med. Assoc., *185:*105, 1984.
89. Nelson, R.W., and Feldman, E.C.: Complications of insulin therapy in canine diabetes mellitus. J. Am. Vet. Med. Assoc., *182:*1321, 1983.
90. Nelson, R.W., Feldman, E.C., and Karam, J.H.: Comparison of immunogenicity of pork insulin versus beef-pork insulin in dogs with spontaneous insulin-dependent diabetes mellitus. Proceedings of the Am. Coll. Vet. Intern. Med. p. 38, 1983.
91. Ninomiya, R., Forbath, N.F., and Hetenyi, G.: Effect of adrenal steroids on glucose kinetics in normal and diabetic dogs. Diabetes, *14:*729, 1965.
92. Olin, D.D., Rogers, W.A., and MacMillan, A.D.: Lipid-laden aqueous humor associated with anterior uveitis and concurrent hyperlipemia in two dogs. J. Am. Vet. Med. Assoc., *168:*861, 1976.

93. O'Toole, D., Miller, G.K., and Hazel, S.: Bilateral retinal microangiopathy in a dog with diabetes and hyperadrenocorticism. Vet Pathol., *21:*120, 1984.
94. Park, R., et al.: Metabolic effects of dichloroacetate in diabetic dogs. Am. J. Physiol., *245:*E94, 1983.
95. Patz, A., et al.: Studies on diabetic retinopathy. II. Retinopathy and nephropathy in spontaneous canine diabetes. Diabetes, *14:*700, 1965.
96. Peiffer, R.L., Gelatt, K.N., and Gwin, R.M.: Diabetic cataracts in the dog. Canine Pract., *4:*18, 1977.
97. Peterson, M.E., and Altszuler, N.: Characterization of the insulin resistance and glucose tolerance of spontaneous canine Cushing's syndrome. Proceedings of the Am. Coll. Vet. Intern. Med., p. 62, 1981.
98. Peterson, M.E., Javanovic, L., and Peterson, C.M.: Insulin resistant diabetes mellitus associated with elevated growth hormone concentrations following megestrol acetate treatment in a cat. Proceedings of the Am. Coll. Vet. Intern. Med., p. 63, 1981.
99. Pogatsa, G., and Dubecz, E.: Effect of hyperglycaemia-induced hyperosmolality on heart function in the dog. Eur. J. Clin. Invest., *9:*147, 1979.
100. Randolph, J.F., and Jorgensen, L.S.: Selected feline endocrinopathies. Vet. Clin. North Am., *14:*1261, 1984.
101. Ricketts, H.T., et al.: Degenerative lesions in dogs with experimental diabetes. Diabetes, *8:*298, 1959.
102. Rogers, W.A., Donovan, E.F., and Kociba, G.J.: Idiopathic hyperlipoproteinemia in dogs. J. Am. Vet. Med. Assoc., *166:*1087, 1975.
103. Rogers, W.A., Dovovan, E.F., and Kociba, G.J.: Lipids and lipoproteins in normal dogs and in dogs with secondary hyperlipoproteinemia. J. Am. Vet. Med. Assoc., *166:*1092, 1975.
104. Root, C.R., and Scott, R.C.: Emphysematous cystitis and other radiographic manifestations of diabetes mellitus in dogs and cats. J. Am. Vet. Med. Assoc., *158:*721, 1971.
105. Rottiers, R., et al.: Spontaneous diabetes mellitus in dogs. Ann. Endocrinol., *40:*253, 1979.
106. Rubarth, S.: Diabetes mellitus in a cat. North Am. Vet., *17:*49, 1936.
107. Ryan, C.P., Walder, E.J., and Howard, E.B.: Diabetes mellitus and islet cell carcinoma in a parakeet. J. Am. Anim. Hosp. Assoc., *18:*139, 1982.
108. Schaer, M.: A clinical survey of thirty cats with diabetes mellitus. J. Am. Anim. Hosp. Assoc., *13:*23, 1977.
109. Schaer, M.: A clinicopathologic survey of acute pancreatitis in 30 dogs and 5 cats. J. Am. Anim. Hosp. Assoc., *15:*681, 1979.
110. Schaer, M.: Diabetic hyperosmolar nonketotic syndrome in a cat. J. Am. Anim. Hosp. Assoc., *11:*42, 1975.
111. Schaer, M.: Diabetes mellitus in the cat. J. Am. Anim. Hosp. Assoc., *9:*548, 1973.
112. Schaer, M.: Insulin treatment for the diabetic dog and cat. Compendium on Continuing Education for the Practicing Vet., *5:*579, 1983.
113. Schaer, M.: Transient insulin response in dogs and cats with diabetes mellitus. J. Am. Vet. Med. Assoc., *168:*417, 1976.
114. Schaer, M., et al.: Hyperosmolar syndrome in the non-ketoacidotic diabetic dog. J. Am. Anim. Hosp. Assoc., *10:*357, 1974.
115. Schall, W.D.: Fluid and electrolyte therapy of diabetic ketoacidosis. J. Am. Anim. Hosp. Assoc., *8:*206, 1972.
116. Sherding, R.G., and Chew, D.J.: Nondiabetic emphysematous cystitis in two dogs. J. Am. Vet. Med. Assoc., *174:*1105, 1979.
117. Sirek, A., et al.: Effect of prolonged administration of tolbutamide in depancreatized dogs. Diabetes, *8:*284, 1959.
118. Sirek, A., et al.: The effect of Orinase upon the insulin requirements and liver function test in depancreatized puppies and adult dogs. Rev. Cand. Biol., *16:*515, 1957.
119. Sloan, J.M., and Oliver, I.M.: Progestogen-induced diabetes in the dog. Diabetes, *24:*337, 1975.
120. Steiss, J.E., Orsher, A.N., and Bowen, J.M.: Electrodiagnostic analysis of peripheral neuropathy in dogs with diabetes mellitus. Am. J. Vet. Res., *42:*2061, 1981.
121. Szabo, T., et al.: Pancreatic atrophy in the canine: an entity of exocrine-endocrine dissociation. Mount Sinai J. Med., *45:*503, 1978.
122. Tasker, J.B., Whiteman, C.E., and Martin, B.R.: Diabetes mellitus in the horse. J. Am. Vet. Med. Assoc., *149:*393, 1966.

123. Teunissen, G.H.B., et al.: Insulin content of the blood of dogs with diabetes and some other disease. Kleintier Praxis, *15:*29, 1970.
124. Tischler, S.A.: The effect of the estrous cycle on diabetes mellitus in the dog. J. Am. Anim. Hosp. Assoc., *10:*122, 1974.
125. Veitch, E.R.: The management of diabetes mellitus in cats and dogs. J. Small Anim. Pract., *13:*629, 1972.
126. Waitzman, M.B., Cornelius, L.M., and Evatt, B.L.: Treatment of canine spontaneous diabetes mellitus with aspirin. Metab. Pediatr. Ophthalmol., *4:*151, 1980.
127. Walker, D.: Diabetes mellitus following steroid therapy in a dog. Vet. Rec., *74:*1543, 1962.
128. Weiss, C.W.: Cat and small dog insulin diluent. Can. Vet. J., *20:*190, 1979.
129. Wilson, R.B., and Wilson, W.D.: Hepatotoxicity of tolbutamide in dogs. J. Am. Vet. Med. Assoc., *156:*1557, 1970.
130. Wood, P.A.: Metabolic complications of diabetes mellitus. Compendium on Continuing Educ. for the Practicing Vet., *3:*218, 1981.
131. Wrenshall, G.A., Hartroft, W.S., and Best, C.H.: Insulin extractable from the pancreas and islet histology—comparative studies in spontaneous diabetes in dogs and human subjects. Diabetes, *3:*444, 1954.
132. Yano, B.L., Hayden, D.W., and Johnson, K.H.: Feline insular amyloid: association with diabetes mellitus. Vet. Pathol., *18:*621, 1981.
133. Yano, B.L., Hayden, D.W., and Johnson, K.H.: Feline insular amyloid: incidence in adult cats with no clinicopathologic evidence of overt diabetes mellitus. Vet. Pathol., *18:*310, 1981.
134. Yano, B.L., Hayden, D.W., and Johnson, K.H.: Occurrence of secondary systemic amyloid in the pancreatic islets of a cat. Am. J. Vet. Res., *44:*338, 1983.
135. Yano, B.L., Johnson, K.H., and Hayden, D.W.: Feline insular amyloid: histochemical distinction from secondary systemic amyloid. Vet. Pathol., *18:*181, 1981.
136. Yoon, J., et al.: Virus-induced diabetes mellitus. Isolation of a virus from the pancreas of a child with diabetic ketoacidosis. N. Engl. J. Med., *300:*1173, 1979.

15

Functional Tumors of the Pancreatic Islets

Most tumors of the pancreatic islets secrete hormones in excess. The two most common of these are tumors that secrete insulin (insulinomas) or gastrin (gastrinomas) in excess. Insulinomas have been reported in the dog, cat, and ferret. Gastrinomas have been reported in the dog and cat. Most reports of insulinomas and gastrinomas in companion animals have involved dogs. Excess secretion of glucagon (glucagonomas) and somatostatin (somatostatinomas), which have been reported in humans, have not been reported in companion animals.

INSULINOMA

An insulinoma in a dog was first reported in 1935.[62] Insulinomas are usually an adenoma or carcinoma of the pancreatic islets, but extra-pancreatic insulinomas are possible. In dogs, most insulinomas are islet cell carcinomas, which are the most common functional tumors of the pancreatic islets, comprising 0.4% of all primary tumors in dogs. An insulinoma has also been reported in a cat[46] and a ferret.[37] None has been described in the horse or birds. Clinical signs are produced by the effects of hypoglycemia (Fig. 15–1).

See also references 8, 11–14, 16, 25, 29, 30, 35, 44, 45, 52, 55, 60, 66, 70, 76, and 78.

Incidence in Dogs

The average age of an affected dog is 9 years (range, 3 to 12 years). There is no predisposition for sex. German shepherd dogs, Irish setters, golden retrievers, collies, standard poodles, boxers, and fox terriers are considered the breeds predisposed for insulinomas. Even though about 40% of canine insulinomas appear histologically benign, metastatic neoplasia and histologically malignant tumors of the islets outnumber benign tumors by more than four to one in dogs. In contrast, insulinomas are uncommonly malignant in humans.

See also references 1, 56, and 64.

Clinical Signs

Abdominal enlargement or signs of encroachment on surrounding organs such as icterus or abdominal pain are not manifestations of insulinomas. The presenting signs are, instead, primarily either those resulting from a defi-

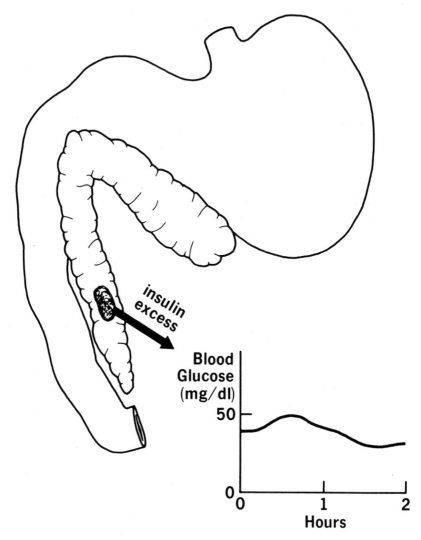

Fig. 15–1. Insulinoma.

cient supply of glucose to the brain (neuroglycopenia) or release of catecholamines (adrenergic).

When the amount of glucose available to the brain is decreased, the
utilization of oxygen by the brain is also decreased. The clinical signs of
neuroglucopenia are the same as those of hypoxia. Presenting clinical signs
and owner complaints are listed in Table 15–1. Unequivocal signs are usually not noticed until blood glucose levels are less than 40 mg/dl. The
expected progression of clinical signs in order of decreasing frequency is
outlined in Table 15–2. Signs may develop during fasting, exercise, periods

Table 15–1. Presenting Clinical Signs Associated With
Insulinomas in Dogs in Approximate Order of
Decreasing Frequency

> Seizures
> Weakness and incoordination
> Depression
> Change in behavior
> Polyphagia
> Syncope

of excitement, or eating a meal. Mild weight gain may occur from hypoglycemia because of the inhibition of the hypothalamic satiety center and unchecked activity of the feeding center in the hypothalamus.

Glucose is the only normal energy source for the brain; moreover, the brain consumes two thirds of the liver's output of glucose when the body is at rest. Low blood glucose levels can cause dysfunction of the brain. Various areas of the central nervous system differ in their susceptibility to hypoglycemia. First and most susceptible is the cerebral cortex. Occipital lobes are more affected than frontal or temporal regions. The diencephalon is intermediate in its sensitivity to low blood glucose, and the medulla is least

Table 15–2. Progression of Clinical Signs
With Hypoglycemia*

Blood Glucose Level (mg/dl)	Response
<60	Parasympathetic response Hunger Nausea Possible bradycardia and hypotension
<50	Cerebral response Decreased mental alertness Lethargy Yawning
<35	Sympathetic (adrenergic) response Increased pulse and blood pressure Increased respiratory rate Muscular weakness
<20	Brain dysfunctions Mental confusion Seizures Coma

* Signs do not correlate directly with blood glucose values, but do progress generally in the above order. Effects of hypoglycemia depend on the rate of blood glucose decline, age of the patient, and each patient's sensitivity to hypoglycemia.

sensitive to low blood glucose. If the hypoglycemia is severe and prolonged, permanent neural damage can result. Acquired epilepsy due to hypoglycemic brain damage should be considered a cause for recurrent seizures after the apparently successful excision of insulinomas.

The degree of hypoglycemia does not always correlate with clinical signs of the neural dysfunction. The brain is able to adapt to low glucose, particularly in periods of rest. The rate of fall of blood glucose and the degree of neural adaptation are important factors governing the clinical signs produced. Chronic hypoglycemia of 20 to 60 mg/dl in a resting patient usually does not cause clinical signs of neural dysfunction in companion animals.

Hypoglycemia stimulates the release of insulin-antagonistic hormones.[19] Initially, the most important antagonistic hormones are epinephrine and glucagon. Epinephrine beneficially decreases glucose use by muscles and the secretion of insulin. It also increases glycogenolysis and the secretion of glucagon. However, it should also be remembered that epinephrine's effects are also responsible for many of the clinical signs of hypoglycemia.

Glucagon corrects hypoglycemia by stimulating hepatic glycogenolysis and gluconeogenesis. Deficiency of either epinephrine or glucagon or adrenergic blockade in adults mildly to moderately increases the activity of developing hypoglycemia. Deficiency of both or deficiency of glucagon with adrenergic blockade results in severe hypoglycemia. The secretion of growth hormone (GH) and cortisol augments recovery from decreasing blood glucose levels by prolonging the stimulation of gluconeogenesis and inhibiting the utilization of peripheral glucose.

Laboratory Findings

Postprandial or fasting hypoglycemia less than 50 mg/dl is the hallmark of insulinomas in older canine patients with muscle weakness, personality changes, and episodic seizures. Insulinoma is the most common cause for hypoglycemia in dogs over 5 years of age. Whipple's diagnostic triad consists of episodes of a neurologic disorder during hypoglycemic periods, which are promptly relieved by the administration of glucose. Fulfillment of Whipple's triad is not pathognomonic of insulinoma. Other possible causes for hypoglycemia exist. Abnormal routine laboratory findings other than hypoglycemia are uncommon. Since insulin inhibits the production of ketones, the finding of ketonemia or ketonuria with hypoglycemia eliminates the diagnosis of insulinoma.[38]

Differential Diagnosis

It is useful to classify hypoglycemia as fasting (Table 15–3) or postprandial (Table 15–4). Hypoglycemia may also be classified as juvenile onset, adult-onset, or unassociated with age.[2–4, 7, 15, 22, 47, 51, 57, 68, 72, 74] Causes of fasting (organic) hypoglycemia generally allow time for some adaptation, so clinical signs may be mild from neuroglycopenia without adrenergic signs.

Table 15–3. Possible Causes of Fasting Hypoglycemia

Juvenile-onset
  Hepatic vascular anomalies
  Ketotic hypoglycemia (alanine deficiency)
  Congenital hypothyroidism
  Glycogen storage diseases
    Type I (Glucose-6-phosphatase deficiency)
    Type III (Amylo-1, 6-glucosidase deficiency)
    Type VI (Hepatophosphorylase deficiency)

Adult-onset
  Insulinoma
  Extrapancreatic tumors
  Diffuse liver disease
  Hypoglycemia of hunting dogs
  Late pregnancy or heavy lactation with cachexia
  Intestinal malabsorption with cachexia

Unassociated with age
  Bacteremia
  Hypopituitarism
  Hypoadrenocorticism
  Drug-related
    Sulfonylureas
    Insulin overdose
    Salicylates
    Ethanol
    Ethylene glycol

Postprandial (reactive) hypoglycemias are more often identified with acute clinical signs of hypoglycemia caused by both adrenergic stimulation and neuroglycopenia. The most common reason for pathologic hypoglycemia in adult dogs is insulinoma. It may cause hypoglycemia both during fasting and postprandially.

SPURIOUS CAUSES OF HYPOGLYCEMIA. Spurious hypoglycemia can occur if blood samples are improperly handled. Plasma or serum should be separated from blood cells within 30 minutes, then refrigerated until measurements of glucose are possible, whereas whole blood should be used as soon as possible for measurement of glucose levels. If whole blood remains at room temperature, blood cells will consume glucose at about 20 mg/dl/hr, depending on cell counts and ambient temperature. Whole blood glucose concentrations are diluted by blood cells. Whole blood glucose levels are approximately 15% lower than plasma or serum levels.

See also reference 26.

EXTRAPANCREATIC TUMORS. Other causes of adult-onset fasting hypoglycemia include extrapancreatic tumors, usually large carcinomas or sarcomas. Hepatomas, lymphatic leukemia, splenic hemangiosarcoma, salivary gland adenocarcinoma, malignant melanomas, and plasma cell dyscrasia have been associated with hypoglycemia in dogs.[20, 21]

There are various means by which extrapancreatic tumors may cause hypoglycemia, including a high rate of anaerobic glycolysis, production of

Table 15–4.   Possible Causes of Postprandial Hypoglycemia

Juvenile-onset
  Glucagon deficiency (Nonketotic hypoglycemia)
  Fructose intolerance (Fructose-1-phosphate aldolase deficiency)
  Galactosemia (Galactose-1-phosphate uridyltransferase)
  Leucine hypersensitivity

Adult-onset
  Insulinoma
  Rapid gastric emptying
    Gastrectomy
    Vagal overstimulation

---

insulin-like peptides, impaired hepatic release of glucose, malnutrition, and adverse effects of chemotherapy.

See also reference 42.

DIFFUSE LIVER DISEASE.   The liver is responsible for the storage of glycogen for immediate mobilization, glycogenolysis, and gluconeogenesis. Normal blood glucose levels can be maintained by the liver with 30% total hepatic functional ability. Diffuse diseases of the liver that impair hepatic function to less than 30% of its normal abilities can cause hypoglycemia. Examples include cirrhosis, inflammation, neoplasia, severe right-sided congestive heart failure, intoxication, fatty infiltration, and vascular anomalies.

See also reference 53.

HYPOGLYCEMIA OF HUNTING DOGS.   Those dogs who hunt by scent, such as pointers and setters, occasionally develop ataxia, disorientation, weakness, or seizures 1 to 3 hours into a hunt. Affected dogs are usually lean and nervous, and have fasted overnight. It is assumed these signs are due to hypoglycemia. Most affected dogs recover with rest or eating, but it is difficult to substantiate hypoglycemia as a primary cause of the signs under clinical conditions. In humans, strenuous exercise can cause hypoglycemia without hypoglycemic symptoms. The limits of normalcy for blood glucose levels that parallel degrees of exercise have not been established for dogs. There is inadequate evidence to support a previously proposed theory that affected dogs have an amylo-1, 6-glucosidase deficiency. Most, perhaps all, affected dogs are infrequently exercised and may develop hypoglycemia because of insufficient conditioning relative to the energy expended during hunting.

PRECIPITATING CAUSES OF HYPOGLYCEMIA WITH CACHEXIA.   Hypoglycemia does not occur in normal dogs fasted for at least 30 days; however, if conditions demanding large amounts of energy (such as late pregnancy or heavy lactation in combination with inanition) are present, hypoglycemia can result.[31] Intestinal malabsorption, if not corrected or correctable, leads to cachexia of the degree that can cause hypoglycemia.

BACTEREMIA.   Overwhelming bacteremia has been associated with hypoglycemia. Mechanisms thought involved include the depletion of glycogen stores, decreased gluconeogenesis, anaerobic glycolysis, and increased peripheral utilization of glucose.

See also reference 9.

HYPOPITUITARISM AND HYPOADRENOCORTICISM. A deficiency in glucocorticoids or GH renders the body more susceptible to hypoglycemia. However, single adenohypophyseal hormone deficiencies usually do not cause hypoglycemia. Primary hypoadrenocorticism in dogs causes hypoglycemia in less than 5% of affected cases. A deficiency in adrenocorticotropic hormone (ACTH), called secondary hypoadrenocorticism, along with a GH deficiency, bacteremia, or other causes of hypoglycemia will more often lead to clinical hypoglycemia.

DRUG-RELATED HYPOGLYCEMIA. Iatrogenic excess of insulin or drugs that cause the secretion of insulin, that increase sensitivity to insulin, that inhibit gluconeogenesis, or that inhibit glycogenolysis can cause hypoglycemia. Examples of such drugs include sulfonylureas, salicylates, ethanol, and ethylene glycol.

RAPID GASTRIC EMPTYING. A postprandial cause of hypoglycemia is rapid gastric emptying from gastrectomy or vagal overstimulation. Rapid entry of carbohydrates into the duodenum can produce an abrupt rise in blood glucose, followed by oversecretion of insulin and rebound hypoglycemia 1 to 3 hours after the ingestion of food.

Diagnosis

Persistent hypoglycemia in an older dog with a history of seizures is not enough to warrant the attempted surgical excision of a suspected insulinoma. It is enough to warrant an insulin assay during fasting and blood glucose measurements to confirm preoperative, inappropriate hyperinsulinemia. In most patients with insulinoma, hypoglycemia is found on the initial measurement of blood glucose. However, the failure to show persistent hypoglycemia does not eliminate the possibility of insulinoma. In some cases, measurements of blood glucose are required every 2 hours during a fast, until a blood glucose level of less than 60 mg/dl is detected. Fasts of more than 8 hours are rarely necessary and could be dangerous. Frequent small meals should be offered after the fast.

Once fasting hypoglycemia is noted, a fasting insulin (IRI) assay should be done. Shipments of serum to reference laboratories require packing with dry ice owing to degradation of insulin in unfrozen serum. The measurement of blood glucose levels should be determined with blood samples drawn at the same time as serum for IRI determination. Several methods of insulin-to-glucose (I/G) or glucose-to-insulin ratios may be used as diagnostic indices (Table 15–5).

The most reliable ratio for the diagnosis of insulinomas is controversial, but the largest published study to date indicated the amended I/G ratio is best. Severe obesity or hyperadrenocorticism alters ratios because of decreased numbers of insulin receptors, although fasting hypoglycemia does not occur with either condition. Normal fasting serum IRI levels in dogs are

Table 15–5. Diagnostic Insulin to Glucose and
Glucose to Insulin Fasting Ratios

Ratio	Normal	Hyperinsulinemia
Insulin (μU/ml) to glucose (mg/dl)	$\leqslant 0.25$	>0.3
Amended insulin to glucose $(\dfrac{IRI \times 100}{BG\text{-}30})$	$\leqslant 30$	>30
Glucose (mg/dl) to insulin (μU/ml)	$\geqslant 5$	<3

IRI = immunoreactive insulin.
BG = blood glucose.

less than 30 μU/ml. The tolbutamide, glucagon, L-leucine, ethanol, and glucose tolerance tests have been advocated for the diagnosis of insulinoma despite serious, even lethal, hazards of induced hypoglycemia. Their clinical indications are now restricted to cases that have equivocal insulin-to-glucose ratios. Even then, their diagnostic accuracy is questionable.

Newer diagnostic tests have been discovered useful in human patients with insulinomas. Proinsulin normally constitutes less than 30% of IRI. Most insulinomas secrete excessive proportions (>40% of IRI) of proinsulin. Unfortunately, proinsulin values are as of yet unreported in the dog and cat. Another test involves the C-peptide response to infused insulin. In humans, the secretion of C-peptide by an insulinoma is frequently unaffected by exogenous insulin-induced hypoglycemia. This test, which has not been evaluated in the dog and cat, is complicated by the fact that C-peptide assays are species specific. Commercial assays of C-peptide in companion animals are not available. Glycohemoglobin assays have not proved sensitive enough for the diagnosis of intermittent hyperglycemia associated with insulinomas.

Computerized tomography or selective arterial angiography has been successfully used to show tumors larger than 2 cm. However, many tumors are smaller than 2 cm, and radiographic proof of the tumor is generally unnecessary for diagnosis or management.

See also references 23, 39, 41, 43, 65, and 73.

Prognosis

Insulinomas in dogs are generally malignant, but slow growing. Two thirds appear histologically malignant. Forty-five percent of insulinomas have metastasis to the liver and regional lymph nodes that is evident at laparotomy. It is not possible to predict liver metastasis by determining that serum liver enzymes are elevated. Virtually all tumors eventually recur after excision, but excision of the primary tumor can eliminate clinical signs in most cases for as long as 3 years. The average life expectancy following excision is about 1 year.

Treatment

SURGICAL TREATMENT. Most pancreatic insulinomas are visible or palpable at surgery. On the rare occasions when they are not visible or palpable, it is not advisable to guess which limb of the pancreas to remove since the frequency is nearly equal in right and left pancreatic limbs. Complete pancreatectomy is not recommended if pancreatic tumors are not visible or palpable because of the possibilities of production of insulin by a nonpancreatic tumor or a presurgical misdiagnosis.

When pancreatic insulinomas are not evident at the time surgical excision of the tumor is being attempted, the entire abdominal cavity should be thoroughly investigated for a nonpancreatic tumor and the tip of the pancreas should be biopsied to determine whether islet cell hyperplasia is present. It is not possible to predict liver metastasis based on elevated levels of serum liver enzymes. Recommended presurgical, surgical, and postsurgical care is listed (Table 15–6). If the insulinoma has been sufficiently excised, the blood glucose should rise to normal levels within 2 hours.

Postsurgical complications include diabetes mellitus and trauma-induced pancreatitis. The pancreas must be handled delicately. The hazard of postsurgical pancreatitis is related to the skill of the surgeon and the size of the insulinoma. Diabetes occurs in 20% to 25% of patients treated surgically. In most, the hyperglycemia is mild and transient, lasting only 3 to 5 days. Treatment for hyperglycemia is not necessary unless the fasting blood glucose level exceeds 250 mg/dl or is above 140 mg more than 1 week after surgery.

If surgical treatment is not possible or not successful, or if hypoglycemic episodes return after surgery, medical therapy is indicated.

Table 15–6. Recommended Surgical Care for Insulinoma Patients

---

Presurgical procedures
1. Feed several small, high-protein meals daily. Give diazoxide in a dose of 5 mg/kg body weight every 8 hours and chlorothiazide in a dose of 20 mg/kg twice daily.
2. No food by mouth for 8 hours before surgery.
3. Give 5% to 10% dextrose intravenously at a constant slow rate beginning 8 hours before anesthesia is induced.
4. Monitor serum potassium and blood glucose every 8 hours after an intravenous infusion is begun.

Surgical procedures
1. Infuse an intravenous solution of 10% dextrose levels during surgery at a constant moderate rate.
2. Monitor blood glucose levels every 30 minutes during surgery.

Postsurgical Procedures (after partial pancreatectomy)
1. Measure blood glucose every 8 hours.
2. Administer 5% to 10% dextrose slowly in an intravenous or balanced electrolyte solution (lactated Ringer's) depending on blood glucose values.
3. No food or water by mouth for 3 days.
4. Monitor serum potassium, urea nitrogen, lipase, and amylase daily for 3 days.

MEDICAL MANAGEMENT.   Medical therapy alone for insulinomas is less desirable than surgical excision. Medical management should not be recommended to owners as an alternative to surgery, only as a supplement.

Initial medical management for hypoglycemia from insulinomas should include giving small, frequent meals high in protein, plus prednisolone in a dose of 0.5 to 1 mg/kg body weight/day in divided doses. Should dietary management and prednisolone be inadequate, diazoxide (Proglycem), 10 mg/kg body weight/day in divided doses, may be tried.[54]

Used to treat hypertension in humans, diazoxide is a benzothiadiazine derivative that has hyperglycemic effects. The dosage may be increased to 40 mg/kg body weight/day in divided doses, if necessary. Its hyperglycemic actions include the inhibition of insulin secretion, enhancement of epinephrine-induced glycolysis, decreased peripheral utilization of glucose, and increased mobilization of glycerol and free fatty acids. Common adverse effects are vomiting and anorexia. Chlorothiazide (Diuril), in twice daily doses of 20 to 40 mg/kg body weight, should be used with diazoxide to reduce sodium retention and potentiate hyperglycemic effects. Phenytoin (Dilantin), in a twice daily dose of 2 to 6 mg/kg body weight in the dog, inhibits insulin secretion, but is less effective than diazoxide.

The management of metastasis from insulinomas is difficult. Streptozotocin (Zanosar) is a nitrosourea antitumor antibiotic produced by *Streptomyces achromogenes.*[6] It is cytotoxic to pancreatic islets. It is also toxic to the liver and kidneys.[36] Administration should be by slow intravenous infusion of a dose of 20 mg/kg body weight once weekly for 4 weeks. Fluorouracil (Fluorouracil Ampuls) or mithramycin (Mithracin) can also be considered. An optimal therapeutic protocol, in which a number of drugs are used, has not been determined for the dog.[48, 49]

See also references 5 and 79.

Special Problems

Hypoglycemia, if severe, can cause acquired epilepsy from focal necrosis of the cerebral cortex. Hypoglycemic brain damage is suggested if improvement of behavior or the incidence of seizures does not accompany normalization of the blood glucose.

Seizures occurring before or after excision of an insulinoma should be considered as resulting from hypoglycemia until it is proved otherwise. When seizures occur, a solution of 50% dextrose should be administered in an intravenous dose of 0.5 to 1 ml/kg body weight over 1 to 3 minutes. If there is no response, cerebral necrosis or cerebral edema may be present. Diazepam (Valium) may be given intravenously in a dose of 2 to 10 mg to control the seizure, and 20% mannitol should be given intravenously in a dose of 0.5 to 2 g/kg body weight to reduce cerebral edema. Dexamethasone may be given, but its usefulness in cytotoxic brain edema is questionable.

See also references 18, 40, 63, and 77.

GASTRINOMA (Zollinger-Ellison-like syndrome)

Gastrinomas have only been reported in humans, dogs, and cats. In 1955, Zollinger and Ellison described the human gastrinoma syndrome. The first reported gastrinoma in the dog was in 1976.[34] Several other spontaneous canine cases have been reported since, and the syndrome has also been experimentally produced in dogs. In addition, a gastrinoma has been found in a cat.[50] Gastrinomas are usually carcinomas arising from "non-B cells" (D cells) of the pancreatic islets that produce gastrin. Gastrin is normally produced by the gastric antrum and mucosa of the upper duodenum. Islet cell D cells normally produce gastrin only during the fetal period. Extrapancreatic gastrinomas of the duodenum, stomach, and hilus of the spleen and antral gastrin-cell hyperplasia have been reported in humans. The resulting hypergastrinemia causes parietal cell hyperplasia leading to hyperchlorhydria and, secondarily, gastroduodenal ulceration (Fig. 15–2).

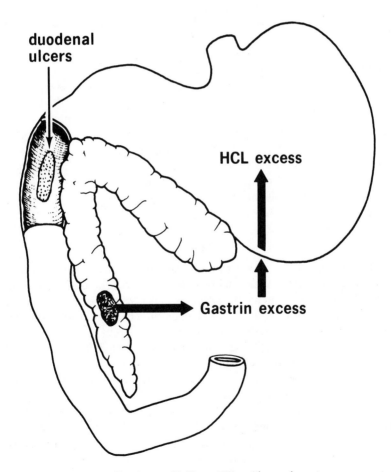

Fig. 15–2. Gastrinoma (Zollinger-Ellison-like syndrome).

In about 30% of human cases of gastrinomas, other endocrine tumors are present, usually in the parathyroids or pituitary. This condition of multiple endocrine adenomas involving the pancreatic islets, parathyroids, and pituitary is called multiple endocrine neoplasia (MEN), Type I. MEN Type I has not been reported in companion animals.

See also references 28, 58, 59, 67, and 75.

Incidence

Owing to the limited number of reported cases, little can be said concerning incidence and predisposing factors. It is presumed that age is a predisposing factor. The youngest dog reported to have a gastrinoma was 6 years old.

Clinical Signs

The clinical signs produced by gastrinomas are related to gastroduodenal ulcerations and malabsorption produced by hypergastrinemia and hyperchlorhydria. Reported clinical signs include vomiting with or without blood in vomitus, diarrhea with or without melena or steatorrhea, anorexia, weight loss, and erosive esophagitis.

Hypergastrinemia causes increased gastric fluid secretions with low pH. The decreased pH of fluid entering the duodenum damages the mucosa and results in submucosal inflammation with partial villous atrophy. In addition, bile salts are precipitated and pancreatic enzymes denatured, leading to malabsorption, particularly of fat. Gastrinoma should be suspected in any patient with prolonged diarrhea or steatorrhea, especially if an abnormal gastric mucosal pattern suggestive of parietal cell hyperplasia is seen on contrast radiographs of the upper gastrointestinal system.

See also reference 32.

Laboratory Findings and Diagnosis

Anemia may occur if gastroduodenal ulceration is severe. No other nonspecific laboratory abnormalities are common. The definitive diagnosis requires the measurement of serum gastrin levels. Normal fasting serum gastrin values in dogs and cats are approximately 30 to 100 pg/ml. Fasting values exceeding 500 pg/ml are diagnostic.

Mild to moderate hypergastrinemia occurs with hypercalcemia, short-bowel syndrome, gastric dilatation-volvulus, immunoproliferative small intestinal disease of basenjis,[10] chronic renal failure,[33,71] and administration of cimetidine, ranitidine, or glucocorticoids.

A stimulation test, involving the administration of Prescription Diet p/d and Swanson's clear beef broth, has been recommended to diagnose gastrinomas in the dog.[24] Antral distention and partially digested protein in contact with the duodenal mucosa are normally stimuli for the secretion of gastrin. Serum gastrin levels should not exceed 200 pg/ml after 30 minutes and should be less than 100 pg/ml after 90 minutes. Gastrinomas do not increase serum gastrin levels postprandially.

Secretin, in an intravenous dose of 2 U/kg body weight, does not normally increase serum gastrin levels. With gastrinomas, secretin can cause marked elevation of serum gastrin levels within 15 minutes. An intravenous dose of calcium also stimulates the release of gastrin from gastrinomas, but according to tests on humans, secretin is safer and more reliable.

Treatment

Gastrinomas should be excised, if at all possible. Most gastrinomas whose primary site is the pancreas are malignant. Metastasis occurs to the liver and regional lymph nodes. In humans, the prognosis is better if the tumor is found in the duodenum or if no tumor is found.

A presurgical trial with cimetidine (Tagamet), in a thrice daily dose of 20 mg/kg body weight, or ranitidine (Zantac), in a twice daily dose of 10 mg/kg body weight, is advisable before the laparotomy is done. Cimetidine is an imidazole H_2 receptor antagonist blocking the gastrin-induced secretion of gastric acid. Ranitidine is a furan H_2 antagonist that is 5 to 12 times more potent than cimetidine on a molar basis. If clinical signs (vomiting and diarrhea) improve, the surgery can be limited to excision of the gastrinoma. If no response to cimetidine or ranitidine occurs, a total gastrectomy is recommended in addition to excision of the gastrinoma. Failure to locate a tumor necessitates a pancreatic biopsy to investigate the possibility of islet hyperplasia. A selective vagotomy should also be done if no tumor is found or metastasis is evident. Immediate postsurgical care is similar to that recommended for insulinomas. Iron supplementation is necessary if a total gastrectomy is done.

Clinical signs may not be corrected by surgery alone. Reasons include the possibilities that all of the tumor was not found or could not be resected and that parietal cell hyperplasia may still be hypersecretory. Postsurgical medical management may be necessary with cimetidine[61] or ranitidine. Isopropamide (Darbid), in a dose of 0.2 mg/kg body weight given twice daily, can be used in addition to the H_2 antagonist when H_2 antagonists alone are not sufficient to control clinical signs.

SOMATOSTATINOMA AND GLUCAGONOMA

Some pancreatic and extrapancreatic tumors, somatostatinomas and glucagonomas, in humans have been shown to produce excessive levels of somatostatin or glucagon, respectively. Both tumors induce a mild state of diabetes mellitus by antagonizing the action of insulin. Somatostatin suppresses several hormones in addition to insulin, including glucagon. The net effect has been a persistent hyperglycemia, plus maldigestion with steatorrhea and cholelithiasis. One canine case of hypoglycemia has been reported in which production of somatostatin by a hepatic tumor was suspected.[69] Verification requires finding elevated plasma somatostatin levels.

In addition to diabetes, glucagonomas have been associated with stomatitis, anemia, and a skin rash of the legs and perineum in affected humans. Catabolic effects of the excessive amounts of glucagon lead to deficiencies in zinc and amino acids responsible for the rash and stomatitis. The rash, migratory necrolytic dermatitis, in a diabetic is the key to a tentative diagnosis that should be confirmed by demonstration of elevated serum glucagon levels and an exploratory laparotomy.

For further information on somatostatinoma and glucagonoma, see references 17 and 27.

PANCREATIC CHOLERA (Verner-Morrison Syndrome, Tumors of Vasoactive Intestinal Peptide, Watery Diarrhea-Hypokalemia-Achlorhydria Syndrome)

Pancreatic cholera in humans is a syndrome of watery diarrhea, hypokalemia, and hypochlorhydria associated with an islet cell tumor of the pancreas. It has not been recognized in companion animals, but veterinary clinicians should consider the possibility in cases of chronic idiopathic watery diarrhea in companion animals. Although gastrin plus glucagon, motilin, secretin, and gastric inhibitory polypeptide has been implicated, oversecretion of a secretin-like hormone, vasoactive intestinal peptide (VIP), is usually considered the cause. The tumors are called VIPomas. VIPomas have secreted adrenocorticotropic hormone, antidiuretic hormone, parathyroid hormone, and cholecystokinin in lesser amounts than VIP. If total excision of the tumor is successfully done, the diarrhea is eliminated.

REFERENCES

1. Anderson, N.V., and Johnson, K.H.: Pancreatic carcinoma in the dog. J. Am. Vet. Med. Assoc., *150:*286, 1967.
2. Atkins, C.E.: Disorders of glucose homeostasis in neonatal and juvenile dogs: hypoglycemia. Part I. Compendium on Continuing Educ. for the Practicing Vet., *6:*197, 1984.
3. Atkins, C.E.: Disorders of glucose homeostasis in neonatal and juvenile dogs: hypoglycemia. Part II. Compendium on Continuing Educ. for the Practicing Vet., *6:*353, 1984.
4. Bardens, J.W.: Glycogen storage disease in puppies. Vet. Med. Small Anim. Clin., *61:*1174, 1966.
5. Beck, A.M., and Krook, L.: Canine insulinoma. Two surgical cases with relapses. Cornell Vet., *55:*330, 1965.
6. Black, H.E., Rosenblum, I.Y., and Capen, C.C.: Chemically induced (streptozotocin-alloxan) diabetes mellitus in the dog. Am. J. Pathol. 98:295, 1980.
7. Bleicher, S.J., et al.: Effect of ethanol on plasma glucose and insulin in the fasted dog. Proc. Soc. Exp. Biol. Med., *115:*369, 1965.
8. Botha, W.S., and Irvine-Smith, C.: Hypoglycemia in a dog with pancreatic islet cell adenomas. J. S. Afr. Vet. Assoc., *49:*67, 1978.
9. Breitschwerdt, E.B., et al.: Hypoglycemia in four dogs with sepsis. J. Am. Vet. Med. Assoc., *178:*1072, 1981.
10. Breitschwerdt, E.B., et al.: Clinical and laboratory characterization of basenjis with immunoproliferative small intestinal disease. Am. J. Vet. Res., *45:*267, 1984.
11. Brady, L.J., et al.: Influence of prolonged fasting in the dog on glucose turnover and blood metabolites. J. Nutr., *107:*1053, 1977.
12. Bullock, L.: Two cases of a functioning islet cell tumor in the canine. Calif. Vet., *19:*14, 1965.
13. Capen, C.C., and Martin, S.L.: Hyperinsulinism in dogs with neoplasia of the pancreatic islets. Pathol. Vet., *6:*309, 1969.

14. Caywood, D.D., et al.: Pancreatic islet cell adenocarcinoma: clinical and diagnostic features of six cases. J. Am. Vet. Med. Assoc., *174:*714, 1979.
15. Ceh, L., et al.: Glycogenosis type III in the dog. Acta Vet. Scand., *17:*210, 1976.
16. Cello, R.M., and Kennedy, P.C.: Hyperinsulinism in dogs due to pancreatic islet cell carcinoma. Cornell Vet., *47:*538, 1957.
17. Chick, W.L., et al.: "Somatostatinoma": a somatostatin-containing tumor of the endocrine pancreas. N. Engl. J. Med., *296:*963, 1977.
18. Chrisman, C.L.: Postoperative results and complications of insulinomas in dogs. J. Am. Anim. Hosp. Assoc., *16:*677, 1980.
19. deBruijne, J.J., et al.: Fat mobilization and hormone levels in fasted dogs. Metabolism, *30:*190, 1981.
20. DeSchepper, J., VanderStock, J., and DeRick, A.: Hypercalcemia and hypoglycemia in a case of lymphatic leukemia in the dog. Vet. Rec., *94:*602, 1974.
21. DiBartola, S.P.: Hypoglycemia and polyclonal gammopathy in a dog with plasma cell dyscrasia. J. Am. Vet. Med. Assoc., *180:*1345, 1982.
22. Fajans, S.S., and Floyd, J.C.: Fasting hypoglycemia in adults. N. Engl. J. Med., *294:*766, 1976.
23. Feldman, E.C., Kruth, S.A., and Kennedy, P.C.: Insulin-secreting islet cell tumors: diagnosis and clinical course in 29 dogs. Proceedings of the 6th Kal Kan Symposium, p. 101, 1982.
24. Gaggert, G.H., et al.: Serum immunoreactive gastrin concentrations in the dog: basal and postprandial values measured by radioimmunoassay. Am. J. Vet. Res., *45:*2351, 1984.
25. Grant, C.A.: Pancreatic insulinoma with clinical manifestations in a dog. J. Comp. Pathol., *70:*450, 1960.
26. Greene, C.E.: Artifactual hypoglycemia (Letter). J. Am. Vet. Med. Assoc., *179:*317, 1981.
27. Greider, M.H., Rosai, J., and McGuigan, J.E.: The human pancreatic islet cells and their tumors. II. Ulcerogenic and diarrheogenic tumors. Cancer, *33:*1423, 1974.
28. Happe, R.P., et al.: Zollinger-Ellison syndrome in three dogs. Vet. Pathol., *17:*177, 1980.
29. Hill, F.W.G., et al.: Functional islet cell tumour in the dog. J. Small Anim. Pract., *15:*119, 1974.
30. Huxtable, C.R., and Farrow, B.R.H.: Functional neoplasms of the canine pancreatic-islet B-cells: a clinico-pathological study of three cases. J. Small Anim. Pract., *20:*737, 1979.
31. Jackson, R.F., et al.: Hypoglycemia-ketonemia in a pregnant bitch. J. Am. Vet. Med. Assoc., *177:*1123, 1980.
32. Jennewein, H.M., et al.: Experimental hypergastrinemia in the dog. Horm. Metab. Res., *8:*455, 1976.
33. Jonas, L.D., and Twedt, D.C.: Serum gastrin concentrations in dogs with acute and chronic renal failure. Proceedings of the Am. Coll. Vet. Intern. Med., p. 79, 1982.
34. Jones, B.R., Nicholls, M.R., and Badman, R.: Peptic ulcerations in a dog associated with an islet cell carcinoma of the pancreas and an elevated plasma gastrin level. J Small Anim. Pract., *17:*593, 1976.
35. Justus, H.A.: Pancreatic insulinoma in a dog. J. Am. Vet. Med. Assoc., *142:*1413, 1963.
36. Kaneko, J.J., et al.: Renal function, insulin secretion, and glucose tolerance in mild streptozotocin diabetes in the dog. Am. J. Vet. Res., *39:*807, 1978.
37. Kaufman, J., and Schwarz, P.: Pancreatic beta cell tumor in a ferret. J. Am. Vet. Med. Assoc., *185:*998, 1984.
38. Keller, U., et al.: The roles of insulin, glucagon, and free fatty acids in the regulation of ketogenesis in dogs. Diabetes, *26:*1040, 1977.
39. Knowlen, G.G., and Schall, W.D.: The amended insulin-glucose ratio. Is it really better? J. Am. Vet. Med. Assoc., *185:*397, 1984.
40. Krook, L., and Kennedy, R.M.: Central nervous system lesions in dogs with metastasizing islet cell carcinoma. Cornell Vet., *52:*385, 1962.
41. Kruth, S.S., Feldman, E.C., and Kennedy, P.C.: Insulin-secreting islet cell tumors: establishing a diagnosis and the clinical course for 25 dogs. J. Am. Vet. Med. Assoc., *181:*54, 1982.
42. Leifer, C.E., et al.: Hypoglycemia associated with nonislet cell tumor in 13 dogs. J. Am. Vet. Med. Assoc., *186:*53, 1985.
43. Magne, M.L., et al.: Serum insulin and glucose concentrations in normal, stressed, and hyperadrenocortical dogs. Proceedings of the Am. Coll. Vet. Intern. Med., p. 42, 1984.

44. Marcus, L.C., Bucci, T.J., and Kramer, K.L.: Pancreatic islet cell tumor in a dog. J. Am. Vet. Med. Assoc., *145:*1198, 1964.
45. Mattheeuws, D., et al.: Hyperinsulinism in the dog due to pancreatic islet-cell tumour: a report on three cases. J. Small Anim. Pract., *17:*313, 1976.
46. McMillan, F.D.: Insulinoma in a cat. Proceedings of the Am. Coll. Vet. Intern. Med., p. 51, 1983.
47. Meyer, D.J.: Fasting hypoglycemia in a pup (Letter). J. Am. Vet. Med. Assoc., *173:*1286, 1978.
48. Meyer, D.J.: Pancreatic islet cell carcinoma in a dog treated with streptozotocin. Am. J. Vet. Res., *37:*1221, 1976.
49. Meyer, D.J.: Temporary remission of hypoglycemia in a dog with an insulinoma after treatment with streptozotocin. Am. J. Vet. Res., *38:*1201, 1977.
50. Middleton, D.J., Watson, A.D.J., and Culvenor, J.E.: Duodenal ulceration associated with gastrin-secreting pancreatic tumor in a cat. J. Am. Vet. Med. Assoc., *183:*461, 1983.
51. Mofstafa, I.E.: A case of glycogenic cardiomegaly in a dog. Acta Vet. Scand., *11:*197, 1970.
52. Njoku, C.O., Strafuss, A.C., and Dennis, S.M.: Canine islet cell neoplasia: a review. J. Am. Anim. Hosp. Assoc., *8:*284, 1972.
53. Nouel, O., et al.: Hypoglycemia: a common complication of septicemia in cirrhosis. Arch. Intern. Med., *141:*1477, 1981.
54. Parker, A.J., Musselman, E.M., and O'Brien, D.: Diazoxide treatment of canine insulinoma. Vet. Rec., *109:*178, 1981.
55. Prescott, C.W., and Thompson, H.L.: Insulinoma in the dog. Aust. Vet. J., *56:*502, 1980.
56. Priester, W.A.: Pancreatic islet cell tumors in domestic animals. J. Natl. Cancer. Inst., *53:*227, 1974.
57. Rafiquzzaman, M., et al.: Glycogenosis in the dog. Acta Vet. Scand., *17:*196, 1976.
58. Regan, P.T., and Malagelade, J.R.: A reappraisal of clinical, roentgenographic, and endoscopic features of the Zollinger-Ellison Syndrome. Mayo Clin. Proc., *53:*19, 1978.
59. Rogers, W.A.: Gut hormone abnormalities in disorders of the pancreas. Proceedings of the 6th Kal Kan Symposium, p. 45, 1982.
60. Rouse, B.T., and Wilson, M.R.: A case of hypoglycemia in a dog associated with neoplasia of the pancreas. Vet. Rec., *79:*454, 1966.
61. Schulman, J.: Control of gastric ulcers in a dog using cimetidine. Canine Pract., *6:*42, 1979.
62. Slye, M., and Wells, H.G.: Tumors of islet tissue with hyperinsulinism in a dog. Arch. Pathol., *10:*537, 1935.
63. Spieth, K.: Epileptiform attacks as a result of hypoglycemia in a dog. Der Praktische Tierarzt, *54:*292, 1973.
64. Steinberg, H.S.: Insulin secreting pancreatic tumors in the dog. J. Am. Anim. Hosp. Assoc., *16:*695, 1980.
65. Stockham, S.L., Nachreiner, R.F., and Krehbiel, J.D.: Radioimmunoassay of canine insulin, glucagon, and C-peptide: a comparison and evaluation of the commercial assays. Vet. Clin. Pathol., *9:*41, 1980.
66. Straufuss, A.C., et al.: Islet cell neoplasms in four dogs. J. Am. Vet. Med. Assoc., *159:*1008, 1971.
67. Straus, E., Johnson, G.F., and Yalow, R.S.: Canine Zollinger-Ellison syndrome. Gastroenterology, *72:*380, 1977.
68. Strombeck, D.R., et al.: Fasting hypoglycemia in a pup. J. Am. Vet. Med. Assoc., *173:*299, 1978.
69. Strombeck, D., et al.: Hypoglycemia and hypoinsulinemia associated with hepatoma in a dog. J. Am. Vet. Med. Assoc., *169:*811, 1976.
70. Teunissen, G.H.B., Hendriks, H.J., and deBruijne, J.J.: Hypoglykamie and Insulinom. Klein. Prax., *25:*477, 1980.
71. Thornhill, J.A., and Bottoms, G.D.: Hypergastrinemia as a proposed mechanism for uremic gastritis in the dog with clinical improvement following cimetidine therapy. Proceedings of the Am. Coll. Vet. Intern. Med., p. 80, 1982.
72. Turner, R.C., Oakley, N.W., and Nabarro, J.D.N.: Changes in plasma insulin during ethanol hypoglycemia. Metabolism, *22:*111, 1973.
73. Turner, R.C., Oakley, N.W., and Nabarro, J.D.N.: Control of basal insulin secretion with special reference to the diagnosis of insulinomas. Br. Med. J., *2:*132, 1971.

74. Turnwald, G.H., and Troy, G.C.: Hypoglycemia. Part I. Carbohydrate metabolism and laboratory evaluation. Compendium on Continuing Educ. for the Practicing Vet., 5:932, 1983.

75. Van Der Gaag, I., Happe, R.P., and Lamers, C.B.H.W.: Zollinger-Ellison syndrome in the dog. Vet. Pathol., 15:573, 1978.

76. Weller, R.E., and Leighton, R.: Islet cell carcinoma: diagnosis and treatment. Canine Pract., 6:26, 1979.

77. Wilkinson, G.T.: Epileptiform convulsions in a cat possibly of hypoglycemia origin. J Small Anim. Pract., 9:555, 1968.

78. Wilson, J.W., and Caywood, D.D.: Functional tumors of the pancreatic beta cells. Compendium on Continuing Educ. for the Practicing Vet., 3:458, 1981.

79. Wilson, J.W., and Hulse, D.A.: Surgical correction of islet cell adenocarcinoma in a dog. J. Am. Vet. Med. Assoc., 164:603, 1974.

16

Gastrointestinal Hormones

Gastrointestinal hormones are polypeptides found in the mucosa of the digestive tract and in the pancreatic islets.[4,6] Their actions are to modify gastrointestinal motility, vascular flow, and the secretion of digestive enzymes. Gastrointestinal hormones include gastrin, secretin, cholecystokinin (CCK), vasoactive intestinal peptide (VIP), gastric inhibitory polypeptide (GIP), glucagon, glicentin, somatostatin, substance P, bombesin, motilin, and neurotensin.

Based on reports in humans, possible syndromes of gastrointestinal hormone excess include gastrinomas, glucagonomas, somatostatinomas, and VIPomas. Only gastrinomas have been well described in the dog and cat. Hypofunctional gastrointestinal hormone disorders have not been recognized.

Many gastrointestinal hormones can be subdivided into either the gastrin family or the secretin family. Chemical structures within a family are similar, and effects within a family overlap. The gastrin family consists of gastrin and CCK. These two hormones share the same five C-terminal amino acids. The secretin family consists of secretin, glucagon, glicentin, GIP, and VIP. Overlapping effects may be the result of pharmacologic doses. Physiologic concentrations seem to have more discreet actions.

Mucosal cells producing gastrointestinal hormones are probably of neural crest origin. Hyperfunctional tumors arising from APUD (*a*mine *p*recursor *u*ptake and *d*ecarboxylation) cells are called *apudomas*.[3] Apudomas may arise along with other tumors of neural crest origin. A variety of tumor combinations and conditions of ectopic polypeptide hormone production have been recognized in humans. Cells involved have included those of the pineal gland, parathyroid (chief cells), autonomic neurons, adrenal medulla, carotid body (and other chemodectomas), thyroid (parafollicular cells), bronchi, pancreatic islets, skin (melanocytes), adenohypophysis, hypothalamus, and mucosa of the digestive tract. Hormones produced in excess have included adrenocorticotropic hormone (ACTH), VIP, follicle stimulating hormone (FSH), calcitonin, insulin, antidiuretic hormone (ADH), glucagon, growth hormone (GH), prolactin, parathyroid hormone (PTH), and gastrin. Excessive secretion of hormones by apudomas are often intermittent and involve multiple hormone excesses.

GASTRIN

Gastrin is a straight-chained polypeptide with a molecular weight of 2178. At least three biologically active forms are known to exist. The most

320

common and most active form is G-17 (consisting of 17 amino acids). G-34, "big gastrin," may be a prohormone for G-17. It is three times less active than G-17. Minigastrin, G-14, is about six times less active than G-17. The C-terminal four amino acids in G-14, G-17, and G-34 are identical and may be the active core structure. The C-terminal fragment is only 10% as effective as G-17. There are few species differences in gastrin structure among humans and companion animals.

Gastrin (G-17, G-34, and G-14) is formed and stored in "G" cells of the mucosa of the gastric antrum and duodenum. G-34 and the C-terminal fragment of gastrin are also produced by "G" cells throughout the stomach and small intestine. Gastrin is present in the pituitary, hypothalamus, medulla oblongata, and peripheral nerves. The serum half-life of gastrin is 2 to 3 minutes. It is inactivated by the liver and kidney.

The actions of gastrin (G-17) are primarily to increase the secretion of hydrochloric acid and pepsin and to stimulate the growth of the gastric mucosa. On a molar basis it is 1500 times more potent than histamine in stimulating the secretion of gastric acid. It may also stimulate contraction of the gastroesophageal junction, and it may be involved in the pathogenesis of esophageal achalasia and gastroesophageal reflux. Gastrin promotes pyloric muscular hypertrophy and delays gastric emptying. It stimulates the secretion of insulin and glucagon after a protein meal. Gastrin also stimulates the secretion of calcitonin, which then inhibits gastrin secretion. Its function in the central and peripheral nervous system is unknown.

The normal regulation of the secretion of gastrin is poorly understood. Stimuli, which increase gastrin secretion, are protein digestion products in the stomach (especially glycine), distention of the gastric antrum, vagal stimulation, ethanol, calcium, and epinephrine. Inhibitors of gastrin secretion are acid in the gastric antrum, secretin, GIP, VIP, glucagon, and calcitonin.

Serum gastrin determination by radioimmunoassay (RIA) is commercially available. Samples should be taken after a 12-hour fast. Samples must be frozen when shipped. Normal fasting values for the dog and cat are approximately 30 to 100 pg/ml.

Pentagastrin (Peptavlon) is a synthetic, C-terminal, tetrapeptide gastrin used in research and for clinical diagnostic response tests in humans. It is used in the diagnosis of hypo- and hypersecretory conditions of gastric acid and as a stimulation test for calcitonin-producing medullary carcinomas of the thyroid.

See also references 2, 9, and 10.

CHOLECYSTOKININ

Once thought to be two separate hormones (one contracting the gallbladder, the other increasing pancreatic secretions rich in digestive enzymes), CCK is now known to be responsible for both actions. A polypeptide of 33 amino acids, CCK has a molecular weight of 3918. Its structure is identical to gastrin's five C-terminal amino acids. Several less active forms are recognized, including CCK-39, CCK-12, and CCK-8. It is produced by mucosal cells in the duodenum, jejunum, ileum, and cerebral cortex. CCK-8 is the predominant form found in the brain. CCK-12 and CCK-8 predominate in the duodenum and jejunum.

The actions of CCK are primarily to increase pancreatic secretions rich in enzymes and to contract the gallbladder. Other actions include augmentation of secretin's actions, inhibition of gastric emptying, stimulation of secretion of enterokinase, and stimulation of the secretion of glucagon. CCK may also enhance the motility of the small intestine and colon and augment the contraction of the pyloric sphincter (with secretin).

The secretion of CCK is stimulated by duodenal fatty acids of more than ten carbons, some amino acids (tryptophan and phenylalanine), calcium, and hydrogen ions. Inhibitors of the secretion of CCK are digestive products in the lower digestive tract.

Assays or stimulation tests for CCK are not used for diagnostic purposes. The clinical importance of CCK is currently limited to the normal physiologic events it modifies. For example, fat meals are administered before liver biopsy to stimulate gallbladder contraction through the action of CCK. A contracted smaller gallbladder is less likely to be damaged by percutaneous hepatic needle biopsy. CCK is not available for clinical use.

SECRETIN

Discovered by Bayliss and Starling in 1902, secretin was the first substance to be called a hormone. It is a 27-amino-acid peptide with a molecular weight of 3055. Fourteen of its 27 amino acids are the same as in glucagon. It is produced by the deep glands in the mucosa of the duodenum and jejunum. Only one form is known. There are no active fragments.

The principal action of secretin is to stimulate the watery secretion of the pancreas rich in bicarbonate. It also stimulates increased bile flow with bicarbonate. These effects are potentiated by the presence of CCK. Other actions include stimulation of the secretion of insulin and pepsinogen, inhibition of the secretion of pancreatic glucagon and gastrin-stimulated hydrochloric acid, and augmentation of the actions of CCK on pancreatic secretions rich in enzymes. It may stimulate contraction of the pyloric sphincter.

The secretion of secretin is stimulated by acid in the duodenum and inhibited by neutralization of duodenal acids. Oversecretion of secretin (as well as other hormones) has been implicated in the "pancreatic cholera" syndrome, a watery diarrhea disorder associated with a pancreatic tumor. Commercial assays of secretin are not available for clinical purposes.

Freeze-dried secretin is commercially available. It is used for the diagnostic testing of pancreatic exocrine secretory reserve and as a provocative test for the diagnosis of gastrinomas. The concentration is expressed in clinical units: 4000 clinical units equals 1 mg.

VASOACTIVE INTESTINAL PEPTIDE

A highly basic, 28-amino-acid peptide with a molecular weight of 3326, VIP is produced by mucosal cells throughout the digestive tract, as well as in the central nervous system and sympathetic ganglia. The principal actions of VIP are to relax the intestinal tract, promote the intestinal secretion of water and electrolytes, dilate peripheral blood vessels, and inhibit secretion of gastric acid and pepsin. Its secretion is stimulated by food in the intestine. Oversecretion of VIP is associated with pancreatic tumors, watery diarrhea (pancreatic cholera), and pheochromocytomas. Commercial assays of VIP are not available. It is not commercially available for clinical administration to patients.

GASTRIC INHIBITORY POLYPEPTIDE

A polypeptide with 43 amino acids and a molecular weight of 5104, GIP is produced by mucosal cells in the duodenum and jejunum. The principal action of GIP is to suppress the secretion and motility of gastric acid. It also stimulates the release of insulin. In fact, it seems to be the major physiologic stimulus produced by digestive mucosal cells for the secretion of insulin. The secretion of GIP is stimulated by fat or glucose in the duodenum.

Excess levels of GIP have been associated with some human cases of pancreatic cholera. An assay for serum GIP or GIP for injection is not commercially available.

SUBSTANCE P

Substance P is produced by mucosal cells throughout the gastrointestinal tract and in the brain and spinal cord. It is a polypeptide with 11 amino acids. Although its physiologic role is unknown, substance P experimentally causes increased motility of the intestines, vasodilation, increased pancreatic exocrine secretions, and gallbladder contraction. Elevated serum levels of substance P have been reported in the carcinoid syndrome in humans.

SOMATOSTATIN

Somatostatin is produced by pancreatic D cells, the mucosa of the stomach and small intestines, central nervous system and peripheral ganglia, and, perhaps, thyroid. Somatostatin has an extremely short serum half-life of about 1 minute. Most degradation occurs in liver and kidneys. Owing to its diverse actions, short half-life, and absence in the general circulation, it is not universally accepted as a hormone.

The principal action of somatostatin is that of a hormone inhibitor. It was first reported to inhibit GH. Now it is also known to inhibit TSH, ACTH, gastrin, CCK, secretin, pancreatic polypeptide, VIP, GIP, motilin, glucagon, insulin, and glicentin. It also directly or indirectly inhibits the secretion of gastric acid, gastric motility, gallbladder contraction, and pancreatic exocrine secretions.

Serum somatostatin assays are difficult since somatostatin is essentially nonexistent in venous blood of the extremities. Somatostatin assays require selective catheterization and are not commercially available. These assays do not have any current clinical uses.

See also references 5 and 7.

GLICENTIN (Glucagon-Like Immunoreactivity) AND GLUCAGON

Glicentin is produced by the mucosa of the entire gastrointestinal tract. Most is secreted by the ileum. Glicentin is a polypeptide composed of 100 amino acids and has a molecular weight of 11,650. Glucagon is contained in the glicentin molecule. The stimulus for glicentin's release is food in the digestive tract. Glicentin promotes the secretion of insulin and the production of hepatic glucose.

Glucagon is produced by A cells located in the antrum of the stomach and upper duodenum, as well as in the pancreatic islets. Its characteristics have been previously described (see Chap. 13).

See also references 1 and 8.

BOMBESIN

Bombesin is present in the brain and throughout the gastrointestinal tract. Highest concentrations are in gastric mucosa. Its structure in frogs has 14 amino acids and a molecular weight of 1620. The structure of bombesin in companion animals is unknown. Its action under laboratory conditions is to stimulate the release of gastrin and CCK. It also increases motility of the digestive tract, contracts the gallbladder, and stimulates the secretion of pancreatic amylase.

MOTILIN

Motilin is a polypeptide of 22 amino acids with a molecular weight of 2698. Its structure is dissimilar to the other gastrointestinal hormones. Production occurs in the mucosa of the intestines after acidification of the duodenum. Actions include stimulation of cyclic peristalsis of the stomach and small intestines, contraction of the gallbladder, and stimulation of the secretion of pepsin.

NEUROTENSIN

"N" cells in the jejunum and ileum produce neurotensin, a 13-amino-acid polypeptide. Neurotensin causes vasodilation, inhibits gastrin effects, and delays gastric emptying. Stimulatory and inhibitory factors are unknown.

REFERENCES

1. Chen, C.L., et al.: Possible source and control of trauma-induced glucagonemia in dogs. Am. J. Vet. Res., *38:*1259, 1977.
2. Leib, M.S., et al.: Plasma gastrin immunoreactivity in dogs with acute gastric dilatation-volvulus. J. Am. Vet. Med. Assoc., *185:*205, 1984.
3. Morrison, W.B.: The clinical relevance of APUD cells. Compendium on Continuing Educ. for the Practicing Vet., *6:*884, 1984.
4. O'Dorisio, T.M., O'Dorisio, M.S., and Cataland, S.: Overview: endocrinology of the gastrointestinal tract. Proceedings of the 6th Kal Kan Symposium, p. 47, 1982.
5. Sakurai, H., Dobbs, R., and Unger, R.H.: Somatostatin-induced changes in insulin and glucagon secretion in normal and diabetic dogs. J. Clin. Invest., *54:*1295, 1974.
6. Straus, E.: The explosion of gastrointestinal hormones: their clinical significance. Med. Clin. North Am., *62:*21, 1978.
7. Strombeck, D.R., et al.: Hypoglycemia and hypoinsulinemia associated with hepatoma in a dog. J. Am. Vet. Med. Assoc., *169:*811, 1976.
8. Vranic, M., et al.: Extrapancreatic glucagon in the dog. Metabolism, *25:*1469, 1976.
9. Walsh, J.H., and Grossman, M.I.: Gastrin. Part I. N. Engl. J. Med., *292:*1324, 1975.
10. Walsh, J.H., and Grossman, M.I.: Gastrin. Part II. N. Engl. J. Med., *292:*1377, 1975.

Section VI

THE ADRENALS

17

The Normal Adrenal Gland and Clinical Tests of Its Function

Adrenals, meaning "next to the kidneys," are endocrine glands composed of a cortex and medulla. The cortex is essential for life; the medulla is not. The most common dysfunctions are hyposecretion of the adrenal cortex, hypoadrenocorticism (Addison's-like disease), and hypersecretion of the cortex, hyperadrenocorticism (Cushing's-like disease or syndrome). Both disorders are potentially fatal and occur frequently in dogs. The most common clinical problem associated with the adrenal medulla are tumors called pheochromocytomas. Adrenal glands also have clinical significance because synthetic analogues of the secretions of the adrenal cortex and medulla are among the most commonly used drugs in veterinary medicine.

REGIONAL ANATOMY AND MICROANATOMY

The normal canine adrenal glands are vascular organs that together weigh about 1 g. They lie cranial to the kidneys in beds of retroperitoneal fat (Fig. 17–1). The left adrenal is slightly larger than the right. Each gland is approximately $20 \times 10 \times 5$ mm in average-sized dogs. The left is oval but flattened dorsoventrally in its cranial end. It is found at the craniomedial border of the left kidney beneath the psoas minor muscle at the level of the 2nd lumbar vertebrae. It is just caudal to the cranial mesenteric artery and cranial to the renal artery and vein. The ventral surface is bisected by the left phrenicoabdominal vein.

The right adrenal gland has an angular bend. It lies near the cranial portion of the hilus of the right kidney. It is ventral to the crus of the diaphragm and the psoas minor muscle beneath the 13th thoracic vertebrae. The right kidney covers the ventrolateral end of the right adrenal gland. The cranial 60% is covered by the caudal end of the right lateral lobe of the liver. Its ventral surface is bisected by the right phrenicoabdominal vein. The caudal vena cava is just ventromedial to the right adrenal. Both adrenal glands receive arterial blood from numerous short arterioles that enter through the glands' dorsal surfaces. Both glands drain into one vein per gland originating from their medullas. Avian adrenal glands are islands of glandular tissue, yellowish in color, and located at the cranial pole of the kidneys.

A cross-section of the canine adrenals shows a pale golden-yellow cortex and dark-brown medulla. The adult mammalian adrenal cortex is composed

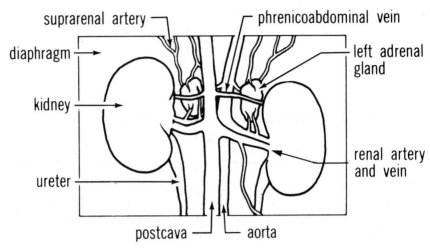

Fig. 17-1. The canine adrenal glands. (Adapted from Evans, H.E., and Christensen, G.C.: Miller's Anatomy of the Dog. 2nd Ed. Philadelphia, W.B. Saunders, 1979).

of radiating cords of cells in three major subdivisions (zones) surrounded by a thick fibrous capsule, which is unique among endocrine organs. The outermost major zone of the adult adrenal cortex is called the *zona arcuata* in dogs and cats because it is composed of cords of cells arranged in an arclike configuration. In humans, this zone is called the *zona glomerulosa* because the cells form clusters resembling glomeruli in the kidney. The second zone inward from the capsule is called the *zona fasciculata* and is composed of long columns of cells. The cortical zone adjacent to the adrenal medulla is the *zona reticularis* comprised of interlacing rows of cells separated by wide blood spaces. In adults, 25% of the volume of the adrenal cortex is *zona arcuata*, 60% is *zona fasciculata,* and 15% is *zona reticularis* (Fig. 17-2). The corticomedullary junction in avians is indistinct, and the cortex is not subdivided into zones.

Smaller, much less distinct zones have been described in the adrenal cortex of the dog and cat. The *zona intermedia* is found in dogs between the zona arcuata and the zona fasciculata. It is most prominent in the young (dogs less than 3 months old) but serves as a blastema for all the other zones throughout life. An "X" zone has been described to exist in the cat between the zona reticularis and the adrenal medulla. It is apparently responsive to gonadotropins but degenerates with puberty.

The adrenal medulla normally composes 10% to 20% of the volume of an adrenal gland. It is characterized microscopically by interlacing cords of cells containing granules that stain dark brown with chromium salts (chromaffin tissue) and are separated by venous sinuses. The adrenal cortex is separated from the medulla by an indistinct septum. The medulla is perfused with blood from the cortex through sinusoidal capillaries that are continuous with the zona fasciculata and reticularis. These drain into

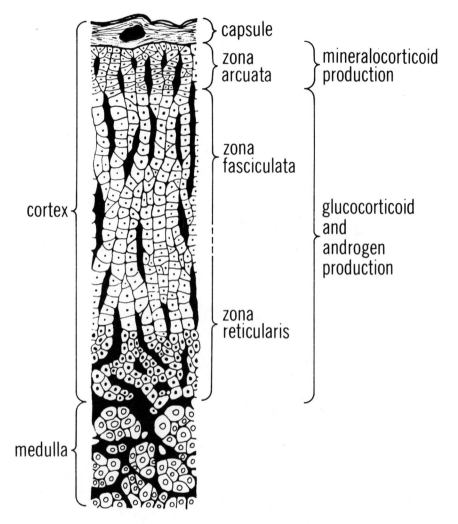

Fig. 17–2.   Cross-section of normal canine adrenal gland.

venules, then into the central vein. The medulla receives a generous supply of preganglionic sympathetic fibers.

DEVELOPMENT, AGING, AND ANOMALIES OF THE ADRENAL GLANDS

The adrenal cortex and medulla develop independently of each other until the medullary precursor cells invade the cluster of cortical precursor cells (Fig. 17–3). The fetal adrenal cortex develops from celomic mesoderm on the dorsal abdominal wall near the genital ridge of the embryo. The fetal cortex is gradually replaced by the adult cortex. In humans, the fetal cortex

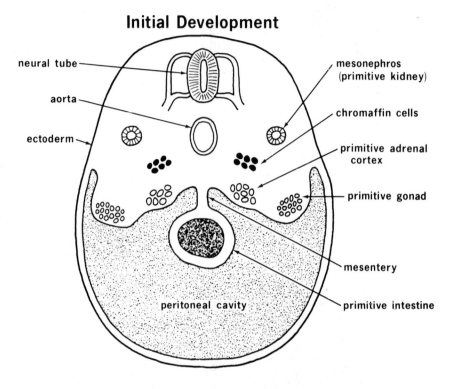

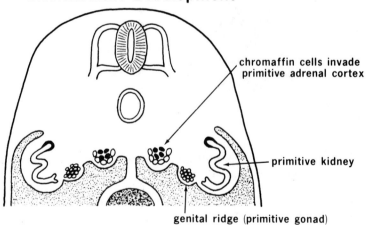

Fig. 17–3. Development of the canine adrenals (cross-section of fetal dorsal abdominal wall).

produces sulfates of adrenal androgens, which are converted into androgens and estrogens by the placenta and enter the maternal circulation in the form of those hormones. Zones in the cortex are not evident at birth, but become well defined by 3 months of age.

Development of the zones begins with the zona arcuata and the zona intermedia. As the inner two zones form, they gain the ability to produce more complex enzymes and thereby additional steroid hormones. The capsule is formed by a condensation of peripheral cortical cells. Thickening of the capsule continues until 6 months of age. The zona intermedia can produce cortical cells by centrifugal and centripetal migration. During normal aging, the zona arcuata is unaffected, but the zona fasciculata and the zona reticularis atrophy with age. In dogs, nodules of cortical cells consisting mostly of zona arcuata cells tend to form during aging in intra- and pericapsular areas. In humans, ectopic adrenal cortical tissue has been found in periadrenal fat, the spleen, and caudal to the kidneys, and has been associated with the ovaries or testes. The occurrence of ectopic adrenal cortical tissue has not been investigated sufficiently in companion animals.

The adrenal medulla originates from the neural crest. Cells from the neural crest normally migrate into the cortex cells near the genital ridge. This migration can produce ectopic chromaffin tissue and continues even after birth. Masses of neural crest cells outside the adrenal medulla are called *paraganglia*. Chromaffin tissue of paraganglia can occur near autonomic ganglia and along the aorta. It gradually involutes after birth, but some persists in adults. After the invasion of the cortex by the medullary cells from the neural crest, the organs separate from the dorsal celomic wall and are situated craniomedial to the kidneys.

See also reference 40.

SECRETIONS OF THE ADRENAL CORTEX

The adrenal cortex produces about 30 different hormones. Many of these hormones have little or no clinical significance. Some have more than one action of clinical importance. All cortical hormones are derivatives of cholesterol with the cyclopentanoperhydrophenanthrene nucleus. Cardiac glycosides, bile acids, vitamin D, and ovarian and testicular steroids are similar in structure. The adrenal cortex takes up some cholesterol from the circulation and synthesizes some from acetate within the adrenal cortex. The adrenal cortex also contains concentrated quantities of ascorbic acid. Although ascorbic acid quantities are diminished by secretions from the adrenal cortex, its action in the adrenal cortex is unknown.

Hormones produced in the adrenal cortex are categorized into three groups based on their major effect on target tissues. These groups include the *mineralocorticoids* (so named because of their effect on sodium and potassium homeostasis), the *glucocorticoids* (which promote gluconeogenesis), and *sex hormones* (particularly male sex hormones with weak androgenicity). Approximate secretion rates are listed in Table 17–1.

Table 17–1. Approximate Corticosteroid Secretion Rates in the Dog

Hormone	Secretion Rate (μg/kg body weight/day)
Cortisol	700–800
Corticosterone	300–400
Deoxycortisol	80–90
Deoxycorticosterone	5–10
Aldosterone	5–10
Total	1.2 mg/kg body weight/day

BIOSYNTHESIS AND SALIENT BIOCHEMISTRY OF ADRENOCORTICAL HORMONES

The most important mineralocorticoid is aldosterone, which is produced in the zona arcuata. The zonas fasciculata and reticularis produce the major glucocorticoid, cortisol, and androgen, dehydroepiandrosterone (DHEA). Synthesis pathways are summarized in Figure 17–4. Adrenal steroid synthesis occurs in the mitochondria (pregnenolone, 11 and 18 hydroxylation) and smooth endoplasmic reticulum (17 and 21 hydroxylation). The major steroids move back and forth between mitochondria and endoplasmic reticula for synthesis.

All adrenal cortical hormones are derivatives of the *cyclopentanoperhydrophenanthrene nucleus* (Fig. 17–5). Carbon numbers and ring letters are illustrated in Figure 17–6. There are three basic groups of steroid structures (Fig. 17–7). The simplest group in structure contains only an additional carbon at the number 18 position. All C-18 compounds exhibit female hormone (estrogenic) activity. C-19 compounds possess additional carbons to the basic steroid nucleus at C-18 and C-19 positions. C-19 compounds exhibit male hormone (androgenic) activity. C-21 compounds have additional carbons at C-18, C-19, C-20, and C-21 positions. C-21 compounds may show glucocorticoid, mineralocorticoid, or progestogen activity. Natural C-21 compounds have actions that overlap the three possible effects of C-21 compounds, but either glucocorticoid, mineralocorticoid, or progestogen effects predominate. Synthetic C-21 compounds have more exclusive effects as a glucocorticoid, mineralocorticoid, or progestogen than natural C-21 compounds. C-21 compounds with an hydroxy group at C-17 are called *17-hydroxycorticosteroids* and have predominantly glucocorticoid effects. C-19 compounds with a keto group at C-17 are called *17-ketosteroids* (oxosteroids) and are androgenic.

Adrenocorticosteroids are catabolized by the liver, kidney, and target organs. The liver metabolizes most adrenal corticosteroids. The steroid nucleus cannot be catabolized. Adrenal corticosteroids are excreted after conjugation to glucuronides or esterified to sulfates.

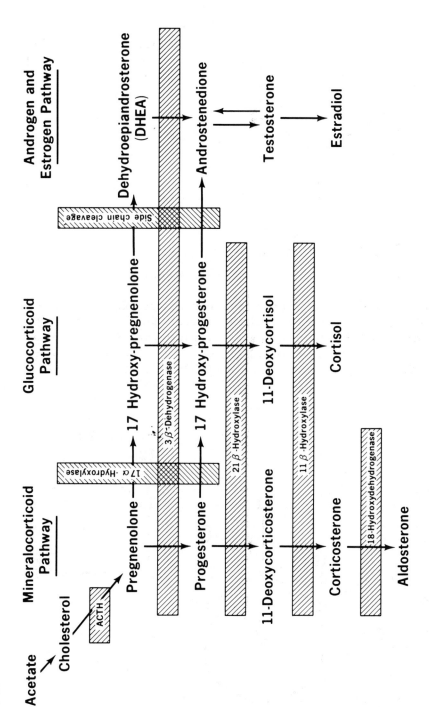

Fig. 17–4. Adrenocortical hormone synthesis.

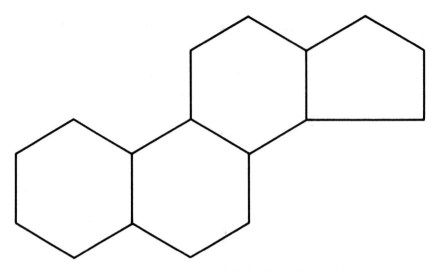

Fig. 17–5. The cyclopentanoperhydrophenanthrene nucleus.

    The conversion of cholesterol to pregnenolone, the immediate precursor of all steroid hormones, is markedly facilitated by adrenocorticotropic hormone (ACTH).[33] Without ACTH, less than 10% of normal adrenal corticosteroid production can occur. Production of adrenal corticosteroids (especially cortisol) inhibits the release of ACTH (Fig. 17–8). Serum levels of

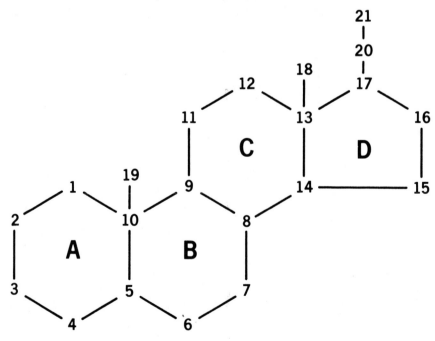

Fig. 17–6. Carbon numbers and ring letters.

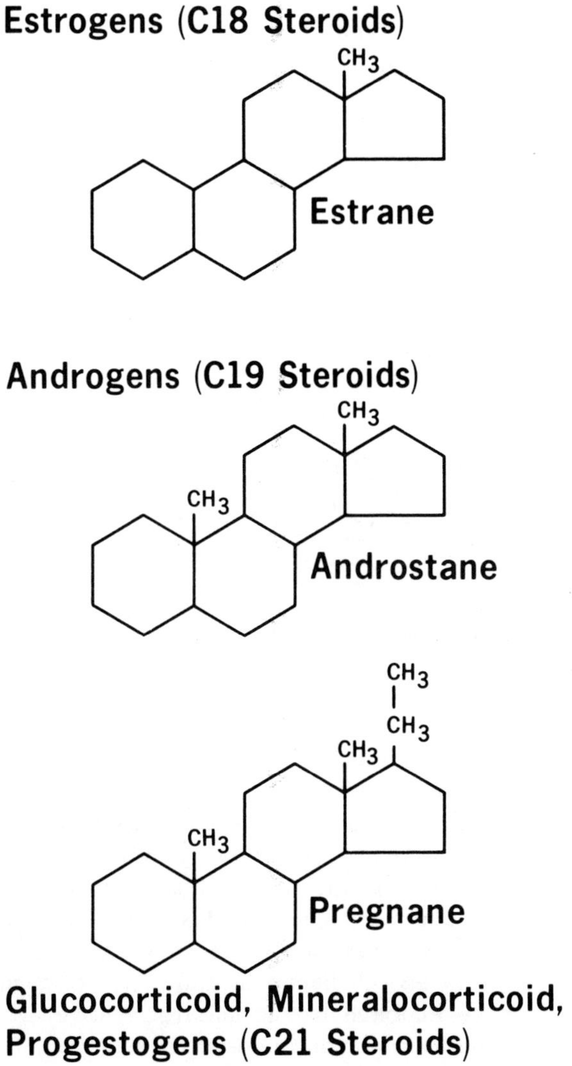

Estrogens (C18 Steroids)

CH₃

Estrane

Androgens (C19 Steroids)

CH₃

CH₃

Androstane

CH₃

CH₃

CH₃

CH₃

Pregnane

Glucocorticoid, Mineralocorticoid, Progestogens (C21 Steroids)

Fig. 17–7. Basic steroid hormone structures.

adrenal corticosteroids fluctuate during the day as a result of the normal episodic bursts of ACTH secretion.

See also references 1, 4, 14, 16, 17, 22, 23, 41, and 93.

Mineralocorticoids and Their Actions

Aldosterone is the most physiologically important mineralocorticoid. Others include corticosterone, 11-deoxycorticosterone, and 18-hydroxydeoxycorticosterone. Aldosterone's main purposes are to protect against

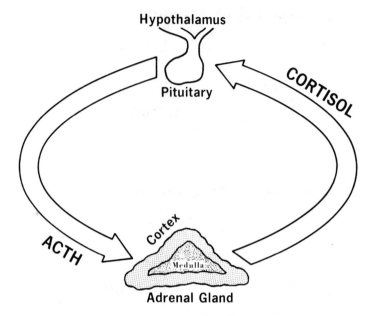

Fig. 17–8. Normal central nervous system-adrenal hormonal feedback. ACTH = adreno-corticotropic hormone.

hypotension and potassium intoxication. Relative mineralocorticoid poten-cies for selected corticosteroids are listed in Table 17–2.

Stimuli for aldosterone secretion are listed in Table 17–3. The major physiologic stimuli for increased aldosterone production is *angiotensin II* and hyperkalemia (Fig. 17–9). Angiotensin II, an octapeptide, is a product of *angiotensin I,* a decapeptide. Angiotensin I is converted to angiotensin II (and III) by converting enzymes found in several tissues, but especially in the pulmonary capillary endothelium. The conversion of angiotensin I to angiotensin II can be inhibited by the antihypertensive drug, captopril (Capoten). In addition to stimulating aldosterone secretion, angiotensin II stimulates the thirst center in the brain and is the most potent endogenous vasoconstrictor known. Its serum half-life is only 1 to 2 minutes. *Angio-tensin III* is a heptapeptide capable of releasing aldosterone, as well as angiotensin II, but possesses only 40% of the vasoconstrictor ability of angiotensin II. Weaker mineralocorticoids such as corticosterone are more affected by increased stimulation of ACTH.

Angiotensin I is a product of renin's action on the circulating α-2 globulin (molecular weight of 57,000) from the liver, *angiotensinogen. Renin* is a proteolytic enzyme with a serum half-life of 80 minutes and a molecular weight of 40,000. It originates from juxtaglomerular apparatus. Normal plasma renin levels in dogs are about 2 to 3 ng/ml/hr. Renin is usually measured as the amount of angiotensin I generated per unit of time. Renin

Table 17-2. Relative Mineralocorticoid Potencies

Adrenal Corticosteroid	Potency
Cortisol	1
Corticosterone	15
Aldosterone	3000
Deoxycorticosterone	100

and growth hormone (GH) are required for their permissive effects on ACTH and angiotensinogen II's stimulation of the adrenal cortex.

The *juxtaglomerular* apparatus consists of special epithelial cells in the distal convoluted tubule adjacent to the afferent glomerular arteriole called the *macula densa* and specialized (juxtaglomerular) myoepithelial cells in the wall of the afferent glomerular arteriole (Fig. 17-10). Renin release may be stimulated by stretch receptors in the juxtaglomerular cells or by a sodium and chloride chemoreceptor in the macula densa. Renin is also released by sympathetic autonomic stimuli. Renin release is inhibited by angiotensin II, ADH, hypertension, and increased reabsorption of renal tubular sodium.

Aldosterone has a negative feedback effect on the juxtaglomerular apparatus. It promotes sodium reabsorption, which expands the intravascular volume (water follows the sodium into the intravascular space), thereby raising the blood pressure in the afferent glomerular arteriole.

Another important basic stimulus for aldosterone secretion is hyperkalemia. An increase in serum potassium of 1 mEq/L can increase the secretion of aldosterone more than threefold. Aldosterone, in turn, is the most potent stimulator of potassium excretion. Hyponatremia is also effective as a direct stimulus for aldosterone secretion, but to a lesser degree. The actions of renin, angiotensin, and aldosterone are illustrated in Figure 17-11.

ACTH can temporarily promote the secretion of aldosterone. Hypophysectomy temporarily decreases the production of aldosterone by about 40% in the dog. The role of ACTH in the production of aldosterone is of little physiologic importance and is short-lived. The ACTH-induced release of aldosterone initiates and augments the secretion of aldosterone in stressful situations, but it does not maintain such secretion.

Table 17-3. Possible Stimuli for Aldosterone Production

Increased intake of potassium
Decreased intake of sodium or sodium depletion resulting from diuretics
Constriction of the caudal vena cava
Renal hypotension (hemorrhage, dehydration, heart failure)
ACTH* (surgery, anxiety, trauma, hemorrhage)
Hepatic cirrhosis
Standing (humans only?)

* ACTH = adrenocorticotropic hormone.

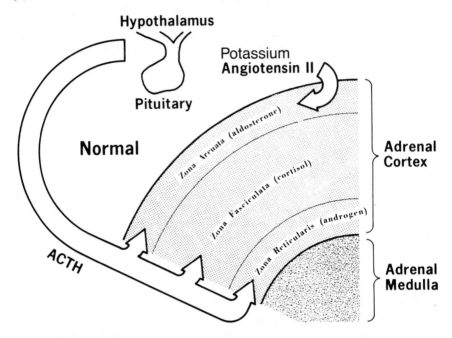

Fig. 17–9. Stimuli for aldosterone secretion.

Aldosterone promotes the reabsorption of sodium from urine, saliva, and gastric juice. Its most important effects are on the distal convoluted tubule and collecting ducts, where it promotes the reabsorption of sodium and secretion of potassium. Aldosterone also stimulates the secretion of ammonia, magnesium, and hydrogen, leading to metabolic alkalosis. Although aldosterone effects the reabsorption of only 2% of the total filtered sodium in the distal tubule and collecting ducts, the absolute quantity effected is large—6 g of sodium in 24 hours in a 20-kg dog. Persistent hyperaldosteronemia normally results in an "escape phenomenon," whereby natriuresis occurs after normal renal blood pressure is re-established. The mechanism of escape is unknown, but prostaglandins of the A series are probably involved.

In comparison to cortisol, aldosterone has one-half to one-third the glucocorticoid potency per mg. Because its normal rate of secretion in mg is slight compared to that of cortisol, aldosterone does not have any significant physiologic glucocorticoid effect. Aldosterone is weakly bound to plasma proteins, mostly albumin, while in circulation. Its serum half-life is approximately 20 minutes. It is inactivated 75% by reduction and conjugation on its first pass through the liver. Spironolactone is a potent competitive antagonist for aldosterone receptors. Progesterone is a mild competitive antagonist.

Aldosterone is not used clinically. A less potent (per mg) mineralocorticoid, deoxycorticosterone, is equally effective in the proper dosages and is

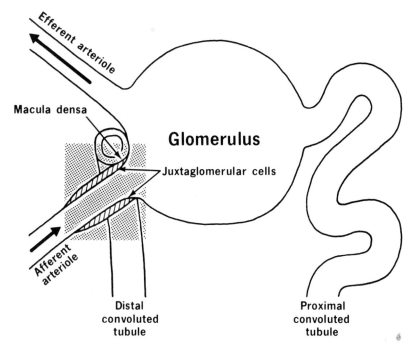

Fig. 17–10. The juxtaglomerular apparatus.

more easily manufactured. Aldosterone can be measured by radioimmuno-assay (RIA). Normal serum levels in fasting dogs and cats on normal sodium-potassium-containing diets are usually less than 1 to 6 ng/dl (as determined by RIA), but normal values have reportedly ranged up to 30 ng/dl.

See also references 24, 31, 34, 37, and 51.

Glucocorticoids and Their Physiologic and Pharmacologic Actions

Cortisol, compound "F," is the major glucocorticoid produced by the body. Corticosterone is the second most physiologically important glucocorticoid. In the dog, cortisol is usually secreted in a 2:1 to 5:1 ratio to corticosterone; in the cat and human, the ratio is about 5:1 to 10:1. Cortisol and corticosterone are occasionally called 11-beta hydroxycorticosteroids in reference to their chemical structure. Synthetic analogues to cortisol are used clinically and are much more potent glucocorticoids than cortisol.

There is only one stimulus for cortisol production, ACTH. The rise in plasma cortisol lags behind ACTH by less than 3 minutes, but peak cortisol values occur about 1 hour after ACTH is administered intravenously as a bolus. ACTH and, therefore, cortisol are secreted in episodic bursts with the greatest quantities released in the early morning hours (peak levels

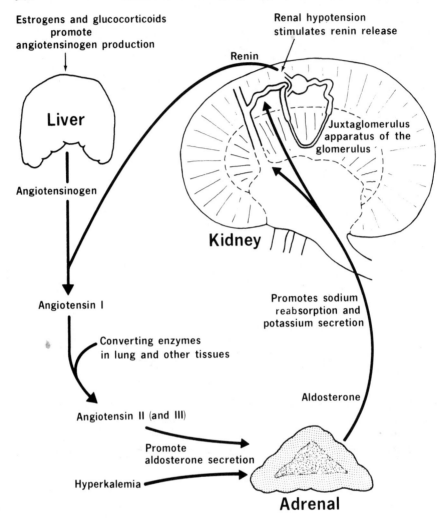

Estrogens and glucocorticoids promote angiotensinogen production

Renal hypotension stimulates renin release

Renin

Liver

Juxtaglomerulus apparatus of the glomerulus

Angiotensinogen

Kidney

Angiotensin I

Promotes sodium reabsorption and potassium secretion

Converting enzymes in lung and other tissues

Aldosterone

Angiotensin II (and III)

Promote aldosterone secretion

Hyperkalemia

Adrenal

Fig. 17–11. Actions of renin, angiotensin, and aldosterone.

occur at 8:00 A.M., lowest levels at 11:00 P.M.) in the dog, horse, and human.[52] In the cat, peak secretion occurs in the evening hours. Diurnal rhythm changes in the secretion of cortisol seem to coincide with ancestral hunting tactics. Dogs, who are day hunters, have elevated levels of ACTH and cortisol in the mornings; cats, who are night hunters, have elevations in the evenings. Possibly owing to domestication, the diurnal changes in domestic companion animals are small and inconsistent.[43] It is interesting to note that modern man, who still must "hunt" for his survival, has retained a marked diurnal variation in the secretion of ACTH and cortisol in comparison to companion animals.

Cortisol has more known diverse effects on the body than any other hormone. Its physiologic effects are not as numerous as its pharmacologic effects. The major physiologic effects of cortisol are to "permit" the action of catecholamines on vascular and bronchial smooth muscle, that of catecholamines on adipose tissue, and that of glucagon on stores of hepatic glycogen. Cortisol's physiologic effects also include maintenance of normal cardiac and skeletal muscle strength, maintenance of normal brain activity, maintenance of normal water compartment distribution in the body, and preparation of target organs to withstand the deleterious effects of certain stresses.

Cortisol's main effect on carbohydrate, protein, and fat metabolism is to promote gluconeogenesis. Gluconeogenesis is the production of blood glucose at the expense of muscle and adipose tissue. Cortisol induces gluconeogenesis by the formation of hepatic gluconeogenic enzymes. The increased secretion of insulin normally counters the tendency toward hyperglycemia (insulin antagonism).[59] Protein is mobilized from nearly all cells except the liver. In the liver, protein synthesis is promoted. Glucocorticoids also mobilize fatty acids and enhance their oxidation. Plasma lipid content (cholesterol and triglycerides) is increased, and ketogenesis occurs if insulin's effects are exceeded. Lactic acid metabolism is increased. Adipose tissue tends to be redistributed from the extremities and subcutaneous abdominal sites to the pelvis, neck, thorax, and omentum. At the same time that gluconeogenesis is occurring, liver glycogen stores are increased (by means of hepatic glycogenesis).

Cortisol's effects on water distribution, electrolytes, and trace minerals include increased diuresis, inhibition of water shift into cells, increased potassium excretion in urine, increased urinary and fecal losses of calcium, and decreased levels of serum zinc.[73, 87] Some of the proposed mechanisms for cortisol-induced diuresis include increased glomerular filtration rate, inhibition of the action of ADH on the renal tubules, and increased antidiuretic hormone (ADH) inactivation.[44]

Supplementation with zinc reduces the delay in healing associated with cortisol excess. Urinary losses of potassium are a pharmacologic, not physiologic, effect of cortisol. Glucocorticoid-induced potassium loss is rarely severe enough to result in hypokalemia in dogs and cats because cortisol is only 1/1000 as potent per mg as aldosterone is in affecting electrolytes. Hypocalcemia does not develop from glucocorticoid excess as long as the parathyroids respond normally, but secondary hyperparathyroidism and depleted bone mineralization may result.

The gastrointestinal effects of cortisol are increased secretion of gastric acid and pepsin, decreased mucosal cell proliferation, and stimulation of pancreatic secretions.[91] The absorption of calcium and iron is inhibited. Hepatic changes associated with pharmacologic amounts of cortisol are vacuolization of hepatocytes with accumulations of glycogen and fat. Hepatic mitochondria are decreased in number. The production of hepatic alkaline phosphatase is induced.[15] Focal centrolobular necrosis can also occur. The intestinal absorption of fat is enhanced by cortisol. Pancreatic secretions become more viscous, and the pancreatic ductal epithelium becomes hyperplastic.

Cardiovascular effects of cortisol include a permissive effect on vascular responses to catecholamines and an antagonistic effect on responses to kinins and histamine, each of which promotes vasoconstriction. Cortisol also has a weak ionotropic effect on the myocardium and facilitates atrioventricular conduction. The action of the myocardial depressant factor is inhibited.

Skeletomuscular effects of pharmacologic amounts of cortisol are physical weakness, muscular atrophy, and osteoporosis. Skeletal effects are caused by the suppression of GH and somatomedin release, inhibition of fibrocartilage growth, catabolism of the collagenous bone matrix, increased calcium excretion in urine and feces, and inhibition of vitamin D activation, which results in poor gastrointestinal absorption of calcium.[11] A deficiency in glucocorticoids also causes muscular weakness. Physiologic quantities of cortisol are essential for normal growth and muscular strength.

The effects of excessive levels of cortisol on the nervous system include decreased seizure threshold, psychoses, decreased response to pyrogens, and stimulation of the appetite. Cortisol psychoses may cause aggression, altered mood, or neurotic self-mutilation. A deficiency in normal quantities of cortisol is also associated with psychoses, slowed α rhythm on an electroencephalogram, and increased sense of smell. Cortisol in physiologic amounts is required for normal cerebral activity.

The hematologic effects of excessive levels of cortisol include neutrophilia resulting from the stimulated production of neutrophils, release from the bone marrow, and release of the marginated pool. Cortisol can cause lymphopenia, eosinopenia, and basopenia by sequestration of cells in the spleen and lungs, decreased efflux, and decreased lymphocyte mitosis. Red blood cell production is promoted by cortisol, whereas removal of old red blood cells is suppressed. Target cells and Howell-Jolly bodies increase. Platelet and monocyte production is also increased by cortisol. Platelet aggregation is inhibited.

Excessive levels of cortisol can cause immunosuppression. Under the influence of cortisol, lymphocytes disappear from circulation, primarily because of redistribution into the bone marrow and other sites. Their DNA synthesis is also inhibited. Glucocorticoid-sensitive species (mice, rats, hamsters, and rabbits) are much more immunologically affected by glucocorticoids than glucocorticoid-resistant species (dogs, cats, and humans). In addition, thymic-derived (T) lymphocytes are more sensitive to glucocorticoids than bursa equivalent (B) lymphocytes. In addition to decreasing T cells in number, cortisol also inhibits the effects of lymphokines produced by sensitized T cells. The production of lymphokines is not directly inhibited. Cortisol in excess can decrease antibody production, but anamnestic antibody production is relatively resistant compared to initial responses.

Nonspecific immune defenses are affected more than specific acquired immunity. Antigen-antibody reactions are not suppressed, but the action of complement is antagonized. Also inhibited by excess levels of cortisol are neutrophil, macrophage, and monocyte migration; chemotactic response; diapedesis; interferon production; processing of antigens; phagocytosis; and intracellular killing. Fibroblastic proliferation to sequester infectious agents and repair tissue is suppressed. Clinical signs of infection such as pain and leukocytosis are masked by excessive amounts of cortisol. Cortisol inhibits formation of leukotrienes, as well as the synthesis of prostacyclin and the febrile response. The febrile response is also lessened because the effects of the endotoxins are decreased, the release of pyrogen from monocytes is decreased, and neutrophil migration is decreased.

Cortisol has detoxifying actions. Lysosomal membranes are stabilized; capillary permeability is decreased; the effects of vasoactive amines, including histamine and mast cell numbers, are suppressed; and cell membranes tend to maintain their integrity. The formation of histamine is not affected, but its release is suppressed.

The secretion of cortisol increases during pregnancy. Bound and free plasma cortisol increases. Hepatic metabolism of cortisol decreases, while excretion of cortisol in the urine increases. Responsiveness to ACTH increases. Administration of glucocorticoids in early pregnancy can cause teratogenicity. Administration of glucocorticoids in late pregnancy can induce parturition in horses.

Glucocorticoids affect the secretion or cellular effects of nearly all other hormones.[47] Effects on thyroid hormones include suppression of serum thyroxine (T_4) and triiodothyronine (T_3) levels. T_3 levels are more affected than T_4 levels. The secretion of thyroid-stimulating hormone (TSH), the thyrotropin-releasing hormone (TRH)-induced release of TSH, and thyroxine-binding globulin serum levels are decreased by glucocorticoids. Serum testosterone levels are decreased by inhibition of the secretion of follicle-stimulating hormone (FSH) and luteinizing hormone (LH) and gonadotropin-releasing-hormone (GnRH)-induced FSH and LH release. Glucocorticoids may also have direct inhibitory effects on the thyroid, testes, and ovaries. Insulin's binding to receptors and post-receptor effects are inhibited by glucocorticoids. Plasma levels of parathyroid hormones (PTH) are increased by glucocorticoids because calcium's absorption from the digestive tract is inhibited and excretion of calcium in the urine is promoted by glucocorticoids. Osteoblast activity may be directly inhibited by glucocorticoids. The secretion of prolactin and GH, as well as the effects of ADH on renal tubules, is inhibited by glucocorticoids. The calorigenic effects of glucagon and catecholamines, and the lipolytic, pressor, and bronchodilation effects of catecholamines require permissive amounts of glucocorticoids.

Cortisol has a strong affinity for a corticosteroid-binding α-globulin (CBG) called transcortin. Transcortin levels are increased by estrogens and decreased by cirrhosis, nephrosis, and multiple myeloma in humans.

Estrogens, progestogens, and other glucocorticoids compete for transcortin binding with cortisol. Cortisol also binds to albumin, but only weakly. Normally, in the dog, it is thought that 40% of cortisol is circulating bound to transcortin, 50% to albumin, and 5% to 10% is free. The serum half-life of cortisol is about 100 minutes.

Cortisol is removed from the circulation by the liver, where it is converted to water-soluble conjugates for excretion in the urine of dogs. Bilirubin, steroid hormones, and some drugs compete with cortisol for the same conjugation pathways. Major cortisol metabolites found in the urine of dogs are cortol, cortolone, and 3-epiallotetrahydrocortisol. Most are glucuronides and are reduced at C-20. Small quantities of free cortisol are also excreted in the urine. There is some enterohepatic recirculation of adrenal steroids. The cat excretes almost no cortisol or any other steroid metabolites in the urine.[88] Steroid excretion in the cat is biliary. The hepatic inactivation of cortisol is impaired in both the dog and cat by some liver diseases.

Cortisol (hydrocortisone) is rarely used clinically because of its mineralocorticoid side effects in pharmacologic doses and its weak glucocorticoid effects relative to its synthetic analogues. Plasma or serum cortisol RIAs are commercially available. Normal values determined by RIA in unstressed dogs and cats are about 1 to 4 μg/dl.

See also references 5, 67, 68, 72, and 89.

Adrenal Sex Hormones and Their Actions

The adrenal cortex produces several weakly androgenic steroids. *Dehydroepiandrosterone (DHEA)* is produced in the greatest quantities. *Androstenedione,* a product of DHEA, is produced in lesser amounts. Etiocholanolone, epiandrosterone, DHEA sulfate, androsterone, adrenosterone, and 11 β-hydroxyandrostenedione are serum and urinary metabolites of adrenal androgens with androgen activity. Testosterone and dihydrotestosterone can be formed peripherally from androstenedione. Most testosterone in males is produced by the testes. Dihydrotestosterone is formed by target organs from circulating testosterone. Relative androgenicity of several steroids is listed (Table 17–4). Adrenal androgens have less than 20% the androgenic activity of testosterone. For example, testosterone is 5 times more active than androstenedione, 10 times more active than androsterone, and 25 times more active than DHEA.

Table 17–4. Relative Androgenicity of Various Steroids in Decreasing Order

Dihydrotestosterone
Testosterone
Androstenedione and androstenediol
Androsterone
Dehydroepiandrosterone

Androgenic steroids have masculinizing and anabolic effects. In women, nearly all the androgenic steroid urinary metabolites are of adrenal origin. In men, 10% of the urinary metabolites of androgens are from the adrenals. Similar situations are presumed to occur in companion animals. In the amounts normally produced, adrenal androgens have little known effects, but in cases of adrenal cortical hyperplasia or neoplasia, sufficient amounts can be produced to cause masculinization. If excessive adrenal androgens are produced in prepubertal men, precocious pseudopuberty occurs. In postpubertal men, moderate excesses of adrenal androgens do not create clinical abnormalities. In women of any age, secretion of excess adrenal androgens causes changes associated with the male gender. This condition is called the *adrenogenital syndrome.*

Estrogens can be formed by irreversible aromatization from the adrenal androgen, androstenedione, at the target organs. Some estrogens are secreted directly from the adrenal glands. Estrogen-secreting adrenocortical tumors have been reported in humans.

Few adrenal androgens and estrogens are produced until the time of puberty. The pubertal period when adrenal secretion of sex hormones increases to adult production levels is called the *adrenarche.*[78] The initiating factor for the adrenarche is not known.

Adrenal androgenic steroids are primarily metabolized (conjugated) by the liver and then excreted in the urine (this is not so in the cat). If one of the metabolites, etiocholanolone, is released into the circulation without conjugation, it can cause fever in humans.

Most of certain androgens, such as testosterone, is bound to a β-globulin, sex-hormone-binding globulin (SHBG) which also binds estrogens. The serum binding of DHEA is unknown.

Adrenal androgens are not routinely assayed for clinical purposes. Serum levels of androstenedione in normal dogs have been reported to be about 50 to 150 ng/dl.

See also reference 77.

SECRETIONS OF THE ADRENAL MEDULLA

Adrenal medullary cells are arranged in interlacing cords, and if they are stimulated by sympathetic preganglionic autonomic nerve fibers, these cells will secrete catecholamines. They are called *chromaffin cells* because of distinctive staining with chromium salts and ferric chloride. They also fluoresce when allowed to react with ethylenediamine. Smaller amounts of other chromaffin tissue can be found adjacent to sympathetic ganglia and near the bifurcation of the carotids.

BIOSYNTHESIS AND SALIENT BIOCHEMISTRY OF ADRENAL MEDULLARY HORMONES

The secretory products of major importance from the adrenal medulla are epinephrine and norepinephrine. (The name Adrenalin is a trade name for synthesized epinephrine and should not be used to refer to the endogenous hormone.) Some dopamine and enkephalins are also produced and released by the adrenal medulla. Norepinephrine is also produced by and liberated into the circulation from adrenergic nerve endings. Norepinephrine is principally a neurotransmitter, whereas epinephrine is a true hormone. The cells of the adrenal medulla are modified postganglionic sympathetic neurons. They are innervated and stimulated by preganglionic sympathetic (cholinergic) nerves. Their secretory products are stored as cytoplasmic granules. Epinephrine-secreting cells contain large, less dense granules. Norepinephrine granules are smaller, but more dense. In the fetus, the adrenal medulla predominantly produces norepinephrine, but in adults, epinephrine predominates. In adult dogs and horses, about one fourth to one fifth of normal adrenal medullary secretion is norepinephrine. In adult cats, about 40% of normal medullary secretions are norepinephrine. In humans, 80% of urine catecholamines are from norepinephrine, mostly from postganglionic sympathetic nerve endings.

Some evidence exists that the ratios of epinephrine to norepinephrine can vary, and differential secretion can occur to different stimuli.[12] The caudal paraventricular area of the hypothalamus affects sympathetic tone. Stimuli for adrenal medullary secretion, mediated through the hypothalamus, that may cause the predominant release of epinephrine include hypoxia, pain, cold, unknown dangers, and hypoglycemia. Stimuli that may cause the predominant release of norepinephrine are hypotension, known dangers, rage, or anxiety. The hypothesis of selective secretion is questionable. Other stimuli of catecholamine release are acetylcholine, serotonin, bradykinin, histamine, tyramine, exercise, and glucagon.

Epinephrine, norepinephrine, and dopamine are called *catecholamines* because their chemical structures are composed of an aromatic ring (catechol) attached to an amine. Catecholamines are synthesized from the amino acids phenylalanine and tyrosine. Tyrosine is available as a dietary nutrient or can be synthesized from phenylalanine. Norepinephrine is a result of the hydroxylation of dopamine, and epinephrine results from the methylation of norepinephrine. Catecholamine synthesis is illustrated in Figure 17–12. Blood to the adrenal medulla normally contains high concentrations of adrenocortical steroid hormones, including glucocorticoids, on which the enzyme necessary for methylation of norepinephrine to epinephrine, *phenylethanolamine-N-methyl transferase,* is dependent. Glucocorticoid deficiency will, therefore, cause a deficiency in epinephrine.

Although some of the actions of epinephrine and norepinephrine overlap, the predominant effects of epinephrine are on carbohydrate metabolism, whereas the predominant effects of norepinephrine are on vascular smooth muscle.

Catecholamines are adrenergic agents. Adrenergic receptor effects are, by tradition, pharmacologically categorized as α effects, those that cause contraction of vascular smooth muscle, and β effects, those that cause relax-

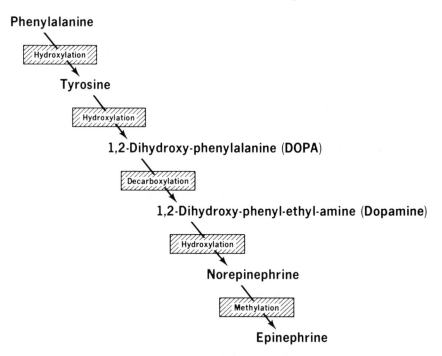

Fig. 17–12. Catecholamine synthesis.

ation of vascular smooth muscle and stimulation of cardiac strength and rate of contraction. Alpha- and beta-adrenergic effects have been further sub-divided into the following categories: α_1, α_2, β_1, and β_2. Alpha- and beta-receptors cannot be identified biochemically or morphologically. Nor-epinephrine has α-adrenergic effects, but epinephrine in supraphysiologic amounts has significant α and β effects. Beta effects are mediated through increased production of cyclic adenosine monophosphate (cAMP) in the target tissues. Alpha (α_2) effects are the result of inhibition of adenyl cyclase. Alpha- and beta-adrenergic effects are summarized in Table 17–5.

Table 17–5. Summary of Alpha- and Beta-Adrenergic Effects

Effects on:	Alpha	Beta
Skeletal muscle vasculature	Constricted	Dilated (β_2)
Strength of cardiac contraction		Increased (β_1)
Heart rate		Increased (β_1)
Gastrointestinal smooth muscle	Relaxed	Relaxed
Gastrointestinal sphincter tone	Increased	Increased
Uterine smooth muscle	Contraction	Relaxation (β_2)
Bronchial smooth muscle		Relaxed (β_2)
Liver	Glycogenolysis	Glycogenolysis
Adipose tissue		Lipolysis
Antagonist	Phentolamine	Propranolol

The cardiovascular effects of epinephrine include increased cardiac output resulting from an increase in the strength of the heart's contractions, increased heart rate, and moderately increased systolic blood pressure. Peripheral circulation is decreased to the skin and viscera (α-adrenergic effect) and increased to the liver, brain, and skeletal muscle (β-adrenergic effect). It decreases peripheral resistance since the net effect is a dilation of skeletal muscle arterioles. Norepinephrine markedly increases systolic and diastolic blood pressure by increasing peripheral resistance. It initially increases heart rate and then causes bradycardia by causing reflexes mediated by increased peripheral blood pressure. As a result, norepinephrine decreases cardiac output, but it has no direct effect on the heart's strength or rate of contraction. Dopamine increases the strength of cardiac contraction, causes vasodilation in the kidneys and mesenteric vessels, and produces vasoconstriction in other vasculature.

Respiratory effects of epinephrine and norepinephrine are similar. Both relax bronchiolar smooth muscle and increase the depth and rate of respiration after a temporary apnea.

The ocular, urinary, and gastrointestinal effects of epinephrine and norepinephrine are also similar. Both relax the pupillary constrictor muscle, resulting in dilation of the pupils, and both relax the smooth muscles of the digestive tract and urinary bladder, with the exception of the sphincters, which are stimulated to constrict. The smooth muscles of the ureters and spleen are stimulated to contract, as are the arrector pili muscles of the skin.

Epinephrine is glycogenolytic to the liver, and also depletes glycogen stored in skeletal muscle. Marked elevation of the blood glucose occurs after the parenteral administration of epinephrine as a result of hepatic glycogenolysis, inhibition of insulin secretion, stimulation of the release of ACTH, and release of lactate from muscle, which is converted to glucose by the liver. Although norepinephrine has similar effects, it is less than 20% as efficient at glycogenolysis as is epinephrine. Epinephrine and norepinephrine increase the consumption of oxygen by the tissues of the body by 30%. This calorigenic effect requires the permissive effect of the presence of thyroid and adrenocortical hormones. Both stimulate a two-phase, mild rise in body temperature. The initial rise is probably due to vasoconstriction of the skin, or increased muscular activity, or both. The delayed phase is due to hepatic oxidation of lactic acid. Despite the fact that the liver can store up to 8% of its weight in glycogen and skeletal muscle can store only 1%, the total quantity of glycogen stored in the muscle exceeds that of the liver. Consequently, conversion of released skeletal muscle glycogen and its transformation to glucose by the liver is also potentially calorigenic.

Epinephrine and norepinephrine have marked lipolytic and ketogenic effects. Free fatty acids increase in the plasma after the administration of either catecholamine. Serum potassium initially increases with the administration of the major catecholamines, then declines slowly. Serum phosphorus also decreases, an effect due primarily to epinephrine.

The actions of epinephrine and norepinephrine on the central nervous system are similar. Both increase impulse transmission in and out of the brain, increasing mental alertness. In humans, epinephrine tends to alter mood toward feelings of anxiety, fear, aggression, or hostility.

The half-life of circulating catecholamines is short. For example, epinephrine's half-life is less than 1 minute. Metabolism of the catecholamines normally occurs primarily in the liver, but peripheral tissues (kidney, brain, adrenergic nerve endings) also degrade catecholamines by oxidation and methylation. The normal degradation of catecholamines is illustrated in Figure 17–13. Most of the circulating catecholamines is norepinephrine, and this is not of adrenal medullary origin. Most originates from postganglionic sympathetic nerve endings; most circulating norepinephrine is again taken up and again used by nerve endings. Only a small amount of norepinephrine is metabolized by the liver, nerve endings, or other tissues. Circulating epinephrine is produced entirely by the adrenal medulla. One half of the circulating dopamine originates in the adrenal medulla.

Excretion of catecholamines is urinary. Most is eliminated as metanephrine, normetanephrine, and vanillylmandelic acid (VMA). Small amounts (about 10% of urine catecholamines) of dopamine, epinephrine, and norepinephrine also normally occur unchanged in the urine. Assays for urinary metabolites of catecholamines provide the most practical means of clinically assessing the function of the adrenal medulla. Some drugs, such as reserpine, amphetamines, and the phenothiazines, augment the excretion of catecholamines.

Epinephrine, norepinephrine, and dopamine are commercially available and used in clinical situations. They cannot be administered by mouth because of destruction in the digestive tract and by rapid hepatic catabolism. Epinephrine (Adrenalin) is used in veterinary medicine to treat anaphylaxis and ventricular asystole, and it is added to local anesthetics to cause delayed absorption through vasoconstriction of local arterioles. Norepinephrine

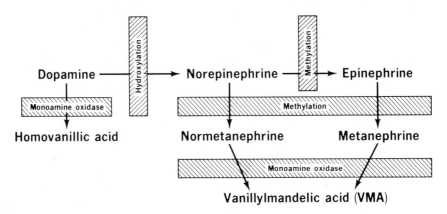

Fig. 17–13. Degradation of catecholamines.

(Levophed) is used to treat shock caused by or associated with trauma, central vasomotor depression, or hemorrhage. Dopamine (Dopamine HCl) is indicated for hypotension with inadequate renal perfusion caused by traumatic or cardiogenic shock.

CLINICAL TESTS OF ADRENOCORTICAL FUNCTION

Baseline Serum Cortisol and Other Glucocorticoids

The most frequently used test of adrenocortical function in veterinary medicine is the serum or plasma cortisol assay. Assay methods still in use include fluorimetry, competitive protein-binding (CPB), and the RIA.

The fluorimetric method (of Mattingly) is based on the formation of fluorescent compounds when 11 β-hydroxycorticosteroids are exposed to ultraviolet light and strong sulfuric acid. It detects both cortisol and corticosterone (11 β-hydroxycorticosteroids), plus other nonspecific fluorescent compounds. Background fluoresence is a problem in dogs and cats because normal 11 β-hydroxycorticosteroid levels are relatively low. The amount of corticosterone is over-represented because its rate of fluorescence is four times greater than that of cortisol. The fluorimetric method is accurate enough for most clinical purposes but is losing favor because of the greater sensitivity of the CPB and especially the RIA methods.

The CPB assay (of Murphy) for cortisol is based on the displacement of radioactively labeled cortisol from cortisol-binding globulin by the patient's serum cortisol after serum proteins have been extracted with ethanol. Minor cross-reactions occur with other glucocorticoids in the circulation, especially corticosterone (60% of corticosterone cross-reacts).

The RIA for cortisol is the most specific assay available, although cross-reactions can occur with pharmacologic doses of prednisone or prednisolone. RIA is a displacement assay similar to the CPB assay, but uses a specific antihormone (cortisol) antibody and radioactively labeled cortisol. Serum and plasma values do not differ significantly. If plasma is used, EDTA is preferred as an anticoagulant to heparin since freezing can sometimes cause clots in heparinized plasma, thus affecting assay methods.

No matter which assay method is used, it is advisable to separate the blood cells from the plasma or serum within 30 minutes, and then to freeze the sample.[69] If the sample is mailed early in the week to prevent unnecessary delays, refrigeration of the shipment is not necessary. Steroid hormones are relatively stable, but degradation by serum enzymes will eventually affect hormone levels, especially the free hormone concentrations. Samples must be analyzed by laboratories prepared to assay cortisol levels of dogs and cats because normal human baseline cortisol values occur in a different range (7 to 27 μg/dl at 9:00 A.M.) than the baseline levels of dogs or cats.

When measured by RIA, normal serum cortisol levels in dogs and cats are less than 1 to 4 μg/dl. In horses, they are slightly higher—2 to 7 μg/dl.

These levels are subject to considerable variation resulting from diurnal rhythms, alterations in serum binding proteins, and stress (both somatic and psychologic). For example, mean baseline levels of serum cortisol in dogs, when the sample is taken in their own household, has been reported to be 1.8 μg/dl; however, after hospitalization in a cage for 4 hours, mean levels rose to 3.8 μg/dl. If kept hospitalized overnight, the mean level was 3.9 μg/dl.[90] Phenylbutazone, a commonly used drug in horses that can decrease concentrations of serum T_4 by competitive binding with plasma proteins, does not alter plasma cortisol concentrations with treatment lasting up to 12 days.[62] Serum cortisol values increase 1 to 4 days before parturition in dogs, horses, and probably cats.

The predominant circulating glucocorticoid in birds is corticosterone. Baseline serum levels for psittacine birds are about 1 to 2 μg/dl. A fluorometric assay or, preferably, an RIA for corticosterone should be done.

High performance liquid chromatography for the determination of serum adrenocortical steroid levels has been advocated by some as superior to RIA.[57, 58] Interspecies differences are supposedly minimized. Resulting cortisol values obtained are about one-half those obtained by RIA.

See also references 2, 8-10, 35, 36, 38, 39, 42, 53, 70, 74, and 83.

Response to Adrenocorticotropic Hormone

Since baseline cortisol levels or changes in normal diurnal rhythm are not reliable diagnostic parameters by themselves, stimulation and suppression tests are generally done to increase diagnostic accuracy. The most frequently used stimulation test is the intramuscular (2.2 U/kg body weight) injection of ACTH gel (H.P. Acthar Gel, Adrenomone, Cortrophin Gel). Peak cortisol elevations normally occur in 2 hours (Fig. 17–14). After stimulation with ACTH, normal cortisol levels in dogs and cats are approximately 7 to 20 μg/dl (as shown by RIA). Alternately, a synthetic N-terminal portion of ACTH, called cosyntropin (Cortrosyn) can be given in an intramuscular or intravenous dose of 0.25 mg with samples drawn 1 hour after administration. The ability of the adrenal cortex to respond to ACTH may decline with age in dogs, but the degree of decline is small enough that any decline has been questioned.[7] An exaggerated adrenocortical response to ACTH can result from some chronic illnesses such as diabetes mellitus and chronic renal disease.[6]

The normal response to cosyntropin has been determined in horses given an intravenous dose of 1.0 mg. Two hours after the administration of cosyntropin, plasma cortisol levels should increase more than 50% above baseline levels, and plasma cortisol levels should exceed 8 μg/dl after the administration of ACTH.

The response of large psittacines to ACTH has been evaluated by administering an intramuscular dose of 0.125 mg of cosyntropin and determining the birds' response 90 minutes afterward. Baseline levels of serum corticos-

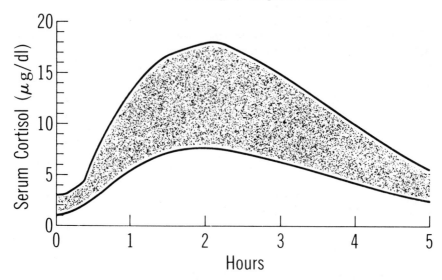

Fig. 17–14. Normal response of dogs in serum cortisol value to stimulation with adrenocorticotropic hormone from an intramuscular dose of 2.2 U/kg body weight.

terone were about 1 to 2 μg/dl, and values determined after the administration of ACTH were approximately 4 to 10 μg/dl.[94]

See also references 18, 28, 29, 48, 54, 56, 64, 66, 79, and 92.

Thorn Test

Another type of adrenocortical stimulation test using ACTH is the Thorn test or a modification of the Thorn test. The Thorn test is based on the effects of endogenous cortisol on the differential blood cell count. Although several methods have been recommended, the most accurate method seems to be the administration of ACTH gel (2.2 U/kg body weight) intramuscularly. Four hours later, the ratio of the absolute neutrophil to lymphocyte (N:L) counts should be compared to the N:L ratio determined before testing. An increase in the N:L ratio of more than 30% suggests normal minimum adrenocortical secretion. Absolute eosinophil counts should decrease 50% by 4 hours. Seven hours after the administration of ACTH, the absolute eosinophil count should have decreased by more than 70% in comparison to the pretest absolute eosinophil count. Modified Thorn tests and cortisol sampling to test for hypoadrenocorticism can be done concurrently.

See also references 60 and 71.

Dexamethasone Suppression Test

Dexamethasone is a potent synthetic glucocorticoid that normally suppresses the release of ACTH and therefore cortisol production. Its structure is sufficiently different from cortisol in that, if it is used in the appropriate amounts, it does not appreciably cross-react with cortisol assays. The ability of dexamethasone to suppress the production of ACTH and cortisol is used clinically to diagnose hyperadrenocorticism and differentiate its various causes.

Numerous dosages and protocols for dexamethasone suppression tests have been described for the dog. Currently, the most popular is the single intravenous administration of dexamethasone in a low dose (0.01 mg/kg body weight) and a high dose (0.1 mg [or more]/kg body weight). Serum cortisol values should decline to their lowest levels in 2 hours. Sampling serum cortisol levels is recommended 3 hours and 8 hours after the injection of dexamethasone. Normal unstressed dogs have serum cortisol values below 1.5 μg/dl at 3 hours and for at least 8 hours after the low-dose administration of dexamethasone. If the animal's production of ACTH and cortisol is insufficiently suppressed by the low-dose administration of dexamethasone, such a response suggests the diagnosis of hyperadrenocorticism. However, inhibition of ACTH by low-dose administration of dexamethasone can be altered by chronic liver and renal disease, diabetes mellitus, malnutrition and weight loss, and recovery from glucocorticoid therapy. A negative response to the high-dose dexamethasone test suggests an autonomous adrenal tumor or, less likely, an autonomous pituitary tumor.

An alternative, high-dose dexamethasone suppression test is an oral administration of dexamethasone (2 mg every 6 hours for 2 days). Failure to suppress plasma cortisol levels after 48 hours of continuous administration of high-dose dexamethasone should be more reliable than the single intravenous dose, assuming there is no problem with absorption from the digestive tract. Horses given a 20-mg, intramuscular dose of dexamethasone normally have plasma cortisol values suppressed to less than 1 μg/dl in 3 hours.

See also references 20 and 65.

Ancillary Serum or Plasma Assays

DHEA, DHEA sulfate, androstenedione, androsterone, aldosterone, renin, and 17-hydroxyprogesterone assays are commercially available RIAs. Their use in clinical veterinary medicine has been curtailed by their expense. Some of, or even all, the assays may have diagnostic value in companion animals in the future.

Uncommon Plasma or Serum Assays and Hazardous Response Tests

Canine and feline assays for ACTH are not commercially available. A modification of the ACTH assay (an RIA) using the 1–24 amino acid (N-terminal) sequence of the known mammalian structure of ACTH has been investigated in dogs. Normal levels have been reported to range from about 20 to 100 pg/ml in dogs and horses and 150 to 850 pg/ml in cats.

Assays for ACTH are expensive. Samples require plastic vials, immediate cooling in ice water, centrifugation during refrigeration, and transport while frozen. It is also secreted in pulsatile fashion, so single samples may not be representative. Multiple plasma samples of ACTH taken before and after provocative stimulation with metyrapone would be an ideal method of taking representative samples. Assays for ACTH may be useful as a diagnostic examination used as an adjunct to cortisol tests, particularly to differentiate primary from secondary hypoadrenocorticism, if it becomes commercially available and economically feasible.[26, 27, 30, 65]

The insulin response test is based on detecting resistance to the action of insulin caused by excessive levels of cortisol or insulin sensitivity caused by a deficiency in cortisol. This test is too dangerous and too insensitive to be routinely used to diagnose adrenal disorders.

The ADH (vasopressin) response test has been recommended to test the ability of the adenohypophysis to produce ACTH in dogs since pharmacologic doses of lysine ADH normally stimulate the release of ACTH.[85] Patients with pituitary-dependent hyperadrenocorticism have serum cortisol values that are higher than normal after the ADH response test. Those with adrenal-dependent hyperadrenocorticism have variable responses. The recommended dosage is 0.2 U/kg body weight, given slowly in an intravenous dose over 5 minutes, with values determined at 15, 30, 60, and 90 minutes after stimulation with ADH. The ADH response test for adrenocortical function can cause vomiting, bradycardia, and ataxia. It is contraindicated if the patient has untreated hypothyroidism or cardiovascular disease.

Urinary Adrenocortical Hormones and Metabolites of Adrenocortical Hormones

The measurement of urinary metabolites requires a 24-hour urine sample, which is difficult to obtain in companion animals. In addition, sensitive assay methods of the steroid urinary metabolites of dogs are not commercially available. Assays for steroid urinary metabolites in cats are probably valueless since steroids are not appreciably eliminated in the urine. The major excretory route for steroid metabolites in the cat is via bile.

In humans, urinary assay for 17-hydroxycorticosteroids is an outmoded clinical diagnostic exam that measures metabolites of C-21 steroids (tetrahydrocortisol and tetrahydrocortisone). Their urinary quantity parallels the production rates of cortisol. The standard assay method (Porter Silber) is a poor method for the quantification of cortisol metabolites in dogs because more than 60% of the cortisol metabolites are reduced at the twentieth position (C-20) on the basic steroid nucleus (see Fig. 17–6). As a result, few metabolites of C-21 steroids are produced in dogs. However, after conversion of metabolites to 17-ketogenic steroids, methods modified for the dog result in the relatively reliable determination of canine cortisol metabolites. Normal values in the dog are about 1.5 to 3.5 mg/24 hr.

Metyrapone inhibits 11 β-hydroxylation of steroids by the adrenal cortex. After its administration, there should be a decrease in serum cortisol, an increased release of ACTH, and an increase in 17-ketogenic steroids in the urine if adrenocortical function is normal. The measurement of plasma ACTH or serum 11-deoxycortisol after the administration of metyrapone can also be used to monitor the response. In humans, the metyrapone test is considered more reliable than high-dose dexamethasone for differentiation of pituitary-dependent from adrenal-dependent hyperadrenocorticism. The administration of phenytoin or untreated hypothyroidism can impair the patient's responsiveness to metyrapone.

Assays for 17-ketosteroids in the urine measure metabolites of C-19 steroids with a ketone group at C-17. C-19 steroids originate from the adrenal cortex, testes, or ovary. There is little increase in urinary 17-ketosteroid values in dogs receiving ACTH, and the values are only slightly increased by the administration of androgens, or by canine hyperadrenocorticism. There is no difference in values between male or female dogs; therefore, urinary 17-ketosteroids are not considered to have any diagnostic value in dogs or cats. Normal values for young postpubertal male dogs are approximately 0 to 8 mg/24 hr, which are lower than those for humans (6 to 21 mg/24 hr).

Assays for adrenocortical hormones in the urine have not been adequately evaluated in companion animals. Urinary corticoids have been measured in the dog, and results indicate this assay is a sensitive index of adrenocortical hyperfunction. Free cortisol in the urine, if it is measuring the cortisol in urine collected over a 24-hour period or if the cortisol is compared with the concentration of urinary creatinine, is considered the most reliable single determinant of hyperadrenocorticism in humans, but urinary free cortisol assays have not yet received attention in veterinary medicine.

See also references 3, 32, 45, 81, 82, and 86.

Salivary Adrenocortical Hormone Assays

Unbound circulating steroidal hormones readily diffuse into the salivary glands. Assays of salivary adrenocortical hormones have the following advantages: salivary levels parallel free circulating hormone levels, and the collection procedure is virtually stress free. Salivary hormone levels have not been evaluated in clinical veterinary medicine. Potentially, they are a better index of adrenal activity than total serum levels of free and bound hormones in patients whose serum protein binding has been altered by certain drugs, liver diseases, pregnancy, and the administration of estrogen.

Glucagon Tolerance Test

Glucocorticoids enhance the deposition of glycogen in the liver. Glycogen can be mobilized by glucagon. Excessively high and prolonged elevations of blood glucose levels occur in response to the intravenous administration of glucagon when hyperadrenocorticism has caused the excessive accumulation of glucagon. The glucagon tolerance test can provide indirect evidence of hyperadrenocorticism.

See also reference 46.

Nuclear Medical Examination

Gamma camera imaging of the adrenal glands has been done in dogs using [131]I-19-iodocholesterol. Adrenals of normal dogs are visible 3 to 4 days after the administration of isotope. Hyperplastic adrenals are visible 2 to 3 days afterward. The best image appears at approximately 8 days. Adrenal tumors may be visible at 5 days.

Gamma camera imaging or rectilinear scanning is available at a few veterinary teaching hospitals. It requires several days' examination, is expensive, and requires special isolation quarters for the patient and special handling of urine and feces. Its potential value is therefore generally outweighed by its disadvantages. Its primary indications would be to substantiate the presence of an adrenal tumor and to determine which side is affected before surgery. See reference 63 for further data on the nuclear medical examination.

For further information on clinical tests of adrenocortical function, see references 19, 21, 25, 49, 50, 55, 57, 75, 76, 80, 84, and 85.

CLINICAL TESTS OF ADRENAL MEDULLARY FUNCTION

Clinical assessment of the function of the adrenal medulla in dogs and horses has rarely been done despite the frequency of pheochromocytomas in those species. In humans, measuring urinary metanephrine per mg creatinine is considered to be the best screening test of the excessive production of catecholamines even though vanillylmandelic acid (VMA) normally comprises the majority of catecholamine metabolites in the urine. If the levels of urinary total metanephrines are excessive, measurement of total metanephrines should be repeated, along with a measurement of VMA. Normal VMA levels in the urine of a young male dog are about 0.6 to 15 mg/24 hr. Because catecholamines and their metabolites are unstable if exposed to a pH of 3 or more, collection of 100 ml of urine should be done in clean bottles containing 30 ml of 6 N HCl. Some diets, particularly those high in cheese or other fermented foods, can elevate urinary catecholamine metabolites.

Several provocative tests have been advocated to increase the diagnostic sensitivity of assessing adrenal medullary function, including the tyramine, glucagon, histamine, and phentolamine response tests. All these provocative tests are potentially hazardous and are best reserved for equivocal screening test results.

A radioenzymatic assay for plasma catecholamines has shown promise in humans with pheochromocytomas. It may be more sensitive than urine metabolite screening tests. After the patient has been resting, an indwelling intravenous catheter is placed. Then, sampling is done 20 to 30 minutes later. The clinical usefulness of this method in dogs and horses has not been determined.

REFERENCES

1. Anderson, J.B., and Clark, D.R.: Pattern of physiologic effect of adrenalectomy in the dog. Am. J. Vet. Res., *36:*1036, 1975.
2. Becker, M.J., Helland, D., and Becker, D.N.: Serum cortisol (hydrocortisone) values in normal dogs as determined by radioimmunoassay. Am. J. Vet. Res., *37:*1101, 1976.
3. Bell, E.T., Christie, D.W., and Parkes, M.R.: Urinary total 17-hydroxycorticosteroid output in intact and ovariectomized bitches. Acta Endocrinol., *68:*387, 1971.
4. Bethune, J.E.: The adrenal cortex. Scope Monograph, pp. 1–68, 1974.
5. Bottoms, G.D., et al.: Circadian variation in plasma cortisol and corticosterone in pigs and mares. Am. J. Vet. Res., *33:*785, 1972.
6. Breitschwerdt, E.G., Ochoa, R., and Waltman, C.: Multiple endocrine abnormalities in basenji dogs with renal tubular dysfunction. J. Am. Vet. Med. Assoc., *182:*1348, 1983.
7. Breznock, E.M., and McQueen, R.D.: Adrenocortical function during aging in the dog. Am. J. Vet. Res., *31:*1269, 1970.
8. Campbell, J.R., and Watts, C.: Assessment of adrenal function in dogs. Br. Vet. J., *129:*134, 1973.
9. Chen, C.L., Gelatt, K.N., and Gum, G.G.: Serum hydrocortisone (cortisol) values in glaucomatous and normotensive beagles. Am. J. Vet. Res., *41:*1516, 1980.
10. Chen, C.L., et al.: Serum hydrocortisone (cortisol) values in normal and adrenopathic dogs as determined by radioimmunoassay. Am. J. Vet. Res., *39:*179, 1978.
11. Collins, E.J., Garrett, E.R., and Johnson, R.L.: Effect of adrenal steroids on radio-calcium metabolism in dogs. Metabolism, *11:*716, 1980.
12. Critchley, J.A.J.H., Ellis, P., and Ungar, A.: The reflex release of adrenaline and noradrenaline from the adrenal glands of cats and dogs. J. Physiol., *298:*71, 1980.
13. Cryer, P.E.: Physiology and pathophysiology of the human sympathoadrenal neuroendocrine system. N. Engl. J. Med., *303:*436, 1980.
14. Dor, P., et al.: Adrenal secretion of estrogens, glucocorticoids, and mineralocorticosteroids in the dog. Eur. J. Cancer, *9:*687, 1973.
15. Dorner, J.L., Hoffman, W.E., and Long, G.B.: Corticosteroid induction of an isoenzyme of alkaline phosphatase in the dog. Am. J. Vet. Res., *35:*1457, 1974.
16. Egdahl, R.H.: The acute effects of steroid administration on pituitary adrenal secretion in the dog. J. Clin. Invest., *43:*2178, 1964.
17. Eigler, N., Sacca, L., and Sherwin, R.S.: Synergistic interactions of physiologic increments of glucagon, epinephrine, and cortisol in the dog. J. Clin. Invest., *63:*114, 1979.
18. Eiler, H., Goble, D., and Oliver, J.: Adrenal gland function in the horses: effects of cosyntropin (synthetic) and corticotropin (natural) stimulation. Am. J. Vet. Res., *40:*724, 1979.
19. Eiler, H., and Oliver, J.: Combined dexamethasone suppression and cosyntropin (synthetic ACTH) stimulation test in the dog: new approach to testing of adrenal gland function. Am. J. Vet. Res., *41:*1243, 1980.
20. Eiler, H., Oliver, J., and Goble, D.: Adrenal gland function in the horse: effect of dexamethasone on hydrocortisone secretion and blood cellularity and plasma electrolyte concentrations. Am. J. Vet. Res., *40:*727, 1979.
21. Eiler, H., Oliver, J., and Goble, D.: Combined dexamethasone-suppression cosyntropin-(synthetic ACTH) stimulation test in the horse: a new approach to testing of adrenal gland function. Am. J. Vet. Res., *41:*430, 1980.
22. Farrell, G.L.: Steroids in adrenal venous blood of the dog: venous-arterial differences across the adrenal. Proc. Soc. Exp. Biol. Med., *86:*338, 1954.
23. Farrell, G.L., and Lamus, B.: Steroids in adrenal venous blood of the dog. Proc. Soc. Exp. Biol. Med., *84:*89, 1955.
24. Farrell, G.L., Rauschkolb, E.W., and Royce, P.C.: Secretion of aldosterone by adrenal of the dog. Effects of hypophysectomy and ACTH. Am. J. Physiol., *182:*269, 1955.
25. Feldman, E.C.: Comparison of ACTH response and dexamethasone suppression as screening tests in canine hyperadrenocorticism. J. Am. Vet. Med. Assoc., *182:*506, 1983.
26. Feldman, E.C.: Effect of functional adrenocortical tumors on plasma cortisol and corticotropin concentrations in dogs. J. Am. Vet. Med. Assoc., *178:*823, 1981.

27. Feldman, E.C., Bohannon, N.V., and Tyrrell, J.B.: Plasma adrenocorticotropin levels in normal dogs. Am. J. Vet. Res., *38:*1643, 1977.
28. Feldman, E.C., et al.: Comparison of aqueous porcine ACTH with synthetic ACTH in adrenal stimulation tests of the female dog. Am. J. Vet. Res., *43:*522, 1982.
29. Feldman, E.C., and Tyrrell, J.B.: Adrenocorticotropin effects of synthetic polypeptide-alpha 1-24 corticotropin in normal dogs. J. Am. Anim. Hosp. Assoc., *13:*494, 1977.
30. Feldman, E.C., Tyrrell, J.B., and Bohannon, N.V.: The synthetic ACTH stimulation test and measurement of endogenous plasma ACTH levels: useful diagnostic indicators for adrenal disease in dogs. J. Am. Anim. Hosp. Assoc., *14:*524, 1978.
31. Fleeman, C.R., Levi, J., and Better, O.: Kidney and adrenocortical hormones. Nephron, *15:*261, 1975.
32. Foss, M.L., Barnard, R.J., and Tipton, C.M.: Free 11-hydroxycorticosteroid levels in working dogs as affected by exercise training. Endocrinology, *89:*96, 1971.
33. Ganong, W.F., Alpert, L.C., and Lee, T.C.: ACTH and the regulation of adrenocortical secretion. N. Engl. J. Med., *290:*1006, 1974.
34. Guthrie, G.P., Cecil, S.G., and Kotchen, T.A.: Renin, aldosterone and cortisol in the thoroughbred horse. J. Endocrinol., *85:*49, 1980.
35. Halliwell, R.E.W., et al.: The value of plasma corticosteroid assays in the diagnosis of Cushing's disease in the dog. J. Small Anim. Pract., *12:*453, 1971.
36. Hechter, O., et al.: Quantitative variations in the adrenocortical secretion of dogs. Am. J. Physiol., *182:*29, 1955.
37. Hiatt, N., et al.: Adrenal hormones and the regulation of serum potassium in potassium loaded adrenalectomized dogs. Endocrinology, *105:*215, 1979.
38. Hoffsis, G.F., and Murdick, P.W.: The plasma concentrations of corticosteroids in normal and diseased horses. J. Am. Vet. Med. Assoc., *157:*1590, 1970.
39. Hoffsis, G.F., et al.: Plasma concentrations of cortisol and corticosterone in the normal horse. Am. J. Vet. Res., *31:*1379, 1970.
40. Hullinger, R.L.: Adrenal cortex of the dog (Canis familiaris) I. Histomorphologic changes during growth, maturity, and aging. Zentrabl. Vet. Med., *7:*1, 1978.
41. James, V.H.T., et al.: Adrenocortical function in the horse. J. Endocrinol., *48:*319, 1970.
42. Johnston, S.D., et al.: Use of radioimmunoassay of plasma cortisol to diagnose adrenal dysfunction in dogs. Minn. Veterinarian, *18:*19, 1978.
43. Johnston, S.D., and Mather, E.C.: Canine plasma cortisol (hydrocortisone) measured by radioimmunoassay: clinical absence of diurnal variations and results of ACTH stimulation and dexamethasone suppression tests. Am. J. Vet. Res., *38:*1766, 1978.
44. Joles, J.A., et al.: Studies on the mechanism of polyuria induced by cortisol excess in the dog. Vet., *2:*199, 1980.
45. Jordan, J.E.: Normal laboratory values in beagle dogs of twelve to eighteen months of age. Am. J. Vet. Res., *38:*409, 1977.
46. Kaufman, J., and Macy, D.W.: The glucagon tolerance test as a screening method for canine hyperadrenocorticism. Proceedings of the Am. Coll. Vet. Intern. Med., p. 30, 1984.
47. Kemppainen, R.J.: Effects of glucocorticoids on endocrine function in the dog. Vet. Clin. North Am. [Small Anim. Pract.], *14:*721, 1984.
48. Kemppainen, R.J., Mansfield, P.D., and Sartin, J.L.: Endocrine responses of normal cats to TSH and synthetic ACTH administration. J. Am. Anim. Hosp. Assoc., *20:*737, 1984.
49. Kemppainen, R.J., and Sartin, J.L.: Effects of single intravenous dose of dexamethasone on base-line plasma cortisol concentrations and responses to synthetic ACTH in healthy dogs. Am. J. Vet. Res., *45:*742, 1984.
50. Kemppainen, R.J., Thompson, F.N., and Lorenz, M.D.: Effects of dexamethasone infusion on the plasma cortisol response to cosyntropin (synthetic ACTH) injection in normal dogs. Res. Vet. Sci., *32:*181, 1982.
51. Knowlen, G.G., et al.: Comparison of plasma aldosterone concentration among clinical status groups of dogs with chronic heart failure. J. Am. Vet. Med. Assoc., *183:*991, 1983.
52. Kumar, M.S.A., Liao, T.F., and Chen, C.L.: Diurnal variation in serum cortisol in ponies. J. Anim. Sci., *42:*1360, 1976.
53. Lester, S.J., et al.: A rapid radioimmunoassay method for the evaluation of plasma cortisol levels and adrenal function in the dog. J. Am. Anim. Hosp. Assoc., *17:*121, 1981.
54. Ling, G.V., et al.: Canine hyperadrenocorticism: pretreatment clinical and laboratory evaluation of 117 cases. J. Am. Vet. Med. Assoc., *174:*1211, 1979.

55. Lorenz, M.D.: Canine hyperadrenocorticism: diagnosis and treatment. Compendium on Continuing Educ. for the Practicing Vet., *1:*315, 1979.
56. Lorenz, M.S., and Cornelius, L.M.: Laboratory diagnosis of endocrinological disease. Vet. Clin. North Am., *6:*687, 1976.
57. Lothrop, C.D., and Oliver, J.W.: Diagnosis of canine Cushing's syndrome based on multiple hormone analysis and dexamethasone turnover kinetics. Am. J. Vet. Res., *45:*2304, 1984.
58. Lothrop, C.D., and Oliver, J.W.: New developments in adrenal function testing in the dog: simultaneous measurement of multiple adrenal hormones by high performance liquid chromatography (HPLC). Proceedings of the Am. Coll. Vet. Intern. Med., p. 88, 1982.
59. Magne, M.L., et al.: Serum insulin and glucose concentrations in normal, stressed, and hyperadrenocorticism. Proceedings of the Am. Coll. Vet. Intern. Med., p. 42, 1984.
60. Martin, J.E., Skillen, R.G., and Deubler, M.J.: The action of adrenocorticotropic hormone on circulating eosinophils in dogs—a proposed screening method for evaluating adrenal cortical function. Am. J. Vet. Res., *15:*489, 1954.
61. Meijer, J.C., et al.: Adrenocortical function tests in dogs with hyperfunctioning adrenocortical tumors. J. Endocrinol., *80:*315, 1979.
62. Morris, D.D., and Garcia, M.C.: Effects of phenylbutazone and anabolic steroids on adrenal and thyroid gland function tests in healthy horses. Am. J. Vet. Res., *46:*359, 1985.
63. Mulnix, J.A., et al.: Gamma camera imaging of bilateral adrenocortical hyperplasia and adrenal tumors in the dog. Am. J. Vet. Res., *37:*1467, 1976.
64. Peterson, M.E., et al.: Adrenal function in the cat: comparison of the effects of cosyntropin (synthetic ACTH) and corticotropin gel stimulation. Res. Vet. Sci. *37:*331, 1984.
65. Peterson, M.E., and Drucker, W.D.: Advances in the diagnosis and management of canine Cushing's syndrome. Proceedings of the 31st Gaines Symposium, p. 17, 1981.
66. Peterson, M.E., Gilbertson, S.R., and Drucker, W.D.: Plasma cortisol response to exogenous ACTH in 22 dogs with hyperadrenocorticism caused by adrenocortical neoplasia. J. Am. Vet. Med. Assoc., *180:*542, 1982.
67. Phillip, E.L.I., and Marotta, S.F.: Cellular variation in the uptake and metabolism of cortisol by canine erythrocytes. Acta Endocrinol., *68:*771, 1971.
68. Plager, J.E., et al.: Cortisol binding by dog plasma. Endocrinology, *73:*353, 1963.
69. Olson, P.N., et al.: Effects of storage on concentration of hydrocortisone (cortisol) in canine serum and plasma. Am. J. Vet. Res., *42:*1618, 1981.
70. Orth, D.N., et al.: Equine Cushing's disease: plasma immunoreactive proopiolipomelanocortin peptide and cortisol levels basally and in response to diagnostic tests. Endocrinology. *110:*1430, 1982.
71. Osbaldiston, G.W., and Greve, T.: Estimating adrenal cortical function in dogs with ACTH. Cornell Vet., *68:*308, 1978.
72. Osbaldiston, G.W., and Johnson, J.H.: Effect of ACTH and selected glucocorticoids on circulating blood cells in horses. J. Am. Vet. Med. Assoc., *161:*53, 1972.
73. Reece, W.O.: Fluid volume changes associated with withdrawal and restoration of steroid therapy in adrenalectomized dogs. Am. J. Vet. Res., *33:*1493, 1972.
74. Riemers, T.J.: Radioimmunoassays and diagnostic tests for thyroid and adrenal disorders. Compendium on Continuing Educ. for the Practicing Vet., *4:*65, 1982.
75. Rijnberk, A., der Kinderen, P.J., and Thijssen, J.H.H.: Investigations on the adrenocortical function of normal dogs. J. Endocrinol., *41:*387, 1968.
76. Rijnberk, A., der Kinderen, P.J., and Thijssen, J.H.H.: Investigations on the adrenocortical function of normal and obese dogs. Acta Physiol. Pharmacol. Néerl., *14:*521, 1967b.
77. Santen, R.J.: Adrenal of male dog secretes androgens and estrogens. Am. J. Physiol., *239:*E109, 1980.
78. Schiebinger, R.J., et al.: Developmental changes in rabbit and dog adrenal function: a possible homologue of adrenarche in the dog. Am. J. Physiol., *240:*E694, 1981.
79. Schwartz-Prosche, E., Weiss, J., and Hollihn, V.: Cortisol concentrations in peripheral blood and renal cortisol excretion in healthy dogs and dogs with adrenal insufficiency before and after ACTH application. Zentralbl. Veterinarmed., *A23:*754, 1976.
80. Siegel, E.T.: Assessment of pituitary-adrenal gland function in the dog. Am. J. Vet. Res., *29:*173, 1968.

81. Siegel, E.T.: Determination of 17-hydroxycorticosteroids in canine urine. Am. J. Vet. Res., 26:1152, 1965.
82. Siegel, E.T.: Urinary excretion of sex steroid catabolites in the dog. Am. J. Vet. Res., 28:287, 1967.
83. Slone, D.E., et al.: Cortisol (hydrocortisone) disappearance rate and pathophysiologic changes after bilateral adrenalectomy in equids. Am. J. Vet. Res., 44:276, 1983.
84. Stabenfeldt, G.H., et al.: Assessment of normal adrenal function in the dog. Calif. Vet., 30:15, 1976.
85. Stolp, R., and Meijer, J.C.: Differential diagnosis and laboratory evaluation of hyperadrenocorticism in dogs. Proceedings of the 6th Kal Kan Symposium, p. 9, 1982.
86. Stolp, R., et al.: Urinary corticoids in the diagnosis of canine hyperadrenocorticism. Res. Vet. Sci., 34:141, 1983.
87. Swingle, W.W., and Swingle, A.J.: Effect of adrenal steroids upon plasma volume of intact and adrenalectomized dogs. Proc. Soc. Exp. Biol. Med., 119:452, 1965.
88. Taylor, W.: The excretion of steroid hormone metabolites in bile and feces. Vitam. Horm., 29:201, 1971.
89. Thompson, E.B., and Lippman, M.E.: Mechanism of action of glucocorticoids. Metabolism, 23:159, 1974.
90. Vial, G.C., et al.: Influence of environment on adrenal cortical response to ACTH stimulation in clinically normal dogs. Am. J. Vet. Res., 40:919, 1979.
91. Watson, L.C., Reeder, D.D., and Thompson, J.C.: Effect of hydrocortisone on gastric secretion and serum gastrin in dogs. Surg. Forum, 24:354, 1973.
92. Weller, R.E., Park, J.F., and Kinnas, T.C.: Responses of plasma cortisol and circulating blood cells to intramuscular injection of adrenocorticotropin in beagle dogs. Proceedings of the Am. Coll. Vet. Intern. Med., p. 52, 1983.
93. Zaffaroni, A., and Burton, R.B.: Corticosteroids present in adrenal vein blood of dogs. Arch. Biochem. Biophys., 42:1, 1953.
94. Zenoble, R.D., and Kemppainen, R.J.: The influence of ACTH on plasma corticosterone and cortisol and influence of TSH on plasma T_4 and T_3 in psittacine birds. Proceedings of the Am. Coll. Vet. Intern. Med., p. 44, 1984.

18

Spontaneous Hyperadrenocorticism

Excessive production of adrenocortical hormones may be predominantly or exclusively mineralocorticoids, glucocorticoids, or sex hormones. Exclusive overproduction of mineralocorticoids or sex hormones is rare in companion animals. When these exclusive excesses do occur, they are the result of rare adrenocortical neoplasms or congenital or acquired enzyme deficiencies in the biosynthesis of the adrenocortical steroids.

The term *hyperadrenocorticism* is often used synonymously with excessive production of glucocorticoids. Most cases of spontaneous hyperadrenocorticism are due to an inappropriate or neoplastic overproduction of adrenocorticotropic hormone (ACTH). ACTH does not selectively stimulate the production of any one of the adrenocortical hormones; however, the effects of ACTH on mineralocorticoid production are too short-lived to cause a clinical disorder due to excessive mineralocorticoids. Since excessive, ACTH-induced production of sex hormone is quite small in comparison to glucocorticoid production, the effects of excessive levels of sex hormones are overshadowed by the simultaneous overproduction of glucocorticoids.

CUSHING'S-LIKE SYNDROME AND DISEASE*

In 1932 Harvey Cushing, a Boston surgeon, published the results of his observations that basophilic tumors of the pituitary were associated with hyperplasia of the adrenal cortices.[11] Tumors of the pituitary with associated hyperadrenocorticism are still called Cushing's disease in humans and *Cushing's-like disease* in animals. The changes that take place as a result of excessive glucocorticoid hormones are called Cushing's syndrome in humans and *Cushing's-like syndrome* in animals, regardless of the cause. Cushing's-like syndrome was first recognized in 1939 in the dog. Now it is known as one of the most commonly diagnosed endocrinopathies in the dog. The incidence in dogs is thought to exceed that in humans. Cushing's-like syndrome is rare in cats.

For further information, see also references 7, 10, 12, 13, 31–34, 37, 52, 53, 60, 63, 72, 73, 83, 84, 87, and 94.

---

* Cushing's-like syndrome will be used to describe all types of hyperadrenocorticism since veterinary clinicians can rarely be certain of a pituitary tumor being the cause.

Causes

Cushing's-like syndrome can be spontaneous or iatrogenic (iatrogenic Cushing's-like syndrome is described in more detail in a later chapter). Possible causes for spontaneous Cushing's-like syndrome in dogs and cats are listed in Table 18–1.

Pituitary-dependent causes are the most frequent reasons for spontaneous Cushing's-like syndrome. Pituitary-dependent causes represent about 80% of the total spontaneous causes in dogs. Reports on the incidence of pituitary neoplasms associated with pituitary-dependent Cushing's-like syndrome in dogs vary widely (from 15% to 80%). ACTH-producing pituitary neoplasms have variable staining characteristics. Most do not stain well with acidic or basic pituitary stains and are therefore classified as chromophobic adenomas or, rarely, carcinomas. ACTH-producing pituitary tumors may or may not compress the remaining adenohypophysis and the area dorsal to the hypophysis, the hypothalamus. In dogs, two thirds of these tumors are situated in the pars distalis; the tumors remaining are found in the pars intermedia. Generally, their growth rate is slow. Brachycephalic breeds have a higher incidence of ACTH-producing pituitary tumors than do other breeds. The most common cause for Cushing's-like syndrome in horses is an adenoma of the pars intermedia of the pituitary.[51, 57, 58] Pituitary-dependent Cushing's-like syndrome has not been reported in the cat.

The defect responsible for pituitary-dependent Cushing's-like syndrome unassociated with pituitary neoplasia is unknown.[50] A primary failure of the feedback response has been proposed. Others suspect an overproduction of corticotropin-releasing hormone (CRH) from the hypothalamus caused by a "serotonin flush."

The true incidence of pituitary-dependent Cushing's-like syndrome in dogs associated with pituitary neoplasia may be higher than suspected. In humans, as many as 80% of pituitary adenomas can be clinically undetectable before surgery. These small, 3- to 10-mm tumors constituting the presurgical undetectable group are usually referred to as pituitary microadenomas. Some microadenomas reported as unassociated with pituitary tumors in dogs with Cushing's syndrome may have gone undetected for various reasons. When immunocytochemical stains for ACTH are used, more than 80% of dogs with pituitary-dependent Cushing's-like syndrome are positive for pituitary adenomas.

Table 18–1. Possible Causes of Cushing's-Like Syndrome (and Disease)

Pituitary-dependent adrenocortical hyperplasia
Associated with pituitary neoplasm
Unassociated with pituitary neoplasm
Adrenal-dependent
Ectopic production of ACTH (possibly CRH)
Iatrogenic

ACTH = adrenocorticotropic hormone; CRH = corticotropin-releasing hormone.

Another cause for Cushing's-like syndrome, and a possible cause for a misclassification of the syndrome as a pituitary-dependent tumor, is the *ectopic production of ACTH* or an ACTH-like peptide by a non-pituitary neoplasm. This cause of Cushing's-like syndrome seems to be rare in companion animals—there are few reports of its occurrence. The production of ectopic ACTH has been associated with lymphosarcoma in a dog that also had a gastrinoma and in another dog with a bronchial carcinoma. Most of the time the production of ectopic ACTH in humans is caused by an anaplastic primary lung, thymic, or pancreatic islet cell carcinoma. Anaplastic primary lung, thymic, and pancreatic islet cell tumors are rare in companion animals; this fact may account for the lack of reports of the production of ectopic ACTH in animals. In humans, 10% to 15% of the cases of Cushing's syndrome are caused by the ectopic production of ACTH. Some carcinomas produce corticotropin-releasing hormone (CRH), and if the tumor or its metastases are located near the pituitary's portal circulation, these tumors can also cause ectopic hyperadrenocorticism.

Adding to the confusion concerning the true incidence of pituitary-dependent adrenocortical hyperplasia unassociated with a pituitary neoplasm is the difficulty in consistently correlating functional ability of the adrenal cortex with its morphology. For example, adrenocortical hyperplasia may be diffuse, or nodular, or both.[2] Nodular hyperplasia of the adrenal cortex is a degenerative change found at necropsy, without associated signs of Cushing's-like syndrome, and is seen in more than one half of dogs over 10 years old. In addition, the histopathologic diagnosis of diffuse adrenocortical hyperplasia is based on subjective judgment. Mild to moderate cases may be overlooked by some pathologists and overdiagnosed by others. Problems with the correct interpretation of clinical laboratory findings may also lead to misdiagnoses.

The remaining 10% to 20% of spontaneous cases of Cushing's-like syndrome in dogs are caused by unilateral or bilateral *adrenocortical neoplasms.* Adrenocortical adenomas are small, well-circumscribed tumors that do not metastasize and are not locally invasive. Adrenocortical carcinomas by the time of diagnosis are large, hemorrhagic, and necrotic. Carcinomas, especially of the right adrenal, frequently invade the caudal vena cava and metastasize to the liver, lungs, kidney, or regional lymph nodes. The occurrence of adrenocortical adenomas and carcinomas in dogs is nearly equal. Adrenocortical neoplasia in the cat is rare.[21, 48]

Incidence

Cushing's-like syndrome occurs frequently in dogs, occasionally in horses, and rarely in cats. Female dogs may have a slightly greater risk than male dogs because of the approximately threefold greater incidence of adrenocortical tumors in female dogs. Boston terriers, dachshunds, boxers, miniature poodles, and toy poodles are the breeds most frequently affected. In one study, two related Yorkshire terriers were affected.[82] Ages affected range from 3 to 15 years; most animals are 7 to 9 years old when Cushing's-like syndrome occurs. Boston terriers and boxers are most often affected with pituitary-tumor-associated, pituitary-dependent hyperadrenocorticism.

Cushing's-like syndrome in dachshunds and poodles is usually caused by bilateral adrenocortical hyperplasia without pituitary tumors demonstrable by conventional means. Adrenocortical neoplasms most frequently occur in large-breed dogs. Adenohypophyseal adenoma of the pars intermedia is the most common cause of spontaneous hyperadrenocorticism in horses.[51,57,58] Affected horses are 7 years of age or older. Cushing's-like syndrome may be more common in mares than stallions or geldings.

See also references 60 and 95.

Clinical Signs

Most of the clinical signs of Cushing's-like syndrome in dogs are caused by excessive levels of cortisol and corticosterone, but in about 30% of the female dogs, clitoral hypertrophy is noted. This effect is caused by excessive levels of adrenocortical androgens. Some signs of hyperglucocorticoidism are more frequently noted than others, but it is important for the clinician to realize that an individual dog or cat with Cushing's-like syndrome can exhibit a variety of possible clinical signs. Maintaining a high index of suspicion for Cushing's-like syndrome is important. Possible clinical signs, in order of their reported occurrence, are listed in Table 18–2.

Most cases of Cushing's-like syndrome in dogs and cats develop a triad of polyuria-polydipsia, pendulous abdomen, and bilateral alopecia (Fig. 18–1). Polyuria-polydipsia is defined as the intake of water in excess of 100 ml/kg body weight/day and production of urine in excess of 50 ml/kg body weight/day. Polyuria-polydipsia of Cushing's-like syndrome is partially responsive to the water deprivation test. Polyuria may be due to an increased glomerular filtration rate, inhibition of the release of antidiuretic hormone (ADH) (neurohypophyseal diabetes insipidus), inhibition of the action of

Table 18–2.   Possible Clinical Signs of Cushing's-Like Syndrome in Dogs and Cats in Approximate Decreasing Order of Occurrence

Polyuria and polydipsia
Pendulous abdomen
Bilateral alopecia
Hepatomegaly
Polyphagia
Muscular weakness and atrophy
Lethargy
Persistent anestrus or atrophied testes
Hyperpigmentation of skin
Calcinosis cutis
Heat intolerance
Hypertrophy of the clitoris
Neurologic deficits or convulsions

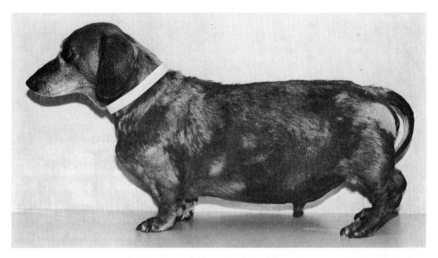

Fig. 18–1. Most dogs with Cushing's-like syndrome exhibit a triad of clinical signs, including polyuria-polydipsia, pendulous abdomen, and bilateral alopecia.

ADH on the renal tubules (nephrogenic diabetes insipidus), or the accelerated inactivation of ADH.[14] The pendulous abdomen is caused by a combination of weakened abdominal muscles, hepatomegaly, and increased omental fat. In addition to increased omental fat, adipose deposits are shifted to the dorsum of the neck and to the gluteal area lateral to the tail.

Alopecia is the apparent result of protein catabolism. It most often first affects the caudal and lateral aspects of the hind legs and then the trunk. The head and distal extremities are little affected, if at all. Poodles seem more likely to develop severe alopecia than other breeds. Another change in the skin, besides alopecia, that may be seen with Cushing's-like syndrome is thinning of the skin, sometimes severe enough to permit abdominal veins to become prominent (Fig. 18–2).

The histologic changes in the skin are degeneration of dermal collagen and fibroelastic tissue, melanosis, atrophy of the adnexal glands, hyperkeratosis of the follicles, and thinning of the epidermis with the exception of the stratum corneum, which becomes hyperkeratotic.[76] Clinically, these changes are manifested as thin, wrinkly, inelastic skin with excessive surface scaling, and small papules or comedones caused by follicular hyperkeratosis (Figs. 18–2, 18–3, and 18–4). Striae (streaks or lines) can form as a result of inelasticity. Comedones are most prominent on the ventral abdomen. Protein catabolism causing atrophic collagen also frequently leads to easy bruising, either spontaneously or after a vein is punctured for blood samples. Bruising is also likely as the result of decreased platelet adhesiveness. Wound healing is extraordinarily slow, presumably because of the inhibition of fibroblast proliferation, synthesis of collagen, and a deficiency in zinc (Fig. 18–5).

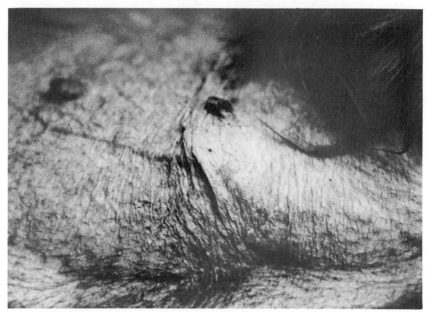

Fig. 18–2. In patients with Cushing's-like syndrome, the skin becomes thinned, abdominal veins are prominent, and the skin's normal elasticity is lost.

Hyperpigmentation may occur in Cushing's-like syndrome. It usually takes the form of pigmented macules rather than diffuse hyperpigmentation. The cause is presumed to be activity of excess ACTH, which contains α melanocyte-stimulating hormone (α MSH) within its structure.

Calcinosis cutis is a cutaneous change that occurs in 25% to 40% of dogs with Cushing's-like syndrome. Humans, horses, and cats with Cushing's-like syndrome are not similarly affected. The development of calcinosis cutis is thought to result from the calcium-attracting alteration of collagen's ionic charge. Serum calcium and phosphorus levels are usually normal. Calcinosis cutis usually appears as a slightly elevated cream-colored plaque surrounded by a ring of bright red erythema (Fig. 18–6). Large plaques tend to crack, become secondarily infected, and then crust.

Hepatomegaly is, in part, the result of increased glycogen synthesis and fatty infiltration caused by gluconeogenesis. Vacuolization also contributes to the hepatomegaly. In many cases the hepatomegaly is palpable. Occasionally, hepatomegaly is only appreciated by radiographic examination of the abdomen. Polyphagia may be the result of a direct effect of glucocorticoids on the appetite center in the hypothalamus or may be caused by hypothalamic compression by a pituitary tumor.

All skeletal muscles are affected by the catabolic action of excessive glucocorticoids. Besides the development of a pendulous abdomen, affected animals may assume a straight- or stiff-legged stance caused by muscular weakness. Owners often notice the patient's reluctance to jump up

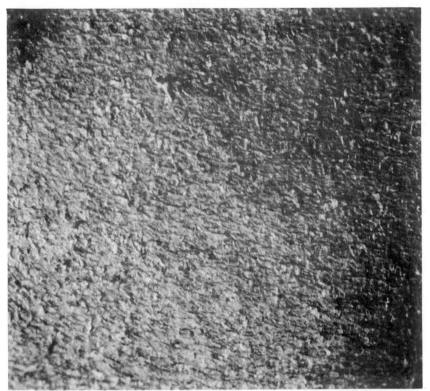

Fig. 18–3. Hyperkeratosis may be grossly evident as a scaly and flaky surface epithelium.

and down from furniture, steps, or pick-up truck beds. Comparison of the adjacent muscle mass with the spine of the scapula, dorsal spinous process of the vertebrae, or sagittal crest of the skull may aid the clinician in detecting more subtle decreases in muscle mass.

Myotonias are continued active contractions that persist after voluntary or involuntary stimuli. Myotonias or pseudomyotonias have been reported in dogs with Cushing's-like syndrome.[5, 15, 22] Percussion of the affected muscle can produce a myotonic dimple. The posture of affected dogs can resemble that of tetanus as a result of extensor rigidity of the proximal appendicular muscles. Rigidity usually begins in one hind leg, then progresses to the other hind leg, and finally affects the front legs. The gait is stiff especially after the animal has rested or has been exposed to cold. Determinations of serum aspartate aminotransferase (SAST) and creatinine phosphokinase (CPK) are usually elevated. Electromyographic (EMG) examination shows spontaneous or evoked bizarre high-frequency discharges that wax and wane. When transformed into auditory waves, the discharges sound like a dive bomber. Pseudomyotonia produces high-frequency discharges that are constant in frequency amplitude but start and end abruptly. If myotonia or pseudomyotonia develops in animals with Cushing's-like

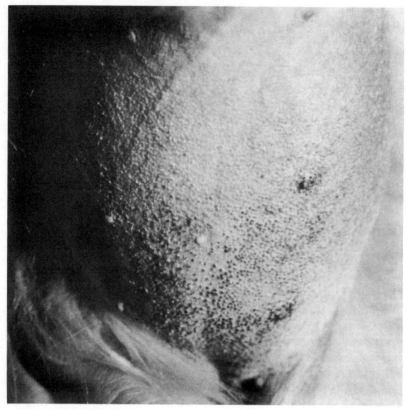

Fig. 18–4. Numerous comedones present on the abdomen of a dog with Cushing's-like syndrome. The central white lesion is a milium or retention cyst caused by follicular hyperkeratosis.

syndrome, and the cause is later controlled or eliminated, the gait may improve, even while the EMG findings persist.

Nearly one in three sexually intact dogs with Cushing's-like syndrome have persistent anestrus or atrophied testes. Possible causes include the production of excessive androgens, a direct negative effect of excessive glucocorticoids on the germinal epithelium, or the decreased production of gonadotropins. Female dogs often develop an enlarged clitoris because of the increased production of adrenal androgens.

Exophthalmos in dogs with Cushing's-like syndrome has been reported by some clinical investigators in Europe. All types of keratitis and corneal ulcerations pose an increased threat to sight because of the impaired healing processes seen in animals with Cushing's-like syndrome.

Intolerance to heat, noted in some patients with Cushing's-like disease or syndrome, may be the result of hypothalamic dysfunction caused by compression from a pituitary tumor or a direct effect of one of the natural adrenocortical steroids or their metabolites that are produced in excess.

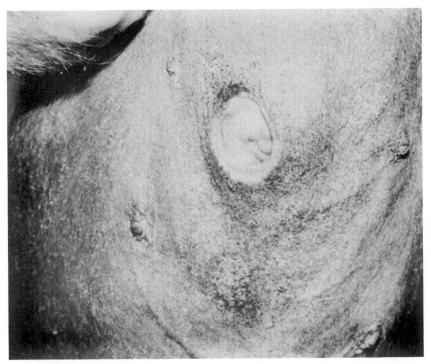

Fig. 18–5. A nonhealing ulcer in a dachshund with Cushing's-like syndrome.

Intolerance to heat has not been reported in iatrogenic Cushing's-like syndrome.

Heat intolerance may lead to respiratory distress. In addition to heat intolerance, congestive heart failure and impaired diaphragmatic movements resulting from obesity and hepatomegaly are common causes for respiratory distress in cases of Cushing's-like syndrome. Sudden development of respiratory distress may be the result of pulmonary thromboemboli.[6, 17] Pulmonary thromboemboli cause hypocapnia, hypoxemia, reflex bronchoconstriction, chest pain, and apprehension. If pulmonary arterial obstruction exceeds 40%, a jugular pulse, second heart sound, and limb edema may occur. Cushing's-like syndrome predisposes the patient to thromboemboli by production of nonfunctional antithrombin III, losses of antithrombin III in the urine from glomerulopathy, and increases in plasma factors V, X, and IX, as well as fibrinogen and plasminogen.

Excessive levels of glucocorticoids can produce behavioral changes, psychoses, depression, and mania.[9] Some neurologic clinical abnormalities are more likely the result of an enlarging pituitary tumor or, possibly, metastasis from an adrenocortical carcinoma. These signs include seizures, somnolence, aimless wandering, blindness, head pressing, anisocoria, and Horner's syndrome. Some behavioral changes may be caused by the hyper-

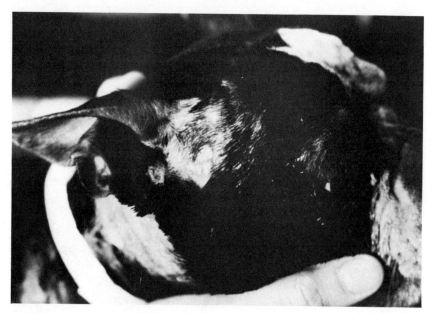

Fig. 18–6. Calcinosis cutis cranial to the ear in a Boston terrier.

tension frequently associated with Cushing's-like syndrome. Peripheral arterial pressures often exceed 180/100 mm Hg (normal range, 130 to 180/60 to 95 mm Hg) in dogs with Cushing's-like disease. Hypertension is presumably the net result of peripheral vasoconstriction, sodium retention, and the glucocorticoids' inotropic effects.

Individual patients with Cushing's-like syndrome will not exhibit all the possible clinical signs of Cushing's-like syndrome. Detection of cases early in their development depends on maintaining a high index of suspicion for the possibility of Cushing's-like syndrome and using appropriate laboratory tests to confirm the diagnosis. Even then, certain types of Cushing's-like syndrome can be easily missed. Cushing's-like syndrome caused by adrenal carcinomas can develop rapidly, precluding development of "classic" clinical signs. In humans, less than half of patients with ectopic ACTH syndrome develop the typical signs seen in Cushing's syndrome.

The clinical signs of equine Cushing's-like disease are similar to canine Cushing's-like syndrome except that alopecia does not occur in horses. Instead, the haircoat becomes dull and long (this condition is called "hirsutism"), as if in preparation for winter weather (Figs. 18–7 and 18–8). The mane and tail hair remain normal. Weight loss, pendulous abdomen, polyuria, polydipsia (more than 30 L/day), laminitis, polyphagia, muscle wasting, hyperhidrosis, hyperglycemia, and chronic infections are common. Blindness from compression of the optic nerve occasionally occurs. There may also be bulging supraorbital fat pads.

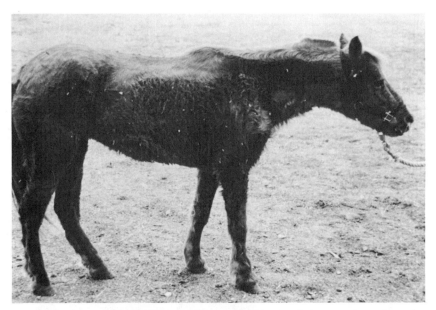

Fig. 18–7. A horse with Cushing's-like disease exhibiting long hair coat and muscle wasting. (Courtesy of Dr. Eleanor Green.)

Routine Laboratory Findings

The most consistent routine hematologic and serum findings with canine Cushing's-like syndrome are relative and absolute lymphopenia (less than 1000/cmm in dogs, 1500/cmm in cats) and increased levels of serum alkaline phosphatase (SAP).

In addition to lymphopenia, common hematologic findings include neutrophilia, eosinopenia (eosinophils, < 100/cmm), and monocytosis. Occasionally, polycythemia, hypersegmented neutrophils, and increased platelets are seen; these findings are thought to result from the stimulating effects of glucocorticoids on the bone marrow's blood cell production and decreased neutrophil margination and diapedesis.

Abnormalities other than increased levels of SAP found in most serum analyses include increases in alanine aminotransferase (SALT), cholesterol, and glucose. SAST, lactic dehydrogenase (LDH), and CPK are also frequently increased. These increases are basically the result of gluconeogenesis. Serum phosphorus levels may be decreased. With the exception of SAP, the increase in serum enzymes is usually mild to moderate. The increase in SAP, which can be greater than 3000 IU/L, generally exceeds all other abnormalities seen in the serum analyses. The origin of the increased SAP is the liver, which responds to excessive levels of glucocorticoids by inducing enzyme production from biliary epithelium.[24, 55, 74, 75, 78] Some of the increase may result from hepatocyte swelling and bile stasis. A marked increase in SAP is not usually seen in cats with Cushing's-like syndrome

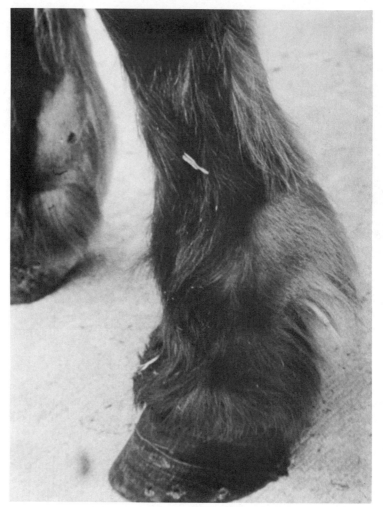

Fig. 18–8. Long hair on the distal limb of a horse with Cushing's-like disease. (Courtesy of Dr. Eleanor Green.)

because cats have the ability to rapidly clear the serum of excess alkaline phosphatase. The half-life of hepatic-origin SAP is 5.8 hours in the cat, compared to 66 hours in the dog.[25, 26] Steroid-induced SAP is less sensitive to heat than other liver-origin SAP. The measurement of steroid-induced SAP elevations has shown that in patients with Cushing's-like syndrome more than 80% of SAP elevations were steroid induced. Sixty to eighty percent of SAP elevations associated with diabetes mellitus are steroid induced. Other causes of SAP elevations, such as the administration of phenobarbital, phenytoin, and primidone, involve less than 60% steroid-induced SAP.

Steroid hepatopathy results in other serum abnormalities. Bromsulphalein retention time becomes slightly increased. Serum urea nitrogen is often decreased by hepatopathy and is lost through polyuria and the resulting serum dilution of remaining urea nitrogen. Liver biopsy shows centrilobular vascuolization and perivacuolar glycogen accumulation with hepatocytes.[3]

Serum glucose is usually in the high normal range, but the response to glucose tolerance tests is abnormal in about two thirds of affected cases. Fasting serum insulin levels are abnormally elevated (greater than 10 μU/L) in more than three fourths of dogs with Cushing's-like syndrome. Approximately 10% to 20% of dogs with Cushing's-like syndrome develop overt diabetes mellitus caused by insulin antagonism and pancreatic islet exhaustion.[30, 59] It seems that overt diabetes mellitus with Cushing's-like syndrome most often affects poodles.

Serum electrolytes (sodium, potassium, calcium, and phosphorus) are usually normal. Hypokalemia with Cushing's-like syndrome is suggestive of an adrenal tumor. Total serum CO_2 levels may be increased, particularly if hypokalemia has developed.

Urinalysis often shows hyposthenuria caused by diuresis. Urine-specific gravity is frequently less than 1.012, unless water is being withheld. The urine should be routinely cultured because the incidence of urinary infections is about 50% in cases of Cushing's-like syndrome; pyuria is inconsistently present because of the anti-inflammatory effects and urine-dilutional effects of excessive glucocorticoids. Proteinuria from glomerulopathy occurs in more than 60% of animals with Cushing's-like syndrome.

The minimal laboratory data to be obtained in patients suspected of having Cushing's-like syndrome cases are listed in Table 18–3. Care must be taken to apply pressure to the venipuncture sites for a minimum of 1 minute to minimize bruising, and to collect urine aseptically by cystocentesis because of the increased susceptibility to urinary tract infections.

Baseline levels of serum thyroxine (T_4) have been reported decreased in approximately 70% of dogs with Cushing's-like syndrome.[68] This is, in part, due to inhibition of the production of thyrotropin-releasing hormone

Table 18–3. Minimal Laboratory Data Base for Suspected Cushing's-Like Syndrome

Collect blood to determine:
  Blood cell counts
  White cell differential count
  Total plasma protein
  Serum albumin
  Serum urea nitrogen
  Serum glucose
  SALT
  SAP
  Serum sodium and potassium

Collect urine via cystocentesis for:
  Complete urinalysis
  Bacterial culture

SALT = serum alanine aminotransferase; SAP = serum alkaline phosphatase.

(TRH). Normal thyroid hormone production is expected to resume if the cause of excessive levels of glucocorticoids is corrected. The response to exogenous stimulation of thyroid-stimulating hormone (TSH) is generally normal.

Plasma testosterone levels tend to be decreased in affected male dogs and increased in affected female dogs.[19] Excessive levels of glucocorticoids can inhibit the secretion of follicle-stimulating hormone (FSH) and luteinizing hormone and may have a direct inhibitory effect on gonadal steroidogenesis.

See also references 39 and 49.

Radiographic Findings

The most consistent radiographic finding of canine Cushing's-like syndrome is hepatomegaly. Other possible findings include soft tissue mineralization (skin, adrenals, bronchi, branches of the abdominal aorta, kidney, gastric mucosa, and liver capsule), osteoporosis, and an enlarged adrenal silhouette (Fig. 18–9). By itself, the bilateral mineralization of the adrenal cortex has no meaning. This is especially true in older cats, 30% of whom develop adrenocortical mineralization.[27, 77] Osteoporosis, if apparent at all, is most likely seen as radiolucent vertebral bodies (relative to their endplate density). Enlarged adrenal shadows suggest adrenal carcinoma. Since pituitary tumors in the dog and cat can increase in a rather unimpeded

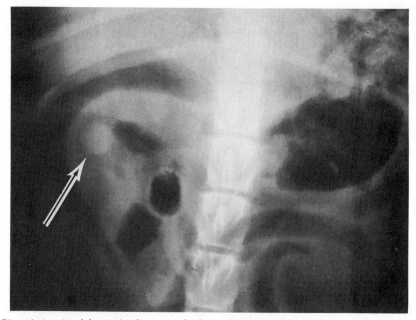

Fig. 18–9.   An abdominal radiograph of a dog with Cushing's-like syndrome and mineralization of the right adrenal gland (*arrow*).

fashion in a dorsal direction, erosion of the sella turcica is not a manifestation of Cushing's-like disease (as it may be in humans with Cushing's disease). Even in humans, pituitary tumors are not often evident unless the examination includes magnification and subtraction techniques after a carotid artery contrast injection or sellar tomography is done.

Only about 15% of adrenocortical neoplasms are visible on routine abdominal radiographs. Unilateral adrenocortical calcification occurs in about 25% of adrenocortical carcinomas. Special radiographic examinations of the adrenals include contrast urography with or without tomography to check for renal compression, arteriography to check for compression of the aorta, retroperitoneal pneumography or adrenal venography to discern better the adrenal size, adrenal imaging with radioisotopes, and computed tomography (CT) scans.

Gamma camera imaging has been described in the dog using ^{131}I-19-iodocholesterol. Bilateral adrenocortical hyperplasia is suspected if both adrenal cortices are visible. Most, but not all, adrenocortical neoplasms are unilateral, and their autonomous production of cortisol results in atrophy of the other adrenal cortex. The limited availability and economic feasibility of gamma camera imaging severely limit its current usefulness.

Pulmonary artery thrombosis may be radiographically visible.[20] Possible indications include pleural effusion, the increased diameter and blunting of pulmonary arteries, decreased vascularity of the affected lobes, increased vascularity of lobes without thrombosis, and elevation of a hemidiaphragm. Many cases may not be evident on thoracic radiographs. Selective or nonselective angiography may be helpful in equivocal cases. Pulmonary perfusion scintigraphy is safer, but it is only available in some referral practices.

See reference 28.

Endocrine Screening Tests

The baseline plasma cortisol value is rarely, if ever, diagnostically useful by itself. Over half the animals with Cushing's-like syndrome have baseline plasma cortisol values within ranges considered normal. Companion animals without Cushing's-like syndrome can have abnormally elevated plasma cortisol values that are caused by the effect of obesity on cortisol metabolism or by the effects of environmental stress on the endocrine brain. The ability to suppress plasma cortisol levels to a significant extent with a low dose of dexamethasone rules out Cushing's-like syndrome. The inability to suppress the plasma cortisol with the low-dose administration of dexamethasone may result from Cushing's-like syndrome, some drugs, and some nonadrenocortical illnesses. Exaggerated responses to the exogenous stimulation of ACTH are seen in most patients with bilateral adrenocortical hyperplasia, more than half of those patients with adrenocortical neoplasms, and in some patients with nonadrenocortical illnesses.[8, 67] Patients with adrenocortical carcinomas have exaggerated plasma cortisol values more

Table 18–4. Initial (Screening) Adrenocortical Function Tests for Glucocorticoid Production and Cushing's-Like Syndrome in Dogs and Cats

9:00 A.M.	Obtain serum or plasma for measuring baseline cortisol levels, then administer 0.01 mg/kg body weight of dexamethasone intravenously* (low-dose suppression test).
12:00 NOON	Obtain serum or plasma for measuring cortisol levels (in response to low-dose dexamethasone suppression test) then intramuscularly administer 2.2 U/kg body weight of ACTH gel (ACTH response test).†
2:00 P.M.	Obtain serum or plasma for measuring cortisol levels (response to ACTH stimulation test).

* Dilution (1:9) of the low-dose of dexamethasone with sterile saline is often required to ensure complete delivery of the dexamethasone.

† An alternative method is to administer 0.25 mg of cosyntropin (Cortrosyn), intravenously or intramuscularly, and obtain post-stimulation plasma cortisol samples in 1 hour.

often and to a greater degree than patients with adrenocortical adenomas. A protocol for screening endocrine tests for Cushing's-like syndrome is listed in Table 18–4, with suggested interpretations of results shown in Table 18–5.

Horses normally have slightly higher baseline plasma cortisol values than do dogs or cats. Normal equine plasma cortisol levels are approximately 2.5 to 6.5 μg/dl. Three hours after a 10-mg, intramuscular dose of dexamethasone has been administered, plasma cortisol levels should be less than 1 μg/dl. Two hours after a 1-mg, intravenous dose of cosyntropin has been administered, plasma cortisol levels should be about 8 to 15 μg/dl. The secretion of ACTH from adenomas of pars intermedia is not well suppressed by the administration of dexamethasone. Failure to suppress plasma cortisol levels in the horse with dexamethasone does not necessarily indicate an adrenal tumor is present.

Table 18–5. Interpretation of Initial Adrenocortical Function Tests

	Baseline Cortisol by RIA (μg/dl)	Cortisol by RIA After Low-Dose Dexamethasone Test	Cortisol by RIA After Stimulation with ACTH
Normal	<1–4*	<1.5	8–20
Spontaneous Cushing's-like syndrome†	Normal or high	>1.5	>20

RIA = radioimmunoassay; ACTH = adrenocorticotropic hormone.

* Baseline cortisol may be normal up to 10 μg/dl depending on laboratory methods and stress at time of sampling.

† Equivocal results, normal low-dose dexamethasone suppression with abnormal ACTH stimulation or vice versa, should be retested at a later date.

Normal dogs continue to have plasma cortisol values suppressed for at least 8 hours after the low-dose administration of dexamethasone. However, plasma cortisol values in dogs without Cushing's-like syndrome who are adapted to chronic illnesses often escape suppression. Adaptation to chronic illnesses such as diabetes mellitus, chronic renal disease, or liver diseases can also lead to ACTH-stimulated plasma cortisol values that exceed otherwise normal limits. The administration of phenytoin, phenobarbital, or the recovery from glucocorticoid therapy can also inhibit the low-dose dexamethasone suppression test. Low plasma cortisol levels after the low-dose administration of dexamethasone exclude a diagnosis of Cushing's-like syndrome. Failure to suppress the plasma cortisol levels with the low-dose administration of dexamethasone in dogs with chronic illnesses is not definitive proof of Cushing's-like syndrome, unless it is determined that the hypercortisolemia is refractory to treatments for the more overt illnesses, is progressive, or is associated with the presence of pituitary or adrenocortical neoplasia. Screening tests with a greater potential for diagnostic accuracy such as free urinary cortisol and salivary cortisol levels need to be investigated in companion animals.

A glucagon tolerance test has been advocated as a screening test for Cushing's-like syndrome in the dog. Normally, blood glucose levels are approximately 200 mg/dl 15 to 30 minutes after the administration of 0.14 mg glucagon/kg body weight. Normoglycemia is attained 90 minutes after the injection of glucagon. Dogs with Cushing's-like syndrome have prolonged hyperglycemia, and blood glucose levels exceed 300 mg/dl 30 minutes after stimulation.

Another screening test for Cushing's-like syndrome that has proved valuable in humans and is potentially useful in companion animals is the metyrapone response test. Metyrapone (Metopirone), given six times daily in an oral 15 mg/kg body weight dose every 4 hours, inhibits 11 β-hydroxylation. This reduces plasma cortisol levels, thereby allowing plasma ACTH levels to rise. Adrenal steroids, such as 11-deoxycortisol, generated before the enzymatic block should increase in the plasma if the adrenal cortices' rate of steroid production is still dependent on ACTH; therefore, the exaggerated elevation of plasma 11-deoxycortisol levels after the administration of metyrapone suggests pituitary-dependent hyperadrenocorticism. No change in plasma 11-deoxycortisol suggests adrenal-dependent hyperadrenocorticisms or the ectopic ACTH syndrome.

See also reference 64.

Endocrine Tests to Differentiate the Inciting Cause of Cushing's-Like Syndrome

Once the diagnosis of spontaneous Cushing's-like syndrome is determined, a high-dose dexamethasone suppression test should be done to determine the cause and to facilitate rendering a prognosis. The protocols for the performance and interpretation of the high-dose dexamethasone

Table 18–6. Adrenocortical Function Test (High-Dose Dexamethasone Suppression Test) for Differentiation of the Cause for Cushing's-Like Syndrome and its Prognosis

9:00 A.M.	Obtain serum or plasma for measurement of baseline cortisol levels, then administer an intravenous dose of 0.1 mg/kg body weight of dexamethasone (high-dose suppression test).
12:00 NOON	Obtain serum or plasma for measurement of cortisol (response to high-dose dexamethasone suppression test).

suppression test are listed in Tables 18–6 and 18–7. The information gathered from high-dose dexamethasone suppression tests should be supplemented by plain abdominal radiographs for an enlarged adrenal gland. Besides autonomous hyperfunctional adrenal neoplasia, high-dose dexamethasone refractoriness could be caused by an ACTH secretory tumor of the pars intermedia or by the ectopic ACTH syndrome.

Additional diagnostic techniques such as adrenal gland imaging, retroperitoneal pneumography, or selective angiography or venography are either not recommended for the inexperienced clinician or not available except at a few teaching or research institutions.

Plasma ACTH assays are expensive. Collection and transport require special handling—that is, avoid the use of glass tubes, use refrigerated centrifugation, and transport with dry ice. Plasma ACTH levels are not useful for the diagnosis for Cushing's-like syndrome but can be useful in differentiating the cause after the diagnosis of the syndrome is made. In the dog, high or normal plasma ACTH levels (20 to 500 pg/ml) with concurrently elevated plasma cortisol levels that can be suppressed with the high-dose administration of dexamethasone are suggestive of pituitary-dependent hyperadrenocorticism. Low plasma ACTH levels (less than 20

Table 18–7. Interpretation of the Results of the High-Dose Dexamethasone Suppression Test

Cortisol Levels After High-Dose Dexamethasone Suppression Test	Probable Cause
<50% of baseline cortisol levels	Pituitary-dependent with or without tumor in pars distalis
>50% of baseline cortisol levels*	Adrenal-dependent (adrenocortical tumor) Pars intermedia tumor Ectopic ACTH syndrome

* Failure to suppress plasma cortisol levels with the intravenous administration of 0.1 mg/kg body weight of dexamethasone can be reconfirmed with the intravenous administration of 1 mg/kg body weight.

pg/ml) with concurrently elevated plasma cortisol levels are suggestive of adrenal-dependent hyperadrenocorticism. Extremely elevated plasma ACTH levels (greater than 1000 pg/ml) that cannot be suppressed by the high-dose administration of dexamethasone would be suggestive of the ectopic ACTH syndrome. Plasma β lipotropin hormone (LPH) levels parallel and nearly equal those of ACTH in the dog.[66]

See also references 18 and 64.

Treatment

The treatment of spontaneous Cushing's-like syndrome can be done by pharmacologic control, surgical correction, or a combination. Without treatment, death from complications should be expected approximately 1 year from the time of diagnosis. Irradiation of the pituitary has been successful in affected humans. For pituitary-dependent Cushing's-like syndrome, the most economical and safest form of treatment for all—with the exception of surgery done by a few excellent surgeons—is the pharmacologic approach with mitotane. For radiographically demonstrable adrenocortical tumors (enlarged carcinomas), attempted surgical excision followed by pharmacologic control of metastasis is preferred. For patients with adrenal-dependent Cushing's-like syndrome who have no visible tumors on abdominal radiography, the most rational approach is to attempt control or suppression of the tumor with mitotane. If the control is less than satisfactory or fear of metastasis is great, excision of the tumor can be attempted. Excision should be attempted quickly if the patient cannot tolerate the drug or if the patient's condition seems to be deteriorating. Pharmacologic trial is sometimes warranted because not all patients whose plasma cortisol levels are not suppressed with the high-dose administration of dexamethasone have adrenocortical tumors and because some adrenal tumors may be relatively sensitive to pharmacologic suppression. If the function of the adrenal cortex can be controlled for 4 to 6 weeks before surgery, the surgical risks (especially delayed healing) are lessened. Treatment regime recommendations are summarized in Table 18–8.

See also references 38, 40–45, 47, and 64.

Table 18–8. Recommended Treatment Regimes for Various Causes of Spontaneous Cushing's-Like Syndrome

Type	Therapeutic Approach
Pituitary-dependent	Treat pharmacologically (with mitotane).
Adrenal-dependent with tumor visible on radiographs	Attempt excision; control metastasis with mitotane and aminoglutethimide.
Adrenal-dependent with no demonstrable tumor	Attempt control or suppression with mitotane; resort to surgery, if necessary.

PHARMACOLOGIC CONTROL.   Several drugs that have suppressive activity on the adrenal cortex have been investigated for their potential clinical usefulness. Aminoglutethimide (Cytadren), an anticonvulsant that blocks the conversion of cholesterol to pregnenolone, is generally undesirable for the treatment of pituitary-dependent hyperadrenocorticism because it results in mineralocorticoid deficiency and has goitrogenic properties. 6-Dehydro-16-methylene-hydrocortisone, an analogue of cortisol, suppresses the release of ACTH but has weak glucocorticoid effects. The results of its trials in the treatment of Cushing's-like disease have been poor. Amphenone B inhibits hydroxylation but leads to adrenocortical hyperplasia and is toxic. Metyrapone inhibits 11 β-hydroxylation and temporarily decreases the production of cortisol. In response to decreased plasma cortisol levels, however, the pituitary releases more ACTH, and soon production of cortisol from the hyperplastic adrenal cortex returns to elevated levels.

The only currently available drug to have therapeutic benefits for Cushing's-like disease from adrenocortical hyperplasia is mitotane (o,p'-DDD, ortho, para prime-DDD, Lysodren).[1] Mitotane is an isomer of the insecticide DDD. During its evaluations as an insecticide, it was discovered to have adrenocorticolytic effects.[4, 54, 90] The exact mechanism of action is unknown, but mitotane seems to block the stimulation of steroidogenesis by ACTH, to hasten the catabolism of cortisol, and to block extra-adrenal cortisol effects. After its administration, mitochondria in adrenocortical cells of the zona fasciculata and zona reticularis swell and rupture. A few hours after the administration of mitotane, microscopic hemorrhage and necrosis occur in the zona fasciculata and zona reticularis. Despite its profound effects in the adrenal cortex, mitotane is not selectively accumulated there. The recommended dose for adrenal hyperplasia in the dog is 50 mg/kg body weight every day until a satisfactory response is noted. The weekly administration of 50 mg/kg body weight is then required indefinitely, because the zona arcuata or zona intermedia will regenerate the hyperplastic zona fasciculata and zona reticularis if not continually suppressed.

The effectiveness of mitotane for the treatment of adrenocortical neoplasia in companion animals is unknown. In humans, adrenocortical adenomas are usually resistant to dosages of mitotane that are effective for hyperplasia.[46] Massive dosages (2500 mg four times daily) are recommended for humans with metastatic adrenocortical carcinomas.

The toxic effects of mitotane are mostly dose dependent. At the recommended dosage for adrenocortical hyperplasia, few toxic effects occur. About 25% of patients treated show mild adverse effects. The most frequent adverse effects are temporary anorexia, weakness, and dizziness for 2 to 12 hours.[36] Rarely, facial nerve paralysis and Horner's syndrome have been associated with mitotane therapy in the dog. If drug-induced, the paralysis usually recovers over a period of a few weeks. Adverse effects can often be reduced by giving mitotane with a meal and dividing the dose into two to four smaller administrations throughout the day. A checklist of the minimum amount of information needed before treatment with mitotane and a recommended protocol for initial therapy with mitotane are listed in Tables 18–9 and 18–10.

If clinical signs of glucocorticoid deficiency such as vomiting, diarrhea, marked depression, or total anorexia develop, replacement glucocorticoid therapy should be initiated. Some clinicians recommend routine replacement glucocorticoid therapy at the initiation of mitotane therapy. However, most patients do not exhibit signs of glucocorticoid deficiency and do not require replacement therapy. In addition, exogenous glucocorticoids eliminate the ability to titrate the length of treatment to improvement in hemograms. When necessary, the dose of 0.22 mg/kg body weight/day of prednisone or prednisolone will replace baseline glucocorticoid effects of normal cortisol levels.

Treatment with mitotane in cats with Cushing's-like syndrome is not recommended. It is suspected that cats are especially susceptible to the toxic effects of mitotane, as they are to the effects of other chlorinated hydrocarbons. Attempts to treat horses with Cushing's-like syndrome with mitotane have not been successful.

The re-examination of treated dogs is recommended 6 weeks after dismissal from the hospital and every 3 to 6 months thereafter. About one half of patients with pituitary-dependent hyperadrenocorticism develop partial resistance to treatment with mitotane because of a compensatory increase in the secretion of ACTH resulting from lowered levels of plasma cortisol. Recommended elements of the recheck examination are listed in Table 18–11. If improvement is less than satisfactory or if a relapse occurs, baseline and ACTH-stimulated measurements of cortisol should be done. Guidelines for dosage adjustments are described in Table 18–12. Hair grown in areas of previous alopecia may be darker and longer than the patient's previous hair coat.

Mitotane is not federally approved in the United States for use in dogs, although it has been extensively investigated and used clinically in dogs since 1969.[80,81] Unfortunately, there have been rare unexplained deaths in dogs receiving mitotane. Some known or possible causes for treatment-related deaths included overwhelming sepsis, rapid enlargement of a pituitary tumor apparently suppressed previously by excessive production of

Table 18–9. Checklist for Minimum Data Needed Before Treatment of Cushing's-Like Syndrome*

Measurement of 24-hour consumption of water for 2 days
Two total lymphocyte counts
Abdominal radiographs to determine size of adrenal glands and liver
General neurologic exam

* In addition to initial laboratory data base (Table 18–3) and endocrine assays (Tables 18–4 and 18–6).

Table 18–10.   Protocol for Initial Mitotane Therapy in Dogs

1. Orally administer 50 mg/kg body weight of mitotane (Lysodren) per day with food.

2. Monitor total lymphocyte counts and 24-hour consumption of water daily.

3. Discontinue daily treatment and begin once-weekly treatment with 50 mg/kg when any of the following occur:

    Total lymphocyte counts are more than 1000/mm 2 days in a row.

    The 24-hour consumption of water is less than 15 ml/kg body weight (1 oz/lb)/day 2 days in a row.

    More than 10 days of continuous daily therapy have been completed.

4. Verify adequate suppression of adrenocortical hyperfunction by repeating the ACTH stimulation test. ACTH-stimulated plasma cortisol levels should not exceed 10 μg/dl.

---

cortisol (Nelson's-like syndrome), and the cessation of the production of mineralocorticoids.

Five to ten percent of the dogs treated with mitotane temporarily or permanently lose sufficient production of mineralocorticoids.[60, 93] The occurrence in most cases is difficult to explain because dosage by kilogram body weight and the length of treatment do not exceed, or even meet, those used in other cases without adverse effects. One possible cause may be a "spillover" of necrotizing enzymes from lyzed adrenocortical cells in the zona fasciculata and the zona reticularis. Overdoses of mitotane can also destroy the zona arcuata, but in normal dogs, death by overdosage on 50 mg/kg body weight/day takes approximately 6 weeks of daily administration.[36]

The prognosis for dogs with pituitary-dependent hyperadrenocorticism treated with mitotane is guarded. About one fourth of those treated survive more than 1 year. If there are no complicating diseases before diagnosis or during initial treatment, survival periods of 3 to 5 years are probable.

Table 18–11.   Recommended Program For Minimum Re-examination of Patients on Mitotane

---

Review owner's observations.
    Patient's 24-hour consumption of water
    Patient's attitude, appetite, and strength

Do a complete physical exam, comparing current findings
    with initial findings.

Compare current laboratory findings with initial laboratory findings.
    Blood cell counts
    White cell differential count
    Serum urea nitrogen
    Serum glucose
    SAP
    Serum sodium and potassium

SAP = serum alkaline phosphatase.

Table 18–12. Possible Treatment Problems and Guidelines for Mitotane Dosage Adjustments

Problem	Adjustment
Dizziness, vomiting, or anorexia on treatment day	Divide dosage into three or four times per day, once per week administrations or give one half of the dose on Monday and one half of the dose on Friday.
Weakness, anorexia, or vomiting throughout week	Check for mineralocorticoid deficiency by measuring serum sodium and potassium levels. Recheck baseline and ACTH-stimulated cortisol levels. Decrease the dose of mitotane by 50%, and add prednisolone or prednisone in a dose of 0.22 mg/kg body weight/day.
Failure to regrow hair	Recheck baseline and ACTH-stimulated cortisol levels. Determine baseline levels of T_4 as well as levels of T_4 after the administration of TSH. Increase the dose of mitotane by 50% if cortisol levels determined after the administration of ACTH >10 μg/dl.
Failure to resume normal consumption of water	Recheck urinalysis and blood urea nitrogen. Recheck baseline and ACTH-stimulated cortisol levels. Increase mitotane by 50% if cortisol levels determined after the administration of cortisol >10 μg/dl.
Rising SAP	Recheck SALT levels. Recheck baseline and ACTH-stimulated cortisol levels. Increase mitotane by 50% if cortisol levels determined after the administration of ACTH > 10 μg/dl.

ACTH = adrenocorticotropic hormone; T_4 = thyroxine; TSH = thyroid-stimulating hormone; SAP = serum alkaline phosphatase; SALT = serum alanine aminotransferase.

Cyproheptadine (Periactin) is an antiserotonin drug with antihistamine and anticholinergic effects that has been found to be effective in the treatment of some patients with pituitary-dependent Cushing's-like syndrome.[65, 70, 88] It has been proposed that cyproheptadine blocks the serotonin-mediated increase in CRH or ACTH and can be effective if pituitary-dependent hyperadrenocorticism is due to a hypothalamic "serotonin flush" or an intermediate lobe pituitary tumor. However, in studies using 0.3 to 3.0 mg/kg body weight/day in dogs with pituitary-dependent hyperadrenocorticism, less than 10% of subjects have shown clinical benefit. The most common adverse effect is a ravenous appetite. Cyproheptadine has been more effective in treating horses with Cushing's-like syndrome than in affected dogs. The recommended dosage for horses is 0.6 mg/kg body weight/day, gradually increased to 1.2 mg/kg body weight/day.

Bromocriptine (Parlodel) is a potent dopamine receptor agonist that may decrease the secretion of ACTH in some animals with pituitary-dependent Cushing's-like syndrome.[70] Limited trials in dogs and a horse with dosages of up to 0.1 mg/kg body weight/day in divided doses (25 to 100 mg/day in horses) indicate that bromocriptine can be effective in treating the occasional patient with the pituitary-dependent form of the condition. Bromocriptine inhibits the secretion of prolactin and frequently causes vomiting, anorexia, depression, and behavior changes.

See also references 23, 35, 38, 56, 61, 62, 71, and 79.

SURGICAL CORRECTION.   Surgical procedures such as adrenalectomy, hypophysectomy, or excision of an ectopic source of ACTH are possible means of correcting Cushing's-like syndrome. Each procedure requires the skill of an experienced surgeon and is expensive in comparison to drug therapy. Adrenalectomy may be done either to remove adrenocortical neoplasms or bilateral adrenocortical hyperplasia. In the dog, the ventral abdominal approach has the advantages that both adrenals are accessible through one incision and that it is the most cosmetic approach. The disadvantages include the risk of pancreatic injury, increased risk of surgical shock, and increased risk of dehiscence. The paracostal approach is generally preferable because of the lack of risk of injury to the pancreas and decreased risk of surgical shock and dehiscence. The medical care for adrenalectomies is outlined in Table 18–13. Possible postsurgical complications include Nelson's-like syndrome (rapid enlargement of a pituitary tumor), shock, dehiscence, and septicemia. Nelson's syndrome occurs in 10% to 30% of human patients with Cushing's syndrome who undergo adrenalectomy.

Were it not for its expense, surgical skill required, and inherent risk, hypophysectomy would be the treatment of choice for pituitary-dependent Cushing's-like disease. Surgical risks include difficult-to-control hemorrhage, hypothalamic or neurohypophyseal damage, and respiratory distress from postsurgical swelling; moreover, surgical difficulty is greatest in

Table 18–13.   Recommended Medical Care for Adrenalectomy

Two hours before surgery administer:
   An intramuscular dose of 0.1 mg/kg body weight of DOCA in oil.
   An intramuscular dose of 5 to 10 mg/kg body weight of hydrocortisone sodium succinate (Solu-Cortef).

At the time of surgery administer:
   100 mg of hydrocortisone sodium succinate diluted in each 500 to 1000 ml of sterile isotonic saline or 5% dextrose slowly in an intravenous dose.

Following adrenalectomy, administer:
   An intravenous dose of hydrocortisone sodium succinate as before, until patient is able to stand unassisted; then give a twice daily, intramuscular dose of 5 to 10 mg/kg body weight of hydrocortisone sodium succinate and daily dose of 0.1 mg/kg body weight of DOCA in oil intramuscularly.

When patient is willing to and capable of eating:
   Discontinue hydrocortisone sodium succinate and give an oral dose of 0.5 mg/kg body weight of prednisone or prednisolone, and an oral dose of 0.1 to 1.0 mg fludrocortisone acetate (Florinef) daily or a dose of 2.5 mg/kg body weight of deoxycorticosterone pivalate (Percorten pivalate) intramuscularly every 3 to 4 weeks. The dose of prednisone or prednisolone should be gradually tapered to 0.11 to 0.22 mg/kg body weight per day.

brachycephalics, the most frequent group with adrenohypophyseal tumors. Postsurgical care routinely requires the life-long replacement of glucocorticoids and thyroid hormones because of the loss of ACTH and TSH. For temporary or permanent diabetes insipidus, ADH is necessary.

See also references 29, 84, 86, and 92.

RADIATION THERAPY. Conventional irradiation with cobalt or heavy particle (cyclotron) and intrasellar implants of yttrium 90 have been successfully used to treat pituitary-dependent Cushing's disease in humans. Reported recovery rates in adult humans are about 20% to 60%. Higher recovery rates occur in children. Regrettably, it may require 6 to 12 months before clinical remission is evident. Attempted pituitary irradiation in dogs or cats for treatment of pituitary-dependent Cushing's-like syndrome has not been reported.

Special Treatment Considerations

The treatment of Cushing's-like syndrome concurrent with insulin-dependent diabetes mellitus requires special considerations. Hypercortisolemia antagonizes the action of insulin, but diabetes mellitus is more immediately life-threatening than is Cushing's-like syndrome. Good results have been obtained by beginning with insulin therapy until the blood glucose has been near normal limits for at least 1 week. Treatment with mitotane is then begun, and the previous insulin dosage is reduced 50% to reduce the risk of hypoglycemia caused by decreasing concentrations of plasma cortisol while still inhibiting ketogenesis and ketoacidosis. After attaining a satisfactory response to mitotane, the insulin dosage is re-adjusted to produce more desirable blood glucose levels. Other clinicians recommend reducing the mitotane dosage and administering exogenous glucocorticoids while maintaining dosages of insulin sufficient to override glucocorticoid-induced insulin resistance.[69]

Animals with Cushing's-like syndrome are predisposed to pulmonary thromboemboli, which are life-threatening and must be treated intensively as soon as their presence is recognized. Heparin, given initially in a dose of 30 to 40 U/kg body weight, should be administered subcutaneously every 8 to 12 hours. Dosages should be gradually increased to prolong the activated partial thromboplastin time or activated clotting time to 150% of normal limits. Heparin potentiates antithrombin III by neutralizing serine proteases. After the patient's respiratory distress is controlled, the administration of heparin can be replaced by 2 to 12 mg/day of crystalline warfarin sodium (Coumadin) and monitored by prothrombin times (PT) to maintain 150% normal PT.

HYPERFUNCTIONAL ADRENOCORTICAL NEOPLASMS

Most primary tumors of the adrenal cortex are hyperfunctional. They are rare in cats and uncommon in dogs. Most adrenocortical adenomas and carcinomas (adenocarcinomas) cause Cushing's-like syndrome. Two thirds of these tumors produce high baseline plasma cortisol values and have an exaggerated response to ACTH. Adrenocortical carcinomas cause higher mean plasma cortisol elevations than do most adenomas of the adrenal cortex. In addition to any of the usual clinical signs of excessive cortisol, adrenocortical carcinomas can produce other clinical signs that are caused by enlargement, encroachment, and invasion of surrounding structures (especially the aorta and kidney), or by metastasis to the regional lymph nodes, lungs, or liver. In fact, carcinomas are often quite large by the time many clinical signs of Cushing's-like syndrome become noticeable. Large adrenocortical carcinomas may also produce hypoglycemia as a result of their large size or of the production of insulin-like hormones. Adrenocortical adenomas may be single, multiple, intracapsular, or extracapsular. Adrenocortical adenomas may or may not be hyperfunctional. Adrenocortical neoplasms may also produce predominant excessive quantities of mineralocorticoids (Conn's-like syndrome), androgens (adrenal virilization), or estrogens (adrenal feminization syndrome).

See also references 8, 10, 18, 48, 60, 85, and 91.

Incidence

Adrenocortical neoplasms are more common in female dogs than male dogs. Older dogs, more than 8 years old, are at greater risk for developing such neoplasms. Large-breed dogs are affected more frequently than small breeds. About 60% of adrenocortical neoplasms are carcinomas; 40% are adenomas. The right adrenal gland is found to be neoplastic three times more often than the left.

Conn's-like Syndrome (Aldosteroma, Primary Aldosteronism)

Hypokalemia in dogs with apparent Cushing's-like syndrome is suggestive of an adrenocortical neoplasm. The probable cause is excessive production of aldosterone, deoxycorticosterone, and corticosterone by an adrenocortical carcinoma. In humans, three fourths of aldosteromas are adrenocortical adenomas. Most of the remaining cases are caused by bilateral adrenocortical hyperplasia.

Conn's-like syndrome has been reported in a cat with an adrenocortical carcinoma.[16] We have noted dogs with adrenocortical carcinomas with elevated plasma aldosterone levels and hypokalemia. Adrenocortical carcinomas may lead to acquired enzyme deficiency, especially a deficiency in 11β-hydroxylase. Such an enzyme deficiency causes excessive plasma concentrations of deoxycorticosterone and testosterone.

Physical and laboratory findings possible with Conn's-like syndrome include hypokalemia and its effects: muscular weakness, polyuria from nephropathy, heart blocks, hyposthenuria, and metabolic alkalosis. Diastolic hypertension from hypervolemia resulting from sodium retention is also likely to occur. Except for pulmonary edema resulting from left heart failure, edema is not to be expected. In addition to hypokalemia and inappropriately elevated concentrations of urine potassium, fasting plasma renin activity (PRA) levels (normally about 1 to 5 ng/ml/hr) should be low, whereas fasting serum aldosterone levels (normally about 10 to 30 ng/dl) should be elevated.

Secondary aldosteronism is much more common than Conn's-like syndrome. Secondary aldosteronism should be suspected in all patients with edematous conditions. In secondary aldosteronism, plasma renin activity is increased, often as a result of hypovolemia to the juxtaglomerular apparatus. This, in turn, increases renin's stimulation of excessive secretion of aldosterone. Possible causes of juxtaglomerular hypovolemia include renal artery occlusion, depletion of sodium, severe depletion of water, hypoalbuminemia, congestive heart failure, glomerulonephritis, sodium-losing nephropathy, hepatic fibrosis with portal hypertension and ascites, juxtaglomerular cell hyperplasia (Bartter's-like syndrome), and juxtaglomerular tumors or other renin-secreting tumors. Serum potassium levels are usually normal. Not all conditions of secondary aldosteronism cause edema.

Liddle's syndrome (pseudohyperaldosteronism) in humans mimics Conn's syndrome, but with Liddle's syndrome, serum aldosterone levels are low. It is suspected that the mechanism involves a primary defect in the transport of renal tubular sodium and potassium.

Bartter's syndrome (juxtaglomerular cell and renomedullary hyperplasia) in humans also mimics Conn's syndrome. Bartter's syndrome seems to be caused by a defect in the reabsorption of chloride in the ascending loop of Henle. Hypertension does not develop, but hypokalemia, increased plasma renin activity, and hyperaldosteronemia do occur.

If fasting PRA and serum aldosterone levels are equivocal, response to provocative tests should be considered. Autonomy of aldosterone secretion can be established by evidence that no decrease has occurred in serum or urine aldosterone levels in response to an intravenous saline infusion or DOCA in oil, given intramuscularly. Autonomous hyperaldosteronemia also inhibits the normal increase in PRA levels that should occur after the administration of furosemide or several days' ingestion of a low-sodium diet.

Adrenal Virilization Caused by Tumor

Adrenal virilization, caused by excessive levels of adrenal androgen, particularly DHEA sulfate, is difficult to detect in postpubertal males. Prepubertal male animals exhibit pseudoprecocious sexual development. Affected female animals, regardless of age, develop an enlarged clitoris and attempt to mount others. Adrenal virilization exclusive of Cushing's-like syndrome has not been reported in the dog or cat.

Adrenal Feminizing Syndrome

Rare cases of adrenal feminization have been reported in humans. Usually they are caused by an adrenocortical carcinoma. It is possible that some of the cases of idiopathic male feminizing syndrome seen in dogs are due to undiagnosed adrenocortical neoplasms. In affected humans, excessive levels of DHEA are produced and are often converted to estriol and estrone. Alopecia and gynecomastia would likely be the predominant clinical signs of excessive estriol or estrone in the dog.

Treatment of Adrenocortical Neoplasms

Surgical excision is the treatment of choice for unmetastasized adrenocortical neoplasia. Treatment of inoperable adrenocortical carcinomas or bilateral adrenocortical hyperplasia can be attempted with the administration of mitotane in a dose of 50 to 150 mg/kg body weight/day and aminoglutethimide (Cytadren) in a dose of 125 to 250 mg three times daily. The excessive mineralocorticoid effects of aldosteromas may be controlled by the competitive antagonist diuretic—spironolactone.

ADRENOCORTICAL ENZYME DEFICIENCIES

Acquired or congenital deficiencies in enzymes necessary to the production of cortisol cause a deficiency in cortisol and thereby stimulate the release of ACTH. This leads to bilateral adrenocortical hyperplasia. Seven types of congenital enzyme deficiencies have been described in humans. None has been proved in companion animals; however, the clinical outcome of congenital adrenal hyperplasia from enzyme deficiencies can be early death, hypernatremia or hyponatremia, hyperkalemia or hypokalemia, masculinization (especially evident in females due to clitoral hypertrophy), or, much less likely, feminization in newborn males. Adequate documentation requires a high index of suspicion, appropriate endocrine assays, and histologic confirmation of adrenocortical hyperplasia. Congenital adrenocortical hyperplasia should be suspected and investigated by endocrine assays in all cases of sibling neonatal deaths, pseudoprecocious puberty, clitoral hypertrophy, idiopathic hypokalemia, and Addison's-like disease in dogs or cats who are less than 1 year old. In humans, the cause is usually an autosomal recessive inheritable trait. The most common in humans is a deficiency in 21 β-hydroxylase.

A deficiency in 21β-hydroxylase is usually incomplete. Plasma cortisol and aldosterone levels tend to be low; 17-hydroxyprogesterone levels are elevated. In 30% of affected humans, mineralocorticoid deficiency is severe enough to cause sodium wasting and sometimes hypotensive shock. Plasma testosterone levels are elevated. Girls have ambiguous genitalia because of enlargement of the clitoris and fusion of the labia. Surviving boys have precocious puberty. Other potential virilizing adrenocortical enzyme deficiencies include 11 β-hydroxylase, 3 β-dehydrogenase, and 17 α-hydroxylase. Other potential sodium wasting enzyme deficiencies include desmolase, 3 β-hydroxysteroid dehydrogenase, 18-hydroxylase, and 18-hydroxycorticosterone dehydrogenase. Deficiencies of 17 α-hydroxylase or 11 β-hydroxylase cause sodium retention.

Acquired enzyme blocks can be created by certain drugs. Metyrapone blocks 11 β-hydroxylation. Ketoconazole, a systemic antifungal agent, and etomidate, an anesthetic, are imidazoles with similar structures. Both drugs inhibit the cholesterol cleavage enzyme and 11 β-hydroxylase resulting in reduction of plasma cortisol and aldosterone levels. Amphenone B blocks 11 β-, 17 α-, and 21 β-hydroxylation.

REFERENCES

1. Anderson, J.G., and Hightower, D.: Residual effects of o,p'DDD on cortisol secretion in dogs. Southwest. Vet., *31:*35, 1978.
2. Appleby, E.C., and Sohrabi-Haghdoosi, I.: Cortical hyperplasia of the adrenal gland in the dog. Res. Vet. Sci., *29:*190, 1980.
3. Badylak, S.F., and Van Vleet, J.F.: Tissue gamma-glutamyl transpeptidase activity and hepatic ultrastructural alterations in dogs with experimentally induced glucocorticoid hepatopathy. Am. J. Vet. Res., *43:*649, 1982.
4. Balazs, T.: Effects of DDD and DDT on the production and metabolism of adrenocortical steroids in guinea pigs and dogs. Am. J. Vet. Res., *30:*1535, 1969.
5. Braund, K.G., et al.: Subclinical myopathy associated with hyperadrenocorticism in the dog. Vet. Pathol., *17:*134, 1980.
6. Burns, M.G., et al.: Pulmonary artery thrombosis in three dogs with hyperadrenocorticism. J. Am. Vet. Med. Assoc., *178:*388, 1981.
7. Capen, C.C., and Martin, S.L.: Hyperadrenocorticism (Cushing's-like syndrome and disease in dogs). Am. J. Pathol., *81:*459, 1975.
8. Chastain, C.B., Mitten, R.W., and Kluge, J.P.: An ACTH-hyperresponsive adrenal carcinoma in a dog. J. Am. Vet. Med. Assoc., *172:*586, 1978.
9. Chastain, C.B.: Hair chewing associated with suspected hyperadrenocorticism in a dog. J. Am. Vet. Med. Assoc., *172:*573, 1978.
10. Cohen, S.J., and Knieser, M.: Hyperadrenocorticism in a dog with adrenal and pituitary neoplasia. J. Am. Anim. Hosp. Assoc., *16:*259, 1980.
11. Cushing, H.: The basophil adenomas of the pituitary body and their clinical manifestations (pituitary basophilism). Bull. Johns Hopkins Hosp., *50:*137, 1932.
12. Dammrich, K.: Die Beeinflussung des Skeletts durch die Hormone der Nebennierenrinde unter besonderer Berucksichtigung des Morbus Cushing beim Hund. Berl. Munch. Tierarztl. Wochensch., *74:*331, 1962.
13. Delmage, D.A.: Three cases of alopecia in the dog related to adrenocortical dysfunction. J. Sm. Anim. Pract., *13:*265, 1972.
14. Dunbar, M., and Ward, B.C.: Hyperadrenocorticism associated with diabetes insipidus and hypothyroidism in a dog. J. Am. Anim. Hosp. Assoc., *18:*737, 1982.
15. Duncan, I.D., Griffiths, I.R., and Nash, A.S.: Myotonia in canine Cushing's disease. Vet. Rec., *100:*30, 1977.
16. Eger, C.E., Robinson, W.F., and Huxtable, C.R.R.: Primary aldosteronism (Conn's syndrome) in a cat: a case report and review of comparative aspects. J. Small Anim. Pract., *24:*293, 1983.
17. Feldman, B.F., Feldman, E.C., and Cowgill, L.D.: Thrombotic disease in canine Cushing's and nephrotic syndromes. Proceedings of the Am. Coll. Vet. Intern. Med., p. 84, 1982.
18. Feldman, E.C.: Distinguishing dogs with functioning adrenocortical tumors from dogs with pituitary-dependent hyperadrenocorticism. J. Am. Vet. Med. Assoc., *183:*195, 1983.
19. Feldman, E.C., and Tyrrell, J.B.: Plasma testosterone, plasma glucose, and plasma insulin concentrations in spontaneous canine Cushing's syndrome. Proceedings of the Am. Coll. Vet. Intern. Med., p. 81, 1982.
20. Fluckiger, M.A., and Gomez, J.A.: Radiographic findings in dogs with spontaneous pulmonary thrombosis or embolism. Vet. Rad., *25:*124, 1984.
21. Fox, J.G., and Beatty, J.O.: A case report of complicated diabetes mellitus in a cat. J. Am. Anim. Hosp. Assoc., *11:*129, 1975.
22. Greene, C.E., et al.: Myopathy associated with hyperadrenocorticism in the dog. J. Am. Vet. Med. Assoc., *174:*1310, 1979.

23. Hart, M.M., Reagan, R.L., and Adamson, R.H.: The effect of isomers of DDD on the ACTH-induced steroid output, histology, and ultrastructure of the dog adrenal cortex. Toxicol. Appl. Pharmacol., 24:101, 1973.

24. Hoffman, W.E.: Diagnostic value of canine serum alkaline phosphatase and alkaline phosphatase isoenzymes. J. Am. Anim. Hosp. Assoc., 13:237, 1977.

25. Hoffman, W.E., and Dorner, J.L.: Disappearance rates of intravenously injected canine alkaline phosphatase isoenzymes. Am. J. Vet. Res., 38:1553, 1977.

26. Hoffman, W.E., Renegar, W.E., and Dorner, J.L.: Serum half-life of intravenously injected intestinal and hepatic alkaline phosphatase isoenzymes in the cat. Am. J. Vet. Res., 38:1637, 1977.

27. Howell, J.M., and Pickering, C.M.: Calcium deposits in the adrenal glands of dogs and cats. J. Comp. Pathol., 74:280, 1964.

28. Huntley, K., et al.: The radiological features of canine Cushing's syndrome: a review of forty-eight cases. J. Small Anim. Pract., 23:369, 1982.

29. Johnston, D.E.: Adrenalectomy via retroperitoneal approach in dogs. J. Am. Vet. Med. Assoc., 170:1092, 1977.

30. Katherman, A.E., et al.: Hyperadrenocorticism and diabetes mellitus in the dog. J. Am. Anim. Hosp. Assoc., 16:705, 1980.

31. Kaufman, J.: Diseases of the adrenal cortex of dogs and cats. Part I. Mod. Vet. Pract., 65:429, 1984.

32. Kaufman, J.: Diseases of the adrenal cortex of dogs and cats. Part 2. Mod. Vet. Pract., 65:513, 1984.

33. Kelly, D.F., and Darke, P.G.G.: Cushing's syndrome in the dog. Vet. Rec., 98:28, 1976.

34. Kelly, D.F., Siegel, E.T., and Berg, P.: The adrenal gland in dogs with hyperadrenocorticalism: a pathologic study. Vet. Pathol., 8:385, 1971.

35. Kirk, G.R., Boyer, S., and Hutchenson, D.P.: Effects of O,P,'DDD on plasma cortisol levels and histology of the adrenal gland in the normal dog. J. Am. Anim. Hosp. Assoc., 10:179, 1974.

36. Kirk, G.R., and Jensen, H.E.: Toxic effects of O,P'-DDD in the normal dog. J. Am. Anim. Hosp. Assoc., 11:765, 1975.

37. Krieger, D.T.: Physiopathology of Cushing's disease. Endocrine Rev., 4:22, 1983.

38. Lavelle, R.B.: The treatment of Cushing's disease in the dog. Vet. Rec., 98:406, 1976.

39. Ling, G.V., Stabenfeldt, G.H., and Comer, K.M.: Canine hyperadrenocorticism: pretreatment clinical and laboratory evaluation of 117 cases. J. Am. Vet. Med. Assoc., 174:1211, 1979.

40. Lorenz, M.D.: Diagnosis and medical management of canine Cushing's syndrome: a study of 57 consecutive cases. J. Am. Anim. Hosp. Assoc., 18:707, 1982.

41. Lorenz, M.D.: Canine hyperadrenocorticism: diagnosis and treatment. Compendium on Continuing Educ. for the Practicing Vet., 1:315, 1979.

42. Lorenz, M.D., and Scott, D.W.: Treatment of canine Cushing's disease with o,p'DDD: a summary. J. Am. Anim. Hosp. Assoc., 8:388, 1972.

43. Lorenz, M.D., Scott, D.W., and Pulley, L.T.: Medical treatment of canine hyperadrenocorticism with o,p'-DDD. Cornell Vet., 63:646, 1973.

44. Lubberink, A.A.M.E.: Diagnosis and treatment of canine Cushing's syndrome. Thesis, Utrecht, Netherlands, 1977.

45. Lubberink, A.A.M.E., et al.: Hyperfunction of the adrenal cortex: a review. Aust. Vet. J., 47:504, 1971.

46. Luton, J.P., et al.: Treatment of Cushing's disease by o,p'-DDD. N. Engl. J. Med., 300:459, 1979.

47. McManus, J.L., Nimmons, G.B., and Buchta, W.: Surgical and medical management of hyperadrenocorticalism in a Boston terrier. Can. Vet. J., 11:78, 1970.

48. Meijer, J.C., Lubberink, A.A.M.E., and Gruys, E.: Cushing's syndrome due to adrenocortical adenoma in a cat. Tijdschr. Diergeneeskd., 103:1048, 1978.

49. Meijer, J.C., et al.: Biochemical characterization of pituitary-dependent hyperadrenocorticism in the dog. J. Endocrinol., 77:111, 1978.

50. Meijer, J.C., et al.: Hypothalamic corticotropin releasing factor activity in dogs with pituitary-dependent hyperadrenocorticism. J. Endocrinol., 79:209, 1978.

51. Moore, J.N., et al.: A case of pituitary adrenocorticotropin-dependent Cushing's syndrome in the horse. Endocrinology, 104:576, 1979.

52. Mulnix, J.A.: Adrenal cortical disease in dogs. Vet. Scope, *19:*12, 1975.
53. Mulnix, J.A., and Smith, K.W.: Hyperadrenocorticism in a dog: a case report. J. Small Anim. Pract., *16:*193, 1975.
54. Nelson, A.A., and Woodard, G.: Severe adrenal cortical atrophy (cytotoxic) and hepatic damage produced in dogs by feeding 2,2 bis (parachlorophenyl)-1, 1-dichorethane, DDD or TDE. Arch. Pathol., *48:*387, 1949.
55. Oluju, M.P., Eckersall, P.D., and Douglas, T.A.: Simple quantitative assay for canine steroid-induced alkaline phosphatase. Vet. Rec., *115:*17, 1984.
56. O'Rourke, M.D.: A medical approach to adrenal gland problems: a report of 3 cases (dogs). J. Am. Anim. Hosp. Assoc., *11:*762, 1975.
57. Orth, D.N., and Nicholson, W.E.: Bioactive and immunoreactive adrenocorticotropin in normal equine pituitary and in pituitary tumors of horses with Cushing's disease. Endocrinology, *111:*559, 1982.
58. Orth, D.N., et al.: Equine Cushing's disease: a variation of the human disease. Clin. Res., *28:*884A, 1980.
59. Peterson, M.E.: Decreased insulin sensitivity and glucose tolerance in spontaneous canine hyperadrenocorticism. Res. Vet. Sci., *36:*177, 1984.
60. Peterson, M.E.: Hyperadrenocorticism. Vet. Clin. North Am. [Small Anim. Pract.], *14:*731, 1984.
61. Peterson, M.E.: Op'-DDD (mitotane) treatment of canine pituitary-dependent hyperadrenocorticism. J. Am. Vet. Med. Assoc., *182:*527, 1983.
62. Peterson, M.E.: Use of o,p'-DDD in treatment of canine hyperadrenocorticism. Proceedings of the 6th Kal Kan Symposium, p. 91, 1982.
63. Peterson, M.E., et al.: Pituitary-dependent canine hyperadrenocorticism with spontaneous remission. Proceedings of the Am. Coll. Vet. Intern. Med., p. 91, 1982.
64. Peterson, M.E., and Drucker, W.D.: Advances in the diagnosis and management of canine Cushing's syndrome. 31st Gaines Veterinary Symposium, p. 17, 1981.
65. Peterson, M.E., and Drucker, W.D.: Cyproheptadine treatment of spontaneous, pituitary ACTH-dependent canine Cushing's disease. Clin. Res., *26:*703A, 1978.
66. Peterson, M.E., Drucker, W.D., and Orth, D.N.: Immunoreactive ACTH and β-lipotropin in spontaneous canine Cushing's and Addison's disease. Clin. Res., *28:*762A, 1980.
67. Peterson, M.E., Gilbertson, S.R., and Drucker, W.D.: Plasma cortisol response to exogenous ACTH in 22 dogs with hyperadrenocorticism caused by adrenocortical neoplasia. J. Am. Vet. Med. Assoc., *180:*542, 1982.
68. Peterson, M.E., et al.: Effects of spontaneous hyperadrenocorticism on serum thyroid hormone concentrations in the dog. Am. J. Vet. Res., *45:*2034, 1984.
69. Peterson, M.E., Nesbitt, G.H., and Schaer, M.: Diagnosis and management of concurrent diabetes mellitus and hyperadrenocorticism in thirty dogs. J. Am. Vet. Med. Assoc., *178:*66, 1981.
70. Richkind, M.: Cushing's syndrome in dogs: treatment with bromocriptine and cyproheptadine. Vet. Med. Small Anim. Clin., *76:*1301, 1981.
71. Richkind, M.: The treatment of unresponsive Cushing's disease after the use of op'-DDD. Canine Pract., *8:*18, 1981.
72. Rijnberk, A., der Kinderen, P.J., and Thijssen, J.H.H.: Canine Cushing's syndrome. Zentralbl. Veterinarmed. [A], *16:*13, 1969.
73. Rijnberk, A., der Kinderen, P.J., and Thijssen, J.H.H.: Spontaneous hyperadrenocorticism in the dog. J. Endocrinol., *41:*397, 1968.
74. Rogers, W.A.: Source of serum alkaline phosphatase in clinically normal and diseased dogs: a clinical study. J. Am. Vet. Med. Assoc., *168:*934, 1976.
75. Rogers, W.A., and Ruebner, B.H.: A retrospective study of probable glucocorticoid-induced hepatopathy in dogs. J. Am. Vet. Med. Assoc., *170:*603, 1977.
76. Rojko, J.L., Hoover, E.A., and Martin, S.L.: Histologic interpretation of cutaneous biopsies from dogs with dermatologic disorders. Vet. Pathol., *15:*579, 1978.
77. Ross, M.A., Gainer, J.H., and Innes, J.R.M.: Dystrophic calcification in the adrenal glands of monkeys, cats, and dogs. Arch. Pathol., *60:*655, 1955.
78. Saini, P.K., and Saini, S.K.: Origin of serum alkaline phosphatase in the dog. Am. J. Vet. Res., *39:*1510, 1978.
79. Schaer, M.: Treatment of canine Cushing's syndrome with op'-DDD. Canine Pract., *6:*38, 1979.

80. Schechter, R.D.: Medical treatment for Cushing's disease in the dog: a clinical report. J. Am. Anim. Hosp. Assoc., *8:*389, 1972.
81. Schecter, R.D., et al.: Treatment of Cushing's syndrome in the dog with an adrenocorticolytic agent (op'-DDD). J. Am. Vet. Med. Assoc., *162:*629, 1973.
82. Schulman, J., and Johnston, S.D.: Hyperadrenocorticism in two related Yorkshire terriers. J. Am. Vet. Med. Assoc., *182:*524, 1983.
83. Scott, D.W.: Hyperadrenocorticism (hyperadrenocorticism, hyperadrenocorticalism, Cushing's disease, Cushing's syndrome). Vet. Clin. North Am. [Small Anim. Pract.], *9:*3, 1979.
84. Siegel, E.T., Kelly, D.F., and Berg, P.: Cushing's syndrome in the dog. J. Am. Vet. Med. Assoc., *157:*2081, 1970.
85. Siegel, E.T., et al.: Functional adrenocortical carcinoma in a dog. J. Am. Vet. Med. Assoc., *150:*760, 1967.
86. Slone, D.E., et al.: Vascular anatomy and surgical technique for bilateral adrenalectomy in the Equid. Am. J. Vet. Res., *41:*829, 1980.
87. Spearman, J.G., and Little, P.B.: Hyperadrenocorticism in dogs: a study of eight cases. Can. Vet. J., *19:*33, 1978.
88. Stolp, R., Croughs, R.J.M., and Rijnberk, A.: Results of cyproheptadine treatment in dogs with pituitary-dependent hyperadrenocorticism. J. Endocrinol., *101:*311, 1984.
89. Swift, G.A., and Brown, R.H.: Surgical treatment of Cushing's syndrome in the cat. Vet. Rec., *99:*374, 1976.
90. Vilar, O., and Tullner, W.W.: Effects of op'-DDD on the histology and 17-hydroxycorticosteroid output of the dog adrenal cortex. Endocrinology, *65:*80, 1959.
91. Vince, M.E., and Watson, A.D.J.: Functioning adrenocortical tumour in a dog. Aust. Vet. J., *58:*156, 1982.
92. Walker, R.G., Halliwell, R.E.W., and Hall, L.W.: The surgical treatment of Cushing's disease in a dog. Vet. Rec., *90:*723, 1972.
93. Willard, M.D., et al.: Hypoadrenocorticism following therapy with o,p'-DDD for hyperadrenocorticism in four dogs. J. Am. Vet. Med. Assoc., *180:*638, 1982.
94. Willeberg, P., and Krogsgaard, O.W.: Some cases of Cushing's syndrome in the dog. Nord. Vet. Med., *24:*113, 1972.
95. Willeberg, P., and Priester, W.A.: Epidemiological aspects of clinical hyperadrenocorticism in dogs (canine Cushing's syndrome). J. Am. Anim. Hosp. Assoc., *18:*717, 1982.

19

Spontaneous Hypoadrenocorticism

Hypoadrenocorticism is most often a deficiency of all adrenocortical hormones. It is occasionally a deficiency of only the adrenocortical hormones most dependent on stimulation by adrenocorticotropic hormone (ACTH), namely, glucocorticoids and adrenal sex hormones, and rarely it can be an exclusive deficiency in mineralocorticoids. A clinical deficiency in all adrenocortical hormones occurs with *primary hypoadrenocorticism,* which requires destruction of more than 95% of both adrenal cortices. Its first description was reported in a human by Thomas Addison in 1855. As a result, primary hypoadrenocorticism in humans is usually referred to as Addison's disease. In companion animals, the appropriate term is *Addison's-like disease.* Although Brown-Sequard reported the fatality of adrenalectomy in dogs in 1856, spontaneous *Addison's-like* disease was not reported in the dog until 1953 and in the cat until 1983.[20]

Secondary hypoadrenocorticism is caused by a deficiency in ACTH. It is usually the result of iatrogenic suppression of ACTH by glucocorticoid therapy, but diseases of the adenohypophysis can also cause a deficiency in ACTH. The production of mineralocorticoids generally remains adequate with secondary hypoadrenocorticism, so it is not as commonly life threatening as Addison's-like disease.

PRIMARY HYPOADRENOCORTICISM (Addison's-Like Disease)

Causes and Incidence

There are numerous possible causes for Addison's-like disease (Table 19–1). The most common cause in the dog and human is idiopathic. Most idiopathic causes of Addison's-like disease are autoimmune in origin. Addison's-like disease has been reported in cats, but the diagnosis of Addison's-like disease is much less frequent in cats than in dogs. Approximately 75% of cases of Addison's disease in humans are apparently autoimmune in origin. Published case reports and our clinical observations indicate that at least 75% of dogs with Addison's-like disease are apparently autoimmune. There are no well-documented reports of dogs whose idiopathic Addison's-like disease was associated with other autoimmune disorders such as chronic lymphocytic thyroiditis (Schmidt's syndrome in humans), diabetes mellitus, vitiligo, hypoparathyroidism, hypogonadism, or atrophic gastritis, as has been noted in humans. However, veterinary clinicians should remain mindful of the possibility.

Table 19–1. Possible Causes of Primary Hypoadrenocorticism (Addison's-Like Disease)

Idiopathic*
Infectious diseases
Extension of granulomatous disease
Toxemia, hemorrhage, necrosis, subsequent to septicemias or viremias†
Infarction
Metastatic neoplasia
Iatrogenic (glucocorticoids or mitotane therapy)
Amyloidosis

  * Most cases of idiopathic primary hypoadrenocorticism are associated with antiadrenocortical antibodies and lymphocytic infiltration suggestive of autoimmunity.
  † Examples include leptospirosis, pyometra, infectious canine hepatitis, and canine distemper.

Addison's-like disease occurs most frequently in middle-aged (2 to 5 years old) bitches. The incidence is three to four times greater in female dogs than in male dogs. There is no predisposition for breed. The progression of Addison's-like disease may be acute or chronic. Chronic Addison's-like disease is more common than acute Addison's-like disease in dogs.

Clinical Signs of Acute Addison's-Like Disease

Acute Addison's-like disease may be caused by a sudden extensive destruction of the adrenal cortices or by acute stress occurring in a patient with chronic Addison's-like disease (Fig. 19–1). The clinical appearance of acute Addison's-like disease is that of hypovolemic shock. The history and physical examination may suggest an acute overwhelming illness, or a chronic idiopathic syndrome of weight loss, anorexia, and weakness. The patient is usually found in a state of collapse or collapses when stressed. Probable clinical signs of acute Addison's-like disease are listed in Table 19–2.

Clinical Signs of Chronic Addison's-Like Disease

Addison's-like disease does not always occur under extreme circumstances. Marginal deficiencies may remain precariously in a state of ill-defined illness for months. Most cases of idiopathic Addison's-like disease have a chronic course, until some stress causes an acute adrenocortical deficiency. Clinical signs of chronic Addison's-like disease are subtle and slow in development. Classic signs are small weak muscles, depression, and anorexia with a history of waxing and waning gastrointestinal upsets (Fig. 19–2). The patient is invariably ectomorphic: thin, spindly, gangly, and frail. The cause of Addison's-like disease may be easily mistaken for chronic renal insufficiency, primary neuromuscular disorders, or various other causes for such symptoms as weight loss, weakness, and anorexia. Possible clinical signs of chronic Addison's-like disease are listed in approximate order of decreasing frequency of occurrences in Table 19–3.

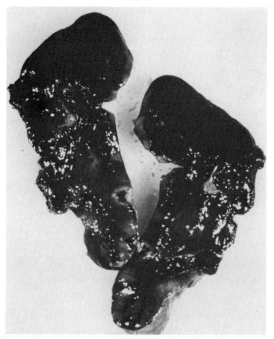

Fig. 19–1. Hemorrhage and necrosis in the adrenals of a horse with acute hypoadrenocorticism.

Cardiovascular examination may show bradycardia or bradyarrhythmias,
primarily effects of mineralocorticoid deficiency. The sinoatrial node is
relatively resistant to hyperkalemic effects. The atrioventricular node, followed by the atrial muscle, is most depressed by hyperkalemia. Electrocardiographic (ECG) examination may show elevation and peaking of the
T wave, a small amplitude or absent P wave, increased PR interval, prolonged QT, decreased R wave amplitude, increased QRS duration, atrioventricular blocks, or ectopic pacemakers (Fig. 19–3). Although the order
of ECG effects is generally uniform, ECG abnormalities do not correlate
directly with serum potassium levels. The detrimental effects of hyperkale-

Table 19–2. Possible Clinical Signs of Acute Primary
Hypoadrenocorticism (Addison's-Like Disease)

Hypotensive collapse
Weak pulse
Bradycardia and bradyarrhythmias
Abdominal pain
Vomiting
Diarrhea, with or without blood, or constipation
Dehydration
Hypothermia

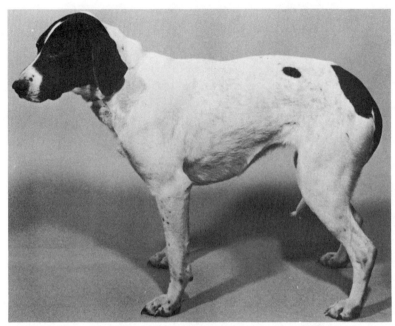

Fig. 19–2. A dog with Addison's-like disease exhibiting ectomorphy, weakness, and depression.

mia on cardiac conduction are aggravated by hyponatremia. Absence of P waves due to depressed atrial conductivity from hyperkalemia should not be misinterpreted as atrial fibrillation. With atrial fibrillation, the ventricular rate is increased and irregular. With hyperkalemia, the ventricular rate is usually regular and slow. Reported peripheral arterial blood pressure in dogs with Addison's-like disease is frequently low—100 to 130/50 to 80 mm Hg (normal ranges, 130 to 180/60 to 95 mm Hg).[43] Cardiac arrest is possible during acute collapse.

Table 19–3.　Possible Clinical Signs of Chronic Primary Hypoadrenocorticism (Addison's-Like Disease) in Approximate Order of Decreasing Occurrence

Depression
Weakness
Anorexia
Periodic vomiting
Periodic diarrhea, with or without blood, or constipation
Weight loss
Polyuria-polydipsia
Dehydration
Syncope
Irritability
Restlessness
Bronzing hyperpigmentation of skin
Decreased libido, impotence, or persistent anestrus

Serum Potassium 8 mEq/L, (heart rate=40 beats per minute)

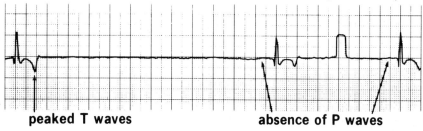

peaked T waves   **absence of P waves**

Serum Potassium 4 mEq/L 48 hours after treatment for Primary Hypoadrenocorticism, (heart rate=100 beats per minute)

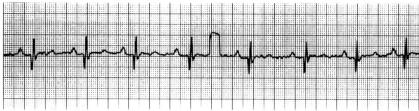

(1mv/cm, 50mm/sec)

Fig. 19–3. Electrocardiogram of a dog with Addison's-like disease before and after supplementation with glucocorticoids and mineralocorticoids.

The cause of gastrointestinal disturbances such as vomiting, abdominal pain, and diarrhea with blood or without blood is not known; however, gastrointestinal upsets can occur in secondary hypoadrenocorticism and are remediable by glucocorticoid replacement.

The pathophysiology involved in causing clinical signs of Addison's-like disease can be explained by the loss of normal glucocorticoid and mineralocorticoid effects. Glucocorticoid deficiency causes decreased mental activity, slowing of the α rhythm on the electroencephalogram (EEG), decreased stress tolerance, increased insulin sensitivity, anorexia, inability to normally excrete a water load, and decreased vascular response to catecholamines. Mineralocorticoid deficiency causes hyponatremia and hyperkalemia. Effects of hyponatremia include lethargy, mental depression, nausea, hypovolemia, hypotension, metabolic acidosis, and prerenal azotemia. Hyperkalemia can cause weakness, hyporeflexia, and slowed cardiac conduction.

Mild hyperpigmentation of the skin or mucous membranes is possible with Addison's-like disease, resulting from either the melanocytic stimulating effects of excessive levels of ACTH and its precursors, or from deficient levels of glucocorticoids. The change in color is a bronzing effect that is difficult to detect in companion animals. It may be most evident at points of trauma such as surgical scars or pressure points such as the elbows.

Laboratory Findings

The most consistent laboratory abnormalities caused by Addison's-like disease are prerenal azotemia (40 to 200 mg/dl), hyponatremia (<137 mEq/L), and hyperkalemia (>5.5 mEq/L). Prerenal azotemia is caused by decreased cardiac output, peripheral vasodilation, shift of body water into cells, and hyponatremia. It is characterized by azotemia concurrent with hypotension and concentrated urine (specific gravity, >1.020). Patients with severe cases of Addison's-like disease may develop impaired urine-concentrating ability because of sodium loss and hypotensive nephrosis.

Mineralocorticoid deficiency causes hyponatremia and hyperkalemia. Other possible causes for hyponatremia and hyperkalemia are listed in Tables 19–4 and 19–5. The ratio of serum sodium to potassium may be more reliable than absolute serum sodium or potassium values. The normal serum sodium to potassium ratio is 27:1 to 32:1, whereas in patients with Addison's-like disease, ratios of ≤23:1 are common. Urine sodium levels are inappropriately high for the patient with hyponatremia, and urine potassium levels are inappropriately low for the patient with hyperkalemia. In addition to hyponatremia and hyperkalemia, possible serum electrolyte changes include hypochloremia, hyperphosphatemia, and hypercalcemia. Hypercalcemia occurs in up to 45% of dogs with Addison's-like disease. This clinical sign is caused by hemoconcentration, increased renal tubular reabsorption, and decreased glomerular filtration. The occurrence of hypercalcemia is greater in more severely affected patients with Addison's-like disease. Approximately 10% of patients with Addison's-like disease have normal serum electrolyte values.

Hematologic changes may include relative neutropenia, lymphocytosis, relative eosinophilia, and mild normocytic, normochromic nonregenerative anemia. Anemia may not be evident until after the replacement of fluids has taken place because of hemoconcentration from dehydration and an intracellular shift in body water. Stress normally causes the increased secretion

Table 19–4. Possible Causes of Hyponatremia Other than Primary Hypoadrenocorticism (Addison's-Like Disease)

Dilutional hyponatremia
  Congestive heart failure
  Hepatic fibrosis
  Nephrotic syndrome
  Psychogenic polydipsia
  Syndrome of inappropriate antidiuretic hormone
  Polyuric end-state renal failure
  Iatrogenic overdose of sodium-free fluids

Sodium-depleted hyponatremia
  Sodium-depleting nephropathy
  Iatrogenic overdosage of some diuretics
  Severe vomiting
  Severe diarrhea

Table 19–5. Possible Causes of Hyperkalemia Other than Primary Hypoadrenocorticism (Addison's-Like Disease)

Acute renal failure
Acute obstructive (post-renal) uropathy
Iatrogenic overdose
Massive soft tissue trauma (crushing injuries or burns)
Severe acidosis
Rapid blood transfusions
Hemolysis

of glucocorticoids, which suppress the number of lymphocytes and eosinophils in circulation. Any clinically stressed patient who does not have a normal hematologic stress—that is, a normal stress response such as relative neutrophilia, lymphopenia, and eosinopenia—should be evaluated for Addison's-like disease or secondary hypoadrenocorticism.

Venous blood from patients with Addison's-like disease often appears abnormally dark because of hemoconcentration and increased deoxygenated hemoglobin.[42] Venous pO_2 is very low because of decreased blood pressure, 2,3-DPG concentration, and the oxygen saturation of hemoglobin. Total venous CO_2 and plasma bicarbonate are usually decreased because of metabolic acidosis and compensatory respiratory alkalosis.

Other routine laboratory parameters are generally normal. Hypoglycemia is possible during stress, but despite impaired gluconeogenesis caused by glucocorticoid deficiency and anorexia, hypoglycemia is rare with primary hypoadrenocorticism. Hypocholesterolemia occurs occasionally.

See also references 32 and 33.

Radiographic Findings

The radiographic findings possible to see in patients with acute Addison's-like disease are caused by hypotension and esophageal asthenia. Possible findings include microcardia, which is best appreciated on the lateral view; decreased size of pulmonary vasculature; decreased size of the caudal vena cava; and dilatation of the esophagus.

See also reference 35.

Diagnostic Examinations

Historical and clinical findings that should alert the veterinary clinician to the possibility of Addison's-like disease are listed in Table 19–6. Addison's-like disease can be ruled out if the history indicates a recent gain in weight, good appetite, and normal vigor. A recommended method of Addison's-like disease confirmation is also listed in Table 19–7. Exogenous administration of ACTH should create a stress response in the leukogram if the adrenal cortices have the reserve capacity to produce cortisol. Even though the ACTH preparation for intravenous injection is more expensive than the ACTH gel, the absorption of ACTH gel (which must be given intramuscu-

Table 19–6. Historical and Clinical Findings Particularly Suggestive of Addison's-Like Disease

---

On-and-off weakness and depression responsive to fluids, or
  adrenocorticosteroids, or both

Unexplained anorexia and weight loss

Sudden collapse during exertion or other stresses

Prerenal azotemia with normal cardiac auscultation findings

Normal or elevated relative lymphocyte and eosinophil counts during stress

Bradycardia or bradyarrhythmia during shock-like collapse

---

larly) should not be relied on if the patient has collapsed or severe hypotension is suspected. If the patient shows normal stressed neutrophil to lymphocyte ratios and eosinophil counts once the ACTH has been administered, the need for treatment of acute Addison's-like disease is eliminated, but not the diagnosis. The interpretation of ACTH responses is outlined in Table 19–8.

Other less valuable or practical tests have been reported. The water-loading test and the insulin response test are insensitive and potentially hazardous. Aldosterone assays are commercially available but are expensive and rarely necessary. ACTH assays in dogs have confirmed elevated ACTH levels in Addison's-like disease. The plasma ACTH assay would help to differentiate primary from secondary hypoadrenocorticism if serum electrolytes are normal. Unfortunately, plasma ACTH assays are expensive and require special handling such as placing the sample in an ice bath after it has been taken, refrigerated centrifugation, and shipment in dry ice. Measuring the patient's plasma cortisol levels, in response to repeated ACTH injections for 3 to 5 days, should also help to differentiate primary from secondary hypoadrenocorticism; moreover, the test is much less expensive.

Table 19–7. Recommended Diagnostic Procedure for Addison's-Like Disease

---

Step 1. Obtain baseline serum or plasma cortisol levels, plus whole blood for total white blood cell count, and differential white blood cell count.

Step 2. Initiate emergency treatment* if patient is in collapse.

Step 3. Intravenously administer 0.25 mg of synthetic ACTH, cosyntropin (Cortrosyn).

Step 4. One hour after the administration of cosyntropin, measure serum or plasma levels of ACTH-stimulated cortisol. If emergency treatment has not been necessary (Step 2), then follow Step 5.

Step 5. Four hours after the administration of cosyntropin, obtain whole blood for total white blood cell count and differential white blood cell count.

ACTH = adrenocorticotropic hormone.
* Use dexamethasone to supplement suspected glucocorticoid deficiency so that there will not be interference in the cortisol assays.

Table 19–8. Interpretation of Diagnostic Data for Addison's-Like Disease

Results	Interpretation
Baseline Samples	
Baseline cortisol levels <1 μg/dl, with clinical signs and history consistent with Addison's-like disease	Probable glucocorticoid deficiency
Samples taken 1 hour after the intravenous administration of cosyntropin	
Cortisol levels <5 μg/dl	Definite glucocorticoid deficiency
Samples taken 4 hours after the intravenous administration of cosyntropin*	
Ratio of neutrophils to lymphocytes (absolute counts) fails to increase at least 30% from the baseline ratio	Probable glucocorticoid deficiency
Absolute eosinophil count fails to decrease 50% from the baseline absolute eosinophil count	Probable glucocorticoid deficiency

* Neutrophil to lymphocyte (N:L) ratios and eosinophil counts can be obtained more readily than cortisol assays. A normal N:L ratio and eosinophil count in response to the administration of cosyntropin may eliminate the need for proceeding with the cortisol assays.

Treatment

Acute Addison's-like disease is life-threatening. Whenever it is suspected, treatment should be begun immediately. Diagnostic tests for confirmation can be done during treatment if dexamethasone is used rather than hydrocortisone during the testing. An electrocardiogram can provide readily available indications of hyperkalemia. In patients who have shock without hyperkalemia, the heart rate is increased. Acute Addison's-like disease characteristically causes tall, peaked T waves, bradycardia, atrial standstill (absent P waves), atrioventricular heart blocks, and other bradyarrhythmias.

The treatment of Addison's-like disease initially involves the replacement of insufficient mineralocorticoids and glucocorticoids, depleted sodium, and intravascular volume deficit. Other considerations include correction of acid-base imbalance, hyperkalemia, and hypoglycemia. Recommended methods of treatment of acute and chronic Addison's-like disease are listed in Tables 19–9 and 19–10.

Hyperkalemia can cause serious cardiotoxicity. Serum potassium levels begin to drop promptly as soon as potassium-free fluids (saline) dilute concentrations of intravascular potassium and increase glomerular filtration. Administered glucocorticoids also enhance the glomerular filtration rate by various means. In the hypoadrenocortical state, glucocorticoids are the most potent kaliuretic, but mineralocorticoids enhance the selective secre-

Table 19–9. Emergency Treatment of Acute Addison's-Like Disease

Step 1. Insert indwelling catheter in jugular vein* and obtain heparinized venous blood to determine pH and total CO_2 or bicarbonate.

Step 2. Intravenously administer sterile isotonic saline.

Step 3. Administer soluble glucocorticoid (select one of the preparations listed below), one third as intravenous bolus, one third intramuscularly, and one third diluted in 5% dextrose for the total initial dose:

   10 mg/kg body weight hydrocortisone sodium succinate (Solu-Cortef)

   5 mg/kg body weight prednisolone sodium succinate (Solu-Delta Cortef)

   0.5 mg/kg body weight dexamethasone sodium phosphate† (Decadron phosphate injection)

Step 4. Intramuscularly administer 0.1 mg/kg body weight of deoxycorticosterone acetate (DOCA) in oil.

Step 5. If blood pH is ≤7.1, administer 50% of the amount of bicarbonate determined deficient by bicarbonate deficit (mEq/L deficit × 0.4 × kg body weight) diluted in a slow intravenous drip of 5% dextrose.

Step 6. If there is no response in 30 minutes, monitor femoral pulse palpability, catheterize urinary bladder, and monitor urine output after establishing a slow intravenous drip of levarterenol (Levophed bitartrate) in a dose of 2 ml (2 mg)/500 ml of 5% dextrose.

Step 7. Give nothing by mouth for the first 24 hours.

Step 8. Maintain patient on a dose of 11 mg/kg body weight of hydrocortisone sodium succinate given intramuscularly three times daily, plus an intramuscular dose of 0.1 mg/kg body weight of deoxycorticosterone acetate (DOCA) in oil daily, until patient is alert and capable of eating without vomiting.

Step 9. Select and begin maintenance treatment for chronic Addison's-like disease.

* Obtain baseline cortisol sample for diagnosis, if necessary.
† If serum cortisol is to be sampled, use dexamethasone to avoid assay interference.

tion of potassium in the renal tubules. Administered bicarbonate facilitates the intracellular shift of potassium if acidosis is present; therefore, it is rarely necessary to resort to additional means to lower serum potassium levels faster than does conventional treatment. Insulin therapy, in an intravenous dose of 0.5 U/kg body weight of regular insulin, and glucose, intravenously administered in a dose of 10 ml/kg body weight of 10% glucose in 30 minutes, has been recommended if serum potassium levels exceed 8 mEq/L. No reported study has substantiated the necessity or safety of insulin therapy to treat hyperkalemia in Addison's-like disease. It should also be remembered that Addison's-like disease renders the patient insulin sensitive.

Which glucocorticoid is administered is not critical; however, it is critical that the glucocorticoid used is water soluble and an intravenous bolus is given before fluid replacements are used. Otherwise, water intoxication is possible. Long-term glucocorticoid replacement is advisable since normal blood pressure, attitude, and appetite may not be maintained with only mineralocorticoid replacement. The replacement dose of glucocorticoid should be increased at least two- to threefold during periods of acute stress.

Table 19–10. Treatment Methods for Chronic Addison's-Like Disease

Step 1. Intramuscularly administer 11 mg/kg body weight of hydrocortisone sodium succinate three times daily, plus 0.1 mg/kg body weight of deoxycorticosterone acetate (DOCA) in oil daily, until serum sodium and potassium levels are normal and until patient is capable of eating without vomiting.

Step 2. If vomiting has not occurred recently, orally administer 1 to 3 g of enteric-coated sodium chloride or lightly sprinkle food with table salt for 1 week.

Step 3. Orally administer 0.5 mg/kg body weight of hydrocortisone twice daily for 1 week, then once daily thereafter.* Double or triple the dose of maintenance glucocorticoids during acute stress.

Step 4. Select one of the following long-term mineralocorticoid replacement methods:

Deoxycorticosterone pivalate (Percorten pivalate) in an intramuscular dose of 2.5 mg/kg body weight every 3 to 4 weeks

Fludrocortisone acetate (Florinef acetate) 0.1 mg/10 kg body weight/day

---

* For long-term maintenance, prednisone (a less expensive drug than hydrocortisone) may be substituted for hydrocortisone to replace glucocorticoid deficiency. The replacement dose of prednisone during periods without stress is 0.1 to 0.2 mg/kg body weight/day.

There are two common methods of long-term mineralocorticoid replacement: intramuscular injections of repositol and tablets. Deoxycorticosterone is available as a pivalate ester for slow, intramuscular absorption. At the recommended dosage, the duration of effect is about 4 weeks. Deoxycorticosterone pivalate is particularly useful in the treatment of temporary Addison's-like disease which may occur in response to the presence of mitotane. Since the pivalate ester leads to gradual tapering of the final absorption of deoxycorticosterone, the endogenous production of mineralocorticoid may resume, blending with the final absorption of deoxycorticosterone pivalate. Usually, clinical signs suggestive of recurring Addison's-like disease occur for several days before the risk of hypoadrenocortical crisis is likely. Owners should be instructed to watch out for weakness, depression, anorexia, or weight loss any time 3 weeks after the deoxycorticosterone has been administered. If the injection is suspected to have become completely absorbed, serum sodium and potassium levels should be determined. If serum potassium exceeds 5.2 mEq/L, or the sodium to potassium ratio is < 27:1, another deoxycorticosterone pivalate injection should be administered.

Fludrocortisone acetate is a synthetic adrenocortical steroid with mineralocorticoid effects. It is absorbed well by the digestive tract and is usually administered once or twice per day. Successful mineralocorticoid replacement with fludrocortisone acetate requires that the administration of the drug is regular, that the patient has a normal gastrointestinal tract, and that the chance of the patient running away is small. Dosages required are higher per kg body weight than those used in humans, and the required dosage tends to increase during the first year of treatment. The cause for the difference is not known. Whatever form of treatment for chronic

Addison's-like disease is chosen, some form of a medical warning attached to the patient's collar is advisable.

See also reference 7.

Atypical Forms of Primary Hypoadrenocorticism

Mineralocorticoid deficiency can occur with adequate production of glucocorticoids and vice versa. Selective hypoaldosteronism can be caused by chronic tubulointerstitial nephropathy, 18-hydroxycorticosterone dehydrogenase deficiency, chronic heparin therapy, or lead poisoning. It is characterized by the clinical findings of muscular weakness, cardiac conduction abnormalities, mental depression, and dehydration. Laboratory findings include hyperkalemia, prerenal azotemia, and hyponatremia. Urine sodium levels are inappropriately high for serum sodium levels, and urine potassium levels are inappropriately low for the serum levels. Diagnosis requires evidence of normal plasma cortisol levels with low plasma aldosterone levels in the presence of low serum sodium levels or low plasma aldosterone levels unresponsive to ACTH, a low-sodium diet, or the administration of furosemide. Treatment is identical to that for Addison's-like disease but glucocorticoid therapy is not necessary.

Glucocorticoid deficiency may become clinically evident before the loss of aldosterone. All forms of congenital adrenal hyperplasia result from the inadequate synthesis of cortisol, which is caused by an enzyme deficiency. With 11 β- or 17 α-hydroxylase and most 21-hydroxylase deficiencies, adequate or excessive levels of mineralocorticoids are produced but the production of cortisol is deficient. Measuring plasma ACTH levels may be necessary to differentiate primary selective glucocorticoid deficiency, which has elevated concurrent plasma ACTH levels, from secondary hypoadrenocorticism, which has low concurrent plasma ACTH levels.

See also reference 36.

For further information on primary hypoadrenocorticism (Addison's-like disease), see also references 1–6, 8–19, 21–31, 34, 37–41, 44, and 45.

SECONDARY HYPOADRENOCORTICISM

Secondary hypoadrenocorticism is the deficiency of glucocorticoid and adrenocortical sex hormones caused by a deficiency in ACTH. Only the deficiency in glucocorticoids produces clinical signs. After an adrenalectomy, the secretion of aldosterone in the dog decreases by about 40%, but clinical findings associated with a mineralocorticoid deficiency do not occur. Compensatory hyperreninemia later restores normal production of mineralocorticoids. Even if the deficiency in adrenocortical sex hormones is complete, no clinical abnormalities occur. Possible causes of the deficiency in ACTH are destructive lesions in the hypothalamus or adenohypophysis or, most likely, prolonged suppression of ACTH by drug therapy with glucocorticoids.

The clinical signs of secondary hypoadrenocorticism are variable. The glucocorticoid deficiency may be partial or complete. Partial glucocorticoid deficiency may only cause signs of glucocorticoid deficiency during times of stress. Clinical signs of glucocorticoid deficiency are depression, anorexia, occasional vomiting or diarrhea, weak pulse, and sudden collapse when stressed. If the deficiency is caused by a hypothalamic or adenohypophyseal lesion, a deficiency in hypothalamic-releasing or -inhibitory factors, as well as adenohypophyseal or even neurohypophyseal hormones, may produce concurrent diabetes insipidus, secondary or tertiary hypothyroidism, dwarfism, secondary or tertiary hypogonadism, or galactorrhea. If the hypothalamic or adenohypophyseal lesion is space-occupying, a wide variety of neurologic clinical signs are possible. If secondary hypoadrenocorticism is caused by previous or current glucocorticoid therapy, clinical findings of iatrogenic hyperadrenocorticism (Cushing's-like syndrome) may be present.

The diagnosis of secondary hypoadrenocorticism is based on the finding that the patient's serum cortisol response to the administration of ACTH is subnormal. Repeated injections of ACTH should eventually cause a stair-step increase in serum cortisol levels. Treatment of secondary hypoadrenocorticism is by glucocorticoid replacement in a dose of 0.1 to 0.2 mg/kg body weight/day of prednisone or prednisolone. Dosages must be increased two- to threefold during stress. The prognosis for secondary hypoadrenocorticism depends on its cause and whether the cause can be eliminated.

REFERENCES

1. Annis, Jr., R.: Adrenal cortical failure in the dog. Vet. Med., 55:35, 1960.
2. Atwell, R.B., Filippich, L.J., and O'Grady, A.: Hypoadrenocorticoidism in a dog. Aust. Vet. Pract., 9:167, 1979.
3. Baarschers, J.J., Hommes, U.E., and Poll, P.H.A.: A case of Addison's disease in a dog. Tijdschr. Diergeneeskd., 100:894, 1975.
4. Bath, M.L., and Hill, F.W.G.: Adrenocortical insufficiency in the dog. Aust. Vet. J., 54:128, 1978.
5. Bonneau, N., and Reed, J.H.: Adrenocortical insufficiency in a dog. Can. Vet. J., 12:100, 1971.
6. Bozzini, C.E., Rendo, M.E.B., and Kofoed, J.A.: Erythrokinetics in adrenalectomized dogs. Acta Physiol. Lat. Am., 18:304, 1968.
7. Byyny, R.L.: Preventing adrenal insufficiency during surgery. Postgrad. Med. J., 67:219, 1980.
8. Cornelius, L.M.: Canine distemper presenting as acute adrenocortical insufficiency: a case report. J. Am. Anim. Hosp. Assoc., 10:153, 1974.
9. Crenshaw, W.E.: A case of adrenocortical hypofunction in a dog. Southwest Vet., 32:125, 1979.
10. DeLahunta, A., et al.: Clinical pathological conference (adrenal cortical atrophy in a dog). Cornell Vet., 62:145, 1972.
11. Ditchfield, J., Archibald, J., and Cawley, A.J.: Adrenal cortical failure in dogs. Can. Vet. J., 2:175, 1961.
12. Feldman, E.C., Ettinger, S.J., and Peters, G.: Hypoadrenocorticism in a dog. Mod. Vet. Pract., 58:433, 1977.
13. Feldman, E.C., and Peterson, M.E.: Hypoadrenocorticism. Vet. Clin. North Am. [Small Anim. Pract.], 14:751, 1984.
14. Feldman, E.C., and Tyrrell, J.B.: Hypoadrenocorticism. Vet. Clin. North Am. [Small Anim. Pract.], 7:555, 1977.

15. Fox, J.G., and Beatty, J.O.: Adrenal insufficiency in the dog: two case reports. J. Small Anim. Pract., *14*:167, 1973.
16. Hadlow, W.J.: Adrenal cortical atrophy in the dog. Report of three cases. Am. J. Pathol., *29*:353, 1953.
17. Harolton, B.W.: Addison's disease in a dog. Vet. Med. Small Anim. Clin., *71*:285, 1976.
18. Hiatt, N., et al.: Adrenal hormones and the regulation of serum potassium in potassium-loaded adrenalectomized dogs. Endocrinology, *105*:215, 1979.
19. Hill, F.W.G.: Adrenocortical insufficiency in the dog. *In* Veterinary Annual. 19th Ed. Bristol, England, John Wright & Sons Ltd., 1979, p. 223.
20. Johnessee, J.S., Peterson, M.E., and Gilbertson, S.R.: Primary hypoadrenocorticism in a cat. J. Am. Vet. Med. Assoc., *183*:881, 1983.
21. Keeton, K.S., Schechter, R.D., and Schalm, O.W.: Adrenocortical insufficiency in dogs. Mod. Vet. Pract., *53*:25, 1972.
22. Kelly, D.F.: Necrosis of the adrenal cortex and adrenal capsular myoarteritis in a dog. Vet. Rec., *77*:998, 1965.
23. Kitchfield, J., Archibald, J., and Cawley, A.J.: Adrenal cortical failure in dogs. Can. Vet. J., *2*:175, 1961.
24. Lorenz, M.D.: Hypoadrenocorticism—diagnosis and treatment. Compendium on Continuing Educ. for the Practicing Vet., *1*:634, 1979.
25. Marshak, R.R., Webster, G.D., and Skelley, J.F.: Observations on a case of primary adrenocortical insufficiency in a dog. J. Am. Vet. Med. Assoc., *136*:274, 1960.
26. Morales, G.A., and Nielsen, S.W.: Canine adrenocortical atrophy: review of literature and a report of 2 cases. J. Small Anim. Pract., *11*:257, 1970.
27. Mulnix, J.A.: Hypoadrenocorticism in the dog. J. Am. Anim. Hosp. Assoc., *7*:220, 1971.
28. Murrell, K.A.: Hypoadrenocorticism in a dog. Mod. Vet. Pract., *61*:625, 1980.
29. Musselman, E.E.: Electrocardiographic signs of adrenocortical insufficiency with hypercalcemia in the dog. Vet. Med. Small Anim. Clin., *70*:1433, 1975.
30. Nimmons, G.B., and McManus, J.L.: Adrenocortical insufficiency in a dog. Can. Vet. J., *9*:252, 1968.
31. O'Rourke, M.D.: A medical approach to adrenal gland problems: a report of 3 cases. J. Am. Anim. Hosp. Assoc., *11*:762, 1975.
32. Peterson, M.E., and Feinman, J.M.: Hypercalcemia associated with hypoadrenocorticism in sixteen dogs. J. Am. Vet. Med. Assoc., *181*:802, 1982.
33. Rakich, P.M., and Lorenz, M.D.: Clinical signs and laboratory abnormalities in 23 dogs with spontaneous hypoadrenocorticism. J. Am. Anim. Hosp. Assoc., *20*:647, 1984.
34. Reimer, N.W., and Dodd, R.R.: Hypoadrenocorticism in the dog. Canine Pract., *5*:61, 1978.
35. Rendano, V.T., and Alexander, J.E.: Heart size changes in experimentally-induced adrenal insufficiency in the dog: a radiographic study. J. Am. Vet. Radiol. Soc., *17*:57, 1976.
36. Rogers, W., Straus, J., and Chew, D.: Atypical hypoadrenocorticism in three dogs. J. Am. Vet. Med. Assoc., *179*:155, 1981.
37. Rothenbacher, H., and Shigley, R.F.: Adrenocortical apoplexy in a dog. J. Am. Vet. Med. Assoc., *149*:406, 1966.
38. Ruben, J.M., Walker, M.J., and Longstaffe, J.A.: Addison's disease in a puppy. Vet. Rec., *116*:91, 1985.
39. Sanger, V.L., Noble, W.E., and Gehrman, R.S.: Adrenal cortical failure in a dog. Vet. Med. Small Anim. Clin., *59*:579, 1974.
40. Schaer, M., and Chen, C.L.: A clinical survey of 48 dogs with adrenocortical hypofunction. J. Am. Anim. Hosp. Assoc., *19*:443, 1983.
41. Siegel, E.T., Schryver, H.F., and Fidler, I.: Clinico-pathologic conference. J. Am. Vet. Med. Assoc., *150*:423, 1967.
42. Thompson, F.N., et al.: Effect of adrenalectomy in the dog on blood gas tensions and oxygen content. Am. J. Vet. Res., *38*:235, 1977.
43. Weiser, M.G., Spangler, W.L., and Gribble, D.H.: Blood pressure measurement in the dog. J. Am. Vet. Med. Assoc., *171*:364, 1977.
44. Willard, M.D.: An unusual case of hypoadrenocorticism in a dog. Mod. Vet. Pract., *61*:830, 1980.
45. Willard, M.D., et al.: Canine hypoadrenocorticism: report of 37 cases and review of 39 previously reported cases. J. Am. Vet. Med. Assoc., *180*:59, 1982.

20

Glucocorticoid Therapeutics, Iatrogenic Secondary Hypoadrenocorticism, and Iatrogenic Hyperadrenocorticism

In 1929, it was recognized that pregnancy and some liver disorders in humans were associated with a remission of arthritis. It is now known that serum cortisol increases in patients with these conditions. Twenty years later, the successful use of compound E (cortisone) was reported in the treatment of arthritis.[27]

In 1952, the first case of fatal iatrogenic adrenocortical atrophy (iatrogenic secondary hypoadrenocorticism) was reported in a human who had been treated with cortisone.[22] Iatrogenic secondary hyperadrenocorticism was described in dogs in 1961, but not in much detail until 1974. It is now recognized that hyperadrenocorticism is iatrogenic in more than half the dogs who have it.

At present, more than 12 generic glucocorticoids are commercially available. These are sold under numerous proprietary (trade) names, as a glucocorticoid preparation to be taken alone or in combination with antibiotics or various other drugs. Some common glucocorticoids and their proprietary names are listed in Table 20–1. Glucocorticoids and antibiotics are the two most frequently used and prescribed classes of drugs in veterinary medicine. Many disease processes are suppressed and controlled economically by glucocorticoids with minimal adverse effects; however, inappropriately used glucocorticoids can be life-threatening, and it is imperative that veterinary clinicians are well informed on the rational use of glucocorticoids as treatment and the potential hazards of glucocorticoid therapy.

RELATIVE POTENCY AND DURATION OF ACTION OF GLUCOCORTICOIDS

The potency of glucocorticoids is assessed by their anti-inflammatory ability. The degree of anti-inflammation produced by hydrocortisone is used to compare the anti-inflammation produced by equal quantities of other adrenocortical steroids. The essential anti-inflammatory groups forming with a cyclopentanoperhydrophenanthrene nucleus are illustrated in Figure 20–1. Steroids with a keto group at C-11 (cortisone and prednisone) do not have an anti-inflammatory action until the keto group is reduced to a hydroxyl group (hydrocortisone and prednisolone) by the liver. Only when liver dysfunction is severe is the patient unable to convert cortisone or

Table 20–1. Common Generic Glucocorticoids and Their Proprietary Names

Generic Name	Proprietary Names
Betamethasone	Betasone
	Betavet
	Celestone
	Diprosone
	Uticort
	Valisone
Cortisone (Compound E)	Cortogen
	Cortone
Dexamethasone	Azium
	Decadron
	Deronil
	Dexameth
	Dexasone
	Dexate
	Gammacorten
	Hexadrol
	Voren
	Zonometh
Flumethasone	Anaprime
	Flucort
	Locorten
	Methagon
Fluocinolone	Fluocin
	Synalar
Fluoroprednisolone	Predef
Hydrocortisone (Compound F, Cortisol)	Cortef
	Cortril
	Hydrocortone
	Hytex
	Kanfosone
	Solu-Cortef
Methylprednisolone	Depo-Medrol
	Medrol
	Pre-Dep 40V
	Solu-Medrol
Prednisolone	Delta-Cortef
	Hydeltra
	Meticortelone
	Paracortol
	Solu-Delta-Cortef
	Sterane
	Sterosone
Prednisone	Deltasone
	Deltra
	Meticorten
	Paracort
	Prednameen
	Veticort
	Zenadrid
Triamcinolone	Aristocort
	Aristospan
	Aristovet
	Kenacort
	Kenalog
	Vetalog

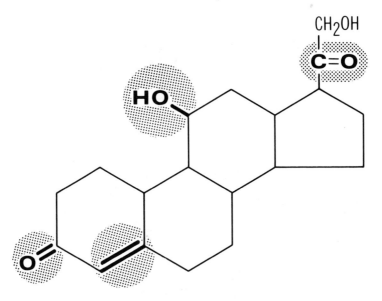

Fig. 20–1. Anti-inflammatory groups.

prednisone to hydrocortisone or prednisolone. C-11 keto compounds (cortisone and prednisone) are not effective topically.

Numerous synthetic glucocorticoids have been developed in an attempt to increase glucocorticoid potency while decreasing or eliminating the mineralocorticoid effects of natural glucocorticoids. Glucocorticoid activity can be increased by the addition of a double bond at C-1–C-2, hydroxylation of C-17 or C-21, or fluorination of C-6, C-9, or C-12 (representative glucocorticoid structures appear in Figure 20–2). Mineralocorticoid activity is decreased by hydroxylation or methylation of C-16. Synthetic analogues of hydrocortisone are derivatives of bovine cholic acid or sapogenins from the Lily family. Synthetic glucocorticoids, in addition to having a greater anti-inflammatory and a lesser mineralocorticoid effect per mg than has cortisol, generally differ from hydrocortisone by binding less to plasma proteins, having a longer duration of action, and being more expensive. Prednisone and prednisolone are the least expensive synthetic glucocorticoids, have an intermediate duration of action, can be administered on an alternate-day program to successfully minimize hypothalamic-pituitary-adrenal (H-P-A) axis suppression, and have little mineralocorticoid effect.[43] Prednisone and prednisolone are the most frequently prescribed orally administered glucocorticoids. It is difficult to justify the routine use of more potent, more expensive glucocorticoids for systemic effects.

The possibility of adverse effects from glucocorticoid therapy is directly proportional to their potency, dosage, duration of action, duration of administration, and systemic absorption. Potency is an inherent quality of each glucocorticoid and a reflection of the dose used. The duration of action

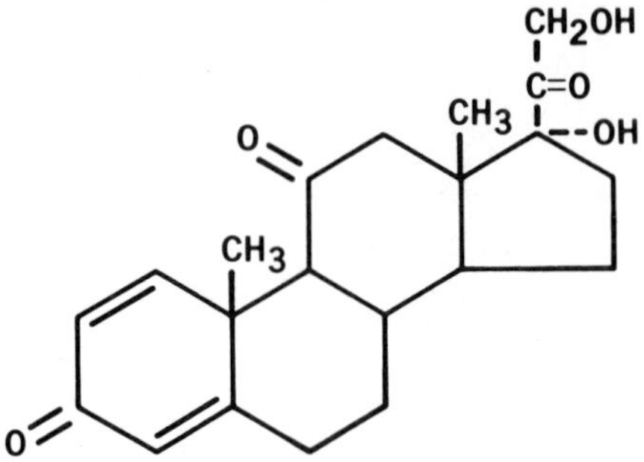

Prednisone

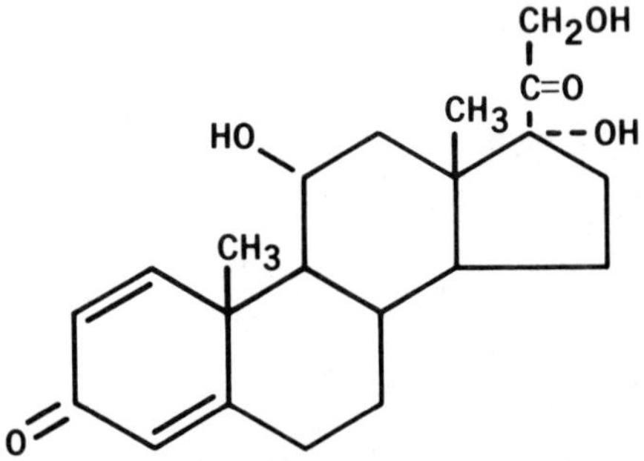

Prednisolone

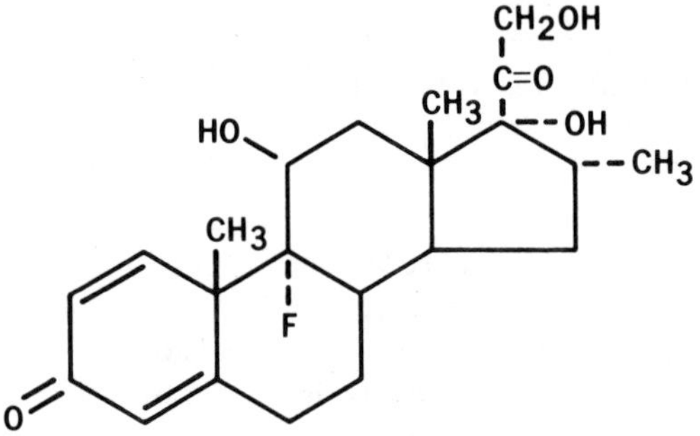

Dexamethasone

Fig. 20–2. Synthetic glucocorticoids.

is affected by the body's ability to metabolize and eliminate the steroid, the dose used, and the rate of absorption. The amount of systemic absorption varies with the route of administration.

Relative Potencies

The relative potencies of various glucocorticoids based on anti-inflammatory effects are listed in Table 20–2. Mineralocorticoid effects of some glucocorticoids may cause adverse effects in patients with certain conditions such as edema and congestive heart failure.

Table 20-2.   Relative Anti-Inflammatory and Mineralocorticoid Potency of Common Glucocorticoids Administered Systemically

Glucocorticoid	Anti-inflammatory Potency (per mg)	Equivalent Dose (mg)	Mineralocorticoid Potency (per mg)
Cortisone	0.8	25	0.8
Hydrocortisone	1.0	20	1.0
Prednisone	4.0	5.0	0.25
Prednisolone	4.0	5.0	0.25
Methylprednisolone	5.0	4.0	0*
Triamcinolone	5.0	4.0	0*
Paramethasone	10.0	2.0	0*
Flumethasone	15.0	1.5	0*
Dexamethasone	30.0	0.75	0*
Betamethasone	35.0	0.6	0*
Fludrocortisone†	10.0		400

* Capable of depleting normal body sodium by induced diuresis.
† An oral mineralocorticoid.

Duration of Action

As with all hormones, the serum half-life of glucocorticoids does not directly correlate with the metabolic duration of their effect. Serum half-lives of nearly all glucocorticoids are within 1 to 3 hours when standard anti-inflammatory doses are used. For practical purposes, glucocorticoids used for systemic effects are classified into three categories—short-, intermediate-, and long-acting, based on their duration of metabolic effects (Table 20–3). Four to five biologic half-lives must lapse before more than 95% of an administered dose of glucocorticoid is eliminated from the body.[12]

The rate of absorption needed to reach and maintain peak systemic effects ranges from minutes for water-soluble esters of glucocorticoids given intravenously to weeks for poorly soluble esters of glucocorticoids given intramuscularly. Examples of glucocortical esters with long duration of effects include methylprednisolone acetate, which in a dose of 2.5 mg/kg body weight in the dog suppresses the adrenal cortex for at least 5 weeks, and triamcinolone acetonide, which in a dose of 0.22 mg/kg body weight in the dog suppresses the adrenal cortex for about 4 weeks.[9, 29, 30] Steroid esters, their relative solubility in water, and the duration of the steroids' release are listed in Table 20–4. The duration of glucocorticoid effects can be decreased by concomitant treatment with hepatic enzyme inducers such as phenobarbital, organochlorines (chlorinated hydrocarbons), phenylbutazone, or phenytoin. The systemic absorption and deleterious effects of glucocorticoids used topically, intralesionally, or by intra-articular injection are slight when conservative doses are used.

Topical glucocorticoids do have the potential of causing adverse systemic effects when given in large amounts. One study in 5- to 7-kg dogs treated with 10% prednisolone acetate ophthalmic solution showed that the adre-

Table 20–3.   Relative Metabolic Duration of Effects for Common Glucocorticoids*

Short-acting (biologic half-life, <12 hours in humans†)
Cortisone
Hydrocortisone
Intermediate-acting (biologic half-life, 12 to 36 hours in humans†)
Prednisone
Prednisolone
Methylprednisone
Triamcinolone (up to 48 hours in humans†)
Long-acting (biologic half-life, >48 hours in humans†)
Dexamethasone
Betamethasone

* Duration of effect is lengthened with increasing dosage.
† Duration of effect may be shorter in dogs and cats.

nocortical response to stimulation with ACTH was suppressed after 2 weeks of treatment using 4 mg of prednisolone daily.[41] Prednisolone acetate is lipid soluble and is readily absorbed by the cornea and conjunctiva. Extra-adrenal effects were also detected by demonstration of excessive storage of hepatic glycogens with the glucagon stimulation test. Succinate or phosphate esters do not penetrate the cornea well, whereas alcoholic forms of ophthalmic glucocorticoids are absorbed even more effectively than acetate esters.

See also references 2, 24, 39, and 45.

CLINICAL USES AND RECOMMENDED DOSAGES FOR GLUCOCORTICOIDS

There are four basic indications for glucocorticoid therapy, each requiring a different dosage. The four basic indications are replacement (of physiologic amounts), anti-inflammation, immunosuppression, and reduction of cerebrospinal edema.

Table 20–4.   Steroid Esters, Compounds, or Vehicles, Solubility, and
*Duration of Steroid Release from Intramuscular Injection

Ester Compound or Vehicle	Relative Solubility (in Water)	Duration of Release	Intravenous Administration
Succinate	Very soluble	Minutes	Yes
Hemisuccinate	Very soluble	Minutes	Yes
Phosphate	Very soluble	Minutes	Yes
Polyethylene glycol	Soluble	Minutes to hours	Yes
Acetate	Moderately insoluble	Days to weeks	No
Diacetate	Moderately insoluble	Days to weeks	No
Acetonide	Markedly insoluble	Weeks	No
Hexacetonide	Markedly insoluble	Weeks	No
Pivalate	Markedly insoluble	Weeks	No
Diproprionate	Markedly insoluble	Weeks	No

Replacement glucocorticoid therapy is necessary to treat hypoadrenocorticism. The normal quantity of cortisol (hydrocortisone) and corticosterone produced by normal dogs is about 1.0 mg/kg body weight/day, the equivalent of 0.25 mg/kg body weight/day of prednisone or prednisolone. If replacement doses of short-acting or intermediate-acting glucocorticoids are used in normal dogs, the administered glucocorticoid will cause inhibition of the production of ACTH, eventual atrophy of the zona fasciculata and the zona reticularis, and decreased production of endogenous glucocorticoids. In stressed animals, decreased ACTH levels and adrenocortical atrophy do not necessarily occur because the negative feedback by glucocorticoids can be overridden by other stimuli for the production of ACTH. Adverse effects on cells outside the hypothalamic-pituitary-adrenal (H-P-A) axis do not occur. The patient's ability to respond to acute stress with an increased production of endogenous glucocorticoids depends on whether adrenocortical atrophy occurred before the acute stress took place. Atrophy of the adrenal cortex resulting from replacement or greater dosages of glucocorticoid is called *iatrogenic secondary hypoadrenocorticism.*

Pharmacologic (supraphysiologic) doses are necessary to suppress inflammation, to suppress immunity, to treat cerebrospinal edema, and perhaps to treat shock. Amounts required to suppress inflammation are less than those necessary to suppress immunity or to treat cerebrospinal edema or shock. Initial anti-inflammatory dosages of prednisone or prednisolone are approximately 0.5 to 1.0 mg/kg body weight/day. The patient's ability to respond adequately to vaccinations while receiving anti-inflammatory doses of glucocorticoids is not impaired, but anamnestic responses may be blunted. If the administration of anti-inflammatory or higher doses of glucocorticoids is extended longer than 2 weeks, tissues outside the H-P-A axis, such as adipose tissue, muscle, and liver, can become adversely affected. The condition with extra-adrenal adverse effects caused by glucocorticoid therapy is called *iatrogenic hyperadrenocorticism.* Iatrogenic hyperadrenocorticism is likely to occur at the same time as iatrogenic secondary hypoadrenocorticism, but in the stressed patient treated with glucocorticoids, it is possible that the H-P-A axis may not be suppressed at the same time that extra-adrenal adverse effects are occurring because of an adaptive inhibition of the suppressive effects of glucocorticoids. Anti-inflammatory doses of the glucocorticoids are also effective in controlling inhalant allergies. Glucocorticoids inhibit the release of histamine, vasodilation, capillary permeability, kinin's actions, and the production of prostaglandins.

Glucocorticoids are often used to suppress immunity and control immune-mediated diseases such as systemic lupus erythematosus, idiopathic thrombocytopenia, pemphigus complex, and others.[53] Different aspects of immunity are affected by different doses of glucocorticoids.[14] Nonspecific immunomechanisms such as trapping and processing of foreign bacteria by macrophages are suppressed by anti-inflammatory doses of glucocorticoids. Neutrophils are stimulated to be released from bone marrow, but margination is inhibited. Glucocorticoids decrease oxidative metabolism in neutrophils. Cell-mediated immunity, inhibition of complement action, and humoral immunity are little affected by anti-inflammatory doses of glucocorticoids. Immunosuppression of cell-mediated immunity, inhibition of complement action, and inhibition of humoral immunity require 2 to 4 mg/kg body weight/day of prednisone or prednisolone.

T-lymphocytes are more sensitive to glucocorticoids than are B-lymphocytes. Several days of therapy may be necessary before clinical improvement is noted in a patient with an autoimmune or immune-mediated disease. Two to four weeks may be necessary before serum IgG levels decrease. Immunosuppressive doses of glucocorticoids are also used as chemotherapy for lymphoreticular neoplasia because of their antimitotic effects on lymphoid tissue. Glucocorticoids may have palliative benefits in some nonlymphoreticular neoplasms, especially intracranial neoplasms, since glucocorticoids pass the blood-brain barrier and relieve associated vasogenic cerebral edema.

Some forms of cerebrospinal edema may be reduced by doses of glucocorticoids that exceed the amounts necessary for anti-inflammation and immunosuppression.[21, 48] Effectiveness has been shown for glucocorticoids in the short-term treatment of interstitial cerebral edema such as occurs in patients with hydrocephalus and tumor-associated vasogenic cerebral edema. Evidence is lacking for the efficacy of glucocorticoid therapy for traumatic cerebral edema or cytotoxic cerebral edema. Recommended dosage for cerebrospinal edema is 15 mg/kg body weight of prednisone or prednisolone. The dosage is repeated as necessary every 8 hours until improvement is apparent. Because dexamethasone does not retain sodium and because of its potency per mg, it is more frequently used (in a dose of 2 mg/kg body weight).

Glucocorticoid therapy may decrease the mortality associated with septic shock by, at least in part, decreasing activation of complement, binding with endotoxin, and inhibiting platelet aggregation.[8, 58] However, in 1981 the Food and Drug Administration removed septic shock as an indication for hydrocortisone because of insufficient proof of efficacy. Evidence obtained experimentally suggests that there may be benefits to glucocorticoid therapy in treating other forms of shock.[15, 18, 19, 34]

To be effective in the treatment of shock, glucocorticoids must be administered at the time of the onset of shock or as early as possible after the onset of shock.[52] They must also be administered with other forms of conventional shock therapy, such as the administration of fluids. Glucocorticoids for the treatment of shock are intravenously administered in large dosages (for example, 40 mg of prednisolone sodium succinate/kg body weight). Administration of glucocorticoids is repeated as necessary, usually every 2.5 to 3 hours.[26] The dosages for replacement, as well as for anti-inflammatory, anti-immunologic, anticerebrospinal edema, and anti-shock therapies, are summarized in Table 20–5.

See also reference 24.

Table 20–5. Basic Indications for Glucocorticoids and Required Dosages

Indication	Initial Required Doses of Prednisone or Prednisolone
Glucocorticoid replacement	0.25 mg/kg body weight/day
Anti-inflammatory (anti-allergic) treatment	0.5–1.0 mg/kg body weight/day
Immunosuppression*	2–4 mg/kg body weight/day
Reduction of cerebrospinal edema	15 mg/kg body weight as necessary†

* Immunosuppressive doses are also used as hormonal chemotherapy for some neoplasias.
† Dexamethasone is more frequently used at an equivalent dose of 2 mg/kg body weight.

PLANNING RATIONAL GLUCOCORTICOID THERAPY

Assessment of the Risk to Benefit Ratio

Regardless of the dose or duration of glucocorticoids used, there are potential hazards. The first consideration before instituting glucocorticoid therapy in a patient is whether the disease to be treated has more potential hazards than the potential hazards of the glucocorticoid therapy being considered. The risks of drug therapy should never exceed the risk of the disease being treated.

Selection of Glucocorticoids and the Appropriate Method of Administration

The prime considerations in selecting the form of glucocorticoid to be used are to determine which route of administration is necessary, which form of glucocorticoid is the least expensive, and whether mineralocorticoid properties could create a problem. If the patient's condition necessitates intravenous administration, a glucocorticoid with a water-soluble ester or in a water-soluble vehicle should be chosen (see Table 20–4). If the patient's condition allows oral administration, the least expensive oral glucocorticoids should be chosen since there is no appreciable difference in the gastrointestinal absorption rates of glucocorticoids (prednisone and prednisolone are the least expensive oral glucocorticoids). The potential adverse effects of prednisone's or prednisolone's mineralocorticoid properties should be considered only if large doses are necessary or edematous disease is present. Water-soluble forms of glucocorticoids may be administered intramuscularly or subcutaneously if the patient's condition or temperament rule out the oral route of administration.

Moderate to markedly insoluble (repositol) forms of glucocorticoids administered intramuscularly have few justifiable indications in veterinary medicine. Their risk to benefit ratio is too high. One 20-mg, intramuscular injection of methylprednisolone acetate much more effectively suppresses the H-P-A axis in 2 weeks than does the oral administration of 40 mg of methylprednisone, divided and administered daily. Such an oral regime is especially safe if given on an alternate-day schedule for 2 weeks. Repositol glucocorticoids are ideal for intra-articular, intralesional, or subconjunctival methods of local administration because the glucocorticoid is released slowly into the local area. With intra-articular, intralesional, or subconjunctival administration, the required dose is small, and the injection is often sequestered.

The systemic distribution and effects of repositol glucocorticoids administered intra-articularly, intralesionally, or subconjunctivally are thought to be little to none. However, when repositol glucocorticoids are deposited in a vascular tissue such as skeletal muscle, and when dosages are used that produce systemic effects, there is the potential for a maximal, constant suppression of the H-P-A axis and no control over its rate or frequency of release into the systemic circulation. The only valid justifications for the use of intramuscular repositol glucocorticoid therapy are lack of owner compliance with other forms of administration or a fractious patient.

The topical, intralesional, intra-articular, or subconjunctival administration of glucocorticoids should be used in place of oral or injectable preparations of glucocorticoids whenever possible to minimize systemic adverse effects. In increasing order of corticosteroid delivery rates to the tissues are the following topical glucocorticoid vehicles: ointments, creams, lotions, foams, gels, and solutions. The selection of synthetic glucocorticoid type, its concentration, its vehicle, and its frequency of administration are based on personal preference, cosmetic considerations, relative expense, and clinical trial and error.

Local absorption of topical corticosteroids can be facilitated, as much as 100-fold, by occlusion with plastic wraps. One method is to apply a corticosteroid cream to a lesion that can be wrapped and tolerated by the patient. A plastic wrapping used to store food is adequate. The lesions only should be covered with plastic. A light gauze and tape bandage is then used to hold the plastic in place. It is best to keep occlusive bandages on the lesion for 12 hours, and then remove the bandages for 12 hours to reduce the risk of occlusion folliculitis and bacterial infection.

Intralesional or sublesional therapy is practical whenever anti-inflammation is desired in a few small external lesions. Intralesional administration is best done by using a tuberculin syringe and intradermal gauge (23 to 25 gauge) needles and injecting up to 0.1 ml per injection site. Larger quantities produce pain and can damage tissue from pressure necrosis. Sublesional injections are practical when larger quantities and fewer injections are desired. High concentrations of relatively insoluble preparations of glucocorticoids should be avoided because of the risk of systemic effects or atrophy of normal tissue. A rule of thumb is to use up to 0.1 ml/cm². Triamcinolone acetonide (Vetalog) in a dose of 2 mg/ml is safe and effective.

The intra-articular administration of glucocorticoids should only be done using a relatively insoluble form of glucocorticoid. Only the joint that has no radiographic evidence of erosion or evidence by arthrocentesis of infection should be injected. One acceptable form and dose of glucocorticoid is triamcinolone acetonide (Kenalog) in a dose of 2.5 to 5.0 mg/joint. Potential hazards are infection, arthropathy, and crystal-injection synovitis.

The subconjunctival injection of relatively insoluble glucocorticoids can have distinct advantages over topical ocular, oral, or parenteral administration in treating some inflammatory ocular diseases. Recommended concentrations of glucocorticoids (40 mg/ml) exceed those recommended for intralesional cutaneous administration. Injected quantities are usually less than 0.25 ml (dose range, 2.5 to 10 mg). The formation of granuloma from the vehicle can result at the site of subconjunctival glucocorticoid injections.

Choice of the Most Appropriate Frequency and Duration of Administration

The most appropriate frequency of administration of parenteral glucocorticoids depends mostly on the duration of effects. The duration of effects varies with the glucocorticoid, its ester, compound, or vehicle, the patient, and the patient's condition. The duration of the administration of glucocorticoids should always be as short as possible. Anticipated duration of treatment is a subjective judgment based on the clinician's experience and the patient's condition.

Since oral glucocorticoids are recommended for conditions requiring more than a few days of systemic effects, oral glucocorticoid therapy has the greatest risk of causing adrenal and extra-adrenal adverse effects. Except during some stressful conditions, any amount of any oral glucocorticoid will suppress the H-P-A axis within 1 week of daily treatment. Greater doses or more frequent administrations are more suppressive. Extra-adrenal adverse effects should not occur unless doses of glucocorticoids exceed equivalent physiologic amounts. Using anti-inflammatory doses, extra-adrenal adverse effects become evident within 2 weeks of daily treatment.

In the early 1960s, it was reported that, in humans, considerable reduction of the risk of suppression of the H-P-A axis could be achieved by administering oral glucocorticoids only after the metabolic duration of effects of the last dose had dissipated and there had been a short period of recovery for the H-P-A axis.[35] The safety of intermittent (alternate-day) oral glucocorticoid therapy has been established in the dog.[10] With intermediate-acting glucocorticoids, administration of anti-inflammatory doses once every 48 hours produces little suppression of the H-P-A axis. For example, a dose of 10 mg of prednisone given every other day for 2 weeks in a 10-kg dog produces much less suppression of the H-P-A axis than 5 mg every day for 2 weeks.

By convention, glucocorticoid therapy is usually terminated by tapering the dose to the amount necessary for replacement or less before total withdrawal. Objective evidence that dose tapering is necessary is lacking.

Guidelines for rational oral glucocorticoid therapy are listed in Table 20–6. Instructions to the owner should be as simple as possible. It is important to make the owner aware of the need to use the lowest possible dose for the shortest possible time.

Precautions Taken in Treatment

There are no absolute contraindications to glucocorticoid therapy, because many conditions requiring glucocorticoid therapy are more serious than the possible adverse effects of glucocorticoids (for example, hypoadrenocortical shock in a patient with viral keratitis should be treated with glucocorticoids since the risk of death from shock outweighs the risk of blindness). However, several conditions do require special consideration—namely, whether glucocorticoid therapy has an advantageous risk to benefit ratio. In some situations, glucocorticoid therapy is still the best treatment the clinician has to offer, but the precaution may warrant reconsidering the type, dose, or form of glucocorticoid therapy. Some precautions requiring special consideration are listed in Table 20–7.

Glucocorticoid therapy is especially hazardous during conditions such as immaturity, bone healing, protein-losing nephropathies, protein-losing enteropathies, diabetes mellitus, and muscle wasting diseases because glucocorticoids inhibit growth and reconstructive anabolism. Survival time is decreased in patients whose amyloidosis is being treated with glucocorticoids.

Table 20–6. Guidelines for Rational Oral Glucocorticoid Therapy in Pharmacologic Doses

---

Short-term therapy (less than 2 weeks)

Establish the necessity of systemic glucocorticoid therapy and consider precautions.

Use an inexpensive intermediate-acting glucocorticoid (prednisone or prednisolone).

Initiate therapy within the appropriate dose range and administer drug in divided doses more than once daily.

Continue initial dose and frequency of administration until condition is controlled for at least 24 hours (usually 4 to 7 days).

Reduce dose at least 50% and administer intermediate-acting glucocorticoid only once daily. If there is no relapse in the condition being treated after the patient has been on the reduced dose for 4 to 7 days, attempt discontinuation of therapy.

Long-term therapy (longer than 2 weeks)

Initiate treatment as if for short-term therapy (as directed above).

Attempt alternate-day therapy by first titrating daily dose to lowest possible single dose per day, then double that dose and give only every other day.

Always try to determine lowest possible dose, no matter whether the patient is on daily therapy or alternate-day therapy.

Try adjunct therapy (antihistamines, salicylates) to keep glucocorticoid dose as low as possible.

If the condition being treated is in remission for at least 1 to 2 weeks, attempt gradual withdrawal of therapy.

Liver disease can pose a special hazard with glucocorticoid therapy since steroid blood transport or steroid inactivation may be affected so that glucocorticoids are more available to target cell receptors for longer than usual periods. Glucocorticoids can also directly cause hepatopathy or aggravate an existing hepatopathy.[36]

Glucocorticoids inhibit the normal inflammatory process, thus suppressing the inactivation, phagocytosis, sequestration, or other immunologic processing of infectious agents. Glucocorticoid therapy may unleash certain infectious disease processes, particularly fungal or viral keratitis, generalized demodectic mange, or chronic bacterial, viral (feline leukemia virus and feline herpesvirus), and deep fungal infections. The administration of glucocorticoids for longer than 6 months to control skin diseases in dogs has been associated with an increased incidence of urinary tract infection, especially in female dogs.[28] Congestive heart failure may be aggravated by glucocorticoid therapy because of the possibility of increased intravascular volume caused by facilitated extracellular shifts of water, sodium retention, and polydipsia.

The fetus may be adversely affected by glucocorticoid therapy during pregnancy. Temporary adrenocortical atrophy is likely, and cleft palate, as reported in rodents and rabbits, is possible. Synthetic glucocorticoids methylated at C-16 (dexamethasone, flumethasone, and betamethasone) given during the last trimester of gestation can induce parturition in the horse, cow, sheep, and human. There is some risk that fetal resorption, abortion, or premature parturition might be induced in the gravid bitch or queen.

Glucocorticoids tend to cause or aggravate psychoses in approximately 20% of humans treated systemically with glucocorticoids. Psychotic manifestations of aggression and hair chewing have been reported in dogs with excesses of endogenous and exogenous glucocorticoids.

Table 20–7. Conditions Requiring Special Considerations before Therapy With Glucocorticoids Is Initiated

Immaturity of the patient
Liver disease
Fungal or viral keratitis
Diabetes mellitus
Muscle wasting
Some protein-losing nephropathies and enteropathies
Congestive heart failure
Healing bone lesions
Chronic bacterial or deep fungal infections
Pregnancy
Psychoses
Gastrointestinal ulcerations
Amyloidosis
Generalized demodectic mange
Acute pancreatitis

Glucocorticoid therapy must be given with special precaution to patients with gastrointestinal ulcerations because fatal colonic perforations have been attributed to glucocorticoid therapy in dogs.[6, 13, 54] Most of the affected dogs have been dachshunds over 5 years of age being treated for intervertebral disk disease. Although dachshunds as a breed have a predisposition for developing intervertebral disk disease, they are probably not predisposed to glucocorticoid-induced colonic perforations. Male dogs are affected more often than female dogs. The risk of perforation of the colon correlates with the severity of the spinal cord injury and the duration of treatment, but not with the dose of glucocorticoid. It has been proposed that spinal cord injury alters the autonomic balance, resulting in decreased mucosal perfusion.

About 15% of dogs with disk disease develop gastrointestinal hemorrhage if treated with high doses of glucocorticoids, and 2% may die from perforation of the colon. Gastric ulcers are also possible because of glucocorticoid-induced increases in plasma gastrin levels, gastric acid and pepsin secretion, decreased gastrointestinal production and viscosity of mucus, and decreased proliferation of mucosal cells. Cimetidine, intestinal protectants, and systemic antibiotics have been recommended for patients at high risk for gastrointestinal ulceration or perforation caused by glucocorticoid therapy. Pancreatic secretions increase in viscosity with glucocorticoid therapy; this can cause or exacerbate acute pancreatitis.[37, 40]

Anti-inflammatory doses of glucocorticoids do not significantly alter the canine patient's ability to respond to distemper vaccinations. Resulting protection withstands challenge with distemper virus.[38] Normal serum titers to rabies vaccinations occur in dogs being treated with anti-inflammatory doses of glucocorticoids.[17] Even so, protection to challenge with rabies virus may not be adequate. It is advisable to avoid treatment with glucocorticoids that is also concurrent with vaccinations whenever possible. Factors to consider during the planning of glucocorticoid therapy are reviewed in Table 20–8.

IATROGENIC SECONDARY HYPOADRENOCORTICISM

Iatrogenic secondary hypoadrenocorticism is adrenocortical atrophy resulting from systemic glucocorticoid therapy (Fig. 20–3). Adrenocortical atrophy initially results from inhibition of the production of ACTH, but large doses of potent glucocorticoids given over extended periods may directly cause adrenocortical atrophy of even the zona arcuata. Adrenocor-

Table 20–8.   Considerations in Planning Rational Glucocorticoid Therapy

1. What is the risk to benefit ratio?
2. Which glucocorticoid and which form?
3. What is the most appropriate frequency and duration of administration?
4. Do any precautions exist?

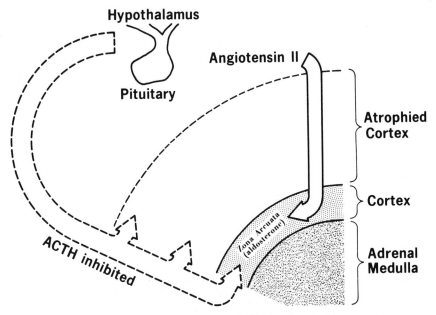

Fig. 20-3. Secondary hypoadrenocorticism. ACTH = adrenocorticotropic hormone.

tical atrophy may result from the administration of all dose ranges, including replacement doses, if therapy is continued for 1 week and no allowance is made for the recovery of the H-P-A axis between dosage administrations. Repositol intramuscular injections of glucocorticoids cause maximum suppression of the H-P-A axis because exogenous glucocorticoids are constantly released into the systemic circulation until the entire repositol injection is absorbed. Iatrogenic secondary hypoadrenocorticism can also result from prolonged administration of megestrol acetate or medroxyprogesterone acetate.[11]

Clinical signs of iatrogenic secondary hypoadrenocorticism do not appear until therapy with glucocorticoids is withdrawn (Fig. 20-4). Then signs are mild under basal conditions because minute amounts of glucocorticoids are necessary for permissive effects on metabolic functions. There may be mental depression and anorexia. If glucocorticoids are again administered during existing atrophy of the adrenal cortex, marked diuresis from intracellular to extracellular fluid shifts may occur. During stressful conditions, glucocorticoid deficiency caused by iatrogenic secondary hypoadrenocorticism can lead to vascular collapse, gastrointestinal hemorrhage, and shock.

The diagnosis of secondary hypoadrenocorticism is based on an inadequate plasma cortisol response to stimulation with ACTH. It has been recommended that the administration of small intravenous doses of 1 μg/kg body weight of cosyntropin is the best means of evaluating the suppression of the adrenocortices by glucocorticoid therapy.[31] Plasma

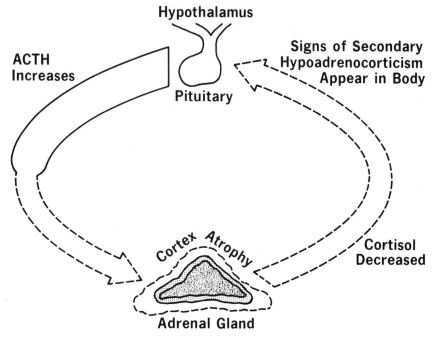

Fig. 20–4. Feedback immediately following withdrawal of corticosteroid therapy. ACTH = adrenocorticotropic hormone.

corticoids should be 6 μg/dl or more 1 hour after the intravenous administration of cosyntropin.

Iatrogenic secondary hypoadrenocorticism always occurs with iatrogenic secondary hyperadrenocorticism (the effect of excessive levels of glucocorticoids on extra-adrenal tissues) whenever daily systemic therapy with glucocorticoids lasts more than 2 weeks at pharmacologic dose levels.

See also references 1, 7, 10, 49, 51, 55, and 56.

IATROGENIC HYPERADRENOCORTICISM

Iatrogenic hyperadrenocorticism occurs when extra-adrenal tissues are persistently exposed to greater than equivalent physiologic amounts of exogenous glucocorticoids (Fig. 20–5). Possible adverse effects associated with iatrogenic hyperadrenocorticism are listed in Table 20–9. Myopathy, glucose intolerance, and osteoporosis may be more common in iatrogenic hyperadrenocorticism than spontaneous hyperadrenocorticism. Cats may be less susceptible than dogs in developing iatrogenic hyperadrenocorticism.[46,47] Cats have not been noted to develop alopecia to the degree of baldness that occurs in dogs affected by excessive glucocorticoids. Cats may not develop polyuria until hyperglycemia and glucosuria occur from steroid diabetes. Since cats have an extremely short serum half-life of alkaline phosphatase, elevations of serum alkaline phosphatase (SAP) are not a reliable indication of iatrogenic hyperadrenocorticism as in dogs.

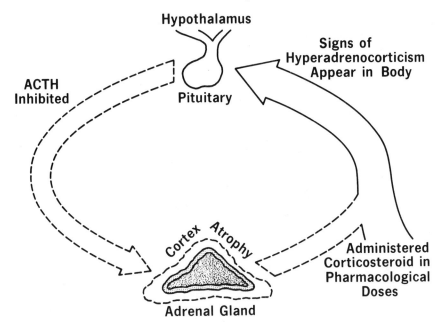

Fig. 20–5. Feedback during systemic corticosteroid therapy. ACTH = adrenocorticotropic hormone.

There are species differences in susceptibility to the adverse effects of glucocorticoids. Humans, monkeys, guinea pigs, and cats are considered relatively "glucocorticoid resistant." Rabbits and rodents are relatively "glucocorticoid sensitive." Dogs are considered "intermediately sensitive" to adverse effects. Some clinical indications of glucocorticoids' adverse effects may be masked by glucocorticoids themselves. For example, the use of glucocorticoids may allow infectious agents to disseminate even while therapy is suppressing pain, fever, and visual signs of inflammation.

The most reliable findings on physical examination indicative of iatrogenic hyperadrenocorticism are thinning of the hair coat on the caudal aspects of the hind legs and in the lateral lumbar area of the abdomen, a pendulous abdomen, inelasticity of the abdominal skin, and increased fat depots on the caudolateral gluteal aspects near the base of the tail. An enlarged clitoris does not occur in iatrogenic hyperadrenocorticism, but it may occur in spontaneous hyperadrenocorticism. The administration of glucocorticoids may cause glucocorticoid myopathy. Synthetic glucocorticoids, particularly those fluorinated at the 9 α-position, have most often been responsible.

Routine laboratory changes to be expected are lymphopenia and elevated SAP values.[3] SAP values are a reasonable indirect measurement of the severity of iatrogenic hyperadrenocorticism in dogs and can be used to monitor extra-adrenal recovery when glucocorticoid therapy is being withdrawn. Levels of SAP and, to a lesser extent, alanine aminotransferase

Table 20–9. Possible Adverse Effects Associated With Iatrogenic Hyperadrenocorticism

Poor wound healing
Excessive appetite
Diarrhea
Polyuria and polydipsia
Alopecia
Obesity
Acne
Muscle weakness and atrophy
Edema
Hepatomegaly
Psychoses and changes in temperament
Easy bruising
Suppressed growth
Glucose intolerance
Fasting hyperlipidemia
Seizures
Acute pancreatitis
Immunosuppression and superinfections
Colonic perforations
Infertility
Birth defects
Abortion
Osteoporosis
Aseptic necrosis of bone*
Benign intracranial hypertension*
Posterior subcapsular cataracts*
Glaucoma*

* Unobserved or unreported effects in companion animals.

(SALT), gamma-glutamyl transpeptidase, and bromsulphalein (BSP) retention may remain elevated 6 weeks after the withdrawal of short-term (less than 2 weeks) glucocorticoid therapy in the dog.[4] Blood ammonia, serum leucine amino peptidase, and serum arginase are not increased by glucocorticoid therapy. Plasma concentrations of triiodothyronine (T_3) and thyroxine (T_4) can be lowered by glucocorticoid therapy.[59] The glucagon response test (in which glucagon is administered in an intravenous dose of 0.14 mg/kg body weight), as determined by blood glucose elevations, may show exaggerated glycogenolysis if iatrogenic hyperadrenocorticism exists.[41] A more objective parameter used to evaluate recovery, the measurement of ACTH-stimulated cortisol levels, should be relied on as an indication of the extent of hypoadrenocorticism. ACTH-stimulated cortisol levels found by radioimmunoassay to be less than 6 μg/dl are definitive for hypoadrenocorticism in dogs, cats, or horses.

When presented with a patient who has been treated with glucocorticoids, is exhibiting clinical signs, and has routine laboratory findings consistent with hyperadrenocorticism, one must not assume that the changes are all due to glucocorticoid therapy. It is not uncommon for patients with spontaneous hyperadrenocorticism to have been placed on therapy with glucocorticoids because of misdiagnosis or as treatment for an unrelated disease. If the signs of Cushing's-like syndrome are present in a female dog who is also exhibiting clitoral hypertrophy, the patient most likely has spontaneous Cushing's-like syndrome. Spontaneous Cushing's-like syndrome cannot be definitively differentiated from iatrogenic hyperadrenocorticism without the measurement of plasma cortisol levels or withdrawal from glucocorticoid therapy.

See also references 2, 3, 5, 6, 16, 20, 25, 32, 33, 42, 44, 45, 50, and 57.

TREATMENT OF IATROGENIC SECONDARY HYPOADRENOCORTICISM AND IATROGENIC HYPERADRENOCORTICISM

The goal of treatment for iatrogenic secondary hypoadrenocorticism is to re-establish normal secretion of adrenocorticotropic hormone (ACTH) and to restore completely the ability of the adrenal glands to respond to ACTH. With iatrogenic hyperadrenocorticism, the initial goal of treatment is to recover normal function of extra-adrenal cells. The means of accomplishing both these goals are to reduce the amount of glucocorticoids used and to attempt withdrawal of therapy in a way that does not leave the patient deficient in both exogenous and endogenous glucocorticoids. Recovery from iatrogenic hyperadrenocorticism can begin once doses of administered glucocorticoids approach replacement levels. It is best to allow 1 to 2 months of extra-adrenal cellular recovery before further withdrawal is attempted.

Once clinical signs of iatrogenic hyperadrenocorticism have disappeared, the daily administration of replacement doses can be discontinued and replaced by double replacement doses as a single administration on alternate days. The alternate-day dose is gradually reduced and all glucocorticoid therapy discontinued 1 month after the beginning of alternate-day therapy. The patient's condition (for which the therapy with glucocorticoids was begun) occasionally requires that some glucocorticoid therapy continue. In that case, the lowest alternate-day dose should be gradually determined and used for continuing therapy. The recommended program for treating iatrogenic secondary hyperadrenocorticism and iatrogenic hyperadrenocorticism is shown in Table 20–10. This program may be unnecessarily long to treat mild cases or hazardously short to treat severe cases, and the clinician should use personal judgment to adapt the recommended program to specific patients.

Recovery of the H-P-A axis occurs first in the recovery of the hypothalamic-pituitary secretion, then in the adrenocortical basal secretion, and finally in normal adrenocortical stress responsiveness. Therapy with ACTH does not hasten the recovery of the H-P-A axis. In gel, ACTH stimulates the production of cortisol and adrenal androgen and promotes adrenocortical hyperplasia for less than 12 hours; therefore, if exogenous ACTH therapy is to be effective in causing recovery of adrenocortical atrophy, twice-a-day

Table 20-10.   Recommended Treatment Regimes for Iatrogenic Secondary Hypoadrenocorticism and Iatrogenic Secondary Hyperadrenocorticism

---

Adrenocortical atrophy only (iatrogenic secondary hypoadrenocorticism)
  Administer 0.50 mg/kg body weight/day of prednisone or prednisolone every other morning.

  Taper dose gradually and withdraw treatment after 1 month.

  Revert to daily treatment with 1 to 2 mg/kg body weight/day of prednisone or prednisolone during severe stress.

Extra-adrenal glucocorticoid-induced changes (iatrogenic hyperadrenocorticism)
  Replace current glucocorticoid with prednisone or prednisolone at equivalent doses.

  Taper current dose down to 0.25 mg/kg body weight/day of prednisone or prednisolone over 1 to 2 months.

  If the original condition being treated with glucocorticoids returns before the tapering of the dose to 0.25 mg/kg body weight/day is reached, double the last effective dose and administer on alternate days.

  If the dose of 0.25 mg/kg body weight/day is given without recurrence of the original condition requiring glucocorticoids, maintain patient on 0.25 mg/kg body weight/day for 1 month, then treat adrenocortical atrophy as described above for adrenocortical atrophy.

---

administration of ACTH would be advisable. Repeated treatment with ACTH of animal origin carries the potential for hypersensitivity reactions.

Mineralocorticoid production is initially increased with ACTH treatment. This could cause problems associated with resulting hypertension. In addition, therapy with ACTH does not stimulate the endogenous production of ACTH. If exogenous ACTH therapy is successful in correcting adrenocortical atrophy, premature endogenous glucocorticoid production would slow or inhibit hypothalamic and pituitary recovery; therefore, therapy with ACTH is not recommended for the treatment of iatrogenic hyperadrenocorticism or iatrogenic secondary hypoadrenocorticism.

See also references 23 and 45.

REFERENCES

1. Anderson, D.C.: Corticosteroid overdosage in dogs. N.Z. Vet. J., *16:*18, 1968.
2. Axelrod, L.: Glucocorticoid therapy. Medicine, *55:*39, 1976.
3. Badylak, S.F., and Van Fleet, J.F.: Sequential morphologic and clinicopathologic alterations in dogs with experimentally induced glucocorticoid hepatopathy. Am. J. Vet. Res., *42:*1310, 1981.
4. Badylak, S.F., and Van Fleet, J.F.: Tissue gamma-glutamyl transpeptidase activity and hepatic ultrastructural alterations in dogs with experimentally induced glucocorticoid hepatopathy. Am. J. Vet. Res., *43:*649, 1982.
5. Bagdade, J.D., Porte, D., Jr., and Bierman, E.L.: Steroid-induced lipidemia. A complication of high-dosage corticosteroid therapy. Arch. Intern. Med., *125:*129, 1970.
6. Bellah, J.R.: Colonic perforation after corticosteroid and surgical treatment of intervertebral disk disease in a dog. J. Am. Vet. Med. Assoc., *183:*1002, 1983.
7. Bhargava, A.S., et al.: Effects of intratracheal and oral application of corticosteroids on the adrenal function tests in beagle dogs after ACTH-stimulation. Arch. Toxicol. Suppl., *2:*425, 1979.

8. Bowen, J.M.: Are corticosteroids useful in shock therapy? J. Am. Vet. Med. Assoc., *177:*453, 1980.

9. Braun, J.P., et al.: Haematological and biochemical effects of a single intramuscular dose of 6 α-methylprednisolone acetate in the dog. Res. Vet. Sci., *31:*236, 1981.

10. Chastain, C.B., and Graham, C.L.: Adrenocortical suppression in dogs on daily and alternate-day prednisone administration. Am. J. Vet. Res., *40:*936, 1979.

11. Chastain, C.B., Graham, C.L., and Nichols, C.E.: Adrenocortical suppression in cats given megestrol acetate. Am. J. Vet. Res., *42:*2029, 1981.

12. Coppoc, G.L.: Relationship of the dosage form of a corticosteroid to its therapeutic efficacy. J. Am. Vet. Med. Assoc., *183:*1098, 1984.

13. Crawford, L.M., and Wilson, R.C.: Melaena associated with dexamethasone therapy in the dog. J. Small Anim. Pract., *23:*91, 1982.

14. Dale, D.C., Fauci, A.S., and Wolff, S.M.: Daily and alternate-day prednisone: leukocyte kinetics and susceptibility to infections. N. Engl. J. Med., *291:*1154, 1974.

15. Dillon, R., et al.: Experimental hemorrhage in dogs: effects of prednisolone sodium succinate. J. Am. Anim. Hosp. Assoc., *14:*673, 1978.

16. Dillon, A.R., Spano, J.S., and Powers, R.D.: Prednisolone induced hematologic, biochemical, and histologic changes in the dog. J. Am. Anim. Hosp. Assoc., *16:*831, 1980.

17. Enright, J.B., et al.: Effects of corticosteroids on rabies virus infections in various animal species. J. Am. Vet. Med. Assoc., *156:*765, 1970.

18. Ferguson, J.L., et al.: Dexamethasone treatment during hemorrhagic shock: effects independent of increased blood pressure. Am. J. Vet. Res., *39:*825, 1978.

19. Ferguson, J.L., Roesel, O.F., and Bottoms, G.D.: Dexamethasone treatment during hemorrhagic shock: blood pressure, tissue perfusion, and plasma enzymes. Am. J. Vet. Res., *39:*817, 1978.

20. Fittschen, C., and Bellamy, J.E.C.: Prednisone-induced morphologic and chemical changes in the liver of dogs. Vet. Pathol., *21:*399, 1984.

21. Franklin, R.T.: The use of glucocorticoids in treating cerebral edema. Compendium on Continuing Educ. for the Practicing Vet., *6:*442, 1984.

22. Fraser, C.G., Preuss, F.S., and Bigford, W.D.: Adrenal atrophy and irreversible shock associated with cortisone therapy. J. Am. Med. Assoc., *149:*1542, 1952.

23. Graber, A.L., et al.: Natural history of pituitary-adrenal recovery following long-term suppression with corticosteroids. J. Clin. Endocrinol., *25:*11, 1965.

24. Greene, C.E.: Glucocorticoids: their use and misuse in veterinary practice. Vet. Med. Small Anim. Clin., *75:*1821, 1980.

25. Hall, S.S.: Iatrogenic hyperadrenocorticism due to prolonged azium therapy. Southwest. Vet., *26:*62, 1972.

26. Hankes, G.H., et al.: Pharmacokinetics of prednisolone sodium succinate and its metabolites in normovolemic and hypovolemic dogs. Am. J. Vet. Res., *46:*476, 1985.

27. Hench, P.S., et al.: The effects of a hormone of the adrenal cortex (17-hydroxy-11-dehydrocorticosterone, Compound E) and of the pituitary adrenocorticotropic hormone on rheumatoid arthritis. Proceedings of Staff Meeting Mayo Clin., *24:*181, 1949.

28. Ihrke, P.J., et al.: Urinary tract infection associated with long-term corticosteroid administration in dogs with chronic skin diseases. J. Am. Vet. Med. Assoc., *186:*43, 1985.

29. Kemppainen, R.J., Lorenz, M.D., and Thompson, F.N.: Adrenocortical suppression in the dog after a single dose of methylprednisolone acetate. Am. J. Vet. Res., *42:*822, 1981.

30. Kemppainen, R.J., Lorenz, M.D., and Thompson, F.N.: Adrenocortical suppression in the dog given a single intramuscular dose of prednisone or triamcinolone acetonide. Am. J. Vet. Res., *42:*204, 1982.

31. Kemppainen, R.J., and Lorenz, M.D.: Use of a low dose synthetic ACTH challenge test in normal and prednisone-treated dogs. Res. Vet. Sci., *35:*240, 1983.

32. Kemppainen, R.J., et al.: Effects of prednisone on thyroid and gonadal endocrine function in dogs. J. Endocrinol., *96:*293, 1983.

33. Knecht, C.D., Henderson, B., and Richardson, R.C.: Central nervous system depression associated with glucocorticoid ingestion in a dog. J. Am. Vet. Med. Assoc., *173:*91, 1978.

34. Kolata, R.J.: The clinical management of circulatory shock based on pathophysiological patterns. Compendium on Continuing Educ. for the Practicing Vet., *2:*314, 1980.

35. MacGregor, R.R., et al.: Alternate-day prednisone therapy. Evaluation of delayed hypersensitivity responses, control of disease and steroid side effects. N. Engl. J. Med., *280:*1427, 1969.

36. Meyer, D.J.: Prolonged liver test abnormalities and adrenocortical suppression in a dog following a single intramuscular glucocorticoid dose. J. Am. Anim. Hosp. Assoc., *18:*725, 1982.
37. Moore, R.W., and Withrow, S.J.: Gastrointestinal hemorrhage and pancreatitis associated with intervertebral disk disease in the dog. J. Am. Vet. Med. Assoc., *180:*1443, 1982.
38. Nara, P.L., Krakowka, S., and Powers, T.E.: Effects of prednisolone on the development of immune responses to canine distemper virus in beagle pups. Am. J. Vet. Res., *40:*1742, 1979.
39. Newsome, H.H., Turley, G.T., and Kennerly, M.: Bioavailability of synthetic steroids for canine adrenal suppression. J. Surg. Res., *23:*315, 1977.
40. Parent, J.: Effects of dexamethasone on pancreatic tissue and on serum amylase and lipase activities in dogs. J. Am. Vet. Med. Assoc., *180:*743, 1982.
41. Roberts, S.M., et al.: Effect of ophthalmic prednisolone acetate on the canine adrenal gland and hepatic function. Am. J. Vet. Res., *45:*1711, 1984.
42. Rojko, J.L., et al.: Influence of adrenal corticosteroids on the susceptibility of cats to feline leukemia virus infection. Cancer Res., *39:*3789, 1979.
43. Schalm, S.W., Summerskill, W.H.J., and Go, V.L.: Development of radioimmunoassay for prednisone and prednisolone. Mayo Clin. Proc., *51:*761, 1976.
44. Scott, D.W.: Iatrogenic calcinosis cutis in a dog. Vet. Med. Small Anim. Clin., *70:*684, 1976.
45. Scott, D.W., and Greene, C.E.: Iatrogenic secondary adrenocortical insufficiency in dogs. J. Am. Anim. Hosp. Assoc., *10:*555, 1974.
46. Scott, D.W., Kirk, R.W., and Bentinck-Smith, J.: Some effect of short-term methylprednisolone therapy in normal cats. Cornell Vet., *69:*104, 1979.
47. Scott, D.W., Manning, T.O., and Reimers, T.J.: Iatrogenic Cushing's syndrome in the cat. Feline Pract., *12:*30, 1982.
48. Sims, M.H., and Redding, R.W.: The use of dexamethasone in the prevention of cerebral edema in dogs. J. Am. Anim. Hosp. Assoc., *11:*439, 1975.
49. Slone, D.E., et al.: Sodium retention and cortisol (hydrocortisone) suppression caused by dexamethasone and triamcinolone in equids. Am. J. Vet. Res., *44:*280, 1983.
50. Sorjonen, D.C., et al.: Effects of dexamethasone and surgical hypotension on the stomach of dogs: clinical, endoscopic, and pathologic evaluations. Am. J. Vet. Res., *44:*1233, 1983.
51. Spencer, K.B., et al.: Adrenal gland function in dogs given methylprednisolone. Am. J. Vet. Res., *41:*1503, 1980.
52. Spring, C.L., et al.: The effects of high-dose corticosteroids in patients with septic shock: a prospective controlled study. N. Engl. J. Med., *311:*1137, 1984.
53. Strombeck, D.R., and Gribble, D.: Chronic active hepatitis in the dog. J. Am. Vet. Med. Assoc., *173:*380, 1978.
54. Toombs, J.P., et al.: Colonic perforation following neurosurgical procedures and corticosteroid therapy in four dogs. J. Am. Vet. Med. Assoc., *177:*68, 1980.
55. Toutain, P.L., Alvinerie, M., and Ruckebusch, Y.: Pharmacokinetics of dexamethasone and its effect on adrenal gland function in the dog. Am. J. Vet. Res., *44:*212, 1983.
56. Toutain, P.L., et al.: Dexamethasone and prednisolone in the horse: pharmacokinetics and action on the adrenal gland. Am. J. Vet. Res., *45:*1750, 1984.
57. Walker, D.: Diabetes mellitus following steroid therapy in a dog. Vet. Rec., *74:*1543, 1962.
58. White, G.L., et al.: Increased survival with methylprednisolone treatment in canine endotoxic shock. J. Surg. Res., *25:*357, 1978.
59. Woltz, H.H., et al.: Effect of prednisone on thyroid gland morphology and plasma thyroxine and triiodothyronine concentrations in the dog. Am. J. Vet. Res., *44:*2000, 1983.

21

Pheochromocytoma

Pheochromocytoma, which means "dusky-colored tumor" in Greek, is usually a slow-growing, well-encapsulated, red-brown tumor of the adrenal medulla or sympathetic paraganglia.[2] The occurrence of adrenal medullary pheochromocytomas is greatest in older dogs. There is no predisposition for sex or breed. The incidence, based on canine necropsies, is about 0.5% of all dogs given a post-mortem examination. Pheochromocytomas in dogs may be associated with tumors of carotid body and aortic body, non-chromophobe paraganglia. Extra-adrenal pheochromocytomas can occur anywhere along the sympathetic ganglia from the neck to the pelvis. Metastasis is rare, but invasion of the caudal vena cava by pheochromocytomas of the right adrenal gland often occurs.[3, 7, 15, 18]

Pheochromocytomas are most common in the right adrenal. Pheochromocytomas have not been described in cats, but do occasionally occur in older horses.[6, 9, 19] In humans, approximately 10% of pheochromocytomas are familial and associated with tumors of the Amine Precursor Uptake and Decarboxylation cells (APUDomas), especially in the case of multiple endocrine neoplasia (MEN), type II, which, in addition to being a pheochromocytoma, consists of medullary carcinomas of the thyroid and parathyroid hyperplasia. MEN, type II, has been reported in the dog.[13] MEN, type III, consists of medullary carcinomas of the thyroid, neuromas, and pheochromocytoma; it has not been reported in dogs.

Most adrenal medullary pheochromocytomas in dogs are thought benign, except for the occasional invasion of the caudal vena cava. Six percent to ten percent are malignant, although their histologic appearance may look misleadingly benign. A few reports on adrenal medullary pheochromocytomas indicate that canine pheochromocytomas, like human pheochromocytomas, can secrete excessive amounts of catecholamines. The true incidence of excess catecholamine-secreting pheochromocytomas in dogs is not currently known because the clinical signs of excessive catecholamines are vague and secretion may be intermittent. In addition, routine screening of peripheral arterial blood pressure and measurements of urinary catecholamine metabolites, the basis of diagnosis of excessive catecholamine secretion by pheochromocytomas in the human, are unfamiliar to most veterinary clinicians. Pheochromocytomas may also produce peptide hormones such as vasoactive intestinal peptide (VIP), adrenocorticotropic hormone (ACTH), calcitonin, or parathyroid hormone (PTH).

CLINICAL SIGNS, ROUTINE LABORATORY FINDINGS, AND RADIOGRAPHIC FINDINGS

Pheochromocytomas can cause clinical signs by compression or invasion of surrounding structures, especially the caudal vena cava, or by secretion of excessive catecholamines. Clinical signs vary, depending on whether an excess of epinephrine or norepinephrine is predominant. More common possible clinical signs and their causes are listed in Table 21–1.[1] The ability to secrete excessive catecholamines is not related to tumor size. Other clinical signs can include palpable abdominal mass, ascites, flushing of mucous membranes, fever, constipation, paresthesias, and various neurologic abnormalities caused by hypertension or cerebral hemorrhage. Affected horses may sweat excessively. Provocation for the secretion of catecholamines from pheochromocytomas include palpation of the tumor, β-adrenergic blockers, induction of anesthesia, exercise, eating, and exposure to cold temperatures.

In humans, most pheochromocytomas secreting excessive amounts of catecholamines secrete excessive amounts of norepinephrine. Reports on dogs with pheochromocytomas thought to have secreted excessive levels of catecholamines indicate that the clinical signs and post-mortem lesions such as cardiomyopathy, arteriolar sclerosis, and tunica media hyperplasia of arterioles are consistent with an excess of norepinephrine.[11] Nearly all the clinical signs caused by pheochromocytomas secreting excessive levels of norepinephrine are the result of persistent or intermittent hypertension.

Table 21–1.   Possible Clinical Signs Caused by Adrenal Medullary Pheochromocytomas

Compression of surrounding structures
Enlarged caudal superficial epigastric (abdominal) veins
Edema of the caudal extremities
Weakness of the hind legs
Secretion of excessive catecholamines*
Predominant epinephrine-secreting
Hypotension
Noncardiac pulmonary edema
Ventricular arrhythmias
Predominant norepinephrine-secreting
Tachycardia and tachyarrhythmias
Congestive heart failure
Excessive panting
Weakness and trembling
Epistaxis
Seizures
Retinal hemorrhage
Head pressing
Weight loss

* Signs caused by excessive catecholamines may be persistent or intermittent.

Conditions with clinical laboratory findings associated persistently or intermittently with pheochromocytomas secreting excessive amounts of catecholamines include hyperglycemia, polycythemia, and hypertriglyceridemia. Packed cell volumes may be increased as a result of decreased plasma volume or decreased as a result of hemorrhage. Urinalysis may show proteinuria and hematuria.

Radiographic examinations of the abdomen may show an enlarged adrenal shadow or adrenal calcification in about one third of the cases. The left adrenal is more easily seen. The right adrenal is normally covered by the liver. Appreciation of the adrenal enlargement may require tomography, retroperitoneal pneumography, intravenous pyelography, contrast venography of the caudal vena cava, or selective angiography. Nonselective vena caval venography can show a tumor thrombus in about 50% of the cases. Selective angiography is the most potentially dangerous procedure because of the risk of vascular rupture. Gamma camera imaging of the adrenal cortex may be helpful if the cortex has been distorted by medullary enlargement. The preferred isotope for scintigraphy of pheochromocytomas is ^{131}I-metaiodobenzylguanidine. It has a structure resembling norepinephrine and is concentrated in the adrenal medulla. If available, computed tomography (CT) scans of the abdomen may be diagnostically useful.

See also references 6, 8, 14, 16, and 17.

DIAGNOSTIC EXAMINATIONS FOR EXCESS CATECHOLAMINE-SECRETING PHEOCHROMOCYTOMAS

Quantitation of the urinary excretion of catecholamines and their metabolites is the standard screening test for the presence of pheochromocytomas secreting excessive amounts of catecholamines in humans. Frequently, a definitive diagnosis can be made without further tests. If the hypersecretion of catecholamines is intermittent, provocative tests may be required.

In humans, the most diagnostically reliable urine component for adrenal medullary pheochromocytomas secreting excessive amounts of catecholamines is the measurement of total metanephrines. Vanillylmandelic acid (VMA) and, occasionally, fractionated free urine catecholamines and homovanillic acid can be helpful. One clinical approach to diagnosis begins with the measurement of the ratio of urinary total metanephrines to urinary creatinine over a 24-hour period. If the total metanephrines to creatinine ratio exceeds 2.2 μg/mg in humans, urinary VMA and fractionated free catecholamines should be measured. Increased urinary epinephrine levels indicate that the site of excessive production is the adrenal medulla. Increased urinary homovanillic acid is suggestive of malignancy. Unfortunately, only normal VMA values have been reported in the dog (0.6 to 15 mg/24 hr).[12] Urine should be collected for 24 hours in a beaker of 15 ml of 6N HCL. Blood pressure response tests to phentolamine, histamine, tyramine, or glucagon are risky and should be reserved for normotensive patients with equivocal urinary catecholamine and catecholamine metabolite values.

Radioenzymatic assays for plasma epinephrine and norepinephrine have been used successfully in humans to diagnose pheochromocytomas.[4,5] Plasma catecholamine assays are expensive, and repeated sampling or provocative tests with glucagon or suppressive tests with clonidine may be necessary to detect intermittent hypersecretion of catecholamines. If catecholamines are being secreted by a pheochromocytoma, plasma catecholamine levels are not suppressed by clonidine. Clonidine blocks the release of neurogenically mediated catecholamines. With pheochromocytomas, plasma catecholamine levels are clearly increased 1 to 3 minutes after the intravenous administration of glucagon. Normal venous norepinephrine levels in horses are about 120 to 300 pg/ml.[10,20] Current costs of plasma catecholamine assays are nearly twice those of the urinary tests.

TREATMENT

Excision is the only satisfactory treatment for pheochromocytomas. An adrenalectomy is done as takes place for adrenocortical neoplasms. Alpha-methyltyrosine (Demser) is an inhibitor of tyrosine hydroxylase and can be used to control the production of catecholamines before excision of the tumors. If tachycardia or tachyarrhythmias are present before surgery, the beta-blocker propranolol hydrochloride (Inderal) may be given in an oral dose of 0.15 to 0.5 mg/kg body weight three times daily, but only after and concurrently with the administration of an oral α_1 and α_2 blocker, phenoxybenzamine hydrochloride (Dibenzyline). Phenoxybenzamine in an oral, twice daily dose of 0.2 to 1.5 mg/kg body weight should be begun 10 to 14 days before surgery to stabilize blood pressure. Otherwise, vasoconstriction and severe hypertension may result from unopposed alpha-adrenergic effects. Prazosin (Minipress) has a shorter duration of activity, is a selective α_1-blocker, and may be preferable to phenoxybenzamine. Preoperative administration of atropine or phenothiazines should be avoided to reduce risks of tachycardia or sudden hypotension. Equipment for measuring the electrocardiogram and blood pressure should be connected to the patient before induction. Induction should be with narcotics or thiobarbiturate combined with glycopyrrolate. Anesthesia should be done with methoxyflurane and nitrous oxide. Halothane can induce arrhythmias and should be avoided. Phentolamine (Regitine), an alpha-blocker for intravenous use, can be used in a dose of 0.02 to 0.1 mg/kg body weight during surgery to lower blood pressure while manipulating the tumor. Propranolol can be given intravenously in a dose of 0.3 to 1 mg/kg body weight, or lidocaine can be administered intravenously as necessary during the surgery to control tachycardia or tachyarrhythmias. Immediately after the adrenalectomy, the rate of fluid administration should be increased. If blood pressure cannot be maintained, norepinephrine (Levophed) should be given carefully in an intravenous dose. Adrenocortical steroids should not be replaced or supplemented unless both adrenals must be removed.

If surgery is not feasible, the administration of phenoxybenzamine or prazosin and α-methyltyrosine may be given to control hypertension. Malignant pheochromocytomas have not been successfully controlled by chemotherapy or irradiation, but treatment with ^{131}I-metaiodobenzylguanidine has shown some promise in humans.

See also references 5, 14, 16, and 17.

REFERENCES

1. Anderson, M.G., and Aitken, M.M.: Biochemical and physiological effects of catecholamine administration in the horse. Res. Vet. Sci., *22:*357, 1977.
2. Appleby, E.C.: Tumors of the adrenal gland and paraganglia. Bull W.H.O., *53:*227, 1976.
3. Berzon, J.L.: A metastatic pheochromocytoma causing progressive paraparesis in a dog. Vet. Med. Small Anim. Clin., 76:675, 1981.
4. Bravo, E.L.: Circulating and urinary catecholamines in pheochromocytoma: diagnostic and pathophysiologic implications. N. Engl. J. Med., *301:*682, 1979.
5. Bravo, E.L., and Gifford, R.W., Jr.: Pheochromocytoma: diagnosis, localization and management. N. Engl. J. Med., *311:*1298, 1984.
6. Buckingham, J.D.E.: Pheochromocytoma in a mare. Can. Vet. J., *11:*205, 1970.
7. Froscher, B.G., and Power, M.T.: Malignant pheochromocytoma in a foal. J. Am. Vet. Med. Assoc., *181:*494, 1982.
8. Frye, F.L., and Clement, E.D.: Sympathicoblastoma in a dog. J. Am. Vet. Med., Assoc., *156:*900, 1970.
9. Gelberg, M., Cockerell, G.L., and Minor, R.R.: A light and electron microscopic study of a normal adrenal medulla and a pheochromocytoma from a horse. Vet. Pathol., *16:*395, 1979.
10. Hardee, G.E., et al.: Catecholamines in equine and bovine plasmas. J. Vet. Pharmacol. Ther., *5:*279, 1983.
11. Howard, E.B., and Nielsen, S.W.: Pheochromocytomas associated with hypertensive lesions in dogs. J. Am. Vet. Med. Assoc., *147:*245, 1965.
12. Jordan, J.E.: Normal laboratory values in beagle dogs of twelve to eighteen months of age. Am. J. Vet. Res., *38:*509, 1977.
13. Peterson, M.E., et al.: Multiple endocrine neoplasia in a dog. J. Am. Vet. Med. Assoc., *180:*1476, 1982.
14. Schaer, M.: Pheochromocytoma in a dog: a case report. J. Am. Anim. Hosp. Assoc., *16:*583, 1980.
15. Stowater, J.L.: Pheochromocytoma metastatic to bone in a dog. Vet. Med. Small Anim. Clin., *74:*343, 1979.
16. Twedt, D.C.: Pheochromocytoma in the canine. J. Am. Anim. Hosp. Assoc., *11:*491, 1975.
17. Twedt, D.C., and Wheeler, S.L.: Pheochromocytoma in the dog. Vet. Clin. North Am. [Small Anim. Pract.], *14:*767, 1984.
18. White, R.A.S., and Cheyne, I.A.: Bone metastases from a phaeochromocytoma in the dog. J. Small Anim. Pract., *18:*579, 1977.
19. Yovich, J.V., and Ducharme, N.G.: Ruptured pheochromocytoma in a mare with colic. J. Am. Vet. Med. Assoc., *183:*462, 1983.
20. Yovich, J.V., Horney, F.D., and Hardee, G.E.: Pheochromocytoma in the horse and measurement of norepinephrine levels in horses. Can. Vet. J., *25:*21, 1984.

Section VII

The Gonads

22

The Normal Gonads, Abnormalities of Sexual Development, and Clinical Tests of Gonadal Function

Except during their earliest stages of development, male gonads are unlike the female gonads. The male gonads are a pair of testes; the female gonads are a pair of ovaries. Gonadal functions are twofold: one function is the secretion of gonadal (sex) hormones; the other function is gametogenesis. Gonadal hormones are androgens, estrogens, progesterone, and relaxin. All but relaxin occur in both males and females. Relaxin, a hormone found in females, facilitates parturition. Male gametes are sperm. Female gametes are ova. Gametogenesis depends on normal gonadal hormonogenesis. Gonadal hormones also prepare the body physically and psychologically for the attraction of the opposite sex and copulation at an appropriate time. In the female, gonadal hormones promote and maintain pregnancy. Then, at the optimal time, they promote the desire and ability to protect and nurse the young.

NORMAL DEVELOPMENT OF THE GONADS AND GENITALIA

Genetic Sex

The testes and ovaries begin as bipotential or indifferent gonads. The type of gonad that ultimately develops is determined at the time of conception by the pairing of the maternal and paternal sex chromosomes. Sex chromosomes are designated X or Y. Maternal sex chromosomes are always X. Paternal sex chromosomes can be X or Y. Offspring with XX-sex-determining chromosomes are genetically female. Genetic males have XY chromosomes. Somatic cells possess paired chromosomes, a diploid number. Two of the diploid number of chromosomes are sex chromosomes. Non-sex-determining chromosomes are called autosomes. Gametes carry unpaired chromosomes, a haploid number (one-half the diploid number), in preparation for joining with the opposite sex's gametes. Normal diploid numbers for companion animals are as follows: the dog, 78; cat, 38; and horse, 64. For example, a normal male dog has a 78 XY genotype. Hybrids have uneven diploid numbers (for example, mules have 63 chromosomes).

The short arm of the Y chromosome normally carries the gene for the testicular organizer, which is associated with a cell surface antigen called the *H-Y antigen*. Before the H-Y antigen's message is activated, primordial indifferent germ cells, originating on the yolk sac near the allantois, migrate up the mesentery of the hindgut to the genital ridge of the embryo. These primordial germ cells become incorporated in the genital ridge with mesenchymal cells and germinal epithelial cells. The three cell lines that result constitute the bipotential indifferent gonad. The H-Y antigen directs the primordial germ cells to become spermatogonia, the mesenchymal cells to become interstitial cells (of Leydig), and the germinal epithelium to become seminiferous tubules and Sertoli's cells of the testes.

An XX genotype is necessary for a normal ovary to develop from the indifferent gonad. In genetic females, primordial germ cells become pri-

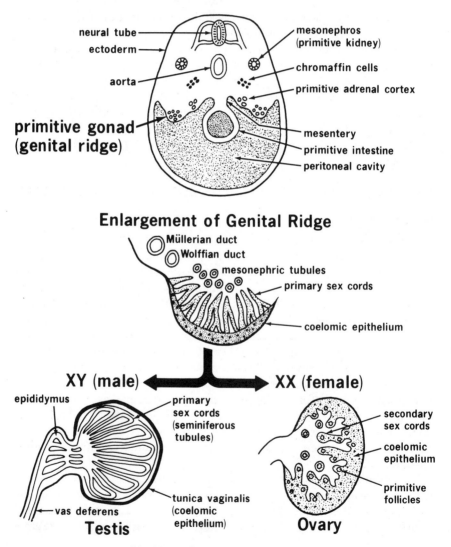

Fig. 22–1. Development of the gonads.

mary ovarian follicles, mesenchymal cells become theca and stromal cells, and germinal epithelial cells become ova.

The indifferent gonad has a cortex and medulla. In genetic males, primary sex cords invade the medulla, forming primordial spermatogonia. The cortex regresses. The medulla regresses in the female while secondary sex cords from the cortex proliferate (development of the gonads is depicted in Figure 22–1).

Differentiation of Internal Genitalia

Unlike the gonads, both male and female internal genitalia are initially present. The male and female internal genitalia are derived from the *Wolffian and Mullerian ducts,* respectively. Both have begun to develop at

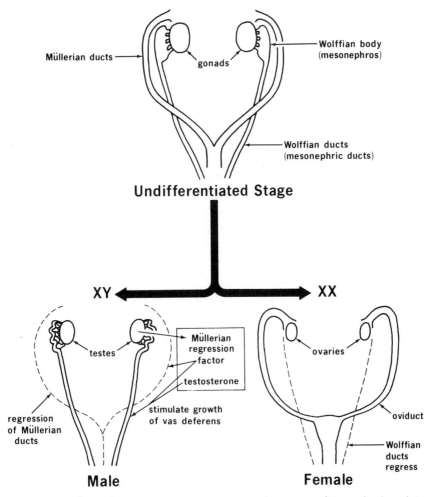

Fig. 22–2. Development of the genital ducts (ventral-dorsal view of the coelomic cavity).

the time the embryonic testes become functional. Normal maintenance and maturation of the Wolffian ducts require testosterone from the interstitial cells of the embryonic testes. Regression of the Mullerian ducts is caused by another fetal testicular hormone, *Mullerian Regression Factor* (MRF), a glycoprotein originating from the Sertoli's cells. Without fetal testosterone and MRF, the Wolffian ducts spontaneously regress and the Mullerian ducts continue to develop and differentiate (Fig. 22–2). Testosterone and MRF exert their effects unilaterally. It is possible for the secretion of testosterone and MRF to be normal on one side of the body with normal male internal genitalia and to be abnormal on the other side with female internal genitalia. Internal genitalia derived from the Wolffian and Mullerian ducts are listed in Table 22–1.

In addition to causing the Wolffian ducts to differentiate into male internal genitalia, testosterone also "organizes" or programs the behavioral centers in the brain so that actions characteristic of males of the species are manifested later in life under further stimulus from testosterone and other stimuli. Testosterone also programs the hypothalamus-adenohypophysis for the noncyclic secretion of gonadotropins.

See also references 94 and 137.

Differentiation of the External Genitalia

After the development of the proper internal genitalia and regression of the unnecessary ductal structures, the external genitalia differentiate (Fig. 22–3). External genitalia spontaneously become female unless actively stimulated to become male-like genitalia. The external genitalia develop from common anlagen: the genital tubercle, urogenital sinus, genital swellings, and genital folds. It is possible for both male and female internal genitalia to persist, but external genitalia must become male, female, or ambiguous.

Table 22–1. Origins of Internal and External Genitalia in Males and Females

| | Differentiated Genitalia | |
Embryonic Structure	Male	Female
Wolffian ducts	Epididymis	
	Vas deferens	
Mullerian ducts		Oviducts
		Uterus
		Cranial vagina
Urogenital sinus	Prostate	Caudal vagina
Genital tubercle	Glans penis	Clitoris
Genital swellings	Scrotum	Labia majora
Genital folds	Penis and penile urethra	Labia minora

Testosterone is indirectly the stimulus for differentiation of external primordia toward male genitalia. More specifically, it is *dihydrotestosterone* (DHT), a potent androgenic metabolite of testosterone that is the stimulus for masculinizing the external genitalia (external genitalia derived from the embryonic primordia are also listed in Table 22–1). The external sexual appearance is called the *phenotype*. Normally, genetic sex, behavioral (psychic) sex, internal genitalia, and phenotype are identical, being either male or female.

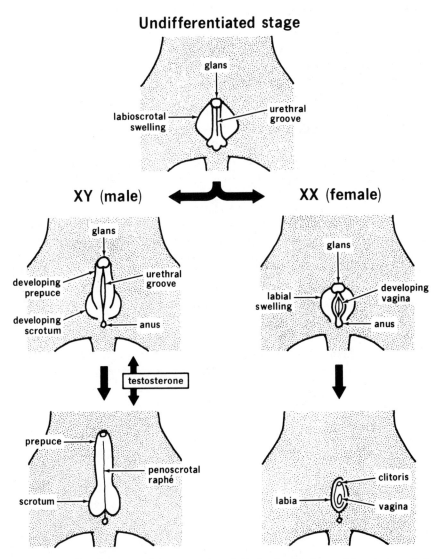

Fig. 22–3. Development of the external genitalia in the dog (ventral-dorsal view of the pubic area).

Descent of the Testes

The last event in completing the male phenotype is the descent of the testes into the scrotum. Their descent is guided and caused by contraction of a fibromuscular cord, the gubernaculum testes, connecting the testes to the scrotal wall. The testes start out caudal to the kidneys, migrate across the abdomen, pass through the inguinal canal, and move subcutaneously (in the dog lateral to the penis) into the scrotum. Testes are normally in the scrotum at the time of birth or before weaning age in companion animals.

ABNORMALITIES OF SEXUAL DEVELOPMENT

Genetic abnormalities of sexual development may result from the defective genetic make-up of the parents, irradiation of the gonads, drugs and other chemicals, aging, or possibly viruses or mycoplasma. If the zygote does not receive the normal diploid number of chromosomes, a heteroploid abnormality develops. Heteroploid abnormalities may be a *monosomy* (the loss of one chromosome from a pair), a *polysomy* (the gain of one or more chromosomes to a normal pair), a *polyploidy* (two or more additional sets of chromosomes), *mosaicism* (two or more cell populations with a different chromosomal make-up derived from faulty cell cleavage in a single zygote), or *chimerism* (two or more cell populations with different chromosomal make-up derived from the fusion of two or more zygotes).

Monosomy and polysomy are the most common disorders. These result from nondisjunction, faulty meiotic cell division of the sperm or ova, or faulty early mitotic cleavage in the zygote. Polyploidy results from fertilization of an ovum with a diploid number of chromosomes, fertilization of the same ovum by two sperm, or division of the chromosomes followed by failure of the cell to divide. The incidence of chromosomal abnormalities in companion animals is not known because of resulting embryonic deaths and

Table 22–2. Clinical Signs Suggestive of Abnormal Sexual Development

---

Males with dysmorphic external genitalia
  Small penis and prepuce
  Hypospadias
  Chordee
Gynecomastia
Cryptorchidism, especially bilateral
Infertility
Primary anestrus
Embryonic and fetal deaths
Attraction of males to another male
Inappropriate psychogender
Virilization in females
  Muscular enlargement
  Enlarged clitoris
  Os clitoris in carnivores
Urinary incontinence
Periodic hematuria

---

the lack of studies surveying chromosomal abnormalities. Suggestive clinical signs of chromosomal and other defects in sexual development are listed in Table 22–2.

Seminiferous Tubule Dysgenesis

The polysomic disorder, XXY (Klinefelter's syndrome), is the most common sex chromosomal abnormality in humans surviving past the neonatal period. It has been reported in the dog,[32] tom cat,[21, 61, 66] and stallion, and is a nondisjunctional defect. Presumably, it is a comparatively common chromosomal abnormality in companion animals.

Klinefelter's syndrome is also called seminiferous tubular dysgenesis. It causes testicular hypoplasia and azoospermia. The Y chromosome overrides the two X chromosomes directing differentiation of the gonads to become testes, at best abnormal ones. Sufficient testosterone and DHT are produced by the fetal testes to allow normal development of male genitalia. Mullerian ducts are normally regressed. The testicular (seminiferous tubule) dysgenesis is progressive. Interstitial cells tend to be hyperplastic and clumped. In humans, gynecomastia may develop at puberty. Serum gonadotropin levels are elevated. Variants include cases with up to four X chromosomes and up to two Y chromosomes in a variety of combinations. The only known predisposing factor for dysgenesis of the seminiferous tubules is maternal aging.

In cats, the gene for orange hair coat and the gene allowing black hair coats are carried by X chromosomes, but only the gene for orange or the gene allowing black in the hair coat, can be carried by one X chromosome.[21] Cats with a tortoise-shell (black and orange) or tricolor (black, orange, and white) hair coat must have two X chromosomes and are generally female ("calico" is also the term used to describe cats with tricolor hair coats). Tom cats with tortoise-shell or calico hair coats also have two X chromosomes. Most of these have feline Klinefelter's syndrome. Some animals are mosaic and have a population of cells with XX genotype. Tom cats with feline Klinefelter's syndrome are infertile from seminiferous tubule dysgenesis. Mosaic cats may have a population of spermatozoa with XY chromosomes and are fertile. Approximately 1 in 3000 tortoise-shell or calico cats are male.

See also references 21, 32, 61, and 66.

Sex Reversal (XX Male)

Phenotypic males with an XX genotype and clinically identical to seminiferous tubule dysgenesis (XXY) have been recognized in cocker spaniels and humans. Such humans and cocker spaniels have the H-Y antigen, which has been translocated to an X chromosome or an autosome. This allows at least partial development of the male internal and external genitalia, and of the psychologic aspects of gender; however, spermatogenesis is impaired.

See also references 77, 155, and 156.

Gonadal Dysgenesis

Another relatively common chromosomal abnormality in humans is the XO genotype (Turner's syndrome), which has been reported in the mare, especially Arabians, and queen. Since two X chromosomes are necessary for normal differentiation of the indifferent gonad into an ovary, an XO pattern prevents ovarian development. The descriptive term for Turner's syndrome is *gonadal dysgenesis,* a nondisjunctional disorder of the first or second meiotic divisions of sperm or ova, or the first mitotic divisions of the zygote. Most are lethal to the fetus. In an analogous nondisjunctional disorder, in which the chromosomes form a YO pattern, all die in utero.

Survivors of the XO genotype are phenotypically female. Some affected women have associated somatic disorders. An affected queen was reported to have coarctation of the aorta, and another had spina bifida. Stunted growth is likely. Secondary sex characteristics and estrus do not occur normally at the usual time for puberty. Unless they are mosaics or chimeras, affected females are infertile with permanent primary anestrus. The ovaries do not develop past the stage of being small bands of tissue ("streaks"). The uterus remains underdeveloped. Serum gonadotropin levels are elevated, and serum estrogen levels are low. Variants of gonadal dysgenesis with normal XX or XY genotypes are possible, but probably less common than XO gonadal dysgenesis. Other similar genetic disorders (XXX and XYY) of the sex chromosomes are more likely to be fertile than the XXY and XO patterns. XXX and XYY incidence is not known.

See also references 10, 17, 18, 61, 86, 111, 123, and 181.

Hermaphroditism (The Intersexes)

Seminiferous tubule dysgenesis and gonadal dysgenesis do not cause ambiguous external genitalia, but many abnormalities of sexual development do. When gonadal sex does not correspond to the sexual phenotype, there is usually ambiguous external genitalia (this condition is called the intersex state or hermaphroditism). Hermaphroditism comes from the mythical Greek god, Hermaphroditos, who was united into one body with the nymph Salmacis. Cocker spaniels, pugs, and beagles may have a greater than expected incidence of hermaphroditism.[47, 54, 80, 169]

See also references 1, 4, 5, 11–16, 47, 48, 52–54, 57–59, 65, 66, 68, 76, 85, 89, 102, 105–107, 116, 120, 140, 141, 149, 153, 158, 175, and 177.

TRUE HERMAPHRODITISM.   True hermaphrodites have an ovary on one side and a testis on the other (a *lateral hermaphrodite*) or an ovotestis on either side (a *unilateral hermaphrodite*) or both sides (a *bilateral hermaphrodite*). True hermaphrodites are comparatively rare, but have been reported in cats, horses, and dogs. They must have cell populations with at least two X chromosomes and a population with a Y chromosome such as XX/XY genotype or have translocated the H-Y antigen to develop both ovarian and testicular tissue from the indifferent gonads. Most true hermaphrodites have an XX sex chromosome constitution, with a translocated H-Y antigen or a mutant autosome. Sexual phenotypes can range from near normal females to near normal males with a wide variety of ambiguous genitalia types in between. Cryptorchidism, hypospadias, and an enlarged clitoris are common. True hermaphrodites are usually infertile, but a successful pregnancy has been reported in a true hermaphroditic cocker spaniel with XX sex chromosomes.

PSEUDOHERMAPHRODITISM. More common than true hermaphroditism, pseudohermaphroditism is classified by the type of gonad present. A *male pseudohermaphrodite* has testes with an ambiguous or near female phenotype. A *female pseudohermaphrodite* has ovaries with an ambiguous or near male phenotype. Male pseudohermaphroditism should be more spontaneously common than female pseudohermaphroditism, but female pseudohermaphroditism is often caused by the use of steroid drugs in pregnant females. Male pseudohermaphroditism can develop from the failure of the fetal testes to secrete testosterone or MRF, the failure to respond to testosterone or DHT, or the failure to convert testosterone to DHT.

Failure to secrete normal amounts of testosterone can result from unresponsiveness to fetal gonadotropins or an inborn error of testosterone biosynthesis. Five enzymes are necessary for the biosynthesis of testosterone: 20, 22-desmolase; 3 β-hydroxysteroid dehydrogenase; 17 α-hydroxylase; 17, 20-desmolase; and 17 β-hydroxysteroid oxidoreductase. Deficiency of any, especially the latter two enzymes, impairs the biosynthesis of testosterone. The first three enzymes are also necessary for the biosynthesis of adrenocortical hormones. None has been reported in companion animals. Based on effects in humans, one would expect bilateral cryptorchidism, absence of Mullerian duct derivative structures, and various degrees of ambiguous external genitalia. Wolffian duct structures develop since enough testosterone is produced by the build-up of precursors, which override the insufficiency of enzymes.

Failure to secrete or respond to normal MRF has been reported in families of miniature schnauzers.[16, 60, 112, 122, 124, 146, 152] Affected miniature schnauzers have unilateral or bilateral cryptorchidism and a small penis and prepuce. They are most often discovered when the cryptorchid testes become neoplastic during middle age. The neoplasm is a Sertoli's cell tumor that typically produces estrogens. The affected dogs most frequently present with depression, anorexia, and gynecomastia. Depression and anorexia are the result of cystic endometritis-pyometra complex, a striking finding in a phenotypic male (Figs. 22–4 and 22–5). It may be that MRF plays a role in the descent of the testes since affected schnauzers also have cryptorchidism. Treatment requires castration and hysterectomy.

Male pseudohermaphroditism caused by defects in androgen-dependent tissues may be caused by end-organ insensitivity or the defective peripheral conversion of testosterone to DHT. *Testicular feminization* is a "complete" androgen insensitivity resulting from a deficiency in testosterone and DHT-

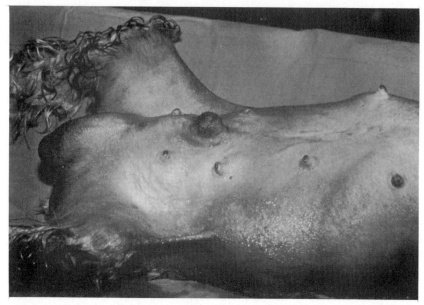

Fig. 22–4. Inguinal area in a male miniature schnauzer with cryptorchidism and gynecomastia. (Courtesy of Dr. M. J. Bojrab.)

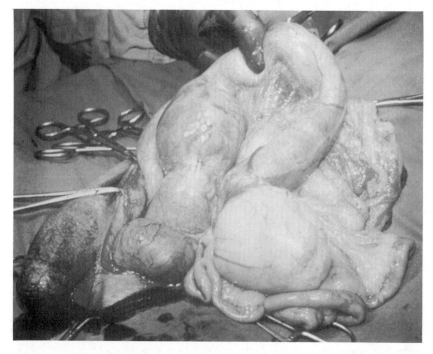

Fig. 22–5. Intra-abdominal Sertoli's cell tumor and pyometra in the same miniature schnauzer as shown in Figure 22–4. (Courtesy of Dr. M. J. Bojrab.)

binding receptors. The secretion and end-organ sensitivity of MRF are normal. Affected males are genotypically male (XY) and phenotypically female, with neither Wolffian nor Mullerian duct derivatives as internal genitalia. Testes are located in the abdomen, inguinal canal, or labioscrotum. The vulva and clitoris are normal. The vagina is short and ends blindly. Secondary sex characteristics of a female occur at puberty because of conversion of testosterone to estradiol, but estrous cycles do not occur. This condition has been reported in the stallion, causing it to appear like a mare.[53, 103]

In humans, testicular feminization is considered an autosomal dominant, sex-linked mutation or an X-linked recessive mutation. The deficiency in receptors may not be complete, allowing some virilization to occur at puberty. In one report, incomplete testicular feminization caused an apparent mare to exhibit aggressive, stallion-like behavior.[103] In animals with testicular feminization, serum levels of gonadotropins, testosterone, and estradiol should be normal to elevated. Cryptorchid testes may become neoplastic and should be excised.

Other forms of incompletely feminized, male pseudohermaphroditism, such as Reifenstein's syndrome in men, have ambiguous genitalia. These are caused by incomplete defective androgen-receptor binding or by a post-receptor activity defect. In addition to male-like ambiguous external genitalia, internal genitalia derived from the Wolffian ducts are present, but hypoplastic. Testes remain small at puberty, gynecomastia often occurs, and there is azoospermia.

The enzyme 5 α-reductase in peripheral tissues is necessary to convert testosterone to DHT. A familial deficiency of 5 α-reductase has been shown in humans to be a cause of male pseudohermaphroditism. Affected men exhibit a female phenotype at birth since DHT is required for masculinization of external genitalia primordia. Mullerian structures regress normally and Wolffian structures differentiate, grow normally, and terminate in a blind-ended vagina. The prostate is absent since it is DHT dependent. At puberty, the testes enlarge, descend into the labioscrotal folds, spermatogenesis begins, secondary sex characteristics of males appear, and virilization of external genitalia occurs. Virilization is presumed to be due to sustained serum elevations of luteinizing hormone (LH) and testosterone. Serum DHT is low. Deficiency of 5 α-reductase has not yet been recognized in companion animals.

Female pseudohermaphroditism is created when a female fetus is exposed to an androgen.[157] The androgen may be of fetal origin or result from the administration of exogenous androgens, progesterone, or certain synthetic progestins. Large doses of progesterone may act as substrate for the synthesis of androgen. Some synthetic progestins are testosterone derivatives. All cases of reported female companion animal pseudohermaphroditism have been caused by exposure of a female fetus to exogenous androgens, progesterone, or progestins.[46]

Another possible cause of female pseudohermaphroditism that has been described well in humans is congenital adrenal hyperplasia caused by deficiencies in adrenocortical enzymes. These deficiencies lead to a shift in the balanced production of adrenocortical steroids toward an excess of adrenocortical androgens. These have not been well documented in companion animals, but we have examined masculinized female dogs with a familial incidence of masculinization and without a history of administered drugs during pregnancy. The degree of masculinization depends on the stage of differentiation at the time the animal is exposed to androgens. Clitoral hypertrophy is the most common abnormality of the external genitalia. Carnivores may develop an os clitoris. Partial fusion of the labioscrotal swelling is possible if exposure is very early in fetal differentiation.

See also references 14, 15, 20, 59, 81, 106, 107, 115, 150, and 183.

THE NORMAL TESTES

Gross Anatomy

The normal canine testes are ovoid organs with compressed sides and are located in the scrotum (Fig. 22–6). The scrotum and testes in the dog and stallion are located below the perineum and between the hind legs. The tom cat's scrotum and testes are in the perineal area immediately beneath the anus. In a 10- to 15-kg dog, the testis is approximately 3 × 2 × 1.8 cm in size and weighs about 8 g.

The testis is surrounded by a capsule composed of two layers (tunics): the outer tunica vaginalis and the inner tunica albuginea. The tunica albuginea extends into the body of the testis and divides it into lobules. Contiguous with the testis is the epididymis, which proximal to the body becomes the vas deferens. The vas deferens and other components of the spermatic cord aid the tunica vaginalis and scrotum in supporting the testis (Fig. 22–7).

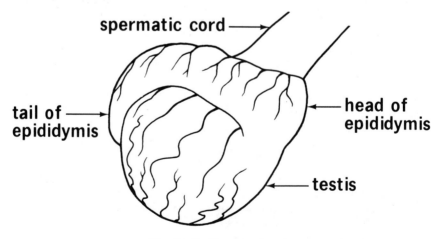

Fig. 22–6. The normal testis.

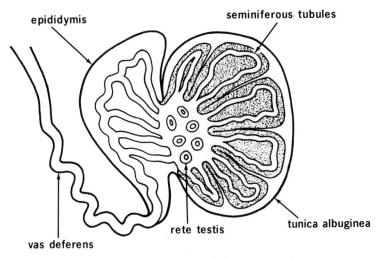

Fig. 22–7. Cross-section of the normal testis.

Microstructure and Function

Testicular lobules are composed of seminiferous tubules that comprise 80% to 90% of the testis (Fig. 22–8). Blood and lymphatic vessels, nerves, fibroblasts, and interstitial (Leydig) cells are located in the loose connective tissues between the seminiferous tubules. The seminiferous tubules contain germ cells and Sertoli's cells. Germ cells are spermatogonia that undergo mitosis to form primary spermatocytes. Primary spermatocytes divide by meiosis to form secondary spermatocytes with the haploid number of chromosomes. A second meiotic division changes secondary spermatocytes to spermatids.

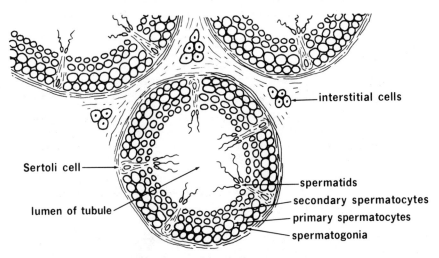

Fig. 22–8. Microstructure of the testis.

Spermatids become spermatozoa by spermiogenesis, a mitotic division. The optimal temperature for spermatogenesis is about 2° C less than normal body temperature. The scrotum and a vascular heat-exchange mechanism provide a favorable temperature for spermatogenesis, a 54- to 55-day process in the dog and a 48- to 49-day process in the stallion.

Sertoli's cells line the basement membrane of seminiferous tubules and form tight junctions with other Sertoli's cells. The junctions are tight enough to act as a protective "blood-testis" barrier, reducing the risk of germinal cell damage by blood-borne elements. Developing sperm are surrounded and nurtured by Sertoli's cells. Sertoli's cells secrete MRF during fetal development. During postnatal life, Sertoli's cells secrete *androgen-binding protein,* which aids in maintaining high intraluminal concentrations of testosterone, and *inhibin,* a polypeptide that inhibits the release of follicle-stimulating hormone (FSH).

After being released from Sertoli's cells, spermatozoa travel the rete testis to the efferent ductules, which lead into the head of the epididymis; then the tubules converge into a single convoluted tube in the body and tail of the epididymis. The tubule of the tail of the epididymis becomes the vas deferens, which empties into the urethra.

Capillaries in the testes have characteristics that are unique for an endocrine organ. In other endocrine organs, capillaries are fenestrated. In the testes, they are not. Spermatic arterioles are tortuous and are paralleled by the pampiniform plexus of veins. This arrangement seems to allow a counter-current exchange of heat and testosterone. The intratesticular concentration of testosterone is 50 to 100 times that of the serum concentration because of this intratesticular testosterone cycle and androgen-binding protein.

Testicular interstitial cells secrete testosterone and small amounts of DHT, dehydroepiandrosterone (DHEA), androstenedione, and estradiol. The biosynthesis of steroid hormones in the testes is similar to the adrenal

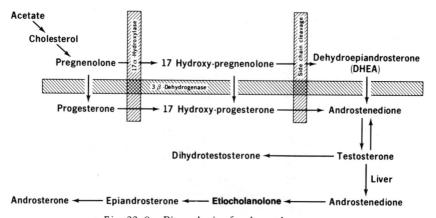

Fig. 22–9. Biosynthesis of male sex hormones.

cortex except that testes do not possess the 11- or 21-hydroxylase enzymes necessary for the production of mineralocorticoids and glucocorticoids (Fig. 22–9). Interstitial cells comprise 5% to 10% of the normal testicular volume. Hyperplasia of the interstitial cells is considered a normal aging process in dogs.

See also references 7, 51, 56, 90, 110, 113, 126, 127, 163, 179, and 191.

Testicular Hormones

Testosterone is a C-19 sex steroidal hormone with a variety of actions (Table 22–3). In the blood, testosterone binds to a high-affinity globulin, *sex hormone binding globulin* (SHBG), produced by the liver, as well as to albumin. Concentrations of SHBG are increased by estrogens and thyroid hormones, and are decreased by growth hormone (GH), obesity, and exogenous androgens. Only about 2% of the total serum testosterone is unbound and enters peripheral cells. Testosterone can be converted in peripheral cells to DHT by 5 α-reductase, to androstenedione, or to 17 β-estradiol. Normal serum testosterone levels in adult male dogs are approximately 0.5 to 6.0 ng/ml. Cats' and horses' serum testosterone levels are about 0.5 to 3.0 ng/ml. Some estrogen is produced by the testes, but most is produced by aromatization of testosterone by peripheral cells. Serum estradiol levels in the male dog and tom cat are about 0.5 to 5 pg/ml and approximately 8 to 12 pg/ml in the stallion.

Testosterone is primarily metabolized by the liver in the dog. Biliary metabolites include androstenedione, androsterone, epiandrosterone, and etiocholanolone. Most is excreted in the bile in the dog, but some is conjugated and excreted in the urine.

See also references 78, 104, 125, 170, 171, and 190.

Table 22–3. Actions of Testosterone

Promotes male secondary sex characteristics
  Enlargement of skeletal musculature
  Aggressive behavior and male libido
  Growth of the penis and scrotum
  Penile spines in tom cats
  Calcification of the os penis in carnivores
  Cresting of the neck in stallions
  Singing in male finches
  Lifting a hind leg to urinate in dogs
  Roaming and urine spraying in tom cats
  Secretion of male pheromones
Promotes protein anabolism
Increases the size of the kidneys and larynx
Maintains spermatogenesis
Promotes growth of long bones initially, then closure of epiphyseal plates
Stimulates erythropoiesis
Causes retention of sodium, potassium, calcium, sulfate, and phosphate

The Hypothalamic-Pituitary-Testes Axis

The hypothalamic-pituitary-testes (H-P-T) axis regulates the serum concentration of free testosterone. Interstitial cell stimulating hormone (known as LH) stimulates the secretion of testosterone. Free testosterone inhibits the adenohypophyseal secretion of LH, and, after being aromatized in the hypothalamus to estrogen, it inhibits the secretion of GnRH. The exogenous administration of progestins in pharmacologic amounts can also inhibit the release of LH. The secretion of LH is pulsatile in males, not cyclic as in females. FSH stimulates the Sertoli's cells to secrete androgen binding protein and inhibin. Inhibin inhibits the secretion of FSH although high concentrations of testosterone or estrogens also inhibit the secretion of FSH. FSH also initiates spermatogenesis and increases interstitial cell LH receptors.

See also references 96, 97, 101, 138, 173, 178, and 182.

Male Puberty

Rapid growth of the testes is induced twice during life. The first period of growth is prenatal, just after gonadal differentiation, during the period of differentiation of the genitalia and imprinting the psychological characteristics of the male gender. In humans, fetal testicular growth is caused by placental gonadotropins. The testes then become relatively quiescent until puberty. Before puberty, the neonatal and juvenile hypothalamus is extremely sensitive to the inhibitory effect of gonadal hormones. Near the time of puberty, the adrenal cortex begins to secrete increased amounts of weak androgens. This period is called the adrenarche. After the adrenarche in males, secretions of LH begin to increase as a result of decreased sensitivity to gonadal hormones. Testosterone secretion is stimulated, and male secondary sex characteristics develop. The secretion of FSH then increases, resulting in the initiation and, with testosterone, the maintenance of spermatogenesis. The initial stimulus for the onset of puberty is not known, but bone age and body weight seem related to its onset. Puberty generally occurs a few months later in male animals than in female animals. Male dogs reach puberty at about 8 to 14 months, tom cats at 6 to 8 months, and stallions at approximately 2 years of age.

THE NORMAL OVARIES

Gross Anatomy

The canine ovaries are paired oval-nodular organs located retroperitoneally 1 to 3 cm caudal to the kidneys (Fig. 22–10). They are held in a peritoneal fold called the mesovarium in the ovarian bursa. The left ovary lies between the abdominal wall and the left colon. The right ovary is more cranial than the left and is dorsal to the descending colon. Pregnancies stretch the suspensory ligaments, and the ovaries migrate caudally and ventrally in parous bitches. In a 10- to 15-kg bitch, an ovary is about 1.5×0.7

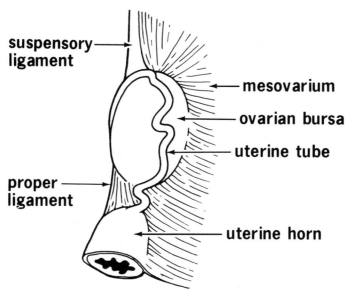

Fig. 22–10. The normal ovary.

× 0.5 cm and weighs about 0.3 g. Changes in ovarian weight occur with the estrous cycle. Its greatest weight occurs before ovulation. The queen's ovary is approximately half the size of that of the 10-kg bitch. Macroscopic regions of the ovary are the cortex, medulla, and hilum.

Microstructure and Function

Columnar cells called the germinal epithelium cover the surface of the ovary. The dense connective tissue of the tunica albuginea lies just beneath the germinal epithelium. The cortex is larger than the medulla. It contains the primary "follicles," which are actually cuboidal granulosa cells surrounding an oocyte. Primary follicles are separated by loose connective tissue and stromal or hilar cells. Hilar cells are similar to testicular interstitial cells in appearance and possibly in function. The medulla is composed of loose connective tissue, blood vessels, nerves, and lymphatics.

In the bitch, primary follicles first develop within the third week after birth. At 15 days of age, it is estimated that the ovaries in a bitch contain 700,000 primordial follicles. Most of these degenerate before puberty, leaving about 250,000. When the animal is 5 years of age, approximately 30,000 follicles are left, and only about 500 remain when the animal has reached the age of 10 years. Stimuli for growth of primordial follicles to primary follicles and primary follicles to secondary follicles are unknown. Stromal cells, which will become theca cells, collect around the basement membrane of the granulosa cells. Gonadotropins induce the growth and maturation of secondary follicles into *tertiary (graafian) follicles*. Granulosa cells of the graafian follicles multiply rapidly into a multilayered band of cells that secrete a fluid and form a fluid-filled cavity, the follicle or antrum. The oocyte and cumulus cells of the granulosa layer are displaced to one side of the follicle. Theca cells proliferate, forming two layers; the *theca interna,* with steroidogenic capabilities; and the *theca externa,* which acts as a vascular and supporting mantle.

FSH induces granulosa cells to produce aromatase that forms estrogens from androstenedione and testosterone and to form LH receptors. Estradiol is secreted into the follicle promoting further proliferation of granulosa cells. LH seems to stimulate the production of androstenedione and testosterone from the theca interna; these then diffuse into the follicular fluid, some of which is converted to estradiol by the granulosa cells. Estradiol is mitogenic to reproductive organs, further inducing proliferation of granulosa cells and their LH receptors. The theca interna also develops the ability to synthesize estradiol, which it releases into the ovarian venous system for systemic effects. Ovarian steroids are concentrated in the follicular fluid to several thousand times those recorded in serum levels.

Although all follicles are exposed to FSH and LH, less than 1% reach full development and ovulation. The exact mechanism involved, in which certain follicles are selected for complete development while others regress (become atretic), is not known. Local factors, including the ratio of estradiol to ovarian androgens in the follicular fluid, are probably important in causing regression of unselected follicles.

In the dog and cat, approximately four to six follicles are usually encouraged to reach the point of ovulation. Mares commonly have one follicle brought to ovulation, although up to 25% of estrus periods may have multiple ovulations. After the release of the oocyte and follicular fluid, the granulosa layer is invaded by vessels from the theca layer. This process, called luteinization, leads to an accumulation of yellow pigment, lutein. The resulting structure created is called the *corpus luteum* (Fig. 22–11). The granulosa and theca cells lose the enzymatic capability of producing androgens and estrogens to the extent they were able to before ovulation. Progesterone is the main secretory product of the corpus luteum.

See also references 34, 67, 109, 136, 163, and 192.

Ovarian Hormones

The ovary produces estrogens, progesterone, androgens, and relaxin. Estrogens and progesterone may also be produced by the placenta. In the pregnant mare, estrogens are produced in large amounts by the placenta after 150 days of gestation. Progesterone is produced by the placenta after 180 to 200 days of gestation. Serum estrogens and progesterone show increases after about 20 days of gestation in the dog and cat. Some of these increases may result from placental production.

17 β-Estradiol (E_2, *estradiol*) is the most potent of estrogens. *Estrone* (E_1) is about one tenth as potent per mg as E_2. E_1 can be converted to E_2, and E_2 can be converted to E_1. *Estriol* (E_3) is a hydroxylated metabolite of estrone.

E₃ competes with estradiol and estrone for binding estrogen receptors, but because the estrogenic effects of estriol are so weak in comparison, E_3 is considered an "impeded" estrogen. Estradiol is the predominant bioactive ovarian hormone released by the ovary, especially during the phase of

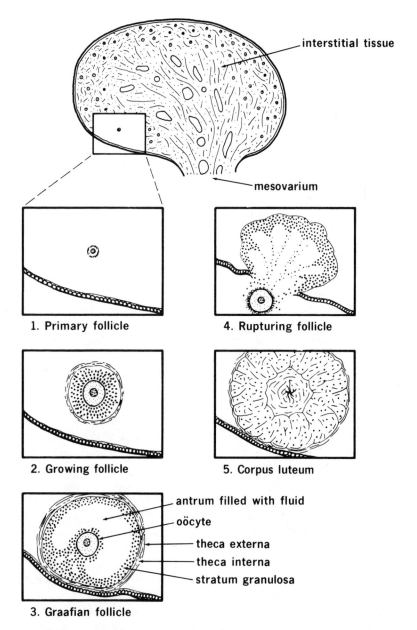

Fig. 22–11. Cross-section of the normal ovary and sequential development of an ovarian follicle.

Table 22–4.   Actions of Estrogens

Promotes female secondary sex characteristics
Growth of the mammary stroma and ducts
Accelerates late prepubertal growth, then closes epiphyseal plates
Facilitates growth of ovarian follicles
Increases motility of oviducts
Opens the cervix
Promotes the growth of straight uterine ducts
Increases size of myometrium and endometrium, and spurs uterine blood flow
Stimulates production of estrogen and progesterone receptors in the uterus
Increases thickness and cornification of vaginal epithelium
Induces oxytocin receptors in uterus
Increases TBG and SHBG levels
Antagonizes PTH effects on bone
Increases the serum concentration of most coagulation factors
Aids in causing estrus-associated behavior
Facilitates loss of intravascular fluid into the extracellular space of the reproductive
  tract
Induces secretion of female pheromones

TBG = Thyroid-binding globulin, SHBG = sex-hormone-binding globulin; PTH = parathyroid hormone.

follicular growth. The actions of estrogens are listed in Table 22–4 and the biosynthesis of female sex hormones is depicted in Figure 22–12. Progesterone is the primary hormone produced by the corpus luteum. As its name implies, it "encourages gestation." Other actions of progesterone are listed in Table 22–5.

Small amounts of androgens (testosterone, androstenedione, DHEA) are secreted into the systemic circulation by the normal ovary. Other important sources of serum androgens in females are the adrenal cortex and peripheral conversion of weak androgens to more potent androgens. Peak serum levels occur at estrus. Small amounts of androgens tend to enhance female libido. Testosterone is the most virilizing androgen produced by the body. Androstenedione is 10% to 20% as virilizing as testosterone per mg. DHEA is 5% as virilizing per mg as testosterone.

Relaxin is a polypeptide hormone (molecular weight, 6,000) from the ovary (and possibly the placenta) with a structure similar to that of insulin. It is secreted during pregnancy to relax the pubic symphysis and pelvic joints and to soften and aid in dilation of the cervix. It may also help coordinate myometrial contractions.

More than 95% of estrogens and progesterone released into the circulation are bound to plasma proteins. Most of those that are bound are bound weakly to albumin. Estradiol and estrone also bind to SHBG. In contrast to estrogens, most testosterone bound to plasma proteins is bound to SHBG. Progesterone binds to corticosteroid-binding globulin in addition to albu-

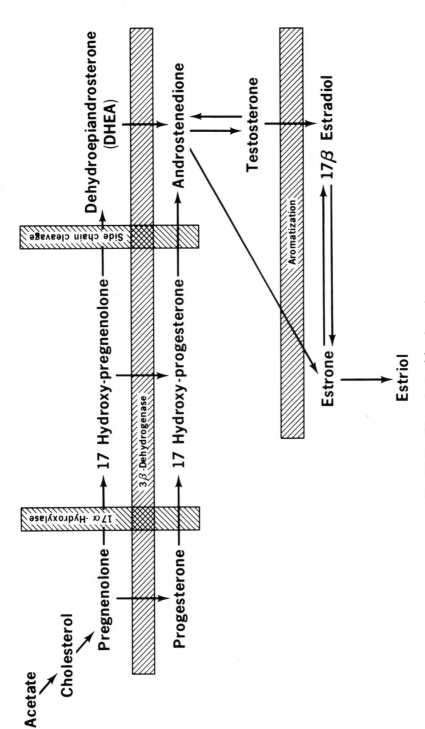

Fig. 22-12. Biosynthesis of female sex hormones.

Table 22–5.   Actions of Progesterone

Inhibits estrogen effects on the myometrium by decreasing estrogen receptors
Decreases estrogen receptors in the endometrium
Increases the excretion of estrogens
Stimulates growth of mammary lobules and alveoli
Antagonizes aldosterone effects on the renal tubules
Promotes estrus-associated behavior in bitches
Increases body temperature (thermogenic)
Promotes a closed cervix and increased viscosity of cervical mucus
Causes hypnotic effects on the brain
Stimulates appetite
Promotes maternal behavior
Inhibits T-lymphocyte function
Stimulates branching and coiling of uterine glands
Stimulates production of fibrinogen

min. Levels of SHBG and corticosteroid-binding globulin (CBG) are increased by estrogens and decreased by androgens and progesterone. Only unbound serum estrogens and progesterone enter peripheral cells to bind with their hormone receptors. A serum globulin with high estrogen affinity may not exist in the dog.

Progesterone and estrogens are metabolized by the liver, conjugated, and eliminated in the bile and urine. Major metabolites excreted in the urine are estriol and pregnanediol. Conjugated estrogens are found in high concentrations in urine. Paradoxically, stallion urine is especially rich in conjugated estrogens. Two estrogens, equilin and equilenin, are found only in urine of pregnant mares.

See also references 6, 63, and 64.

The Hypothalamic-Pituitary-Ovarian Axis

The hypothalamic-pituitary-ovarian (H-P-O) axis regulates the free hormone plasma levels of estrogen and progesterone. Unlike the control of relatively constant day-to-day free testosterone levels in males, plasma levels of free estradiol and progesterone must fluctuate in cycles to bring about coordinated changes in the female's reproductive tract and female receptivity to males. These coordinated cyclic events are necessary for successful mating, conception, implantation, gestation, and lactation.

Gonadotropin-releasing hormone (GnRH) may be stored in the cranial portion of the hypothalamus for surges of secretion and secreted in basal amounts by the ventral portion of the hypothalamus. In response to GnRH's stimulation from the hypothalamus, the secretion of FSH increases slowly, beginning about 5 weeks before ovulation in the bitch. The secretion of LH increases approximately 2 weeks before ovulation of the growing ovarian follicles. Inhibin released from the growing layers of granulosa

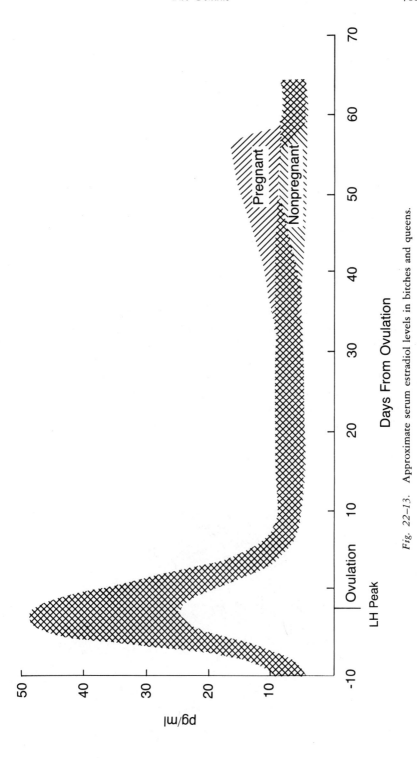

Fig. 22–13. Approximate serum estradiol levels in bitches and queens.

cells begins to suppress FSH levels for several days. As the follicles mature, serum estrogens rise to a peak and then begin to decline, stimulating the cranial hypothalamus, possibly with the aid of rising levels of progesterone in the bitch, to release stored GnRH. A burst in the secretion of LH is closely followed by the peak of another, but more rapid, rise in serum levels of FSH. Serum estrogen levels peak a day or two before the serum levels of LH peak (Fig. 22–13). The burst of LH in most species occurs over a period of 12 hours. In the bitch, however, such a burst lasts 1 to 4 days. Levels of LH decline rapidly after its peak. Levels of FSH decline more gradually. The rise and decline of serum estrogen levels are paralleled by testosterone levels in the bitch. Basal serum testosterone level in bitches is about 100 pg/ml. Before ovulation, levels are near 500 pg/ml.

Twenty-four to seventy-two hours after the LH reaches peak levels in bitches, ovulation occurs and corpora lutea form. Serum progesterone levels begin to rise in bitches before ovulation. After the corpora lutea form, the production of progesterone increases to reach peak serum levels about 15 to 20 days after ovulation. Serum progesterone levels decline slowly, reaching near basal levels 80 to 100 days after ovulation (Fig. 22–14). Another cycle of rising levels of FSH then begins. In mares, the uterus produces prostaglandin $F_{2\alpha}$, which terminates the corpus luteum. In dogs and cats, there does not seem to be a luteolytic prostaglandin of uterine origin that lyses the corpus luteum.

The most significant difference between the H-P-O axis in the bitch and queen is that LH is released spontaneously in the bitch, whereas in the queen, it must be induced by a neurogenic reflex associated with the stimuli

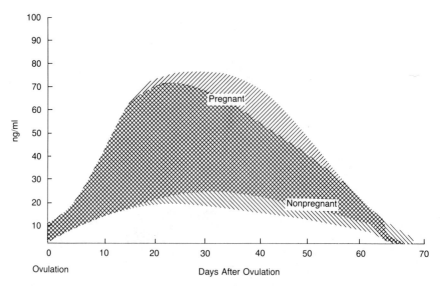

Fig. 22–14. Approximate serum progesterone levels in bitches after ovulation.

of copulation. For most queens, more than one copulation is necessary for the release of LH, but more than half of mated queens release LH after three copulations. Rarely, some older queens may ovulate from being stroked on the back. If the release of LH does not occur, the ovarian follicles regress temporarily for a few days, then follicular growth and increases in serum estrogens resume. If the release of LH does occur spontaneously from sterile mating or from sham copulation, the ovulated queen's serum progesterone levels and the size of the corpora lutea reach peak levels about 3 weeks later. If ovulation occurs, the decline in serum progesterone in nonpregnant queens is more rapid (reaching levels of less than 1 ng/ml about 40 days after ovulation) than the decline of progesterone in nonpregnant bitches, which drops to less than 1 ng/ml about 80 days after ovulation (Fig. 22–15).

See also references 2, 9, 23, 25, 27, 30, 33, 35, 37–42, 71, 72, 74, 92, 95, 100, 108, 114, 117, 121, 129, 130, 164, 176, 180, and 185–189.

Endocrine Levels During Pregnancy

Serum levels of estradiol and progesterone recorded after ovulation in pregnant bitches and queens differ slightly from those in nonpregnant bitches and queens. The degree of differences in bitches may be masked by hemodilution associated with an increase in blood volume during the latter part of pregnancy. Serum estrogen levels are usually higher in the last third of pregnancy. The rise is slow, terminating just before parturition, when serum estrogen levels drop sharply to basal levels (see Fig. 22–13). Serum progesterone levels tend to be higher in pregnant bitches and queens than nonpregnant bitches and queens during approximately 20 to 60 days after

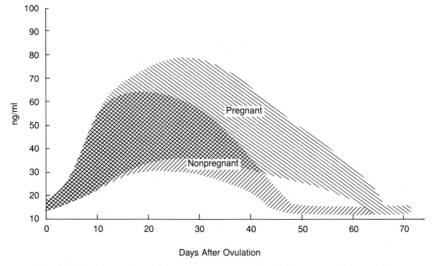

Fig. 22–15. Approximate serum progesterone levels in queens after ovulation.

ovulation (see Figs. 22–14 and 22–15). Serum progesterone levels also sharply decline to near basal levels just before parturition. Approximately 12 hours after the decline in serum progesterone levels, the body temperature drops about 1° to 1.5° C because of the sudden withdrawal from the thermogenic effects of progesterone. Parturition depends on the withdrawal from progesterone, so that the cervix will dilate and motility of the uterus can increase. Such a withdrawal from progesterone's effects is facilitated by the drop in estrogen levels since the withdrawal of estrogen reduces the number of progesterone receptors. In the bitch, serum cortisol levels increase 24 to 36 hours before parturition. It is thought that the rise in cortisol in late pregnancy is produced by the fetal adrenal cortex.

Little is known of the role of the placenta in the endocrine changes of pregnancy in dogs and cats. In women and mares, the placenta produces the following chorionic gonadotropins: human chorionic gonadotropin (HCG) and pregnant mare serum gonadotropin (PMSG), respectively. Laboratory pregnancy tests are based on detecting placental gonadotropins. HCG is predominantly LH-like and supports the corpus luteum; PMSG is FSH-like and induces secondary follicles and, then, secondary corpora lutea. HCG originates from the chorion; PMSG comes from the endometrial cups. HCG passes into the urine in pregnant women; PMSG is not filtered into the urine in pregnant mares. The detection of PMSG by a hemagglutination-inhibition test (the mare immunologic pregnancy test [MIP]) serves as a pregnancy marker in mares between the fortieth and one-hundred-twentieth day of gestation. Immunoreactive levels of FSH in the serum increase in the latter half of pregnancy in the dog. This might reflect an FSH-like placental gonadotropin.

After uterine implantation of the zygote, serum progesterone levels rise in the bitch and queen. Some of this increase may be of placental origin. In the queen, an ovariectomy after 45 days' gestation does not result in abortion, because there are sufficient levels of progesterone, apparently of placental origin. An ovariectomy at any stage of gestation in the bitch results in abortion.[166] If placental progesterone is responsible for the rise in serum progesterone levels after the implantation of the zygote in bitches, the degree of secretion is not enough alone to maintain pregnancy. The placenta in the mare begins to secrete progesterone at 60 to 90 days of pregnancy, becoming the principal source of progesterone at 150 to 180 days of pregnancy, when the secondary corpora lutea induced by PMSG regress.

The rise in estrogen in late pregnancy could also be of placental origin. In pregnant women, the placenta produces estrogens from fetal androgens. Plasma estrogens in mares rise after 120 days of gestation and peak at 180 to 270 days.

See also references 35, 36, 43, 45, 55, 70, 73, 98, 99, 118, and 135.

The Ovarian and Estrous Cycles

Ovarian activities cycle through three phases: the *follicular, luteal,* and, sometimes, a *quiescent* phase. Ovarian phases and associated changes in endocrine secretions are clinically recognized by changes in behavior, male receptivity, and appearance of the external genitalia. Ovarian phases also cause cyclic changes in the size and morphology of the uterus. Cyclic changes in the external genitalia and uterine morphology caused by ovarian phases are collectively called the *estrous cycle.* The estrous cycle is divided into *proestrus, estrus* (Gr., "mad desire"), *metestrus,* and *anestrus.*

Common usage has made diestrus (Gr., "double" estrus) nearly synonymous with metestrus (Gr., "after" estrus). Metestrus has been used to refer only to the period of the corpus luteum or the initial establishment of the corpus luteum. Diestrus has come to represent the period between estrous cycles in polyestrous animals or the period during which the mature corpus luteum functions. The literal meaning of metestrus seems more appropriate than the obscure translation of diestrus. To reduce confusion, only the term *metestrus* will be used here to refer to the period of corpus luteum activity. Clinical characteristics and durations of the estrous cycle of the bitch, queen, and mare are provided in Table 22–6.

The period of the estrous cycle when females are attractive to males is referred to by owners as the female being "in heat" or "in season." Sexual attractiveness in companion animals is signaled by auditory, visual, and tactile stimuli, and by secreted odors called pheromones. Methyl p-hydroxybenzoate is an estrogen-induced pheromone in vaginal secretions of the bitch produced during the follicular phases of the estrous cycle.

The ovarian and estrous cycles are influenced by diseases outside the H-P-O axis and by stresses from the external environment. Environmental stresses include extremes in temperature, humidity, nutritional deficiencies or excesses, duration of daylight, and other real or even imagined threats. These influencing factors are perceived by the nervous system and mediated through the hypothalamus and its production of GnRH.

Ovarian and estrous cycles differ among species of companion animals. The estrous cycle in the bitch is monestral. Only one or two estrous cycles occur per year. The canine interestrous (estrus to estrus) period is about 7 months (4 to 12 months). The season of year has no effect on the incidence of estrus in companion dogs. Kenneled dogs without artificial lighting may have estrus more often during the late winter and late summer months. Other factors affecting interestrous periods in dogs are their breed and age. The interestrous periods of German shepherd dogs are approximately 5 months, 1 to 2 months shorter than the normal average for other breeds. Basenjis cycle only once per year, usually in the fall. After 5 years of age, canine interestrous periods tend to lengthen. In bitches, the length of these periods is unaffected by pregnancy.

Clinical signs of an estrous cycle in the bitch begin with vulvar swelling in early proestrus. Soon after the swelling is noticed, a hemorrhagic discharge appears from the vulva. The blood arises from diapedesis from the rapidly proliferating endometrium and the vaginal wall. During estrus, the period of male receptivity, the vulva becomes less turgid and more flaccid. The hemorrhagic discharge usually subsides by the third day of estrus. In

Table 22-6.   Clinical Characteristics and Durations of the Estrous Cycle

Estrous Period	Predominate Gonadal Hormone in Circulation	Ovarian Phase	Behavioral Characteristics	Duration in Days		
				Bitch	Queen	Mare
Proestrus	Rising estrogen	Follicular	Increased attractiveness to males. Female unreceptive.	9 (2–14)	1 (0–2)	2 (1–3)
Estrus	Estrogen peak*	Follicular	Attractive to males. Female receptive to copulation.	9 (2–14)	7 (3–16)	6 (4–9)
Metestrus	Declining estrogens Rise and fall of progesterone	Luteal	Declining attractiveness to males. Female unreceptive.	60 (50–80)	40 (30–50)†	15 (12–17)
Anestrus	Baseline levels of estrogen and progesterone	Quiescent	Sexually unattractive to males.	120 (60–240)	Seasonal in winter	Seasonal in winter

* Bitch receptivity to male dogs requires declining serum estrogen levels and rising preovulatory serum progesterone levels.
† The queen does not usually ovulate without pregnancy resulting unless she has mated with sterile male or has engaged in sham copulation with a glass rod. Early fetal death or the administration of luteinizing hormone or gonadotropin-releasing hormone can also result in ovulation without pregnancy.

metestrus, the vulvar swelling continues to abate, and the vaginal discharge becomes mucoid and scant. The mammary glands often secrete a clear to mildly cloudy discharge during metestrus. This is a physiologic change called *covert pseudopregnancy* (pseudocyesis). Occasionally in metestrus the mammae will become enlarged and secrete more milk-like secretions than normal; also, behavioral abnormalities occur, including such actions as becoming protective of toys, reclusive behavior, and nest making. This is clinical or *overt pseudopregnancy*. It is thought to coincide with decreasing serum progesterone levels and rising serum prolactin levels.

Queens and mares are seasonally polyestrous. Both have a winter anestrual period (October through December for queens and September through March for mares in the northern hemisphere) caused by decreased daylight hours. The length of daylight is detected by the retinas. Neural pathways transmit information about the length of daylight from the retinas to the pineal gland, affecting its secretion of a GnRH inhibitory factor, probably melatonin. The inhibitory factor acts on hypothalamic function via the suprachiasmic nucleus. Increasing daylight after the winter solstice removes the pineal inhibition of GnRH, and estrous cycles begin 20 to 60 days later. Not all queens have a winter anestrus. Long-haired breeds are more likely to have winter anestrus than short-haired breeds. If the hours of combined daylight and sufficiently bright artificial illumination exceed 14 hours daily, estrous cycles can be induced year-round.

Interestrous periods are approximately 16 days (range, 10 to 22 days) in queens. Unless they have mated, queens have 13 (range, 4 to 25) repeated cycles of proestrus-estrus-atretic follicles with subsiding estrous behavior, proestrous behavior, etc., until the breeding season ends. The intensity of estrus is greatest in February and April (Fig. 22–16). Some Siamese may have persistent estrous behavior until they have mated. An ovulation without subsequent pregnancy delays the next estrus 45 (range, 35 to 70) days. Ovulations occur approximately 24 hours after copulation.

The clinical signs of the estrous period in queens are unlike the clinical signs in bitches. Proestrus in queens is not noticeable unless a tom cat is

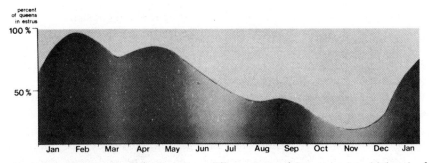

Fig. 22–16. Percent of queens in estrus at different times of the year varies with length of exposure to daylight. (From Lofstedt, R.M.: The estrous cycle of the domestic cat. Compendium on Continuing Educ. for the Practicing Vet., 4:52, 1982).

present. Vulvar swelling may not be detectable, and blood spotting does not occur. Estrus in the queen may cause bizarre behavior such as pacing, vocalizing, rubbing against objects, persistent stretching and rolling, anorexia, and treading on the hind legs while in sternal recumbency. Such behavior is often mistaken by an unsuspecting owner or clinician as ingested foreign bodies, seizures, intoxication, and other illnesses. Pregnancy and lactation delay the onset of the next estrous cycle for the duration of pregnancy and for 2 to 8 weeks after lactation ends, depending on the length of lactation. Lactation suppresses the return to estrus in queens and prolongs the period of anestrus between lactation and subsequent estrus. Overt pseudopregnancy from an ovulation without pregnancy is rare in the queen.

Interestrual periods of mares are approximately 22 (range, 19 to 24) days, depending on the time of year. Early in their breeding season, estrus may persist longer than later in the year, and psychic manifestations of heat may not be accompanied by ovulation. This is called the *transitional period*. Proestrus is difficult to identify unless the mare is unreceptive to teasing with a stallion. No hemorrhage from the vulva occurs with the mare's estrous cycle. Estrus is clinically characterized by frequent urination, whinnies, raised tail, and spontaneous contractions ("winking") of the vulva. Receptivity may temporarily abate for a few days after it begins during estrus, and then it may return; this condition is referred to as *split estrus*. Metestrus is typified by cessation of male receptivity. Lactation does not inhibit regular cycles after parturition. In fact, an estrus called "foal heat" usually occurs 6 to 12 days after foaling. Subsequent estrous periods may be delayed after foal heat.

See also references 8, 19, 24, 28, 29, 44, 45, 69, 70, 83, 84, 91, 93, 134, 139, 142, 144, 147, 148, 151, 161, 162, 165, 167, and 168.

The Uterine and Vaginal Cycle

The ovarian cycle causes cyclic changes in the morphology of the uterus and vagina. Cytologic examination of vaginal smears in bitches and queens and endometrial biopsy in the mare can be clinically useful in determining the stage of the ovarian cycle.

The vaginal mucosa is stratified squamous epithelium consisting of *superficial, intermediate,* and *basal-parabasal* cells. Before puberty or during anestrus, the vaginal epithelium is only 2 to 3 basal-parabasal cells deep. Estrogen has mitogenic effects on the vaginal epithelium, inducing a process of modified cornification. During the follicular phase of the ovarian cycle when serum estrogen concentrations are high, the vaginal epithelium proliferates to 10 to 20 cell layers and produces intermediate and superficial cells.

The endometrial cycle can be divided into three phases: *proliferative, secretory,* and *involutive.* The proliferative phase occurs under the influence of estrogens during the ovarian follicular phase. The endometrial epithelium and stroma increase in size and depth. The uterus becomes hyperemic and edematous. Endometrial glands become elongated and straight. After luteinization of the granulosa cells and the rise of serum progesterone level, the endometrial glands become tortuous and secretory. Secretion subsides and the uterus involutes concurrently with the fall in serum progesterone levels in mid- to late metestrus. The bitch's uterus requires a minimum of approximately 150 days after ovulation for complete involution to occur. Uteri of all other companion animals involute more rapidly than does that of the bitch.

Female Puberty

Female companion animals generally reach puberty at least 2 months earlier than do male companion animals. Bitches usually begin puberty at 6 to 12 months. The first estrus may be split, meaning a temporary loss of male receptivity after a normal onset of estrus. Silent estrus, an estrus with few signs in behavior or the external genitalia, is also common in the first estrous period.

Because of the effects of their seasonal anestrus, the onset of puberty in queens and mares is more variable than in bitches. Queens may begin puberty at 4 to 21 months of age. Late normal puberty is likely to occur in a queen reaching the usual body weight associated with the onset of puberty in early winter. Psychic stimuli of other females in estrus stimulate other queens to come into estrus early in the breeding season. In cats, there are also breed differences. Most short-haired breeds go through puberty earlier than long-haired breeds. The manx is one short-haired breed in whom puberty occurs late. The mare reaches puberty at 15 to 24 months of age.

Puberty in female animals, like that in male animals, is thought to result from an unexplained decrease in the hypothalamic or pituitary sensitivity to negative feedback with gonadal steroids. A rise in FSH occurs first in the onset of puberty in females. The cause for this change is not known, but it seems to correlate with bone age and a particular body weight. For example, queens usually begin puberty at a body weight of 2.3 to 2.5 kg. Small breeds of dogs attain body weights approximating the body weight of normal adults earlier than do large dog breeds. Small breeds also begin puberty earlier than do large breeds. Other factors known to influence the onset of puberty in companion animals are nutrition; climate; season of year; environmental, physical, and psychic stresses; and interaction with postpubertal male and female animals of the same species.

CLINICAL TESTS OF GONADAL FUNCTION

The usefulness of a complete pertinent history and physical examination in clinical assessments of gonadal function cannot be overemphasized. No laboratory test is as singularly helpful; however, laboratory examinations done in series or combinations can frequently substantiate and supplement the findings of a physical examination and a complete pertinent history.

Semen Evaluation

Normal spermatogenesis cannot occur if the H-P-T axis is abnormal. Finding normal mature sperm in a semen sample rules out an endocrine disorder of the H-P-T axis. Semen is collected in dogs by gentle but firm manual compression caudal to the bulb of the penis. The presence of a bitch in proestrus or estrus helps the male to achieve an erection and ejaculation. An artificial vagina may be used, but it is usually less efficient.

Semen of tom cats is difficult to collect. Electroejaculation while under general anesthesia is the most useful method. Weeks of training are necessary to adjust a tom cat to an artificial vagina. The least desirable but most practical means of collecting a tom cat's semen is by vaginal irrigation immediately following mating.

The sperm of a stallion is collected in an artificial vagina when the stallion is mounting a teaser mare. The collection of a stallion's semen is a hazardous procedure that should be attempted only by trained personnel with adequate restraint facilities.

The concentration, motility, and morphology of spermatozoa indicate whether the H-P-T axis may be normal or abnormal. Oligospermia should be reassessed twice at monthly intervals. Normal semen values for the dog, tom cat, and stallion are listed in Table 22–7.

See also reference 172.

Testicular Biopsy

Testicular biopsies can be done by fine needle aspiration, excisional biopsy needles, or surgical excisional biopsy. Fine needle aspirates can differentiate an outflow obstruction from impaired spermatogenesis as the cause for oligospermia or azoospermia. Excisional biopsy needles are not advisable because of risk of vascular injury and unavoidable distortion of the sample's morphology. Incisional slice biopsies are most practical in the dog. The procedure is done with the patient under general anesthesia after normal blood coagulation times are confirmed. The testis to be biopsied is pushed cranial to the scrotum. Careful incision allows the large blood vessels of the testis to be located and avoided. An incision is then made through the tunica albuginea and into the testis. Superficial lobules nor-

Table 22–7. Normal Semen Values in the Dog, Tom Cat, and Stallion

	Dog	Tom Cat*	Stallion
Volume (ml)	2–10	0.08–0.7	20–300
Concentration (10^6/ml)	100–200	100–5,000	30–800
Motility (% progressive)	80–100	60–100	50–100
Morphology (% normal heads and mid-pieces)	60–100	80–100	60–100

* Collection by electroejaculation.

mally bulge through the incision. The bulging testicular lobules can be best excised with a cold-sterilized razor blade. The preferred fixatives are Bouin's, Zenker's, or Stieve's. These fixatives cause less distortion of the testicular architecture than does 10% buffered formalin. The potential usefulness of having cell preparations taken from biopsy material to determine the testicular karyotype should be considered before doing a testicular biopsy to prevent the necessity of a second biopsy.

Gonadal Hormone Assays

Testosterone, estradiol, and progesterone radioimmunoassays are done commercially by reference laboratories. Normal serum values for some gonadal hormones are listed in Table 22–8. Testosterone values fluctuate widely throughout the day. Three samples taken 20 to 30 minutes apart should be pooled for measuring baseline levels. Some hormones such as progesterone can be degraded if plasma is not separated from red blood cells soon after the collection of blood. The degradation of progesterone is a glycolytic process that can be avoided if whole blood is collected in potassium oxalate-sodium fluoride tubes and refrigerated immediately after collection. Assays for gonadal hormone serum concentrations should not be affected if the serum is separated and refrigerated just after the clot forms. Serum that will not be assayed within a few days should be frozen.

See also references 9, 22, 24, 30, 35, 38, 45, 55, 62, 70, 72–74, 79, 88, 96, 101, 114, 128–130, 133, 135, 147, 148, 159, 160, 174, 176, 180, 184, and 187.

Table 22–8. Approximate Normal Serum Gonadal Hormone Values in the Dog, Cat, and Horse

	Dog		Cat		Horse	
	Dog	Bitch	Tom	Queen	Stallion	Mare
Testosterone (ng/ml)	0.5–6		0.5–3		0.5–3	<0.1
Follicular phase		>0.3				
Luteal phase		<0.3		<0.3		
Estradiol (pg/ml)	0.5–5		0.5–5		8–12	
Follicular phase		>20		>20		
Luteal phase		<15		<15		
Progesterone (ng/ml)	<1		<2		<1	
Follicular phase		<5		<5		<1
Luteal phase		>15		>15		>5

The Luteinizing Hormone (Human Chorionic Gonadotropin) Stimulation Test in Males

The response in serum testosterone levels to exogenous LH stimulation can be useful in assessing the presence of cryptorchid testes in a possibly castrated male and in differentiating whether the cause of the lower serum testosterone values is primary (from testicular origin) or secondary (from pituitary origin). Serum testosterone levels rise when cryptorchid testes are stimulated with LH. Low testosterone values in testicular failure secondary to pituitary disease may rise after multiple injections of LH, but primary bilateral testicular failure will not respond to LH with increasing serum testosterone values.

Gonadotropin-releasing Hormone and Clomiphene Stimulation Tests

GnRH and clomiphene, a nonsteroid that binds to estrogen receptors, induce the release of gonadotropins. A stimulated response in plasma gonadotropin or serum testosterone levels could be useful in assessing the ability of the adenohypophysis to produce and release LH. Protocols and normal responses have not yet been well established in companion animals.

See also reference 96.

Plasma Gonadotropins and Prolactin

Although they have been developed and used for research, plasma LH, FSH, and prolactin assays for companion animals are not yet commercially available. Their value in evaluating hypogonadism in humans is well established. Commercial assays will develop as veterinary clinicians become more aware of the usefulness of such assays for gonadotropins and prolactin in companion animals. If the plasma gonadotropin and prolactin assays were available and economically feasible, there is no doubt they would enable veterinary clinicians to markedly improve their noninvasive diagnostic abilities concerning hypogonadism.

See also references 25, 32, 35–38, 40, 41, 45, 50, 56, 70, 91, 98–100, 117, 121, 133, 164, 185, 186, and 189.

Urine Estrogen Assays

An assay for estrogens in the urine of bitches has been advocated for the diagnosis of pregnancy. Urine estrogen values, determined by the Kober-Ittrich fluorescence reaction using the Brown method, may show a significant difference between values of pregnant and nonpregnant bitches at 14 to 25 days of gestation. The difference is reportedly most evident at 19 to 22 days of gestation. This test is not yet in common use.

Urine estriol determinations have been used in pregnant women to monitor the health of the fetus. Urine estriol values increase during a healthy pregnancy due to fetal conversion of DHEA by the placenta to estradiol. Measurement of urine estriol is not yet used in the clinical assessment of companion animals.

See also reference 143.

Vaginal Cytology

Vaginal smears may be used to determine the stage of the ovarian cycle in the bitch and queen. They are not helpful in the mare. Smears of the vagina can be obtained with a cotton-tipped applicator or spatula. Care must be taken not to make smears of the clitoral fossa. Smears should instead be obtained from the cranial vagina. If cotton-tipped applicators are used, they should be applied to the slide as a rolling impression, not in the manner of painting the slide.

Cytologic material can also be obtained with a bulb pipette flush and aspiration using sterile isotonic saline. After the slides are made and fixed by dipping in 95% methanol, a variety of stains may be used, such as Wrights, Wrights-Giemsa, Diff-Quik, new methylene blue, or trichrome stains. Slides stained with trichrome are technically the most difficult to prepare, but they produce sharper contrast between cell types. With trichrome stains, superficial cells stain orange and parabasal cells stain blue-green. The percentage of cells staining orange is referred to as the *eosinophilic index.* Trichrome stains include Shorr's and Sano-Pollack stains.

Cells found in vaginal smear preparations are parabasal cells (basal cells are not shed) and intermediate and superficial cells. Parabasal cells are small, round-to-oval cells with smooth cytoplasmic borders. Intermediate cells are much larger than parabasal cells and have irregular cytoplasmic borders. Superficial cells are even larger than intermediate cells. Superficial cells have a small dark pyknotic nucleus or are anuclear. Their cytoplasmic

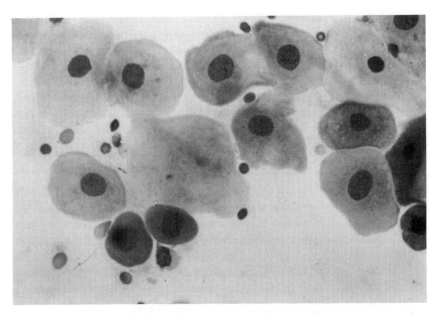

Fig. 22–17. Vaginal smear from a bitch in proestrus showing red blood cells, intermediate cells, and superficial cells. (Courtesy of Dr. Don Schmidt, University of Missouri, College of Veterinary Medicine.)

borders are irregular and often folded. Two other epithelial cells, metestrual and foam cells, may be found during metestrus in the bitch. Metestrual cells are parabasal cells containing a neutrophil. Foam cells are parabasal cells with cytoplasmic vacuoles. Red blood cells, neutrophils, and bacteria also occur, depending on the stage of the estrous cycle.

The percentage of superficial cells present has a direct relationship with concentrations of serum estradiol. There is a lag of 1 to 2 days in the rise and fall of superficial cell concentrations behind the rise and fall of the serum estrogen levels. In proestrus, the bitch's vaginal smear shows numerous red blood cells, a few neutrophils, and bacteria. More than 60% of the epithelial cells are superficial cells (Fig. 22–17). Proestrual vaginal smears in queens are virtually devoid of red blood cells. During estrus, there are no neutrophils. The background is clear of debris. More than 90% of the epithelial cells are superficial cells, which can occur in sheets (Figs. 22–18 and 22–19). Metestrual changes are abrupt. Superficial epithelial cells decrease to number less than 80% of the epithelial cells present, and neutrophils appear (Figs. 22–20 and 22–21). Foam cells and metestrual cells may be evident in bitches, but not queens. Anestrual smears show predominantly parabasal and intermediate epithelial cells.

See also references 3, 31, 82, 119, 131–133, 145, 147, and 159.

Endometrial Biopsy

Endometrial biopsies are rarely done in bitches or queens because a laparotomy is required. In mares, endometrial biopsy forceps can be used to

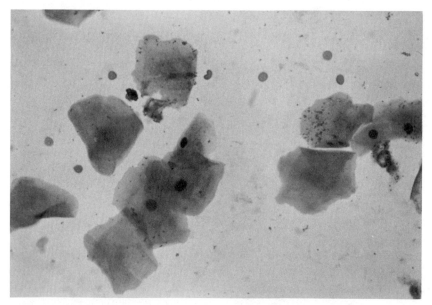

Fig. 22–18. Vaginal smear from a bitch in estrus showing predominantly superficial cells. (Courtesy of Dr. Don Schmidt, University of Missouri, College of Veterinary Medicine.)

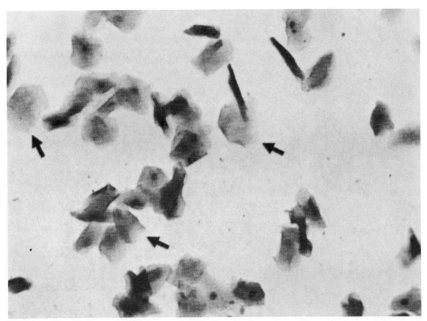

Fig. 22–19. Vaginal smear from a queen in estrus showing predominantly superficial cells (*arrows*). (From Lofstedt, R.M.: The estrous cycle of the domestic cat. Compendium on Continuing Educ. for the Practicing Vet., 4:52, 1982.)

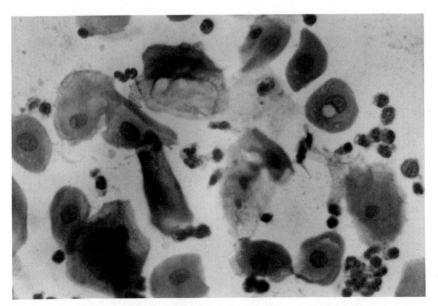

Fig. 22–20. Vaginal smear from a bitch in metestrus showing neutrophils and intermediate cells. (Courtesy of Dr. Don Schmidt, University of Missouri, College of Veterinary Medicine.)

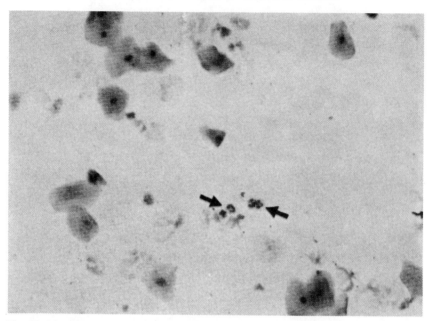

Fig. 22–21.   Vaginal smear from a queen in metestrus showing neutrophils (*arrows*) and intermediate cells. (From Loftstedt, R.M.: The estrous cycle of the domestic cat. Compendium on Continuing Educ. for the Practicing Vet., 4:52, 1982.)

obtain biopsy material through an open cervix. Endometrial biopsy can be useful in staging the ovarian cycle and in the diagnosis of primary uterine diseases. Samples should be fixed in Bouin's solution.

Chromosome Analyses

Chromosome analyses are at present underused in clinical veterinary medicine. Chromosomal abnormalities causing gonadal dysfunction may be presented as cases of unexplained male or female infertility, ambiguous genitalia, cryptorchidism, hypospadias, inguinal hernia, enlarged clitoris, gynecomastia, repeated abortions, or behavioral or training problems.

Buccal smears can be prepared for the identification of Barr bodies. *Barr bodies* are the inactivated X chromatin found in genetic females. The X chromosome-to-be-inactivated condenses and becomes heterochromatic in interphase and early prophase. It appears as a small dark mass next to the nuclear membrane in more than 15% of buccal cells of genetic females. In neutrophils, the Barr body appears like a drumstick (Fig. 22–22). They are less common (accounting for only 1% to 5% of the neutrophils) than Barr bodies in buccal smears. There is one Barr body per cell in all cells in interphase for each X chromosome in excess of the one that does not become inactivated. Normally, there is only one Barr body per cell, but not all cells are in interphase so some cells will have none. If samples are taken from a site of buccal inflammation, the mitotic rate will be increased so less

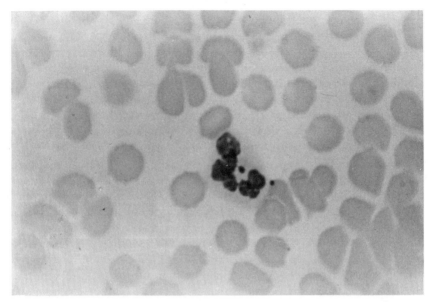

Fig. 22–22. Blood smear of a female dog with a neutrophil containing a Barr body. (Courtesy of Dr. Don Schmidt, University of Missouri, College of Veterinary Medicine.)

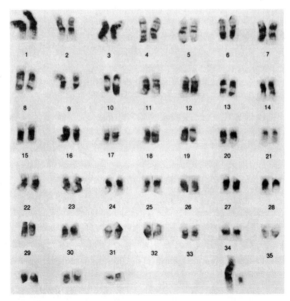

Fig. 22–23. G-banded karyotype of a normal male dog. (From Hare, W.C.D.: Cytogenetics. *In* Current Therapy in Theriogenology. Edited by D.A. Morrow. Philadelphia, W.B. Saunders, 1980, p. 149.)

cells will be in interphase and fewer will have Barr bodies. Artifacts may be mistaken for Barr bodies in genetic males in 1% to 3% of buccal cells.

Karyotyping facilitates thorough examination of the sex chromosomes and also permits examination of the autosomes. Tissues that are generally examined are circulating lymphocytes, splenic lymphocytes, dermal fibroblasts, testes, or ovaries. Tissue samples are grown in cell culture. Cultured lymphocytes are stimulated to divide with phytohemagglutinin. Replication of other cell cultures is a slower process. Cell division is arrested in metaphase with colchicine because chromosome pairing is most evident during metaphase. Cells are then swollen with a hypotonic solution, squashed, stained, photographed, paired in homologous pairs, and arranged in groups (Fig. 22–23). Stains are used to aid the identification and pairing of chromosomes. Staining of chromosomes occurs irregularly creating "bands," typical of a particular chromosome. Banding is done with either quinacrine hydrochloride (Q-banding), Giemsa (G-banding), Giemsa after pretreatment of the chromosomes to alter their staining (Reverse, R-banding), or Giemsa after DNA is extracted to permit staining of centromeric heterochromatin (C-banding). Autoradiography has also been used to aid in doing karyotyping.

See also references 26, 75, 87, and 154.

REFERENCES

1. Allen, W.E., Daker, M.G., and Hancock, J.L.: Three intersexual dogs. Vet. Rec., *109:*468, 1981.
2. Austad, R., Lunde, A., and Sjaastad, O.V.: Peripheral plasma levels of oestradiol-17 β and progesterone in the bitch during the oestrous cycle, in normal pregnancy and after dexamethasone treatment. J. Reprod. Fertil., *46:*129, 1976.
3. Barrett, R.P.: Exfoliative vaginal cytology of the dog using Wright's stain. Vet. Med. Small Anim. Clin., *71:*1236, 1976.
4. Basrur, P.K., Kanagawa, H., and Gilman, J.P.W.: An equine intersex with unilateral gonadal agenesis. Can. J. Comp. Med., *33:*297, 1969.
5. Basrur, P.K., Kanagawa, H., and Podliachouk, L.: Further studies on the cell populations of an intersex horse. Can. J. Comp. Med., *34:*294, 1970.
6. Batchelor, A., Bell, E.T., and Christie, D.W.: Urinary oestrogen excretion in the beagle bitch. Br. Vet. J., *128:*560, 1972.
7. Bedrak, E., and Samuels, L.T.: Steroid biosynthesis by the equine testis. Endocrinology, *85:*1186, 1969.
8. Bell, E.T., and Christie, D.W.: Duration of proestrus, oestrus, and vulval bleeding in the beagle bitch. Br. Vet. J., *127:*25, 1971.
9. Bell, E.T., Christie, D.W., and Younglai, E.V.: Plasma oestrogen levels during the canine oestrous cycle. J. Endocrinol., *51:*225, 1971.
10. Blue, M.G., Bruere, A.N., and Dewes, H.F.: The significance of the XO syndrome in infertility of the mare. N.Z. Vet. J., *26:*137, 1978.
11. Bornstein, S.: The genetic sex of two intersexual horses and some notes on the karyotype of normal horses. Acta Vet. Scand., *8:*291, 1967.
12. Bosu, W.T.K., Chick, B.F., and Basrur, P.K.: Clinical, pathologic and cytogenic observations on two intersex dogs. Cornell Vet., *68:*376, 1978.
13. Bouters, R., Vandeplassche, M., and de Moor, A.: An intersex (male pseudohermaphrodite) horse with 64XX/65XXY mosaicism. Equine Vet. J., *4:*150, 1972.
14. Brodey, R.S., Martin, J.D., and Lee, D.G.: Male pseudohermaphroditism in a toy terrier. J. Am. Vet. Med. Assoc., *125:*368, 1954.
15. Brown, R.D., Swanton, M.C., and Brinkhous, K.M.: Canine hemophilia and male pseudohermaphroditism: cytogenetic studies. Lab Invest., *12:*961, 1963.
16. Brown, T.T., Burek, J.D., and McEntee, S.: Male pseudohermaphoroditism, cryptorchi-

dism, and Sertoli cell neoplasia in three miniature schnauzers. J. Am. Vet. Med. Assoc., *169:*821, 1976.

17. Bruere, A.N., et al.: Preliminary observations on the occurrence of the equine XO syndrome. N.Z. Vet. J., *26:*145, 1978.
18. Buoen, L.C., et al.: Sterility associated with an XO karyotype in a Belgian mare. J. Am. Vet. Med. Assoc., *182:*1120, 1983.
19. Burke, T.J.: Feline reproduction. Vet. Clin. North Am., *6:*317, 1976.
20. Carillo, J.M., and Burk, R.L.: Male pseudohermaphrodism associated with urinary incontinence in an Afghan. J. Am. Anim. Hosp. Assoc., *13:*80, 1977.
21. Centerwall, W.R., and Benirschke, K.: An animal model for the XXY Klinefelter's syndrome in man: tortoiseshell and calico male cats. Am. J. Vet. Res., *36:*1275, 1975.
22. Chaffaux, S., and Thibier, M.: Effects of hysterectomy in bitches in terms of plasma progesterone concentrations. Recueil de Medecine Veterinaire d'Alfort, *154:*933, 1978.
23. Chakraborty, P.K., Wildt, D.E., and Seager, S.W.J.: Induction of estrus and ovulation in the cat and dog. Vet. Clin. North Am., *12:*85, 1982.
24. Chakraborty, P.K., Panko, W.B., and Fletcher, W.S.: Serum hormone concentrations and their relationships to sexual relationships to sexual behavior at the first and second estrous cycles of the Labrador bitch. Biol. Reprod., *22:*227, 1980.
25. Chakraborty, R.K., Wildt, D.G., and Seager, S.W.J.: Serum luteinizing hormone-releasing hormone in the estrous and anestrous domestic cat. Lab. Anim. Sci., *27:*338, 1979.
26. Chandley, A.C., et al.: Chromosome abnormalities as a cause of infertility in mares. J. Reprod. Fertil. [Suppl.], *23:*337, 1975.
27. Christie, D.W., and Bell, E.T.: Endocrinology of the oestrus cycle in the bitch. J. Small Anim. Pract., *12:*383, 1971.
28. Christie, D.W., and Bell, E.T.: Some observations on the seasonal incidence and frequency of estrus in breeding bitches in Britain. J. Small Anim. Pract., *12:*159, 1971.
29. Christie, D.W., and Bell, E.T.: Studies on canine reproductive behavior during the normal estrous cycle. Anim. Behav., *20:*621, 1972.
30. Christie, D.W., et al.: Peripheral plasma progesterone levels during the canine oestrous cycle. Acta Endocrinol., *68:*543, 1971.
31. Cline, E.M., Jennings, L.L., and Sojka, N.J.: Analysis of the feline vaginal epithelial cycle. Feline Pract., *10:*47, 1980.
32. Clough, E., et al.: An XXY sex chromosome constitution in a dog with testicular hypoplasia and congenital heart disease. Cytogenetics, *9:*71, 1970.
33. Colby, E.D.: Induced estrus and timed pregnancies in cats. Lab. Anim. Care, *20:*1075, 1970.
34. Collins, D.C., Musey, P.I., and Preedy, J.R.: Identification of conjugated estrogen metabolities in dog plasma following administration of estriol-2, 4, 6, 7-3H. Steroids, *28:*67, 1976.
35. Concannon, P.W.: Reproductive physiology and endocrine patterns of the bitch. *In* Current Veterinary Therapy. Vol. VIII. Edited by R.W. Kirk. Philadelphia, W.B. Saunders, 1983, pp. 886–901.
36. Concannon, P.W., et al.: Parturition and lactation in the bitch: serum progesterone, cortisol and prolactin. Biol. Reprod., *19:*1113, 1978.
37. Concannon, P.W., Cowan, R., and Hansel, W.: LH release in ovariectomized dogs in response to estrogen withdrawal and its facilitation by progesterone. Biol. Reprod., *20:*523, 1979.
38. Concannon, P.W., and Hansel, W.: Changes in plasma progesterone and corticoids at parturition in the bitch. Biol. Reprod., *9:*104, 1973.
39. Concannon, P.W., and Hansel, W.: Effects of estrogen and progesterone on plasma LH, sexual behavior, and pregnancy in Beagle bitches. Fed. Proc., *34:*323, 1975.
40. Concannon, P.W., Hansel, W., and McEntree, K.: Changes in LH, progesterone, and sexual behavior associated with preovulatory luteinization in the bitch. Biol. Reprod., *17:*604, 1977.
41. Concannon, P.W., Hansel, W., and Visek, W.J.: The ovarian cycle of the bitch: plasma estrogen, LH, and progesterone. Biol. Reprod., *13:*112, 1975.
42. Concannon, P., Hodgson, B., and Lein, D.: Reflex LH release in estrous cats following single and multiple copulations. Biol. Reprod., *23:*111, 1980.
43. Concannon, P.W., et al.: Pregnancy and parturition in the bitch. Biol. Reprod., *16:*517, 1977.
44. Concannon, P.W., et al.: Sexual behavior in ovariectomized bitches in response to estrogen and progesterone treatments. Biol. Reprod., *20:*799, 1979.

45. Concannon, P.W., and Lein, D.H.: Feline reproduction. *In* Current Veterinary Therapy Vol. VIII. Philadelphia, W.B. Saunders Co., 1983, pp. 932–936.

46. Curtis, E.M., and Grant, R.P.: Masculinization of female pups by progesterone. J. Am. Vet. Med. Assoc., *144:*395, 1964.

47. Dain, A.R.: Intersexuality in a cocker spaniel dog. J. Reprod. Fertil., *39:*365, 1974.

48. Dain, A.R., and Walker, R.G.: Two intersex dogs with mosaicism. J. Reprod. Fertil., *56:*239, 1979.

49. Dawson, A.B.: Early estrus in the cat following increased illumination. Endocrinology, *28:*907, 1941.

50. DePalatis, L., Moore, J., and Falvo, R.E.: Plasma concentrations of testosterone and LH in the male dog. J. Reprod. Fertil., *52:*201, 1978.

51. Deykin, D., Balko, C., and Wilson, J.D.: Recent studies on the mechanism of action of testosterone. N. Engl. J. Med., *287:*1284, 1972.

52. Dunn, H.O., et al.: Two equine true hermaphrodites with 64,XX/64,XY and 63,XO/64,XY chimerism. Cornell Vet., *71:*123, 1981.

53. Dunn, H.O., Vaughan, J.T., and McEntee, K.: Bilaterally cryptorchid stallion with female karyotype. Cornell Vet., *64:*265, 1974.

54. Edols, J.H., and Allan G.S.: A case of male pseudohermaphroditism in a cocker spaniel. Aust. Vet. J., *44:*287, 1968.

55. Edquist, L.E., et al.: Blood plasma levels of progesterone and oestradiol in the dog during the oestrous cycle and pregnancy. Acta Endocrinol., *78:*554, 1975.

56. Falvo, R.E., et al.: Annual variation in plasma levels of testosterone and luteinizing hormone in the laboratory male mongrel dog. J. Endocrinol., *86:*425, 1980.

57. Felts, J.F., et al.: Hermaphroditism in a cat. J. Am. Vet. Med. Assoc., *181:*925, 1982.

58. Fischer, K.: Pseudohermaphroditism in a dog. Vet. Med. Small Anim. Clin., *78:*683, 1983.

59. Fretz, P.B., and Hare, W.C.D.: A male pseudohermaphrodite horse with 63XO?/64XX/65XXY mixoploidy. Equine Vet. J., *8:*130, 1976.

60. Frey, D.C., Tyler, D.E., and Ramsey, F.K.: Pyometra associated with bilateral cryptorchism and Sertoli's cell tumor in a male pseudohermaphrodite dog. J. Am. Vet. Med. Assoc., *146:*723, 1965.

61. Frota-Pessoa, O.: XO and XXY karyotypes in cats. Lancet, *1:*1304, 1962.

62. Ganjam, V.K., and Kenney, R.M.: Androgens and oestrogens in normal and cryptochid stallions. J. Reprod. Fertil., *23:*67, 1975.

63. Gentry, P.A., and Liptrap, R.M.: Influence of progesterone and pregnancy on canine fibrinogen values. J. Small Anim. Pract., *22:*185, 1981.

64. Gentry, P.A., and Liptrap, R.M.: Plasma levels of specific coagulation factors and oestrogens in the bitch during pregnancy. J. Small Anim. Pract., *18:*267, 1977.

65. Gerneke, W.H., and Courbrough, R.I.: Intersexuality in the horse. Onderstepoort J. Vet. Res., *37:*211, 1970.

66. Gilbride, A.P.: A quick review of the genetics of the male calico cat. Feline Pract., *2:*33, 1972.

67. Ginther, O.J., and First, N.L.: Maintenance of the corpus luteum in hysterectomized mares. Am. J. Vet. Res., *32:*1687, 1971.

68. Gluhovschi, N., et al.: A case of intersexuality in the horse with type 2 A+ XXXY chromosome formula. Br. Vet. J., *126:*522, 1970.

69. Goodwin, M., Gooding, K.M., and Regnier, F.: Sex pheromones in the dog. Science, *203:*559, 1979.

70. Graf, K.J.: Serum oestrogen, progesterone and prolactin concentrations in cyclic, pregnant and lactating beagle dogs. J. Reprod. Fertil., *52:*9, 1978.

71. Hadley, J.C.: The effect of serial uterine biopsies and hysterectomy on peripheral blood levels of total unconjugated oestrogen and progesterone in the bitch. J. Reprod. Fertil., *45:*389, 1975.

72. Hadley, J.C.: Total unconjugated estrogen and progesterone concentration in peripheral blood during the oestrous cycle of the dog. J. Reprod. Fertil., *44:*445, 1975.

73. Hadley, J.C.: Total unconjugated estrogen and progesterone concentration in peripheral blood during pregnancy in the dog. J. Reprod. Fertil., *44:*453, 1975.

74. Hadley, J.C.: Unconjugated oestrogen and progesterone concentrations in the blood of bitches with false pregnancy and pyometra. Vet. Rec., *95:*545, 1975.

75. Hare, W.C.D., et al.: Cytogenetics in the dog and cat. J. Small Anim. Pract., *7:*575, 1966.

76. Hare, W.C.D.: Intersexuality in the dog. Can. Vet. J., *17:*7, 1976.
77. Hare,W.C.D., McFeely, R.A., and Kelly, D.F.: Familial 78XX male pseudohermaphroditism in three dogs. J. Reprod. Fertil., *36:*207, 1974.
78. Hart, B.L., and Barrett, R.E.: Effects of castration on fighting, roaming, and urine spraying in adult male cats. J. Am. Vet. Med. Assoc., *163:*290, 1973.
79. Hart, B.L., and Ladewig, J.: Serum testosterone of neonatal male and female dogs. Biol. Reprod., *21:*289, 1979.
80. Herraman-Johnson, K.: Complex hermaphrodism in a cocker. Vet. Rec., *15:*1099, 1935.
81. Herron, M.A., and Boehringer, B.T.: Male pseudohermaphroditism in a cat. Feline Pract., *5:*30, 1975.
82. Herron, M.A.: Feline vaginal cytologic examination. Feline Pract., *7:*36, 1977.
83. Holst, P.A., and Phemister, R.D.: Onset of diestrus in the beagle bitch: definition and significance. Am. J. Vet. Res., *35:*401, 1974.
84. Holst, P.A., and Phemister, R.D.: Temporal sequence of events in the estrous cycle of the bitch. Am. J. Vet. Res., *36:*705, 1975.
85. Holt, P.E., Long, S.E., and Gibbs, C.: Disorders of urination associated with canine intersexuality. J. Small Anim. Pract., *24:*475, 1983.
86. Hughes, J.P., et al.: Gonadal dysgenesis in the mare. J. Reprod. Fertil. [Suppl.], *23:*385, 1975.
87. Hughes, J.P., and Trommerhausen-Smith, A.: Infertility in the horse associated with chromosomal abnormalities. Aust. Vet. J., *53:*253, 1977.
88. Inaba, T., Shimizu, R., and Imori, T.: Radioimmunoassay for male canine plasma 4-androstenedione, testosterone, and 5-alpha-dihydrotestosterone. Jpn. J. Anim. Reprod., *23:*63, 1977.
89. Jackson, D.A., et al.: Non-neurogenic urinary incontinence in a canine female pseudohermaphrodite. J. Am. Vet. Med. Assoc., *172:*926, 1978.
90. James, R.W., and Heywood, R.: Age-related variations in the testes and prostate of beagle dogs. Toxicology, *12:*273, 1979.
91. Jemmet, J.E., and Evans, J.M.: A survey of sexual behavior and reproduction in female cats. J. Small Anim. Pract., *18:*31, 1977.
92. Jochle, W.: Current research in coitus-induced ovulation: a review. J. Reprod. Fertil. [Suppl.], *22:*165, 1975.
93. Jochle, W., and Andersen, A.C.: The estrous cycle in the dog: a review. Theriogenology, *7:*113, 1977.
94. Johnson, C.A.: The role of the fetal testicle in sexual differentiation. Compendium on Continuing Educ. for the Practicing Vet., *5:*129, 1983.
95. Johnson, L.M., and Gay, V.L.: Luteinizing hormone in the cat. II. Mating-induced secretion. Endocrinology, *109:*247, 1981.
96. Jones, G.E., et al.: Effect of luteinizing hormone releasing hormone on plasma levels of luteinizing hormone, oestradiol, and testosterone in the male dog. J. Endocrinol., *68:*469, 1976.
97. Jones, G.E., and Boyns, A.R.: Effect of gonadal steroids on the pituitary responsiveness to synthetic luteinizing hormone releasing hormone in the male dog. J. Endocrinol., *61:*123, 1974.
98. Jones, G.E., et al.: Immunoreactive luteinizing hormone and progesterone during pregnancy and following gonadotrophin administration in beagle bitches. Acta Endocrinol., *72:*573, 1973.
99. Jones, G.E., et al.: Plasma oestradiol, luteinizing hormone and progesterone during pregnancy in the beagle bitch. J. Reprod. Fertil., *35:*187, 1973.
100. Jones, G.E., et al.: Plasma oestradiol, luteinizing hormone and progesterone during the oestrous cycle in the beagle bitch. J. Endocrinol., *57:*331, 1973.
101. Jones, G.E., et al.: Effect of sex steroids on testosterone, oestradiol-17β and luteinizing hormone secretion after the injection of synthetic luteinizing hormone releasing hormone into male dogs. J. Endocrinol., *61:*123, 1974.
102. Kelly, D.F., Long, S.E., and Strohmenger, G.D.: Testicular neoplasia in an intersex dog. J. Small Anim. Pract., *17:*247, 1976.
103. Kieffer, N.M., Burns, S.J., and Judge, N.G.: Male pseudohermaphroditism of the testicular feminizing type in a horse. Equine Vet. J., *8:*38, 1976.
104. Klempiem, E.J., Voigt, R.D., and Tamm J.: The metabolism of dehydroepiandrosterone in dog liver. Acta Endocrinol., *36:*498, 1961.

105. Lawrence, J., and Meisels, R.: A lateral canine hermaphrodite. J. Am. Vet. Med. Assoc., *121:*171, 1952.
106. Lee, J.: Paraphimosis in a pseudohermaphrodite dog. Vet. Med. Small Anim. Clin., *71:*1076, 1976.
107. Leighton, R.L.: Ablation of the penis and castration in a male pseudohermaphrodite dog. J. Am. Anim. Hosp. Assoc., *12:*664, 1976.
108. LeRoux, P.H.: The use of a teaser tom to terminate oestrum in female cats. J. S. Afr. Vet. Med. Assoc., *42:*95, 1971.
109. Lessey, B.A., Wahawisan, R., and Gorell, T.A.: Hormonal regulation of cytoplasmic estrogen and progesterone receptors in the beagle uterus and oviduct. Mol. Cell Endocrinol., *21:*171, 1981.
110. Lipsett, M.B.: Physiology and pathology of the Leydig cell. N. Engl. J. Med., *303:*682, 1980.
111. Long, S.E., and Berepubo, N.A.: A 37, XO chromosome complement in a kitten. J. Small Anim. Pract., *21:*627, 1980.
112. Marshall, L.S., et al.: Persistent Mullerian duct syndrome in miniature schnauzers. J. Am. Vet. Med. Assoc., *181:*798, 1982.
113. Martin, R.P., Loriaux, D.L., and Farnham, G.S.: Enterohepatic cycling of metabolized testosterone in the male dog. Steroids [Suppl.], *2:*149, 1965.
114. Masken, J.F.: Circulating hormone levels in the cycling beagle. *In* 22nd Gaines Veterinary Symposium. White Plains, New York, Gaines Dog Research Center, 1972, p. 33.
115. McFeely, R.A., and Biggers, J.D.: A rare case of female pseudohermaphroditism in the dog. Vet. Rec., *77:*696, 1965.
116. McIlwraith, C.W., Owen, R.Ap.R., and Basrur, P.K.: An equine cryptorchid with testicular and ovarian tissues. Equine Vet. J., *8:*156, 1976.
117. Mellin, T.N., et al.: Serum profiles of luteinizing hormone, progesterone, and total estrogens during the canine estrous cycle. Theriogenology, *5:*175, 1976.
118. Metzler, F., Eleftherion, B.E., and Fox, M.: Free estrogens in dog plasma during the estrous cycle and pregnancy. Proc. Soc. Exp. Biol. Med., *121:*374, 1966.
119. Mowrer, R.T., Conti, P.A., and Rossow, C.F.: Vaginal cytology. An approach to improvement of cat breeding. Vet. Med. Small Anim. Clin., *75:*691, 1975.
120. Murti, G.S., Gilbert, D.L., and Borgmann, A.R.: Canine intersex states. J. Am. Vet. Med. Assoc., *149:*1183, 1966.
121. Nett, T.M., et al.: Levels of luteinizing hormone, estradiol, and progesterone in serum during the estrous cycle and pregnancy in the beagle bitch. Proc. Soc. Exp. Biol. Med., *148:*134, 1975.
122. Newman, R.H.: Pyometra and a Sertoli cell tumor in a hemaphroditic dog. Vet. Med. Small Anim. Clin., *74:*1757, 1979.
123. Norby, D.E., et al.: An XO cat. Cytogenet. Cell Genet., *13:*448, 1974.
124. Norrdin, R.W., and Baum, A.C.: A male pseudohermaphrodite dog with a Sertoli cell tumor, mucometra, and vaginal glands. J. Am. Vet. Med. Assoc., *156:*204, 1970.
125. Oertel, G.W., and Eik-Nes, K.B.: Plasma levels of dehydroepiandrosterone in the dog. Endocrinology, *65:*766, 1959.
126. Oh, R., and Tamaoki, B.: In vitro biosynthesis of androgens in canine testes. Acta Endocrinol., *74:*615, 1973.
127. Oh, R., and Tamaoki, B.I.: In vitro steroidogenesis in feline testes. Biochim. Biophys. Acta, *316:*395, 1973.
128. Olson, P.N., et al.: Concentrations of testosterone in canine serum during late anestrus, proestrus, estrus, and early diestrus. Am. J. Vet. Res., *45:*145, 1984.
129. Olson, P.N., et al.: Concentrations of progesterone and luteinizing hormone in the serum of diestrous bitches before and after hysterectomy. Am. J. Vet. Res., *45:*149, 1984.
130. Olson, P.N., et al.: Concentrations of reproductive hormones in canine serum throughout late anestrus, proestrus and estrus. Biol. Reprod., *27:*1196, 1982.
131. Olson, P.N., et al.: Vaginal cytology. Part I. A useful tool for staging the canine estrous cycle. Compendium on Continuing Educ. for the Practicing Vet., *6:*288, 1984.
132. Olson, P.N., et al.: Vaginal cytology. Part II. Its use in diagnosing canine reproductive disorders. Compendium on Continuing Educ. for the Practicing Vet., *6:*385, 1984.
133. Olson, P.N., et al.: Reproductive endocrinology and physiology of the bitch and queen. Vet. Clin. North Am., *14:*927, 1984.
134. Paape, S.R., et al.: Luteal activity in the pseudopregnant cat. Biol. Reprod., *13:*470, 1975.

135. Parkes, M.R., Bell, E.T., and Christie, D.W.: Plasma progesterone levels during pregnancy in the beagle bitch. Br. Vet. J., *128:*15, 1972.
136. Phemister, R.D., et al.: Time of ovulation in the Beagle bitch. Biol. Reprod., *8:*74, 1973.
137. Picon, R., et al.: Effects of canine fetal testicles and testicular tumors on mullerian ducts. Biol. Reprod., *18:*459, 1978.
138. Post, K.: Effects of human chorionic gonadotropin and castration on plasma gonadal steroid hormones of the dog. Can. Vet. J., *23:*98, 1982.
139. Prescott, C.W.: Reproductive patterns in the domestic cat. Aust. Vet. J., *49:*126, 1973.
140. Pullen, C.M.: True bilateral hemaphroditism in a beagle: a case report. Am. J. Vet. Res., *31:*1113, 1970.
141. Rhoades, J.D., and Foley, C.W.: Cryptorchidism and intersexuality. Vet. Clin. North Am., *7:*798, 1977.
142. Richkind, M.: The reproductive endocrinology of the domestic cat. Feline Pract., *8:*28, 1978.
143. Richkind, M.: Possible use of early morning urine for detection of pregnancy in dogs. Vet. Med. Small Anim. Clin., *78:*1067, 1983.
144. Rogers, A.L., Templeton, J.H., and Stewart, A.P.: Preliminary observations of estrous changes in large, colony raised laboratory dogs. Lab. Anim. Care, *20:*11133, 1970.
145. Roszel, J.F.: Genital cytology of the bitch. Vet. Scope, *19:*2, 1975.
146. Salkin, M.S.: Pyometra in a male pseudohermaphrodite dog. J. Am. Vet. Med. Assoc., *172:*913, 1978.
147. Schille, V.M., Lundstrom, K.E., and Stabenfeldt, G.H.: Follicular function in the domestic cat is determined by estradiol-17β concentrations in plasma: relation to estrous behavior and cornification of exfoliated vaginal epithelium. Biol. Reprod., *21:*953, 1979.
148. Schmidt, P.M., Chakraborty, P.K., and Wildt, D.E.: Ovarian activity, circulating hormones and sexual behavior in the cat. Biol. Reprod., *28:*657, 1983.
149. Schneck, G.W.: Hermaphroditism in a Shetland sheepdog. Vet. Rec., *96:*323, 1975.
150. Schultz, M.G.: Male pseudohermaphroditism diagnosed with aid of sex chromatin technique. J. Am. Vet. Med. Assoc., *140:*241, 1962.
151. Scott, P.P., and Lloyd-Jacob, M.A.: Reduction in the anoestrus period of laboratory cats by increased illumination. Nature, *184:*2022, 1959.
152. Selden, G.: Pyometra in a male pseudohermaphrodite dog. J. Am. Vet. Med. Assoc., *172:*913, 1978.
153. Selden, J.R.: The intersex dog: classification, clinical presentation, and etiology. Compendium on Continuing Educ. for the Practicing Vet., *1:*435, 1979.
154. Selden, J.R., et al.: The Giemsa-banding pattern of the canine karyotype. Cytogenet. Cell Genet., *15:*380, 1975.
155. Selden, J.R., et al.: Inherited XX sex reversal in the cocker spaniel dog. Hum. Genet., *67:*62, 1984.
156. Selden, J.R., et al.: Genetic basis of XX male syndrome and XX true hermaphroditism: evidence in the dog. Science, *201:*644, 1978.
157. Shane, B.S., et al.: Methyl testosterone-induced female pseudohermaphroditism in dogs. Biol. Reprod., *1:*41, 1969.
158. Sharp, A.J., Wachtel, S.S., and Benirschke, K.: H-Y antigen in a fertile XY female horse. J. Reprod. Fertil., *58:*157, 1980.
159. Shille, V.M., Lundstrom, K.E., and Stabenfeldt, G.H.: Follicular function in the domestic cat as determined by estradiol-17β concentrations in plasma: relation to estrous behavior and cornification of exfoliated vaginal epithelium. Biol. Reprod., *21:*953, 1979.
160. Shille, V.M., and Stabenfeldt, G.H.: Luteal function in the domestic cat during pseudopregnancy and after treatment with prostaglandin $F_{2\alpha}$. Biol. Reprod., *21:*1217, 1979
161. Shille, V.M., and Stabenfeldt, G.H.: Current concepts in reproduction of the dog and cat. Adv. Vet. Sci. Comp. Med., *24:*211, 1980.
162. Shille, V.M., Stabenfeldt, G.H., and Andersen, A.C.: The estrous cycle of the bitch. Canine Pract., *1:*29, 1974.
163. Siegel, E.T.: Urinary excretion of sex steroid catabolites in the dog. Am. J. Vet. Res., *28:*287, 1967.
164. Smith, M.S., and McDonald, L.E.: Serum levels of luteinizing hormone and progesterone during the estrous cycle, pseudopregnancy, and pregnancy in the dog. Endocrinology, *94:*404, 1974.

165. Smith, W.C., and Reese, W.C., Jr.: Characteristics of a Beagle colony. I. Estrous cycle. Lab. Anim. Care, *18:*602, 1968.
166. Sokolowski, J.H.: The effects of ovariectomy on pregnancy maintenance in the bitch. Lab. Anim. Sci., *21:*696, 1971.
167. Sokolowski, J.H.: Reproductive features and patterns in the bitch. J. Am. Anim. Hosp. Assoc., *9:*71, 1973.
168. Sokolowski, J.H., Stover, D.G., and Van Ravenswaay, F.: Seasonal incidence of estrus and interestrous interval for bitches of seven breeds. J. Am. Vet. Med. Assoc., *171:*271, 1977.
169. Stewart, R.W., et al.: Canine intersexuality in a pug breeding kennel. Cornell Vet., *62:*464, 1962.
170. Suzuki, Y., Okumura, Y., and Sinohara, H.: Purification and characterization of testosterone-binding globulin of canine serum. J. Biochem., *85:*1195, 1979.
171. Tabei, T., et al.: Sex steroid binding protein (SBP) in dog plasma. J. Steroid Biochem., *9:*983, 1978.
172. Taha, M.B., Noakes, D.E., and Allen, W.E.: The effect of season of the year on the characteristics and composition of dog semen. J. Small Anim. Pract., *22:*177, 1981.
173. Taha, M.B., Noakes, D.E., and Allen, W.E.: The effect of some exogenous hormones on seminal characteristics, libido and peripheral plasma testosterone concentration in the male beagle. J. Small Anim. Pract., *22:*587, 1981.
174. Taha, M.B., and Noakes, D.E.: The effect of age and season of the year on testicular function in the dog, as determined by histological examination of the seminiferous tubules and the estimation of peripheral plasma testosterone concentrations. J. Small Anim. Pract., *23:*351, 1982.
175. Tangner, C.H., Breider, M.A., and Amoss, M.S.: Lateral hemaphroditism in a dog. J. Am. Vet. Med. Assoc., *181:*70, 1982.
176. Telegdy, G., Endroczi, E., and Lissak, K.: Ovarian progesterone secretion during the oestrous cycle, pregnancy and lactation in dogs. Acta Endocrinol., *44:*461, 1963.
177. Todoroff, R.J.: Congenital urogenital anomalies. Compendium on Continuing Educ. for the Practicing Vet., *1:*780, 1979.
178. Tremblay, R.R., et al.: Studies on the dynamics of plasma androgens and on origin of dihydrotestosterone in dogs. Endocrinology, *91:*556, 1972.
179. Van Der Molen, H.J., and Eik-Nes, K.B.: Biosynthesis and secretion of steroids by the canine testis. Biochem. Biophys. Acta, *248:*343, 1971.
180. Verhage, H.G., Beamer, N.B., and Breener, R.M.: Plasma levels of estradiol and progesterone in the cat during polyestrus, pregnancy, and pseudopregnancy. Biol. Reprod., *14:*579, 1976.
181. Walker, K.S., and Bruere, A.N.: XO condition in mares. N.Z. Vet. J., *27:*18, 1979.
182. Wassermann, G.F., and Eik-Nes, K.B.: Interrelation between adrenal function and formation of testosterone *in vivo* in the testis of the dog. Acta Endocrinol., *61:*33, 1969.
183. Weaver, A.D., et al.: Phenotypic intersex (female pseudohermaphroditism) in a dachshund dog. Vet. Rec., *105:*230, 1979.
184. Wichmann, U., Wichmann, G., and Krause, W.: Serum levels of testosterone precursors, testosterone and estradiol in 10 animal species. Exp. Clin. Endocrinol., *83:*283, 1984.
185. Wildt, D.E., et al.: Relationship of reproductive behavior, serum luteinizing hormone and time of ovulation in the bitch. Biol. Reprod., *18:*561, 1978.
186. Wildt, D.E., et al.: Relationship of serum estrone, estradiol 17-beta, and progesterone to LH, sexual behavior and time of ovulation in the bitch. Biol. Reprod., *20:*648, 1979.
187. Wildt, D.E., et al.: Ovarian activity, circulating hormones, and sexual behavior in the cat. Part I. Biol. Reprod., *25:*15, 1981.
188. Wildt, D.E., Seager, S.W., and Chakraborty, P.K.: Behavioral, ovarian and endocrine relationships in the pubertal bitch. J. Anim. Sci., *53:*182, 1981.
189. Wildt, D.E., Seager, S.W.J., and Chakraborty, P.K.: Effect of copulatory stimuli on incidence of ovulation and on serum luteinizing hormone in the cat. Endocrinology, *107:*1212, 1980.
190. Wilson, J.D.: Recent studies on the mechanism of action of testosterone. N. Engl. J. Med., *287:*1284, 1972.
191. Yamamoto, Y., et al.: Testosterone metabolites in dog bile. Steroids, *31:*233, 1978.
192. Younglai, E.V., et al.: Testosterone production by ovarian follicles of the domestic cat (*Felis catus*). Hormone Res., *7:*91, 1976.

23

Clinical Disorders Related to
Testicular Endocrine Function

Endocrine disorders of the testes can be of primary testicular or secondary/tertiary (pituitary/hypothalamic) origin. Endocrine disorders may also be prepubertal or postpubertal. Some are neoplastic; others cause hypogonadism, infertility, gynecomastia, or precocious sexual development.

Additional testicular hormone clinical disorders may be caused or enhanced by the stimulation of androgens, excessive production of testicular estrogen, or imbalances in the normal androgen to estrogen ratio. Foremost among clinical disorders related to testicular function in companion animals are male infertility, perineal hernias, benign prostatic hypertrophy, perianal gland adenomas, galactorrhea, and alopecia in dogs. Gonadal-hormone-related alopecias begin in the perineal and genital regions, presumably because gonadal hormone receptors and 5 α-reductase predominate in these regions.

MALE HYPOGONADISM

Male hypogonadism is deficient function of the testes. Possible causes are listed in Table 23–1.

Male Hypogonadism of Hypothalamic-Pituitary Origin (Hypogonadotropic Hypogonadism)

Male hypogonadism of hypothalamic-pituitary origin is associated with deficient testicular function as a result of gonadotropin deficiencies. Follicle-stimulating hormone (FSH) and luteinizing hormone (LH) levels are decreased along with serum testosterone levels. In theory, there would be no significant increase in serum testosterone levels in response to the administration of gonadotropin-releasing hormone (GnRH), but repeated injections of human chorionic gonadotropin (HCG) would lead to normal serum testosterone levels. Testicular biopsy should show prepubertal morphology. When available, plasma prolactin levels should be investigated since hyperprolactinemia can inhibit the release of gonadotropins. Exogenous androgens, estrogens, or progestins can also inhibit the secretion of gonadotropins. Sources of excessive androgens and estrogens of endogenous origin include adrenocortical hyperplasia and neoplasia, as well as hepatic failure.

Prepubertal hypogonadotropic hypogonadism would prevent puberty, the attainment of normal stature, and the normal development of male

Table 23–1. Possible Causes of Male Hypogonadism

Hypothalamic-pituitary origin (Hypogonadotropic)
    Primary or metastasized neoplasia
    Cystic Rathke's pouch
    Administration of exogenous gonadal steroid hormones
    Starvation
    Hemorrhage, infarction, or infection
    Hyperprolactinemia
    Adrenocortical hyperplasia or neoplasia
    Hepatic failure
Gonadal origin (Hypergonadotropic)
    Seminiferous tubule dysgenesis and other chromosomal abnormalities
    Cryptorchidism
    Defects in the biosynthesis of androgen
    Acquired seminiferous tubule failure
    Bilateral anorchia
Defects in androgen's action
    Complete or incomplete androgen insensitivity
    Drug-induced causes

---

secondary sex characteristics such as leg lifting to urinate in dogs, urine spraying in tom cats, and a crested neck in stallions.

Postpubertal hypogonadism is more subtle in appearance. Infertility and impotence usually occur, but few secondary sex characteristics regress (they are often normal). If there is selected LH deficiency, but normal levels of plasma FSH are present, fertility may remain (such characteristics of postpubertal hypogonadism are seen in the "fertile eunuch syndrome" in humans).

Replacement therapy with gonadotropins would require repeated parenteral administrations. The treatment would be sensitizing and expensive and is, therefore, impractical. Treatment of hypogonadotropic hypogonadism involves eliminating the cause, if possible, and providing replacement androgen therapy.

Hypogonadism of Gonadal Origin and Defects in Androgen Action (Hypergonadotropic Hypogonadism)

Gonadal-origin hypogonadism and defects in androgen action lead to male hypogonadism with insufficient negative feedback on the hypothalamus and pituitary. Plasma gonadotropin levels are elevated. There should be no increase in serum testosterone levels in response to repeated administration of GnRH or LH (HCG). Testicular biopsy may show primary destructive lesions or an abnormal testicular karyotype. Karyotypes of other tissues may also show abnormalities. Plasma prolactin levels should be normal. A history of administered drugs may disclose the use of a drug that impairs the synthesis of testosterone or its peripheral effects. The clinical features of prepubertal and postpubertal hypergonadotropic hypogonadism are identical to those of prepubertal and postpubertal hypogonadotropic hypogonadism, respectively.

See also reference 36.

Seminiferous Tubule Dysgenesis (Klinefelter's Syndrome)

The most common cause of hypogonadism in men, seminiferous tubule dysgenesis, is a nondisjunctional chromosomal abnormality (XXY) with several less common variant syndromes possible (XX male, XY/XXY, XX/XXY, XXXY, XXXXY, XXYY, and XYY). It is probably a common cause of idiopathic hypogonadism in male companion animals. It has been reported in the dog, tom cat, and stallion. Clinical signs include infertility, decreased libido, small but firm testes, subnormal development of secondary sex characteristics, and possibly gynecomastia. Serum testosterone levels should be normal to low. Plasma FSH and LH levels should be elevated. Semen evaluation shows azoospermia, and buccal smears are "chromatin-positive," that is, an inactive X chromosome is found in the nuclei as if the animal were a genetic female. Treatment will not correct Klinefelter's syndrome, but normal secondary sex characteristics can be stimulated with androgen therapy.

Cryptorchidism

Cryptorchidism (Gr., "hidden testes") is maldescent of one or both testes. Unilateral cryptorchidism is maldescent of one testis, a common abnormality. Monorchidism is the term for the rare situation in which one testis fails to develop; as a term, it should not mistakenly be used to refer to a unilateral cryptorchid. Unilateral cryptochidism is much more common than bilateral cryptorchidism. Cryptorchid testes are described according to the level at which their descent to the scrotum ended. Possible locations are abdominal, inguinal, prescrotal, and rarely, ectopic (a location outside the normal descent path).

The cause for cryptorchidism is not known. It is suspected that a major cause is genetic. Several chromosomal abnormalities have a high frequency of bilateral cryptorchidism. Experimental studies have indicated that dihydrotestosterone (DHT) is necessary for normal testicular descent. Prenatal androgen deficiency may be part of the pathophysiology. Cryptorchid male animals are not recommended to be used for breeding.

The incidence of cryptorchidism in dogs is about 9% (range, 0.5% to 12.9%), and in stallions it is less than 2%. In tom cats, it is rarer than in stallions. Canine breeds reported to have a higher than expected risk for cryptorchidism are the Chihuahua, miniature schnauzer, Pomeranian, poodles (miniature, toy, and standard), Shetland sheepdogs, Siberian husky, and Yorkshire terrier. Mongrels, beagles, and Labrador retrievers are thought to have a lower than expected risk of cryptorchidism. The right side is involved in dogs almost twice as often as the left side. Cryptorchidism in stallions occurs on either side with equal frequency.

Cryptorchid testes are nearly always sterile. A decrease in seminiferous tubules and spermatogenesis may be the cause or effect. Exposure to normal body temperature, 1° to 2° C higher than scrotal temperature, is at least a contributing factor to the sterility. Interstitial cells are relatively unaffected.

Canine testicular neoplasia is at least ten times more common in cryptorchid testes than in scrotal testes. The average age of onset of cryptorchid testicular neoplasms in dogs is 2.5 years earlier than the average age of onset in most scrotal testicular neoplasms in dogs. Although the overall risk of canine cryptorchidism is approximately 9% of males, more than one half of all Sertoli's cell tumors and one third of seminomas occur in cryptorchid testes. The incidence of interstitial cell tumors is not affected by cryptorchidism. Torsion of the testes occurs more easily and frequently in cryptorchid testes, particularly cryptorchid testes in the abdomen, than in scrotal testes. Seventy percent of torsional testes are neoplastic and are usually abdominal.

Cryptorchidism in stallions is not always easily discerned from anorchidism by history or physical examination. Serum testosterone levels above 0.1 ng/ml in a possible castrate (gelding) have been said to be consistent with the presence of testicular tissue. Levels of serum testosterone below 0.04 ng/ml suggest a gelding. An HCG response test has been recommended for further evaluation of stallions with equivocal serum testosterone levels of 0.04 to 0.1 ng/ml. Cryptorchid stallions should have a significant rise in serum testosterone levels by 30 to 60 minutes after the intravenous administration of 12,000 IU of HCG. Another differential evaluation for geldings and cryptorchid stallions is the assay of serum total estrogens. Normal serum total estrogen values in stallions are about 40 to 50 pg/ml. In cryptorchid stallions, the estrogen/testosterone ratio is elevated.

Medical correction of cryptorchid testes has been attempted with multiple injections of HCG or GnRH. Although some testes have descended after therapy was instituted, there is insufficient evidence to prove that these testes would not have descended without medical therapy. Because of the risk of testicular neoplasia in cryptorchid testes, it is recommended that all dogs, tom cats, and stallions that are still cryptorchid by 6 months of age be castrated.

See also references 2, 16, 18, 19, 26, 33, 45, 48, 71, 75, 77, 78, 87, and 90.

Defects in the Synthesis of Androgens

Congenital deficiencies of any of the five necessary enzymes for the biosynthesis of testosterone can cause male hypogonadism. Congenital deficiency of enzymes required for the biosynthesis of androgens has not yet been reported in companion animals; however, inhibition of androgenic biosynthesis can be achieved with the administration of spironolactone and the antifungal agent, ketoconazole.

Acquired Seminiferous Tubule Failure

Some of the possible causes for canine acquired seminiferous tubule failure, or interstitial cell failure, or both, are listed in Table 23–2. Spermatogonia rapidly divide and are therefore more susceptible to injury than Sertoli's cells and interstitial cells. Semen evaluation will show oligospermia or azoospermia. Serum testosterone and plasma LH levels are normal. Plasma FSH levels become elevated since Sertoli's cell secretion of inhibin is affected.

Treatments that may be tried for acquired seminiferous tubule failure include removal of the cause—if possible—and hormonal therapy. Testosterone rebound therapy, the administration of GnRH, and injections of gonadotropins can stimulate regeneration of spermatogonia and eventually spermatozoa in some cases of oligospermia. Testosterone rebound therapy consists of 6 to 10 weeks of testosterone administration or until azoospermia occurs; then therapy is discontinued. Treatment with testosterone enanthate (Delatestryl) or testosterone cypionate (Depo-Testosterone) is preferred in intramuscular doses of 2.2 to 4.4 mg/kg body weight every 2 to 3 weeks. Long-term therapy with GnRH is prohibitively expensive. Gonadotropin therapy may cause hypersensitivity or refractoriness to desired effect and is also expensive.

Bilateral Anorchia

Congenital bilateral anorchia, a condition not resulting from castration, can occur in phenotypic males; however, functional testicular tissue must be present in utero to produce Mullerian duct regression factor (MRF) and testosterone so that internal and external genitalia can differentiate toward a male phenotype. Congenital bilateral anorchia in a phenotypic male results from a destructive or atrophic process. Another term for congenital bilateral anorchia in a phenotypic male is the "vanishing testes syndrome."

The cause for spontaneous anorchia is unknown. It may be unilateral or bilateral. The possibility of castration causing anorchia should always be

Table 23–2.   Possible Causes for Acquired Seminiferous Tubule Failure in Dogs

---

Orchitis
   Brucella canis
   Trauma
Uremia
Irradiation
Lead poisoning
Drugs
   Cyclophosphamide
   Chlorambucil
   Vincristine
   Methotrexate

---

investigated when recording the history. Increased serum testosterone levels in response to injections of HCG could be used to differentiate bilateral anorchia from bilateral cryptorchidism.

Other than the lack of scrotal testes, no clinical signs are evident until the lack of development of secondary sexual characteristics is noted at the normal time for puberty. Treatment consists of the administration of androgen replacement drugs.

Complete or Incomplete Androgen Insensitivity

Complete androgen insensitivity (testicular feminization) is caused by testosterone receptor defects or deficiency. It results in a female phenotype. Incomplete androgen insensitivity can be caused by a post-receptor defect in androgen action or by a deficiency in 5 α-reductase. Incomplete androgen insensitivities result in ambiguous genitalia. Cryptorchid testes should be excised because of the risk of torsion or neoplasia.

See also reference 36.

PRECOCIOUS MALE SEXUAL DEVELOPMENT

Precocious (premature) sexual development may be defined as the occurrence of secondary sexual characteristics in dogs younger than 6 months of age, tom cats younger than 4 months of age, and stallions under 1 year of age. True precocious puberty is caused by early activation of the hypothalamus and subsequent gonadotropin secretion from the pituitary.

Precocious pseudopuberty is caused in male dogs by prepubertal treatment with an androgenic drug, by autonomous secretion of androgens from the adrenal cortex or testes, or by ectopic production of gonadotropins. However, prepubertal androgenic drug treatment is the most common cause.

Clinical signs of precocious male puberty or pseudopuberty are an increased muscular mass, rapid growth followed by premature epiphyseal closure, enlargement of the penis, and other, more species-specific secondary sexual characteristics such as dogs' leg lifting to urinate. The testes may be unusually large or small for the animal's age, depending on the cause for precocious sexual development.

If semen can be collected and mature spermatozoa are present, secretion of gonadotropins has occurred. Sources of gonadotropins are the pituitary or ectopic gonadotropin production by a tumor outside the pituitary (true precocious puberty). Aspermia and atrophic testes are suggestive of treatment with androgen, or of the autonomous secretion of androgens from the testes or adrenals (precocious pseudopuberty).

True precocious puberty may respond to the administration of medroxyprogesterone acetate, which inhibits the release of gonadotropins. Treatment of precocious pseudopuberty is directed at eliminating the cause, for example, by ceasing treatment with androgens, removal of an underlying tumor, or suppression of the adrenocortical hyperactivity of congenital adrenocortical hyperplasia.

MALE INFERTILITY

Table 23–3 lists possible causes of male infertility. Systemic illnesses are undoubtedly the most common cause in male companion animals. Hypothyroidism is the most frequently diagnosed endocrine cause in dogs. Disorders of the H-P-T axis, adrenals, and thyroid are suspected to cause less than 25% of all male infertility in companion animals. Conversely, virtually all H-P-T axis disorders lead to male infertility.

Evaluations of infertile male dogs should begin with a complete pertinent history of known illnesses, breeding tactics, and breeding results. Physical examinations should not be limited to the reproductive tract. Assuming that the history and general physical examination do not lead to the possibility of systemic illness as the cause for infertility, laboratory examinations should begin with an evaluation of semen. If the evaluation is normal, another breeding trial with a parous female, supervised by experienced personnel, is recommended. If the evaluation shows oligospermia or azoospermia with the presence of blood or cells of inflammation, semen samples should be collected for bacterial cultures. Dogs should be tested for brucellosis. Oligospermia with no signs of inflammation of the gonads or genitalia should be reconfirmed twice more at 2- to 4-week intervals because systemic stresses can temporarily halt spermatogenesis.

Dogs require 54 to 55 days to complete spermatogenesis, and stallions require 48 to 49 days. Affected dogs should be tested for the possible occurrence of hypothyroidism and adrenocortical dysfunction. Measurement of serum testosterone, buccal smear examinations for X chromatin, and testicular biopsy may be useful if oligospermia without inflammation of the gonads or genitalia is persistent and thyroid and adrenal function tests are normal. Additional tests that could be considered on selected animals are gonadotropin assays, prolactin assay, a GnRH stimulation test, and a HCG stimulation test.

See also reference 80.

Table 23–3. Possible Causes of Male Infertility

Endocrine
    Hypothalamic-pituitary disorders
    Hypothyroidism
    Hypoadrenocorticism
    Hyperadrenocorticism
    Testicular disorders
    Defects in androgen action
Defects in spermatogenesis
Systemic illnesses
Ductal obstructions
Prostatic disease
Antisperm antibodies
Penis deformities
Improper breeding techniques

GYNECOMASTIA

Gynecomastia is the excessive development of mammary tissue in a male. The earliest sign of gynecomastia in the dog is elongation of the nipples, but generalized mammary gland enlargement and even lactation can occur (Fig. 23–1). Possible causes of gynecomastia are listed in Table 23–4. All causes are mediated by increased levels of serum estrogens or an increased serum estrogen to androgen ratio affecting the mammary gland.

Drugs can induce gynecomastia by several means. Androgens can cause gynecomastia by being converted at the mammae to estrogens. Cimetidine and spironolactone compete with androgens for androgen receptors. Spironolactone also inhibits the synthesis of testosterone. Digitalis glycosides have a steroid structure that can bind to estrogen receptors and produce weak estrogenic effects. Phenothiazines cause gynecomastia by increasing circulating levels of prolactin.

Endocrine causes of gynecomastia may act by directly decreasing free serum testosterone (hypogonadism), increasing sex-hormone-binding-globulin (SHBG), indirectly decreasing free serum testosterone (hyperthyroidism), or increasing prolactin's secretion (hypothyroidism).

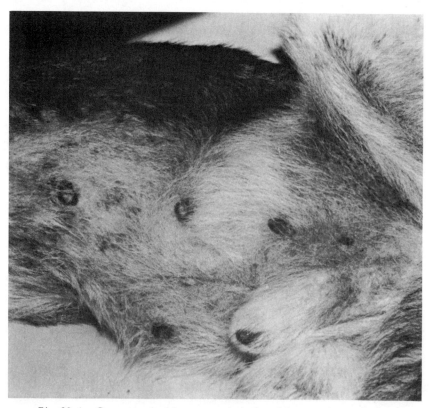

Fig. 23–1. Gynecomastia. Mammary and nipple enlargement in a male dog.

Table 23–4. Possible Causes of Gynecomastia

Drug-induced
  Androgens
  Cimetidine
  Digitalis glycosides
  Estrogens
  Vincristine
  Phenothiazines
  Spironolactone
Endocrine
  Hypogonadism (interstitial cell defects)
  Hyperprolactinemia
  Hyperthyroidism
  Hypothyroidism
Neoplasms
  Sertoli's cell tumor
  Interstitial cell tumor
  Seminomas
  Adrenocortical neoplasia
Systemic diseases
  Hepatic failure
  Renal failure
  Recovery from malnutrition

Hyperprolactinemia can impair the secretion of LH and diminish peripheral actions of testosterone. Hypergonadotropic hypogonadism is associated with high plasma gonadotropin levels, and excessive stimulation by gonadotropins of interstitial cells of the testes favors production of estrogen relative to production of androgens.

Neoplasms of the testes and adrenals may be autonomously secreting estrogen or secreting weak androgens that are converted to estrogens at the peripheral tissues. A testicular tumor could also produce LH, stimulating the contralateral testes to hypersecrete estrogens or weak androgens. Systemic diseases (hepatic and renal failure) and malnutrition are often accompanied by the decreased secretion of plasma gonadotropins. Partial or complete recovery from inanition or malnutrition may cause an acute and prolonged secretion of gonadotropins that favors synthesis of estrogen relative to the synthesis of androgens sufficient to produce gynecomastia.

In addition to a complete medical history, including questions about the drugs that have been administered and a general physical examination, the attempt to find out the cause of gynecomastia should include serum endocrine assays and an evaluation for genotype. Buccal smears and tissue karyotyping are indicated when the cause is not made evident by the history or physical examination. Measuring serum or plasma levels for estrogens, testosterone, and prolactin can also be considered.

The ideal treatment for gynecomastia is to eliminate the cause. If the cause remains idiopathic or is not amenable to correction, empiric management may be tried. The antiestrogens, tamoxifen (Nolvadex) or clomiphene

(Clomid), might alter the estrogen/androgen ratio enough to reverse gynecomastia in some cases. If a biopsy of the mammae shows fibrosis, reduction mammoplasty should be considered.

Several idiopathic cases of canine gynecomastia have been noted in association with a dermatosis. The condition has been termed the *canine male feminizing syndrome*. The syndrome affects middle-aged male dogs with scrotal testes of symmetrical size. Despite a lack of libido, some affected dogs are reported to have normal semen evaluations. Dogs with male feminizing syndrome may be sexually attractive to other male dogs. Alopecia, hyperpigmentation, seborrhea, hyperkeratosis, and lichenification occur beginning in the perineal and genital regions. Ceruminous otitis externa may be present. Serum testosterone and estrogen levels are within normal limits. Suggested treatments have included castration or the administration of androgens.

It is probable that canine male feminizing syndrome is not caused by one disease; therefore, one treatment may not be effective for all. Further information needed to be known on this syndrome includes confirmation of the genotype, plasma gonadotropin levels, measurement of plasma prolactin levels, quantification of androgen and estrogen receptors in the mammae, and histopathology of involved testes.

See also references 10, 20, 49, 53, 59, and 65.

ANDROGEN-ENHANCED DISORDERS

Benign prostatic hypertrophy, prostatic adenocarcinoma, perianal gland adenoma and adenocarcinoma, and perineal hernia occur more frequently in sexually intact male dogs than in female dogs or castrated male dogs. Castration of a sexually intact male dog with one of these disorders often results in the disorder's regression, stagnation, or reduced incidence of relapse after the utilization of adjunct treatment methods. Administration of androgens to male dogs does not reliably produce any of these disorders; however, if androgens are administered to an affected male, they will enhance the development of the disorder.

Canine Benign Prostatic Hypertrophy and Prostatism

Canine benign prostatic hypertrophy (BPH) occurs in more than 60% of male dogs over 5 years of age. Since most older dogs develop BPH, it must be considered a normal aging process. However, in some dogs BPH progresses, causing the prostrate to enlarge sufficiently to cause duct obstructions and cystic dilations. At that stage, *prostatism,* which is considered a clinical disease, may occur. Patients with prostatism exhibit the clinical signs of tenesmus, constipation, hematuria, or dysuria.

Size alone cannot be the only criterion for the diagnosis of benign prostatic hypertrophy. Normal prostatic size varies among canine breeds. The Scottish terrier normally has the largest prostate on the basis of prostatic weight to body weight. Even though glandular hyperplasia in dogs becomes microscopically evident as early as 2.5 years of age, cystic hyperplasia with prostatism is rare in dogs younger than 4 years of age. Prostatism may be precipitated by prostatic engorgement with blood when the male dog is sexually stimulated by a bitch in estrus.

Canine BPH is different from the disease in humans. Canine BPH is a diffuse epithelial-glandular proliferation. In humans, BPH results from hypertrophy of the stroma, especially in the periurethral area. Stranguria is more common in human patients with BPH than in canine patients with BPH (stranguria may not occur at all in dogs).

The exact mechanism of BPH's androgen dependency is unknown. DHT and its metabolites, 5 α-androstanediols, are particularly concentrated in patients with BPH. Plasma and prostatic estradiol and estrone concentrations are also increased. Experimentally, androgens alone induce diffuse hyperplasia of the prostate; androgens plus estrogens alter the normal order of morphology, cause metaplasia, and increase prostatic weight. Serum androgen levels decrease with advancing age, but serum estradiol levels remain the same. BPH may be caused by the animal's increased sensitivity to androgens, which, in turn, may be caused by increased androgen receptors induced by estradiol or a decreased androgen to estrogen ratio.

The most economical, effective, and safe treatment of canine BPH is castration. Estrogens have been advocated for many years, but in our opinion, they are the least desirable form of medical management. In addition to estrogens' toxicity to the bone marrow of the dog, estrogens cause squamous metaplasia of the prostate, desquamation of cells that obstruct prostatic ducts, and inhibit prostatic secretion.

High doses of estrogen cause prostatic enlargement resulting from squamous metaplasia, predisposing the prostate to prostatitis. Megestrol acetate (Ovaban) is a progestin with antigonadotropin and antiandrogen effects. When it is given in doses of 0.55 mg/kg body weight per day, prostatic size is noticeably reduced within 1 to 3 weeks.

See also references 7, 13, 25, 28, 32, 37, 39, 46, 50, 58, 82, 83, 91, and 93.

Perineal Hernia in Dogs

Perineal hernias are a protrusion of the abdominal or pelvic viscera through the muscles lateral to the anus and tailhead and dorsal to the ischium, especially the levator ani and coccygeus muscles (Fig. 23–2). Tenesmus may be a precipitating factor in at least some cases. More than 90% of affected animals are sexually intact male dogs. The average age of onset is 8 years (range, 6 to 13 years). Breeds with a greater than average risk are the Boston terrier, collie, boxer, Pekingese, Welsh corgi, and dachshund. Two thirds of those affected are unilaterally involved. The right side is affected more than the left. The rectum is found in the hernia in most cases. Less often, the urinary bladder, prostate, small intestine, and retroperitoneal fat become included in the hernia.

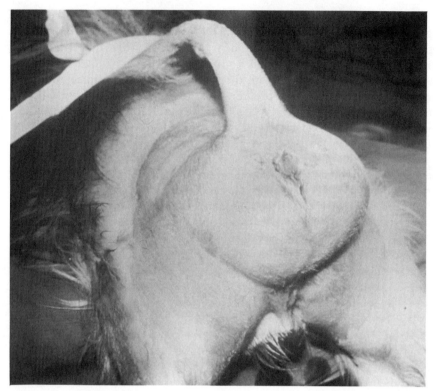

Fig. 23–2. Bilateral perineal hernias in an older male dog. (From Bojrab, M.J., and Toomey, A.: Perineal herniorrhapy. Compendium on Continuing Educ. for the Practicing Vet., *3*:8, 1981.)

Androgens do not induce perineal hernias. Male dogs are predisposed because they do not possess the perineal support most female dogs have to withstand the pressures during parturition. Bitches have larger levator ani muscles and sacrotuberous ligaments than do male dogs. Approximately one third of affected male animals have a recurrence of perineal hernia after reconstructive surgery. If castrated at the time of perineal hernia repair, the risk of recurrence is reduced two to three times. The reason for this apparent paradox is that the precipitating tenesmus in many cases may be due to prostatomegaly, testicular disease, or perineal adenomas. All these precipitating factors are reduced or eliminated by castration.

See also references 5, 6, 9, 22, 23, 38, 41, 42, 98, and 99.

Perianal Gland Adenoma in Dogs

Perianal gland adenoma is a neoplasm of the circumanal glands, which are modified sebaceous glands found adjacent to the anus. Occasionally, circumanal glands can be located on the tail, prepuce, or dorsal pelvic area. Dogs are the only companion animals possessing circumanal glands.

Nothing is known about the purpose of the circumanal glands. They are modified sebaceous glands that after birth lose all connections with the follicles and surface of the body. Significant growth in the gland then occurs at puberty. It has been suggested that circumanal glands may be endocrine glands. Excision of the glands causes no discernible ill effects.

Perianal gland adenomas are common tumors of male dogs 8 years of age or older. They comprise approximately 5% of all canine tumors and are the third most common neoplasm in male dogs. In general, male dogs have a five- to sixfold greater risk than female dogs of having a perianal gland adenoma. The ratio of sexually intact male dogs to sexually intact bitches who have adenomas is about 12 to 1. Breeds most affected are the cocker spaniel, English bulldog, Samoyed, and beagle. Female cocker spaniels are more frequently affected than the female dogs of other breeds. Spayed bitches develop perianal gland adenomas three times more often than do sexually intact bitches. Androgen receptors have been shown in perianal gland tumors. One survey found that one third of affected male dogs had testicular interstitial cell tumors (which may have been secreting androgen). About 10% of male dogs with perianal gland tumors develop perineal hernias.

Ten percent to twenty percent of perianal gland tumors are adenocarcinomas. Perianal gland adenocarcinomas are invasive. They rapidly occlude the rectum and spread to the sublumbar lymph nodes. Castration does not alter the growth of perianal gland adenocarcinomas.

The treatment of choice for perianal gland adenomas is castration. If the tumors are ulcerated or the patient is female, the tumors should be excised. Because perianal gland adenomas are also radiosensitive, radiation therapy can be considered as an adjunct to surgery. Patients with poor anesthetic risk may be managed with an antiandrogenic progestin such as megestrol acetate (Ovaban) in a dose of 0.55 mg/kg body weight/day and an intratumor injection of estradiol (ECP) in a dose of 0.2 mg per tumor. The intratumor administration of estradiol is believed to be able to displace bound androgen. It is also possible that adrenal androgens may enhance the growth of perianal gland adenomas. Affected bitches might benefit from minimal adrenocortical suppressive doses of a glucocorticoid such as prednisone or prednisolone in a dose of 0.22 mg/kg body weight/day.

See also references 12, 29, 31, and 100.

Acne

Acne is a disease of the hair follicles resulting in papules, pustules, and comedones (blackheads). Dogs and cats are affected, male animals more often than female animals. The incidence of acne in dogs is greatest during and just after puberty. Cats tend to develop acne as adults. Lesions are most evident on the chin, but in dogs the upper lips may also be involved. In short-haired, large-bodied dog breeds, a generalized superficial folliculitis sometimes accompanies acne.

Levels of free serum testosterone and dehydroepiandrosterone (DHEA) sulfate correlate with the incidence and severity of acne in humans. DHEA sulfate can be converted to DHEA, testosterone, and DHT at the hair follicle. Improvement has been noted in women with acne after treatment with low-dose dexamethasone and is related to a decrease in serum DHEA sulfate. Cyproterone acetate, an antiandrogen not commercially available in the United States, competitively inhibits androgen binding and has also produced improvement in human acne.

Canine and feline acne may or may not be infected with bacteria. In our experience, response to systemic antibiotics and topical medications in the early stages of acne is not as good as the response to short-term, low-dose corticosteroids or an antiandrogenic progestin such as megestrol acetate.

TESTICULAR NEOPLASIA

Testicular neoplasms in companion animals are primarily interstitial cell tumors, seminomas, Sertoli's cell tumors, or teratomas. Embryonal carcinomas and other tumor types are rare. The incidence of testicular tumors in dogs exceeds that of all other companion and domestic animals. The incidence in dogs peaks when the animals are about 10 years old. Canine testicular tumors are rare in animals younger than 6 years of age. They are the second most common neoplasm in male dogs; the most common is neoplasia of the skin.

Cryptorchidism influences the incidence of testicular tumors in dogs. Cryptorchid testes are 13 times more likely to develop Sertoli's cell tumors and seminomas than are scrotal testes. Canine breeds at increased risk for cryptorchidism are also at increased risk for testicular neoplasia—these include the poodles, Chihuahua, Yorkshire terrier, miniature schnauzer, Pomeranian, Shetland sheepdog, and Siberian husky. Testicular tumors occur more commonly on the right side of the animal, as does cryptorchidism, which occurs twice as commonly on the right side than the left. The mean age of animals who develop Sertoli's cell tumors and seminomas in cryptorchid testes is 2 years earlier than the average age of animals who develop the tumors in scrotal testes. The occurrence of inguinal hernia is also linked to the risk of seminomas and Sertoli's cell tumors. Testicular tumors occur four to five times more often if an inguinal hernia is present.

Male boxer dogs are predisposed to developing all three of the common canine testicular tumors (the Sertoli's cell tumor, interstitial cell tumor, and seminoma). These three testicular tumor types are diagnosed in about equal numbers in dogs. Interstitial cell tumors may actually be the most common; they are often overlooked because of their small size. About 10% to 20% of dogs with a testicular tumor have more than one cell type. Malignancy occurs less often with canine testicular tumors than with the common testicular tumors in humans (teratomas and embryonal carcinomas in children and seminomas in adults).

The enlarged size of a neoplastic testis or testicular production of estrogenic or androgenic substances may be responsible for clinical signs of testicular tumors in dogs (Table 23–5). Acute abdominal or inguinal pain with or without hypotensive shock may also be a clinical sign of testicular neoplasia if the enlarged testis undergoes torsion and strangulates the vascular supply in the spermatic cord.

Tom cats rarely develop testicular neoplasia. Sertoli's cell tumors and an embryonic carcinoma have been reported. There have not been any signs of feminization. The rate of malignancy has been noted as being higher than that of dogs. The few reports of feline testicular neoplasia may not represent the tom cats' true risk since most tom cats kept as companion pets are castrated early in life.

Most stallions are also castrated early in life. This might explain why they too seem to be at low risk for developing testicular neoplasia. If one considers the equine testicular tumors that have been reported, there is no breed predisposition. Seminomas are the most frequently reported tumors, followed by teratomas. Sertoli's cell tumors, interstitial cell tumors, and other possible testicular tumors are rare in stallions.

Bilateral castration is indicated in all cases of testicular neoplasia. Bilateral involvement occurs too frequently for the clinician to chance leaving the other testis thought to be uninvolved. Drugs used for metastatic testicular neoplasia have not yet been evaluated in companion animals. In

Table 23–5.   Possible Clinical Signs of Testicular Neoplasms in the Dog

Signs of enlarged testicular size
  Lameness
  Abdominal pain
  Wide stance of hind legs
  Licking scrotum
  Palpable testicular enlargement
  Cryptorchidism

Signs of estrogenic effects (feminization)
  Loss of libido
  Gynecomastia
  Atrophy of contralateral testis
  Alopecia with hyperpigmentation, especially of perineal and genital regions
  Attractiveness to other males
  Behavioral changes—lethargy and irritability
  Pendulous prepuce
  Atrophy of penis
  Squamous metaplasia of prostate, prostatomegaly, and bacterial prostatitis
  Hypoplasia of the bone marrow
  Squatting to urinate
  Infertility

Signs of androgenic effects
  Perianal gland adenomas
  Perineal hernia
  Benign prostatic hypertrophy
  Behavioral changes—lethargy, irritability, aggression

humans, cisplatin, vincristine, and bleomycin have been recommended. Seminomas are radiosensitive. Treatment with mitotane has caused the remission of interstitial cell tumors in humans.

See also references 1, 11, 15, 17, 21, 24, 30, 40, 43, 44, 57, 67–70, 79, 81, 85, 88, 94, 95, 101, and 102.

Sertoli's Cell Tumors

Canine Sertoli's cell tumors most often affect the boxer, Cairn terrier, Labrador retriever, border collie, German shepherd dog, rough collie, Weimaraner, Shetland sheepdog, and Pekingese. The boxer, Shetland sheepdog, and Weimaraner are statistically at high risk. The dachshund and mongrel breeds are at low risk. On the average, onset occurs in animals who are 9.7 years old; this average age of incidence is the earliest of all testicular tumors.

More than one half (53%) of all canine Sertoli's cell tumors occur in cryptorchid testes. One in ten to twenty affected dogs has Sertoli's cell tumors in both testes, and nearly one in five has other tumors present. The mean age of onset for animals with these tumors is earlier for affected cryptorchid testes than for affected scrotal testes. The average age of incidence for abdominal cryptorchid Sertoli's cell tumors is 8 years, and the average age of onset for inguinal cryptorchid is around 9 years. The mean age of onset for Sertoli's cell tumors in scrotal testes is greater: 11 years. The right testis is involved more frequently than the left, even if both testes are in the scrotum.

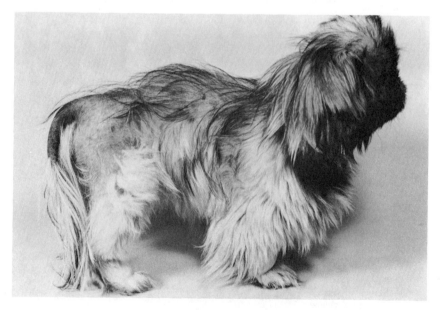

Fig. 23–3. Alopecia in a male dog with a feminizing Sertoli's cell tumor.

Overall, about one third of all Sertoli's cell tumors are feminizing in dogs (Figs. 23–3 and 23–4). In the horse, Sertoli's cell tumors have also been suspected to cause feminization, but there have not been signs of feminization reported in tom cats with Sertoli's cell tumors. Feminizing Sertoli's cell tumors occur in budgerigars. In male budgerigars, the cere is blue, and in the female, it is brown. Feminization of a male budgerigar changes the normally blue cere to brown. Production of excess estrogenic substances in birds can also cause hyperostosis. Enlargement of the avian testis can cause unilateral paralysis from pressure on a sciatic nerve.

In dogs, feminization from Sertoli's cell tumors is correlated with the tumor's size and location. If the tumor is a large Sertoli's cell tumor or occurs in a cryptorchid testis, the chance is greater that the tumors are feminizing. Feminization occurs in 15% of animals whose scrotal testes have Sertoli's cell tumors, 50% of animals whose inguinal testes have Sertoli's cell tumors, and 70% of animals whose abdominal testes have Sertoli's cell tumors. Serum estradiol levels are not always elevated in cases of feminizing Sertoli's cell tumors. This may be because some of the tumors can produce a weaker estrogen, such as estrone, or some may produce a weak androgen, such as androstenedione, which is converted to estrogens when it has reached the peripheral target cells. Sertoli's cell tumors are hard, lobulated, greasy tumors with golden specks on their cut surface. They are white to gray in color (Fig. 23–5).

Metastasis occurs in 10% to 14% of dogs with Sertoli's cell tumors. The route of spread is lymphatic and hematogenous. Lymphatic spread to the

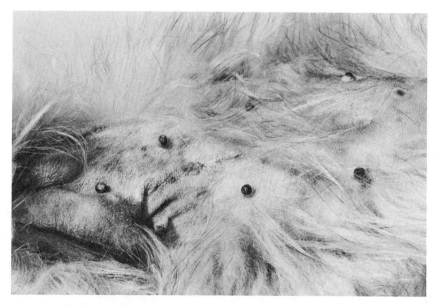

Fig. 23–4. Gynecomastia in the same dog as seen in Figure 23–3.

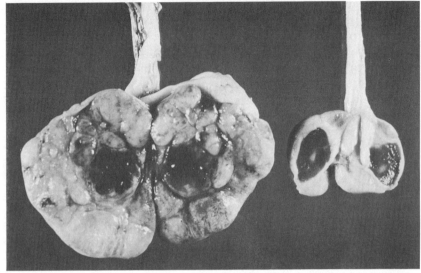

Fig. 23-5. A large Sertoli's cell tumor involving the left testicle. The contralateral testicle at right is atrophied.

internal iliac and sublumbar lymph nodes usually occurs first. Metastasized foci can also produce estrogenic substances. If signs of feminization do not regress within 3 months of castration, metastasis is probably present.

See also references 8, 14, 27, 35, 52, 54–56, 60–66, 72–74, 84, and 97.

Interstitial (Leydig's) Cell Tumors

According to statistics, the boxer is at elevated risk for developing interstitial cell tumors. Cryptorchidism does not influence the risk of developing interstitial cell tumors. About 95% of canine interstitial cell tumors involve scrotal testes. The incidence of these tumors in the right and left testes is equal. In 30% to 40% of animals, the tumors occur in both testes. The average age when the animal is diagnosed is 11 years. Malignancy is rare.

Interstitial cell tumors may produce feminization or androgenic hormones. Feminization is less frequently due to interstitial cell tumors than to Sertoli's cell tumors. Feminization from interstitial cell tumors is probably due to the increased production of weak androgens that are converted peripherally to estrogens. The increased occurrence of androgen-enhanced disorders that occur with interstitial cell tumors gives evidence of their ability to produce excessive androgens. About one third of dogs with these tumors have concurrent prostatic hyperplasia and perianal gland adenomas. Approximately 15% of the dogs affected have perineal hernias. In stallions, interstitial cell tumors have been associated with increased aggressiveness.

Most canine interstitial cell tumors are soft and small, 1 to 2 cm in diameter. Many may go clinically undetected. The color of their cut surface is orange or brown. Large tumors may be cystic and contain a clear or hemorrhagic fluid.

See also reference 47.

Seminomas

The boxer and German shepherd dog are statistically predisposed to seminomas. Mongrels are at low risk. The average age of onset in dogs is 10 years. Seminomas are the most common testicular tumor in adult stallions. In dogs, but not stallions, cryptorchidism increases the risk of developing seminomas. One third (36%) of canine seminomas occur in cryptorchid testes. They are more commonly found in the right testis than the left.

There have been reports of feminization associated with seminomas in dogs.[3] It is unlikely that seminomas are involved in steroidogenesis. The more probable explanation is that another tumor of a different cell type may have been present but existed undetected in the testis with the seminoma or the contralateral testis. Seminomas and interstitial cell tumors, as well as seminomas and Sertoli's cell tumors, are common multiple tumor combinations.

Seminomas are soft and slightly lobulated. The cut surface is creamy and sometimes mottled by necrosis (gray in color) and hemorrhaging (pink in color). Most tumors in dogs are 1 to 3 cm in diameter.

It is difficult to predict a seminoma's malignancy based on histologic criteria; therefore, all seminomas must be considered potentially malignant. It should be remembered, however, that less than 10% of the tumors in dogs are clinically malignant. Malignant seminomas are more common in stallions than in dogs.

See also references 4, 34, 51, 86, 92, and 96.

Teratomas

Teratomas are benign tumors of well-differentiated cells from all three germ layers. Occasionally malignant cells are found—for these the term "teratocarcinoma" may be applied. Since the teratomas can be large before birth, their size can impair the descent of the involved testis. Cryptorchidism with teratomas is presumably a result of the tumor, not a cause. The most common testicular tumor in prepubertal stallions, teratomas are rare in other male companion animals.

See also references 76 and 89.

REFERENCES

1. Aronsohn, M.: Canine testicular neoplasia. Compendium on Continuing Educ. for the Practicing Vet., *1:*925, 1979.
2. Ashdown, R.R.: The diagnosis of cryptorchidism in young dogs: a review of the problem. J. Small Anim. Pract., *4:*261, 1963.
3. Barsanti, J.A., Duncan, J.R., and Nachreiner, R.F.: Alopecia associated with a seminoma. J. Am. Anim. Hosp. Assoc., *15:*33, 1979.
4. Becht, J.L., Thacker, H.L., and Page, E.H.: Malignant seminoma in a stallion. J. Am. Vet. Med. Assoc., *175:*292, 1979.

5. Bellenger, C.R.: Perineal hernia in dogs. Aust. Vet. J., *56:*434, 1980.
6. Bojrab, M.J., and Toomey, A.: Perineal herniorrhaphy. Compendium on Continuing Educ. for the Practicing Vet., *3:*8, 1981.
7. Brendler, C.B., et al.: Spontaneous benign prostatic hyperplasia in the beagle. J. Clin. Invest., *71:*1114, 1983.
8. Brodey, R.S., and Martin, J.E.: Sertoli cell neoplasma in the dog. The clinico-pathological and endocrinological findings in thirty-seven dogs. J. Am. Vet. Med. Assoc., *133:*249, 1958.
9. Burrows, C.F., and Harvey, C.E.: Perineal hernia in the dog. J. Small Anim. Pract., *14:*315, 1973.
10. Carlson, H.E.: Gynecomastia. N. Engl. J. Med., *303:*795, 1980.
11. Caron, J.P., Barber, S.M., and Bailey, J.V.: Equine testicular neoplasia. Compendium on Continuing Educ. for the Practicing Vet., *7:*553, 1985.
12. Chaisiri, N., and Pierrepoint, C.G.: Steroid-receptor interaction in a canine anal adenoma. J. Small Anim. Pract., *20:*405, 1979.
13. Chaisiri, N., et al.: Demonstration of a cytoplasmic receptor protein for oestrogen in the canine prostate gland. J. Endocrinol., *78:*131, 1978.
14. Coffin, D.L., Munson, T.O., and Scully, R.E.: Functional Sertoli cell tumor with metastasis in a dog. J. Am. Vet. Med. Assoc., *121:*352, 1952.
15. Comhaire, F., Matthews, D., and Vermeulen, A.: Testosterone and oestradiol in dogs with testicular tumours. Acta Endocrinol., *77:*408, 1974.
16. Coryn, M., et al.: Clinical, morphological and endocrinological aspects of cryptorchidism in the horse. Theriogenology, *16:*489, 1981.
17. Cotchin, E.: Testicular neoplasms in dogs. J. Comp. Pathol., *60:*232, 1960.
18. Cox, J.E., et al.: An analysis of 500 cases of equine cryptorchidism. Equine Vet. J., *11:*113, 1979.
19. Cox, V.S., Wallace, L.J., and Jessen, C.R.: An anatomic and genetic study of canine cryptorchidism. Teratology, *18:*233, 1978.
20. Davis, G.: A report on three cases of feminising syndrome in the dog. J. S. Afr. Vet. Assoc., *55:*33, 1984.
21. Daykin, P.W., and Smythe, R.H.: Testicular neoplasm associated with sex inversion in the dog. Vet. Rec., *61:*325, 1949.
22. Desai, R.: An anatomical study of the canine male and female pelvic diaphragm and the effect of testosterone on the status of levator ani of male dogs. J. Am. Anim. Hosp. Assoc., *18:*195, 1982.
23. Dorn, A.S., Cartee, R.E., and Richardson, D.C.: A preliminary comparison of perineal hernia in the dog and man. J. Am. Anim. Hosp. Assoc., *18:*624, 1982.
24. Dow, C.: Testicular tumours in dogs. J. Comp. Pathol., *72:*247, 1962.
25. Dule, J.Y., Lesage, R., and Tremblay, R.R.: Estradiol and progesterone receptors in dog prostate cytosol. J. Steroid Biochem., *10:*459, 1979.
26. Dunn, M.L., Foster, W.J., and Goddard, K.M.: Cryptorchidism in the dog: a clinical survey. J. Am. Anim. Hosp. Assoc., *4:*180, 1968.
27. Edwards, D.F.: Bone marrow hypoplasia in a feminized dog with a Sertoli cell tumor. J. Am. Vet. Med. Assoc., *178:*494, 1981.
28. El Etreby, M.F., et al.: Role of the pituitary gland in experimental hormonal induction and prevention of benign prostatic hyperplasia in the dog. Cell Tissue Res., *204:*367, 1979.
29. Elling, H., and Ungemach, F.R.: Demonstration of oestrogen receptors in peri-anal tumours in dogs. Zentralbl. Veterinarmed. [A], *27:*758, 1980.
30. Eskew, N.E., and Kuh, E.F.: Abdominal pain due to torsion of a retained testicle. Vet. Med., *56:*212, 1961.
31. Evans, C.R., and Pierrepoint, C.G.: Tissue-steroid interactions in canine hormone dependent tumours. Vet. Rec., *97:*464, 1975.
32. Ewing, L.L., et al.: Testicular androgen and estrogen secretion and benign prostatic hyperplasia in the Beagle. Endocrinology, *114:*1308, 1984.
33. Genetzky, R.M., et al.: Equine cryptorchidism: pathogenesis, diagnosis, and treatment. Compendium on Continuing Educ. for the Practicing Vet., *6:*S577, 1984.
34. Gibson, G.W.: Malignant seminoma in a Welsh pony stallion. Compendium on Continuing Educ. for the Practicing Vet., *6:*S296, 1984.
35. Gill, C.W.: Prostatic adenocarcinoma with concurrent Sertoli cell tumor in a dog. Can. Vet. J., *22:*230, 1981.

36. Griffin, J.E., and Wilson, J.D.: The syndromes of androgen resistance. N. Engl. J. Med., *302:*198, 1980.
37. Harper, M.E., et al.: The metabolism of steroids in the canine prostate and testes. J. Endocrinol., *49:*213, 1971.
38. Harvey, C.E.: Treatment of perineal hernia in the dog—a reassessment. J. Small Anim. Pract., *18:*505, 1977.
39. Hawkins, E.F., et al.: Androgen and estrogen receptors in the canine prostate. J. Androl., *1:*234, 1980.
40. Hayes, H.M., Jr., and Pendergrass, T.W.: Canine testicular tumors: epidemiologic features of 410 dogs. Int. J. Cancer, *18:*482, 1976.
41. Hayes, H.M., Jr., and Wilson, G.P.: Hormone-dependent neoplasms of the canine perianal gland. Cancer Res., *37:*2068, 1977.
42. Hayes, H.M., Jr., Wilson, G.P., and Tarone, R.P.: The epidemiological features of perineal hernia in 771 dogs. J. Am. Anim. Hosp. Assoc., *14:*703, 1978.
43. Horsey, J.R.: Testicular torsion in the dog. Vet. Rec., *107:*495, 1980.
44. Hulse, D.A.: Intrascrotal torsion of the testicle in a dog. Vet. Med., *68:*658, 1973.
45. Humke, R.: Treatment results after application of the LH-FSH releasing hormone on mal des census testis of the male dog. Kleintier-Praxis, *22:*315, 1977.
46. Isaacs, J.T., and Coffey, D.S.: Changes in dihydrotestosterone metabolism associated with the development of canine benign prostatic hyperplasia. Endocrinology, *108:*445, 1981.
47. Kahan, I.H.: An atypical case of interstitial cell tumor of the testicle in a dog. J. Am. Vet. Med. Assoc., *126:*471, 1955.
48. Kawakami, E., et al.: Cryptorchidism in the dog: occurrences of cryptorchidism and semen quality in the cryptorchid dog. Jpn. J. Vet. Sci., *46:*303, 1984.
49. Kelch, R.P., et al.: Estradiol and testosterone secretion by human, simian, and canine testes, in males with hypogonadism and in male pseudohermaphrodites with the feminizing testes syndrome. J. Clin. Invest., *51:*824, 1972.
50. Knecht, D.C.: Diseases of the canine prostate gland (Part I). Compendium on Continuing Educ. for the Practicing Vet., *1:*385, 1979.
51. Knudsen, O., and Schantz, B.: Seminoma in a stallion. A clinical, cytological and pathologicoanatomical investigation. Cornell Vet., *53:*395, 1963.
52. Krahwinkel, D.J., and Bierit, W.B.: Torsion of an abdominal testicle with Sertoli cell tumor. Mod. Vet. Pract., *48:*74, 1967.
53. Kravis, E.M., and Lorber, J.H.: Feminization syndrome associated with epididymitis in a dog. J. Am. Vet. Med. Assoc., *140:*803, 1962.
54. Laing, E.J., Harari, J., and Smith, C.W.: Spermatic cord torsion and Sertoli cell tumor in a dog. J. Am. Vet. Med. Assoc., *183:*879, 1983.
55. Lindberg, R., Jonsson, O.-J., and Kasstrom, H.: Sertoli cell tumours associated with feminization, prostatitis and squamous metaplasia of the renal tubular epithelium in a dog. J. Small Anim. Pract., *17:*451, 1976.
56. Lindo, D.E., and Grenn, H.H.: Case report: bilateral Sertoli cell tumor in a canine cryptorchid with accompanying pathological lesions. Can. Vet. J., *10:*145, 1969.
57. Lipowitz, A.J., et al.: Testicular neoplasms and concomitant clinical changes in the dog. J. Am. Vet. Med. Assoc., *163:*1364, 1973.
58. Lloyd, J.W., Thomas, J.A., and Mawhinney, M.G.: Androgens and estrogens in the plasma and prostatic tissue of normal dogs and dogs with benign prostatic hypertrophy. Invest. Urol., *13:*220, 1975.
59. Mattheeuws, D., and Comhaire, F.: Oestradiol and testosterone in male dogs with alopecia and feminization without testicular neoplasia. Br. Vet. J., *131:*65, 1975.
60. McNeil, P.E., and Weaver, A.D.: Massive scrotal swelling in two unusual cases of canine Sertoli-cell tumour. Vet. Rec., *106:*144, 1980.
61. McQueen, S.D., Directo, A.C., and Olsen, G.: An unusual case of Sertoli cell neoplasia in a dog. Vet. Med. Small Anim. Pract., *69:*1449, 1974.
62. Meier, H.: Sertoli cell tumor in the cat. North Am. Vet., *37:*979, 1956.
63. Morgan, R.V.: Blood dyscrasias associated with testicular tumors in the dog. J. Am. Anim. Hosp. Assoc., *18:*970, 1982.
64. Morris, B.J.: Fatal bone marrow depression as a result of Sertoli cell tumor. Vet. Med. Small Anim. Pract., *78:*1070, 1983.
65. Muller, G.H., Kirk, R.W., and Scott, D.W.: Small Animal Dermatology. 3rd Ed. Philadelphia, W.B. Saunders, 1983, pp. 531–546.

66. Mulligan, R.M.: Feminization in male dogs. A syndrome associated with carcinoma of the testis and mimicked by administration of estrogens. Am. J. Pathol., *20:*865, 1944.
67. Mulligan, R.M.: Some endocrinologic considerations of canine neoplastic diseases. Arch. Pathol., *39:*162, 1945.
68. Naylor, R.W., and Thompson, S.M.R.: Intra-abdominal testicular torsion—a report of two cases. J. Am. Anim. Hosp. Assoc., *15:*763, 1979.
69. Pearson, H., and Kelly, D.F.: Testicular torsion in the dog: a review of 13 cases. Vet. Rec., *97:*200, 1975.
70. Peduzzi, R.J., and Carlson, D.J.: Testicular torsion. Canine Pract., *7:*79, 1980.
71. Pendergrass, T.W., and Hayes, H.M.: Cryptorchidism and related defects in dogs: epidemiologic comparisons with man. Teratology, *12:*51, 1975.
72. Pierrepoint, C.G.: The metabolism *in vitro* of dehydroepiandrosterone and dehydroepiandrosterone sulfate by Sertoli cell tumors of the testis of two dogs with clinical signs of hyperestrogenism. J. Endocrinol., *42:*99, 1968.
73. Pierrepoint, C.G., et al.: Steroid metabolism of a Sertoli cell tumour of the testis of a dog with feminization and alopecia and of the normal canine testis. J. Endocrinol., *38:*61, 1967.
74. Pulley, L.T.: Sertoli cell tumor. Vet. Clin. North Am., *9:*145, 1979.
75. Pullig, T.: Cryptorchidism in cocker spaniels. J. Hered., *44:*250, 1953.
76. Rebar, A., et al.: Testicular teratoma in a horse: a case report and endocrinologic study. J. Equine Med. Surg., *3:*361, 1979.
77. Rehfeld, C.E.: Cryptorchidism in a large beagle colony. J. Am. Vet. Med. Assoc., *158:*1864, 1971.
78. Reif, J.S., and Brodey, R.S.: The relationship between cryptorchidism and canine testicular neoplasia. J. Am. Vet. Med. Assoc., *155:*2005, 1969.
79. Reif, J.S., et al.: A cohort study of canine testicular neoplasia. J. Am. Vet. Med. Assoc., *175:*719, 1979.
80. Rosenthal, R.C.: Infertility in the male dog. Compendium on Continuing Educ. for the Practicing Vet., *12:*983, 1983.
81. Schollmeyer, M.P., and DeYoung, D.W.: Torsion of a neoplastic intra-abdominal testicle. J. Am. Anim. Hosp. Assoc., *10:*484, 1974.
82. Shain, S., and Boesel, R.: Androgen receptor content of the normal and hyperplastic canine prostate. J. Clin. Invest., *654,* 1978.
83. Shain, S.A., and Nitchuk, W.M.: Testosterone metabolism by the prostate of the aging canine. Mech. Aging Dev., *11:*23, 1979.
84. Sherding, R.G., Wilson, G.P., and Kociba, G.J.: Bone marrow hypoplasia in eight dogs with Sertoli cell tumor. J. Am. Vet. Med. Assoc., *178:*497, 1981.
85. Siegel, E.T., et al.: An estrogen study in the feminized dog with testicular neoplasia. Endocrinology, *80:*272, 1967.
86. Simon, J., and Rubin, S.B.: Metastatic seminoma in a dog. Vet. Med. Small Anim. Clin., *74:*941, 1979.
87. Stabenfeldt, G.H., and Hughes, J.P.: Diagnostic endocrinology of the horse. Vet. Clin. North Am., *2:*253, 1980.
88. Steele, W.B., et al.: Testicular tumours in dogs. Vet. Rec., *101:*142, 1977.
89. Stick, J.A.: Teratoma and cyst formation of the equine cryptorchid testicle. J. Am. Vet. Med. Assoc., *176:*211, 1980.
90. Stickle, R.L., and Fesler, J.F.: Retrospective study of 350 cases of equine cryptorchidism. J. Am. Vet. Med. Assoc., *172:*343, 1978.
91. Trachtenberg, J., Hicks, L.L., and Walsh, P.C.: Androgen- and estrogen-receptor content in spontaneous and experimentally induced canine prostatic hyperplasia. J. Clin. Invest., *65:*1051, 1980.
92. Trigo, F.J., Miller, R.A., and Torbeck, R.L.: Metastatic equine seminoma: report of two cases. Vet. Pathol., *21:*259, 1984.
93. Tunn, U., et al.: Biochemical and histological studies on prostates in castrated dogs after treatment with androstanediol, oestradiol, and cyproterone acetate. Acta Endocrinol., *91:*373, 1979.
94. Turk, J.R., Turk, M.A.M., and Gallina, A.M.: A canine testicular tumor resembling gonadoblastoma. Vet. Pathol., *18:*201, 1981.
95. Turner, T.: Torsion of the retained testicle in the dog. J. Small Anim. Pract., *11:*436, 1970.

96. Vaillancourt, D., Frete, P., and Orr, J.P.: Seminoma in the horse: report of two cases. J. Equine Med. Surg., *3:*213, 1979.
97. Weaver, A.D.: Survey with follow-up of 67 dogs with testicular Sertoli cell tumours. Vet. Rec., *113:*105, 1983.
98. Weaver, A.D., and Omamegbe, J.O.: Surgical treatment of perineal hernia in the dog. J. Small Anim. Pract., *22:*749, 1981.
99. Whittlestone, J.F.: Perineal hernia. J. Small Anim. Pract., *14:*828, 1973.
100. Wilson, G.P., and Hayes, H.M.: Castration for treatment of perianal gland neoplasms in the dog. J. Am. Vet. Med. Assoc., *174:*1301, 1979.
101. Young, A.C.B.: Two cases of intrascrotal torsion of a normal testicle. J. Small Anim. Pract., *20:*229, 1979.
102. Zymet, C.L.: Intrascrotal testicular torsion in a sexually aggressive dog. Vet. Med. Small Anim. Clin., *70:*1330, 1975.

24

Clinical Disorders Related to
Ovarian Endocrine Function

Endocrine disorders of the ovaries can be of ovarian origin or pituitary/ hypothalamic origin. They may also be prepubertal (primary anestrus) or postpubertal (secondary anestrus). Some disorders cause premature sexual development, and others cause delayed sexual development. Some disorders are caused by ovarian neoplasia. Functional ovarian disorders alter or prevent the ovarian cycle. They may cause masculinization or galactorrhea in addition to persistent anestrus. Certain diseases such as vaginal hyperplasia and prolapse, cystic endometritis/hyperplasia, alopecia syndromes, bone marrow hypoplasia, and mammary tumors can be caused or enhanced by ovarian hormones in certain companion animal species.

FEMALE HYPOGONADISM

Female hypogonadism is the deficient function of the ovaries. Possible causes are listed in Table 24–1.

Hypothalamic-Pituitary Origin Hypogonadism (Hypogonadotropic Hypogonadism)

Hypothalamic-pituitary female hypogonadism is characterized by deficient ovarian function caused by gonadotropin deficiencies. Serum estrogen, progesterone, and androgen levels are subnormal. There should not be a significant increase in serum estrogen levels after stimulation of gonadotropin-releasing hormone (GnRH), but repeated injections of follicle-stimulating hormone (FSH) should lead to an increase in concentrations of serum estrogen.

The cause for gonadotropin deficiency may be a lesion in the hypothalamus-pituitary, or it may be something that alters the functional activity of the hypothalamus-pituitary. Exogenous gonadal steroid hormones inhibit the release of gonadotropins. Starvation inhibits the production of GnRH. Hyperprolactinemia from drugs (cimetidine and phenothiazines), pituitary adenomas, or hypothyroidism can inhibit the release of gonadotropins as well as cause galactorrhea. Excessive gonadal steroids may be secreted from adrenocortical hyperplasia or neoplasia and inhibit the release of gonadotropins. A wide variety of severe systemic illnesses, such as unregulated diabetes mellitus, hypoadrenocorticism, pneumonia, and others, suppress the release of GnRH. Psychologic stresses such as those caused by new

Table 24–1. Possible Causes of Female Hypogonadism

Hypothalamic-pituitary origin
  Neoplasms and cysts
  Hemorrhage, infarction, or infection
  Administration of exogenous gonadal steroid hormones
  Starvation
  Hyperprolactinemia
  Adrenocortical hyperplasia, neoplasia, or hypofunction
  Systemic illnesses
  Psychic stress
Gonadal origin
  Gonadal dysgenesis and other chromosomal abnormalities
  Testicular feminization
  Defects in estrogen biosynthesis

surroundings, intimidation from people or other animals, or from over-crowding can inhibit the release of GnRH.

Hypogonadotropic hypogonadism of the ovaries occurring before puberty prevents the development of secondary sexual characteristics such as mammary development and impairs the normal prepubertal growth spurt. Postpubertal hypogonadism is evident only by its association with failure of the ovarian cycle.

The cause for hypothalamic-pituitary hypogonadism should be sought and eliminated when possible. When the cause cannot be found or eliminated, induction of estrus and ovulation can be considered. The decision to use exogenous gonadotropins is not trivial. The exogenous administration of gonadotropins is expensive and time consuming, yields inconsistent results, induces hypofunctional corpora lutea that tend to regress prematurely, and is potentially hazardous. Adverse effects can include superovulation, cystic follicles, hypersensitivity reactions, and hyperestrogenism. Stimulation of excessive estrogen production in bitches may lead to vaginal prolapse, vaginal hyperplasia, cystic endometritis, or enhanced growth of some ovarian, mammary, or uterine neoplasia. Schedules for two methods of induction of estrus and three methods of induction of ovulation in dogs and cats are provided in Table 24–2. The authors' orders of preference for the methods are also provided in Table 24–2.

There are very few female companion animals whose hypogonadism responds to therapy with gonadotropins without the identification and elimination of the cause. Hypogonadism of gonadal origin has already been exposed to high levels of endogenous gonadotropins without effect and therefore is refractory to exogenous therapy with gonadotropins. GnRH may be used as a substitute for human chorionic gonadotropin (HCG), but only if the adenohypophysis is structurally intact and functional. In the anestrous season of cats, the adenohypophyseal stores of luteinizing hormone (LH) may not be present in adequate amounts to cause ovulation, and GnRH would probably be ineffective during this time.

Table 24-2. Induction of Estrus and Ovulation in Bitches and Queens

	Bitches		Queens	
Product	Option Preferences	Method*	Option Preference	Method*
Induction of Follicle Maturation†				
FSH		0.75 mg/kg body weight/day for 10 days	#1	Expose to 14 hours or more of bright light and other queens in heat
			#2	2 mg/day for 5 days
Induction of Ovulation				
HCG	#1	500–1000 IU for 2 successive days	#1	Multiple matings with tom cat
			#2	250–500 IU for 2 successive days
GnRH	#2	50 µg twice in 1 day	#3	25 µg on 2nd day of estrus (February to August only)

FSH (FSH-P) = follicle-stimulating hormone; HCG (Pregnyl) = human chorionic gonadotropin; IU = international units; GnRH (Cystorelin) = gonadotropin-releasing hormone.
* All injections given intramuscularly.
† Discontinue FSH whenever vaginal cytology indicates that more than 90% of the epithelial cells are superficial cells.

Clomiphene (Clomid, Serophene) is a nonsteroidal competitive antagonist of estrogen frequently used in women as a fertility agent. By binding estrogen receptors in the hypothalamus and adenohypophysis, clomiphene can block estrogen's inhibitory effects on the release of gonadotropins. Its ability to result in the release of endogenous gonadotropins requires normal to high serum estrogen levels and an intact hypothalamus and pituitary. Clomiphene has been used successfully in the mare to induce estrus.

Gonadal-origin Hypogonadism (Hypergonadotropic Hypogonadism)

Ovarian diseases can result in hypogonadism, a condition characterized by elevated serum gonadotropin levels. Serum estrogen, progesterone, and androgen levels are subnormal. There is no change in levels of serum gonadal hormones after the exogenous administration of gonadotropins.

The causes of hypogonadism of gonadal origin are uncommon (Table 24–1). Chromosomal defects are more likely to cause hypogonadism than defects in the biosynthesis of estrogen. Hypogonadism of ovarian origin has a prepubertal onset; therefore, it impairs the prepubertal growth spurt and delays epiphyseal closures. Secondary sex characteristics do not develop at the normal time for puberty. Primary anestrus results. The cause of hypogonadism of ovarian origin can be investigated by buccal smears or karyotyping, by assays of serum estrogen precursor hormones, and by exploratory laparoscopy or laparotomy.

There is no treatment for hypogonadism of ovarian origin that produces normal reproductive capabilities. Secondary sexual characteristics can be created with the administration of estrogens, but in companion animals, there is no good reason to produce female secondary sexual characteristics in affected animals.

INAPPROPRIATE ANESTRUS

Anestrus may be part of the normal estrous cycle. Bitches experience anestrus between each metestrus and the next proestrus. Queens and mares have a physiologic seasonal anestrus. Anestrus is also normal during pregnancy. However, some queens and mares may exhibit estrus during pregnancy. Inappropriate anestrus is thought to occur during any other period when postpubertal estrous cycles have ceased.

Causes of inappropriate anestrus can be classified as *primary anestrus* (an estrus that has never been seen) or *secondary anestrus* (estrous cycles noted before the period of inappropriate anestrus). Possible causes are listed in Table 24–3.

Primary anestrus should be considered in bitches, queens, and mares who have not shown signs of estrus by the time they reach 2 years of age. If the anestrus is caused by hypothalamic or pituitary disease, other signs of pituitary deficiencies, especially dwarfism, may be present. Congenital adrenal hyperplasia should be accompanied by signs of masculinization. Testicular feminization should be suspected if the vagina is short and ends blindly

Table 24–3. Possible Causes of Inappropriate Anestrus

Primary Anestrus
  Cystic Rathke's pouch
  Craniopharyngioma
  Ovarian dysgenesis
  Congenital adrenal hyperplasia
  Testicular feminization
  Psychic stress
Secondary Anestrus
  Drug-induced hypogonadotropic hypogonadism
  Polycystic ovarian syndrome
  Adrenocortical hyperplasia, neoplasia, or hypofunction
  Hypothyroidism
  Chronic debilitating illnesses
  Obesity or severe malnutrition
  Acquired hypothalamic-pituitary disease
  Ovarian neoplasia
  Ovariectomy
  Psychic stress

---

without a cervix. Buccal smears or karotyping would show an XY genotype. The possibility of ovarian dysgenesis (XO genotype) must also be investigated by buccal smears or karyotyping. The diagnosis of psychic stress is made according to the animal's history, exclusion of other causes, and response to modifying the environment and handling of the female animal.

Secondary anestrus may occur at any time after puberty. The case history is helpful in diagnosing or eliminating the possibility of ovariectomy or drug-induced anestrus. Any steroidal drug, even glucocorticoids, could be a cause of inhibited release of gonadotropins. Chronic debilitating illnesses, obesity, or severe malnutrition would be evident on physical examination. These act on the hypothalamus to suppress the release of GnRH. Inappropriate anestrus often occurs with hypoadrenocorticism, and this combination may be due to the weight loss associated with it or its effects on cerebral activity and the hypothalamus. Marked obesity increases the conversion of androstenedione to estrone and decreases the binding of estradiol to sex-hormone-binding globulin (SHBG).

Advanced hypothyroidism and some hypothalamic-pituitary disorders cause hyperprolactinemia, which inhibits the release of gonadotropins. Destructive hypothalamic-pituitary disorders impair the production and release of gonadotropins. Clinical signs of hypothyroidism or hypothalamic-pituitary disease such as alopecia, polyuria, polydipsia, mental depression, lethargy, and others should be disclosed in the history or found on physical examination. Psychic stress may be suggested by the history. It, too, would inhibit the release of GnRH. Sources of excessive endogenous steroids that may inhibit the release of gonadotropins are hyperadrenocorticism resulting from adrenocortical hyperplasia or neoplasia, ovarian neoplasia, or the polycystic ovarian syndrome.

The diagnostic evaluation of inappropriate anestrus should begin with verification of the problem, followed by evaluation of the history, physical examination of the patient, and then laboratory investigations. Laboratory investigations should not be run as a battery of unrelated tests; they are, instead, to be selected according to their potential value as indicated by the findings of the history and physical examination (Table 24-4).

See also references 5, 10, 79, 118, and 133.

ABNORMAL ESTROUS CYCLES

Abnormal estrous cycles may be manifested by prolonged interestrous intervals, shortened interestrous intervals, prolonged estrus, silent estrus, or split estrus.

See also references 74 and 76.

Prolonged Interestrous Intervals

Interestrual periods exceeding 12 months in the bitch (except basenjis), 3 weeks during the breeding season in the queen, and 4 weeks during the breeding season in the mare are considered excessively long. Common causes of prolonged interestrus are hypothyroidism in bitches and persist-

Table 24-4. Approach to the Diagnosis of Inappropriate Anestrus

1. Verify the problem:
   Is the patient old enough for estrous cycles?
   Is the patient exposed to sufficient light?
   Is the patient observed closely for signs of estrus?
   Could the patient be pregnant?

2. Evaluate the history:
   Have drugs been administered that could inhibit the H-P-O axis?
   Have any other signs of illness been noted?
   Have female relatives of the patient been similarly affected?

3. Examine the patient:
   Are the external genitalia normal?
   Are there signs of systemic illness?

4. Select appropriate laboratory investigation:

Physical Exam Findings	Appropriate Laboratory Exams
Normal	Plasma FSH, LH, and prolactin levels; serum estradiol and progesterone levels
Alopecia	Serum estradiol, cortisol, and T_4 levels
Blind vagina	Buccal smear
Enlarged clitoris	Buccal smear; serum testosterone assay
Swollen vulva	Vaginal cytology; serum estradiol
Galactorrhea	Plasma prolactin; serum progesterone

H-P-O = hypothalamic-pituitary-ovarian; FSH = follicle-stimulating hormone; LH = luteinizing hormone; T_4 = thyroxine.

ent corpora lutea in mares. Queens rarely have prolonged interestrual periods. Persistent corpora lutea in mares may be due to insufficient levels of prostaglandin $F_{2\alpha}$ and can sometimes be successfully treated by the administration of $F_{2\alpha}$ to lyse the corpora lutea or by the intrauterine infusion of 500 to 1000 ml of normal saline to stimulate the release of endogenous prostaglandins. Serum progesterone levels in excess of 5 ng/ml are indicative of a functional corpora lutea. Hypothyroidism in bitches is managed by administering replacement thyroid hormone.

Short Interestrous Intervals

Abnormally short interestrous periods are less than 4 months in the bitch, less than 10 days during the breeding season in queens, and less than 18 days during the breeding season in mares. In spontaneous ovulators (bitches and mares), short interestrous periods can be caused by inadequate formation or function of corpora lutea. Rapid estrous cycles prevent adequate endometrial repair sufficient to maintain fertility. Interestrous periods can be prolonged by either progestins or androgens. Androgens are preferred in the bitch because of her susceptibility for developing endometritis when under the effects of progestins.

Prolonged Estrus (or Proestrus)

Estrus should be considered abnormally prolonged if it exceeds 2 weeks in the bitch, 16 days in the queen, or 10 days in the mare. Prolonged estrus is caused by ovulatory failure or functional ovarian neoplasia. Failure to ovulate is normal in the unmated queen, but follicles should temporarily regress along with behavioral signs of estrus, except in some Siamese queens. Possible causes of prolonged estrus are polycystic ovarian syndrome and granulosa-theca cell tumors.

POLYCYSTIC OVARIAN SYNDROME.   Failure to ovulate without regression of follicles and without waning of serum estrogen levels is called the *polycystic ovarian syndrome (PCOS),* a heterogenous disorder affecting both ovaries. Histologic features include multiple follicular and atretic cysts, hyperplastic theca and stromal cells, and thickening of the capsule. Serum levels of estradiol or its weak androgenic precursors are elevated. In affected women, plasma LH levels are elevated; plasma FSH levels are normal to suppressed. The defect in the hypothalamic-pituitary-ovarian (H-P-O) axis that prevents ovulation may be in the hypothalamus-pituitary or in the ovary; there seems to be more than one cause. One form of PCOS in women is familial. Another type, *hyperthecosis,* is characterized histologically by luteinized theca-like stromal cells.

Behavior is altered in patients with PCOS. In bitches, signs of nymphomania and other estrogen-induced disorders predominate. In queens and mares, male-like aggression is more common. Treatment may be attempted with human chorionic gonadotropin (HCG) or GnRH (Cystorelin) in hopes of causing ovulation. The increased endogenous release of LH and ovulation might be achieved by using glucocorticoids to suppress ovarian biosynthesis of androgens, by administration of clomiphene, or by wedge section of the ovaries to debulk the androgen-producing stromal cells. Administration of progesterone can inhibit the secretion of LH and, in turn, ovarian production of androgens. Treatment with progesterone can suppress behavioral abnormalities, but it will prevent recurrence of estrus as long as it is continued to be used. Ovariectomy may be the only satisfactory treatment.

See also references 113, 117, and 127.

GRANULOSA-THECA CELL TUMORS. Usually secreting estrogens, granulosa-theca cell tumors may cause prolonged estrus and, in bitches, other estrogen-induced disorders such as bone marrow aplasia or alopecia.

Silent Estrus

Silent estrus is the failure to exhibit behavioral signs of estrus even though estrous cycles are occurring. Silent estrus is most common in young bitches. Serum progesterone levels in excess of 1 ng/ml indicate that ovulations have occurred recently. If serum progesterone levels are less than 1 ng/ml, close observation of bitches to detect any signs suggestive of proestrus or estrus should be practiced for 6 months. If there are no signs of either after 6 months, the diagnosis of silent estrus should be changed to inappropriate anestrus and treated accordingly. Signs noted in bitches suggestive of proestrus or estrus should be further examined by vaginal cytology to confirm whether estrus is occurring. Treatment is not necessary for silent estrus, but affected females may not allow the male to mate. Artificial insemination may be required.

Split Estrus

Young postpubertal bitches and mares in the transitional period of late winter-early spring may show a split estrus. Split estrus is said to occur whenever signs of estrus subside without ovulation and then return within a few days. Split estrus is usually a temporary abnormality of the estrous cycle and does not require any treatment. It can be due to pain resulting from attempted mating, intimidation during early estrus, or idiopathic temporary atresia of the follicles.

PRECOCIOUS SEXUAL DEVELOPMENT

Secondary sexual characteristics appearing in bitches before 6 months of age, queens before 4 months of age, and mares before 1 year of age are indicative of precocious (premature) sexual development. Secondary sexual characteristics in female companion animals are difficult to detect, but can include mammary development and mounting of the other animals. If precocious secondary sexual development is accompanied by estrus, premature activation of the H-P-O axis has occurred. This is termed *true precocious puberty,* which may be caused by congenital anomalies of the central nervous system, inflammation, trauma, or tumors, particularly involving the hypothalamus or pineal gland.

Precocious pseudopuberty is the premature development of secondary sexual characteristics in female companion animals without the occurrence of estrus. It is caused by the premature occurrence of increased serum levels of estrogens. The source of estrogen may be due to the exogenous administration or endogenous production of the hormone from ovarian tumors or adrenal carcinomas.

VIRILISM (Masculinization)

Virilism is the presence of male characteristics in a female animal. It is mediated by the endogenous production or exogenous administration of an excess of androgens, or, less commonly, exogenous progestins. Possible causes are listed in Table 24–5. The most obvious physical change in virilism is the enlargement of the clitoris (Fig. 24–1). Affected mares may develop crested necks. Behavioral changes may include aggression and mounting other females. Bitches may lift a hind leg to urinate. Queens in anestrus may spray urine to mark territorial limits. Virilism is generally associated with inappropriate anestrus in sexually intact females.

Virilism should be treated by eliminating the cause. If due to drug administration, the use of the drugs should be eliminated. For example, mibolerone (Cheque) is an androgenic steroid used to prevent estrus in bitches. Clitoral hypertrophy frequently occurs with its use. If clitoral hypertrophy is great enough to result in protrusion of the clitoris from the vulva, the drug should be discontinued. Endogenous sources of excessive androgens are the ovaries or the adrenal cortex. Both the ovaries and the adrenals should be evaluated for possible hyperplasia or neoplasia by endocrinologic assays, radiographic examinations, or ultrasonography. Exploratory laparotomy and, in some cases, ovariectomy may be necessary to determine the source of excessive androgens.

ESTROGEN- AND PROGESTERONE-ENHANCED DISORDERS

Estrogen- and progesterone-enhanced disorders in dogs and cats are cystic endometrial hyperplasia, mammary tumors, and mammary hyperpla-

Table 24–5. Possible Causes of Virilism

Exogenous origin
   Administration of androgens
   Administration of progestins

Endogenous origin
   Ovarian sources
      Polycystic ovarian syndrome
      Stromal or hilus cell hyperplasia
      Ovarian neoplasia (arrhenoblastoma)
   Adrenocortical sources
      Congenital adrenal hyperplasia
      Adrenocortical neoplasia
      Bilateral acquired adrenocortical hyperplasia

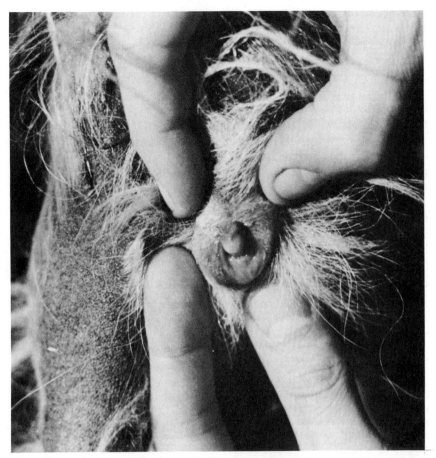

Fig. 24–1. Enlargement of the clitoris in a bitch with virilism.

sia. Additionally in dogs, vaginal hyperplasia and prolapse, alopecia, and bone marrow hypoplasia-aplasia can be induced or enhanced by excessive estrogenic effects.

Cystic Endometrial Hyperplasia

Cystic endometrial hyperplasia (CEH) is the most common disease of the uterus of the bitch and queen. It can be produced experimentally in sexually intact bitches with repeated administration of progestins. A permissive amount of estrogens must be present, and increased stimulation by estrogens potentiates progesterone effects leading to CEH. The spontaneous disease begins during metestrus. For that reason, CEH occurs less frequently in queens than in bitches. Most cases in queens result from the administration of progestins, but spontaneous ovulation, sham mating, treatment with HCG, or infertile matings can also lead to metestrus and CEH in queens. Mares are rarely affected, probably because of the short luteal phase of their ovarian cycle, which is due to prostaglandin lysis of the corpus luteum.

In the United States, CEH is usually a spontaneous disease in bitches over 5 years of age. Most are nulliparous. The risk of CEH is increased by the administration of progestins or estrogens. The practice of giving estrogens to prevent unwanted pregnancies especially predisposes the animal to CEH because the administered estrogens increase uterine progesterone receptors while serum progesterone levels are rising. Estrogens promote the growth of the endometrium, increase progesterone receptors in the uterus, and stimulate the elongation of uterine glands. Progesterone promotes maturation of the uterine glands, stimulating them to become tortuous, secretory, and eventually cystic. Intraluminal secretions accumulate. If bacteriologically sterile, a uterus with CEH and intraluminal secretions is called mucometra. The secretions of the uterine glands readily support bacterial growth, and progesterone has immunosuppressive effects. As a result, the endometrium with CEH and uterine intraluminal secretions easily becomes infected. Involved pathogens are generally gram-negative rods, especially *Escherichia coli*. When the intraluminal contents have become purulent, the condition is called pyometra.

Mucometra is asymptomatic, but pyometra is life-threatening. Pyometra can be associated with drainage of the reddish-brown purulent intraluminal exudate through an open cervix, or it can be an abscessation, that is, purulent uterine contents entrapped behind a closed cervix. Pyometra stimulates production of circulating antigen-antibody complexes which, in turn, frequently causes immune complex glomerulonephritis.

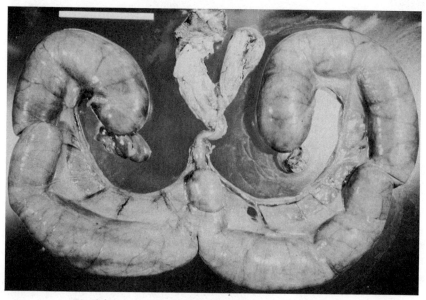

Fig. 24–2. A canine uterus affected by "closed" pyometra.

"Open" pyometra is a febrile illness that may not be noticed by owners of companion animals until a copious discharge from the vagina is noticed. Laboratory examinations usually show poorly regenerative anemia and leukocytosis.

Owners present bitches with *"closed" pyometra* for examination because of the complaints of their pets having polyuria, polydipsia, depression, and anorexia. Physical examination is rarely informative. Pyometra distends the uterus so that the uterine wall becomes thin (Fig. 24–2) and intraluminal contents have a thick liquid consistency; therefore, pyometra can rarely be palpated transabdominally (it is also unwise to attempt to palpate a case of suspected pyometra because of the risk of uterine rupture). Laboratory findings often include leukocytosis with a marked left shift. It is not uncommon for the demand for neutrophils to exceed the supply. At that point, an abnormally low neutrophil count occurs, with a large percentage of those present being bands. This is a degenerative left shift, an ominous sign of exhaustion of the body's defenses. Serum globulins and blood urea nitrogen are usually elevated. The urinalysis may show isosthenuria or hyposthenuria since *Escherichia coli* toxins can impair renal tubular concentrating ability. Abdominal radiographs or ultrasonography are diagnostically useful.

The treatment of choice for pyometra is an ovariohysterectomy. For bitches or queens whose primary value is their ability to produce litters, antibiotics plus prostaglandin $F_{2\alpha}$ (Lutalyse), in a dose of 25 to 50 μg/kg body weight given intramuscularly, twice daily for 3 to 5 days, has been used to expel the uterine contents. This treatment was used successfully to treat pyometra. Transient emesis, anxiety, salivation, dyspnea, and diarrhea often occur. Because bronchial constriction occurs with the administration of $PGF_{2\alpha}$, it should not be used in patients with respiratory disorders. When $PGF_{2\alpha}$ is used to treat closed pyometra, there are additional risks, including the rupture of the uterus, retrograde flow of septic exudate up the uterine ducts, and bacteremia.

See also references 8, 13, 24, 25, 35–37, 48, 55, 58, and 77.

Vaginal Hyperplasia and Prolapse in Bitches

Vaginal hyperplasia is an edematous hyperplastic polypoid growth that originates from the floor of the vagina just cranial to the vaginal urethral meatus. Most often, it occurs in young large breed bitches during their first or second proestrus and estrus. Spontaneous regression occurs during metestrus. On occasion, the proliferated edematous mucosa can be severe enough to protrude from the vulva (Fig. 24–3) or even progress to a circumferential, donut-like protrusion of the vagina wall, called vaginal prolapse (Fig. 24–4).

Unless the vaginal mucosa protrudes from the vulva and is easily traumatized, treatment may not be necessary. In one third of the affected animals, subsequent estrous cycles are not to be accompanied by vaginal hyperplasia or prolapse. When vaginal hyperplasia or prolapse does recur, it is usually

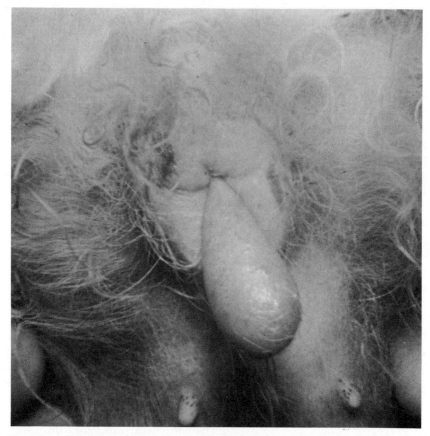

Fig. 24–3. Protrusion of polypoid vaginal hyperplasia from the vulva in a bitch in estrus.

less severe. Ovariectomy prevents spontaneous recurrences. Administration of estrogen can reproduce the condition in susceptible bitches. When the severity is great enough to result in or risk vaginal mucosal trauma, vaginoplasty is necessary.

Estrogen-Induced Alopecia in Bitches (Ovarian Imbalance I)

Prolonged hyperestrogenism in dogs causes alopecia. Bitches with ovarian disorders that cause prolonged estrus can cause alopecia. Estrogen-induced alopecia begins in the perineal, ventral abdominal, and genital region. It is accompanied by seborrheic changes and sometimes ceruminous external otitis. Pruritus may or may not occur. Affected female dogs are usually older than 5 years of age, have enlarged vulvas, and attract male dogs. Although most have never nursed a litter, affected female dogs have well-developed mammae and may lactate (Fig. 24–5). The ventral abdomen often has numerous comedones. Treatment consists of removing the endogenous or exogenous source of excessive estrogens.

See also references 22 and 119.

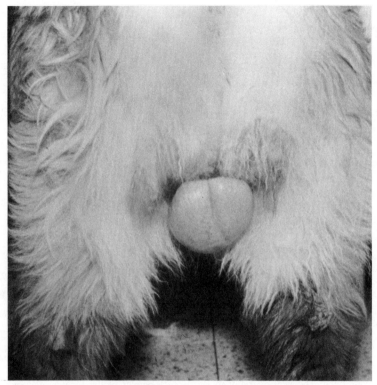

Fig. 24–4. Vaginal prolapse in a bitch in estrus.

Estrogen-Induced Bone Marrow Hypoplasia/Aplasia in Bitches and Jills

Excessive and prolonged estrogenic stimulation of the bone marrow in bitches and jills (female ferrets) may cause hypoplastic or aplastic anemia. Bone marrow cells of bitches are not adversely affected by elevated serum estrogen levels occurring during normal estrus. Jills are induced ovulators like queens. Because their serum estrogen levels are elevated during estrus and remain elevated until ovulation is induced by copulation, 20% to 30% of jills develop bone marrow depression subsequent to a normal but unmated estrus. This usually happens in spring or early summer. Estrogen-induced bone marrow aplasia has not been reported in queens or mares.

Conditions producing estrogens in amounts sufficiently excessive and for a period of time long enough to cause bone marrow hypoplasia in dogs are estrogen-secreting ovarian neoplasia, feminizing testicular tumors, and the administration of exogenous natural or synthetic estrogens. Risk factors to consider include advanced patient age (the number of stem cells decreases naturally with age), duration of exposure to excessive estrogens, as well as the type and dosage of exposure to exogenous estrogens. The initial effect of excessive amounts of estrogen on the bone marrow of bitches is myeloid

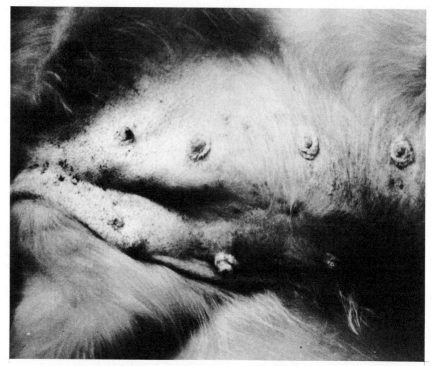

Fig. 24–5. Estrogen-induced alopecia (Ovarian Imbalance I) in an older, sexually intact nulliparous bitch. The ventral abdomen shows enlargement of the nipples, mammae, and comedones, and thinning of the haircoat.

hyperplasia resulting from stimulating committed stem cell lines. Uncommitted stem cell numbers are suppressed. Thrombocytosis occurs within the first 2 weeks and leukocytosis within the first 3 weeks of exposure to excess levels of estrogens followed by thrombocytopenia and granulocytopenia. Clinical signs include petechial hemorrhage, melena, anemia, and other signs resulting from secondary infections. Anemia develops slowly, unless the thrombocytopenia leads to hemorrhage. The immediate cause of death usually results from fulminating infection secondary to neutropenia.

Treatment is mainly supportive. If possible, the source of estrogens should be removed. Jills should be mated or induced to ovulate with the intramuscular administration of 100 IU of HCG. Signs of estrus subside for 21 to 30 days. Then, estrus returns in 40 to 60 days. If these conditions are caused in dogs by an ovarian tumor or feminizing testicular tumor, these tumors should be excised. Broad-spectrum antibiotics are indicated if total white blood cell counts are less than 3000/cmm.

Platelet-rich plasma or compatible whole-blood transfusions are given as necessary. Stimulation of the remaining uncommitted stem cells has been attempted with the administration of androgenic steroids, glucocorticoids, and lithium citrate. It is unclear whether any improvement in bone marrow cellularity can be attributed to these drugs or to time. When recovery occurs, the order of reappearance of blood cells are reticulocytes, granulo-·cytes, and, finally, platelets. Reticulocyte numbers should return to normal within 2 weeks after the decrease—that is, 4 weeks after the administration of exogenous estrogen—or the prognosis is grave. Weak estrogenic anti-estrogens such as tamoxifen may be detrimental since estrogen receptors can be bound and further stimulate bone marrow cells by their inherent weak estrogenic effects.

Canine and Feline Mammary Gland Neoplasias and Hyperplasias

Estrogens and progesterone can unquestionably enhance the growth of certain mammary neoplasias. The role estrogens and progesterone play in initiating mammary tumors in bitches and queens is unclear. Mammary tumors are common in sexually intact bitches and queens. Few mammary tumors have been reported in mares.

See also reference 80.

CANINE MAMMARY GLAND NEOPLASIA.   One fourth to one half of all neoplasia in the bitch are mammary gland neoplasms. The incidence of mammary neoplasia in sexually intact bitches is considered to be three times that in women. Just under one half of canine mammary neoplasms are malignant. Twenty-five percent to fifty percent of malignant mammary tumors have metastasized by the time of initial detection of the primary tumor. Fox terriers, pointers, cocker spaniels, Boston terriers, poodles, and dachshunds may have an elevated risk for developing mammary gland neoplasia. Chihuahuas, collies, and boxers are possibly at low risk.

Advancing age increases the risk of mammary gland neoplasia and increases the percentage that are malignant. The incidence of mammary gland neoplasia rises rapidly in bitches older than 5 years of age and peaks in animals between 10 and 12 years old. Approximately 65% of the tumors occur in the caudal pairs of mammary glands, gland pair numbers 4 and 5. Benign canine mammary neoplasms are papillomas, fibroadenomas, benign mixed tumors, and adenomas. Malignant canine mammary tumors include squamous cell carcinomas, solid carcinomas, tubular adenocarcinomas, papillary adenocarcinomas, anaplastic carcinomas, malignant mixed carcinomas, and sarcomas. Histologic classifications vary somewhat. There is no uniformly accepted classification system. Benign mixed mammary gland tumors are the most common type in the bitch. Over one half of affected bitches have more than one mammary tumor at the time the first tumor is detected.

The evidence is overwhelming that the risk of mammary gland neoplasia in bitches is enhanced by exposure to estrogen and progesterone. If bitches are ovariectomized before their first estrus occurs, the risk of developing mammary gland neoplasia is no greater than that in male animals—0.05% that of sexually intact bitches over 2.5 years old. If an ovariectomy is done after the first or second estrus, the risk is 8% and 26%, respectively. An ovariectomy done in animals older than 2.5 years has no effect on reducing the incidence of developing mammary neoplasia. Most of the male dogs that develop mammary gland neoplasia have feminizing testicular neoplasms. Malignant mammary gland neoplasia is apparently not induced by gonadal steroid hormones in bitches as are some benign mammary gland neoplasms; however, the rate of growth of both can be enhanced by estrogens and progesterone. The neoplasm's rate of growth in some mammary glands is obviously accelerated during estrus, metestrus, or pregnancy.

Benign mammary gland tumors have been induced in dogs on long-term toxicologic studies of progestin. Basaloid adenomas are nearly exclusively associated with prolonged exposure to progestins. Progestins stimulate the secretion of growth hormone (GH) in bitches. It may be the effects of GH, not the direct effects by progestins on the mammary glands, that promote the development of mammary tumors in bitches treated with progestin. Furthermore, there is evidence that the secretion of prolactin increases with mammary tumors in bitches. Since progestins increase the binding of prolactin, it might be that the effect of progestins on mammary tumor growth is a synergistic effect with prolactin.

Several factors have been proposed to contribute to the risk of bitches developing mammary gland neoplasia. Among these are polycystic ovarian syndrome, persistent corporum luteum, pseudopregnancy, and irregular estrous cycles. The possibility that pregnancies have a protective influence has been considered. There is insufficient evidence to substantiate any of these factors proposed to incite or protect from mammary gland neoplasms.

Studies to detect the presence of estrogen and progesterone receptors in mammary tumors yield information on which tumors can be affected by estrogens and progesterone. Receptor assays are now routinely done on breast carcinomas in women to identify those who might respond to hormonal therapy. Such studies have also been done on bitches. In bitches, 40% to 60% of mammary tumors (carcinomas) are estrogen-receptor positive. Sarcomas and large tumors over 10 cm in diameter are estrogen- and progesterone-receptor poor. The production of progesterone receptors is believed usually to be dependent on the presence of estrogen receptors. Most estrogen-receptor-positive mammary tumors in bitches are also progesterone-receptor positive, but occasionally, tumors are progesterone-receptor positive and estrogen-receptor negative (according to present assay methods, which may underrepresent the true incidence of estrogen receptors). Other hormones may also directly affect the growth of mammary tumors. For instance, over one third of canine mammary tumors have dihydrotestosterone receptors.

The treatment of canine mammary neoplasia is generally limited to surgical excision. About one third of breast carcinomas in women regress with hormonal therapy, which is designed to block estrogen effects or to eliminate endogenous sources of estrogen. Fifty percent to sixty-five percent of the tumors respond if they are estrogen-receptor positive. If the tumors are estrogen-receptor negative, no more than 10% respond. The best response to hormonal therapy occurs in tumors that are both estrogen-receptor positive and progesterone-receptor positive. Of these tumors, 80% respond to hormonal therapy.

Endogenous sources of estrogen are the ovaries and adrenal cortex. Means of reducing the production of estrogen or its effects are ovariectomy; the administration of antiestrogens such as tamoxifen (Nolvadex); androgens such as testolactone (Teslac), fluoxymesterone (Fluoxymesterone), or dromostanolone (Drolban); or glucocorticoids. Evaluations of various estrogen-reducing or -blocking protocols have not been done on selected estrogen-receptor-positive mammary tumors. It is reasonable to assume one or more such approaches could cause remission of some metastatic mammary gland tumors, permitting prolonged life of good quality.

See also references 7, 15–17, 19, 20, 28, 38, 40–46, 49, 50, 56, 59, 60, 67, 70, 73, 82, 86–99, 106, 107, 109, 114–117, 123, 124, 128, and 129.

FELINE MAMMARY GLAND NEOPLASIA AND HYPERPLASIA. Mammary gland neoplasia is not as frequent in queens as it is in bitches. Still, it is the third most common feline neoplasia and is responsible for about 20% of all neoplasia in queens. More than 80% of feline mammary neoplasms are malignant. Nearly all malignant mammary gland neoplasms in queens are adenocarcinomas. The average age of the affected animal is approximately 11 years. The first and second cranial pair of mammae are more often affected than the caudal two pair (gland pairs 3 and 4) in the queen. Siamese cats have a greater-than-average risk of developing mammary gland neoplasia and have an earlier-than-average age of onset.

Ovarian-origin hormones can program the queen's mammary gland to later develop neoplasia just as they do in bitches. If the ovaries are excised early in life, the risk of queens having mammary gland neoplasia is reduced sevenfold. Tom cats are virtually free of the risk of spontaneous mammary gland neoplasia.

Progestins, medroxyprogesterone acetate, and megestrol acetate can induce mammary gland adenocarcinomas in cats. Feline mammary gland adenocarcinomas are progesterone-receptor positive. Only about 10% are estrogen-receptor positive. The predominance of progesterone-receptor tumors over estrogen-receptor tumors is difficult to understand since progesterone receptors are generally believed to be dependent on estrogen and estrogen receptors. Hormonal manipulation to reduce estrogen or its effects would not be expected to cause tumor regression in most cases.

Feline fibroadenomatous hyperplasia is a progesterone-induced dysplasia of the feline mammary glands. It was first called feline mammary hypertrophy in 1973. This name and several other synonyms are still used, but the term feline fibroadenomatous hyperplasia, based on the condition's histologic appearance, is the best descriptive name. Young, sexually intact queens under 2 years of age make up at least three fourths of the involved cases. Spontaneous feline fibroadenomatous hyperplasia appears after estrus or during pregnancy as a rapid firm painless growth of all mammae (Fig. 24–6). Spontaneous regression occurs slowly, unless an ovariectomy is done.

The spontaneous form of feline fibroadenomatous hyperplasia in young female animals is a proliferation of ductal and stromal elements. A variant form can be produced in queens or toms by some exogenous progestins such as megestrol acetate. With the progestin-induced form, the hyperplasia is mostly intraductular, papillary, and cystic. It is important to differentiate the benign and transient feline fibroadenomatous hyperplasia from feline adenocarcinomas. The mean survival time for queens with multiple adenocarcinoma is less than 6 months.

See also references 2, 3, 12, 18, 23, 34, 39, 51, 57, 61–64, 66, 68, 69, 75, 78, 81, 100, 101, 105, 110, 116, 125, and 130–132.

OVARIAN NEOPLASIA

Ovarian neoplasms may originate from germinal epithelium, sex cord stroma, germ cells, or supporting tissue (Table 24–6). Most are unilateral. Many are functional and cause syndromes of hormone excess. Other possible clinical signs include those of an abdominal mass or ascites, but detection of ovarian tumors is frequently by chance. Sex cord stromatic origin ovarian tumors are the most common in the queen and mare. Tumors of epithelial origin are slightly more common than other ovarian tumors in bitches. Ovarian neoplasia cause 6.25% of neoplasms in sexually intact bitches examined at necropsy. Reports of ovarian neoplasia in queens, mares, and budgerigar are less than those noted in bitches.

See also references 14, 21, 26, 30, 80, 83, 103, 120, and 121.

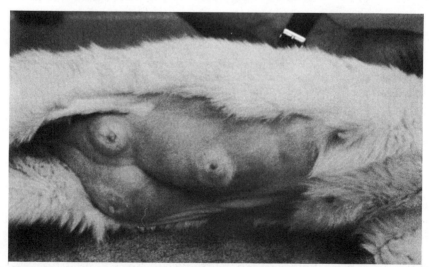

Fig. 24–6. Spontaneous feline fibroadenomatosis hyperplasia in a young pregnant queen.

Table 24–6.   Classification of Ovarian Neoplasia

Sex cord stroma origin
  Granulosa-theca cell
  Sertoli's-Leydig cell
Germ cell origin
  Germinoma
  Gonadoblastoma
  Teratoma
Germinal epithelial origin
  Adenocarcinomas
  Cyst-adenocarcinoma
  Cyst-adenoma
  Adenoma
  Papillary adenocarcinoma
Supporting tissue origin
  Fibroma
  Fibrosarcoma

Tumors of Sex Cord Stromatic Origin

Granulosa-theca cell tumors are the most frequently diagnosed ovarian neoplasm in queens and mares and constitute over 25% of all canine ovarian neoplasia. Most are hormone (particularly estrogen)-producing neoplasms. A few, called luteomas, undergo luteinization and produce progesterone. Others produce excesses of androgens.

Granulosa-theca cell tumors are mixed cell type, solid, or partly cystic unilateral ovarian tumors that occur in middle-aged and older adult bitches. In animals older than 5 to 6 years, the incidence of granulosa-theca cell tumors does not increase. English bulldogs may be predisposed to have these tumors. Syndromes of estrogen or progesterone excess are associated with most canine granulosa cell tumors. Manifestations of granulosa cell tumors can be persistent estrus, bilateral alopecia (ovarian imbalance I), estrogen-induced bone marrow hyperplasia/aplasia, and cystic endometrial hyperplasia. Between 10% to 20% are malignant in bitches. One third are less than 1 cm in diameter, but some reach a size of more than 10 cm. Detection in suspected cases can be aided by hysterography, laparoscopy, or laparotomy.[47]

In queens, granulosa-theca cell tumors cause signs of persistent estrus. Some queens may become aggressive in behavior. Unlike the tumors found in bitches, 70% to 80% of granulosa-theca cell tumors in queens are malignant.

Granulosa-theca cell tumors in mares produce nymphomania with enlarged mammary glands, or anestrus with stallion-like behavior and virilism. In one half of affected mares, virilism and male-like behavior become evident. Serum testosterone levels are more than five times normal. Metastasis of granulosa-theca cell tumors is rare in mares. Sertoli's-Leydig cell tumors secrete estrogens or androgens. If the secretion of androgen and virilization occur, the tumors are called arrhenoblastomas.

See also references 1, 4, 6, 9, 11, 29, 65, 84, 85, 102, 104, 122, and 126.

Tumors of Germ Cell Origin

Germinomas (dysgerminomas) are the most common ovarian tumors of germ-cell origin in bitches and queens. Their histologic appearance resembles the seminoma in male animals. Germinomas account for about 5% to 15% of ovarian tumors in dogs and cats. They are unilateral tumors that occur at or after 10 years of age. Clinical signs of disease are unusual unless they are related to the increasing occupation of space in the abdomen. The average tumor size at the time of excision in bitches is 5 cm. All must be considered potentially malignant since the histologic appearance is that of primitive, rapidly dividing cells. However, only 10% to 30% metastasize in dogs and cats. Some germinomas have been associated with the effects of excessive levels of estrogens.

Gonadoblastomas (gynandroblastomas) are rare tumors of dysgenetic gonads. They occur in phenotypic females with a Y chromosome. The tumor is composed of cells like germinomas and sex cord-origin cells. Some of these cells can differentiate enough to produce estrogens or androgens.

Teratomas (Gr., monster tumor) are the second most common ovarian tumor in the mare. Teratomas are neoplasms of cells foreign to the organ in which they are found. Detection of teratomas usually occurs in young mares because of signs indicating an abdominal mass.

In bitches, teratomas account for 2% to 3% of all ovarian tumors. The left ovary is affected more commonly than the right. Bitches are usually about 4 years old when the teratoma is detected. The recognition of the tumor is usually the result of palpating an abdominal mass or finding an abdominal mass (which may be mineralized) evident on abdominal radiographs. The average tumor size at excision is 8.5 cm. Based on the incidence of metastasis, about 30% of teratomas are malignant in dogs. Some teratomas in women contain thyroid tissue (struma ovarii) and can cause thyrotoxicosis or contain carcinoid tumors. Thyroid tissue and carcinoid tumors in teratomas of companion animals have not yet been reported.

See also references 27, 31–33, 53, 54, 108, and 134.

Tumors of Epithelial Origin

Epithelial-origin tumors are the most common ovarian tumors in the bitch. Their incidence increases with age, peaking at about 9 years. The risk of the occurrence of these tumors is greater than average in pointers. Ovarian carcinomas have been induced in bitches with the prolonged administration of diethylstilbestrol.[71,72] Epithelial-origin tumors may be bilateral; if they are malignant, they can shed neoplastic cells into the abdomen. Ascites may develop with ovarian carcinomas. Tumors of the ovarian supporting tissues are rare in companion animals.

See also reference 52.

REFERENCES

1. Aliakbrai, S., and Ivoghli, B.: Granulosa cell tumor in a cat. J. Am. Vet. Med. Assoc., *174:*1306, 1979.
2. Allen, H.L.: Feline mammary hypertrophy. Vet. Pathol., *10:*501, 1973.
3. Allen, H.L.: Feline mammary hypertrophy. Vet. Pathol., *11:*561, 1974.
4. Allen, H.L., and Franklin, G.A.: Malignant granulosa cell tumor in a bitch. J. Am. Vet. Med. Assoc., *166:*447, 1975.
5. Allen, W.E., and Renton, J.P.: Infertility in the dog and bitch. Br. Vet. J., *138:*185, 1982.
6. Arnbjerg, J.: Extra-ovarian granulosa cell tumor in a cat. Feline Pract., *10:*26, 1980.
7. Attia, M.A.: Cytological study on the anterior pituitary of senile untreated beagle bitches with spontaneous mammary tumours. Arch. Toxicol., *50:*35, 1982.
8. Austad, R., Blom, A.K., and Borresen, B.: Pyometra in the dog. III. A pathophysiological investigation. Nord. Vet. Med., *31:*258, 1979.
9. Baker, E.: Malignant granulosa cell tumor in a cat. J. Am. Vet. Med. Assoc., *129:*322, 1956.
10. Barta, M., Archbald, L.F., and Godke, R.A.: Luteal function of induced corpora lutea in the bitch. Theriogenology, *18:*541, 1982.
11. Bergeron, H., Crouch, G.M., and Bowen, J.M.: Granulosa theca cell tumor in a mare. Compendium on Continuing Educ. for the Practicing Vet., *5:*5141, 1983.
12. Bloom, F.: Feline mammary hypertrophy. Vet. Pathol., *11:*561, 1974.
13. Borresen, B.: Pyometra in the dog—pathophysiological investigation. II. An amnestic, clinical, and reproductive aspects. Nord. Vet. Med., *31:*251, 1979.
14. Bosu, W.T.K., et al.: Ovarian disorders: clinical and morphological observations in 30 mares. Can. Vet. J., *23:*6, 1982.
15. Briggs, M.H.: Progestogens and mammary tumours in the beagle bitch. Res. Vet. Sci., *28:*199, 1980.
16. Bright, R.M., and Aberle, S.: Mammary neoplasia. Compendium on Continuing Educ. for the Practicing Vet., *1:*774, 1979.
17. Britt, J.O., Jr., and Howard, E.B.: An ovarian teratoma in a dog. Canine Pract., *8:*41, 1981.
18. Britt, J.O., Jr., Howard, E.B., and Ryan, C.P.: Simultaneous mixed mammary tumor and adenocarcinoma in a cat. Feline Pract., *9:*41, 1979.
19. Brodey, R.S., Goldschmidt, M.H., and Roszel, J.R.: Canine mammary gland neoplasms. J. Am. Anim. Hosp. Assoc., *19:*61, 1983.
20. Cameron, A.M., and Faulkin, I.J.: Hyperplastic and inflammatory nodules in the canine mammary gland. J. Natl. Cancer Inst., *47:*1277, 1971.
21. Campbell, T.W., and Stuart, L.D.: Ovarian neoplasia in the budgerigar (Melopsittacus undulatus). Vet. Med. Small Anim. Clin., *78:*215, 1984.
22. Cassel, S.E.: Ovarian imbalance in a German shepherd dwarf. Vet. Med. Small Anim. Clin., *73:*162, 1978.
23. Center, S.A., and Randolph, J.F.: Lactation and spontaneous remission of feline mammary hyperplasia following pregnancy. J. Am. Anim. Hosp., Assoc., *21:*56, 1985.
24. Christie, D.W., Bell, E.T., and Parkes, M.F.: Plasma progesterone levels in canine uterine disease. Vet. Rec., *90:*704, 1972.
25. Christie, D.W., et al.: Plasma progesterone levels in canine uterine disease. Vet. Rec., *90:*704, 1971.
26. Clark, T.L.: Clinical management of equine ovarian neoplasms. J. Reprod. Fertil. [Suppl.], *23:*331, 1975.
27. Clayton, H.M.: A canine ovarian teratoma. Vet. Rec., *96:*567, 1975.
28. Concannon, P., et al.: Growth hormone, prolactin, and cortisol in dogs developing mammary nodules and an acromegaly-like appearance during treatment with medroxyprogesterone acetate. Endocrinology, *106:*1173, 1980.
29. Cordes, D.V.: Equine granulosa tumors. Vet. Rec., *85:*186, 1969.
30. Cotchin, E.: Canine ovarian neoplasms. Res. Vet. Sci., *2:*133, 1961.
31. Crane, S.W., et al.: Malignant ovarian teratoma in a bitch. J. Am. Vet. Med. Assoc., *167:*72, 1975.
32. Damodaran, S., and Parthasarathy, K.R.: Mammary neoplasms in male dogs. Indian J. Vet. Pathol., *1:*21, 1976.

33. D'Arville, C.N., and Pierrepoint, C.G.: The demonstration of oestrogen, androgen, and progestagen receptors in the cytosol fraction of canine mammary tumours. Eur. J. Cancer, *15:*875, 1979.
34. Dorn, A.S., Legendre, A.M., and McGavin, M.D.: Mammary hyperplasia in a male cat receiving progesterone. J. Am. Vet. Med. Assoc., *182:*621, 1983.
35. Dow, C.: Experimental reproduction of the cystic hyperplasia-pyometra complex in the bitch. J. Pathol. Bacteriol., *78:*267, 1959.
36. Dow, C.: The cystic hyperplasia-pyometra complex in the bitch. Vet. Rec., *70:*1102, 1958.
37. Dow, C.: The cystic hyperplasia-pyometra complex in the cat. Vet. Rec., *74:*141, 1962.
38. El Etreby, M.F., et al.: The role of the pituitary gland in spontaneous canine mammary tumorigenesis. Vet. Pathol., *17:*2, 1980.
39. Elling, H., and Ungemach, F.R.: Progesterone receptors in feline mammary cancer cytosol. J. Cancer Res. Clin. Oncol., *100:*325, 1981.
40. Elling, H., and Ungemach, F.R.: Simultaneous occurrence of receptors for estradiol, progesterone, and dihydrotestosterone in canine mammary tumors. J. Cancer Res. Clin. Oncol., *105:*231, 1983.
41. Else, R.W., and Hannant, D.: Some epidemiological aspects of mammary neoplasia in the bitch. Vet. Rec., *104:*296, 1979.
42. Evans, B.A.J., et al.: Steroid metabolism and oestradiol-17-β binding in canine mammary tumours. J. Endocrinol., *77:*64, 1978.
43. Evans, C.R., and Pierrepoint, C.G.: Tissue-steroid interactions in canine hormone-dependent tumours. Vet. Rec., *13:*464, 1975.
44. Fanton, J.W., and Withrow, S.J.: Canine mammary neoplasia: an overview. Calif. Vet., *7:*2, 1981.
45. Fowler, E.H., Wilson, G.P., and Koestner, A.: Biologic behavior of canine mammary neoplasms based on a histogenetic classification. Vet. Pathol., *11:*212, 1974.
46. Frank, D.W., et al.: Mammary tumors and serum hormones in the bitch treated with medroxyprogesterone acetate or progesterone for four years. Fertil. Steril., *31:*340, 1979.
47. Funkquist, B., et al.: Hysterography in the bitch. Vet. Radiol., *26:*12, 1985.
48. Ganjam, V.K., et al.: Effect of ovarian hormones on the phagocytic response of ovariectomized mares. J. Reprod. Fertil. [Suppl.], *32:*169, 1982.
49. Graf, K.J., and El Etreby, M.F.: Endocrinology of reproduction in the female beagle dog and its significance in mammary gland tumour-genesis. Acta Endocrinol., *89:*1, 1979.
50. Graf, K.J., and El Etreby, M.F.: The role of the anterior pituitary gland in progestagen-induced proliferative mammary gland changes in the beagle. Drug Res., *28:*54, 1978.
51. Graham, T.C., and Wilson, J.: Mammary adenoma associated with pregnancy in the cat. Vet. Med. Small Anim. Clin., *67:*82, 1972.
52. Greene, J.A., et al.: Ovarian papillary cystadenocarcinoma in a bitch: case report and literature review. J. Am. Anim. Hosp. Assoc., *15:*351, 1979.
53. Greenlee, P.G., and Patnaik, A.K.: Canine ovarian tumors of germ cell origin. Vet. Pathol., *22:*117, 1985.
54. Gruys, E., et al.: Four canine ovarian teratomas and a non-ovarian feline teratoma. Vet. Pathol., *13:*455, 1976.
55. Hadley, J.C.: Unconjugated oestrogen and progesterone concentrations in the blood of bitches with false pregnancy and pyometra. Vet. Rec., *96:*545, 1975.
56. Hamilton, J.M.: Oestrogen receptors in canine mammary tumours. Vet. Rec., *101:*258, 1977.
57. Hamilton, J.M., Else, R.W., and Forshaw, P.: Oestrogen receptors in feline mammary carcinomas. Vet. Rec., *99:*477, 1976.
58. Hardy, R.M., and Osborne, C.A.: Canine pyometra: pathophysiology, diagnosis, and treatment of uterine and extrauterine lesions. J. Am. Anim. Hosp. Assoc., *10:*245, 1974.
59. Harvey, H.J., and Gilbertson, S.R.: Canine mammary gland tumors. Vet. Clin. North Am., *7:*213, 1977.
60. Hasan, S.H., et al.: Growth hormone and prolactin binding in dog mammary gland. Gen. Comp. Endocrinol. *40:*322, 1980.
61. Hayden, D.W., et al.: Feline mammary hypertrophy/fibroadenoma complex: clinical and hormonal aspects. Am. J. Vet. Res., *42:*1699, 1981.
62. Hayden, D.W., and Neilsen, S.W.: Feline mammary tumor. J. Small Anim. Pract., *12:*687, 1971.

63. Hayes, A.: Feline mammary tumors. Vet. Clin. North Am., 7:205, 1977.
64. Hayes, A.A., Hardy, W.D., and McClelland, A.J.: The prevention of canine and feline tumor development. J. Am. Anim. Hosp. Assoc., 12:381, 1976.
65. Hayes, A., and Harvey, H.J.: Treatment of metastatic granulosa cell tumor in a dog. J. Am. Vet. Med. Assoc., 174:1304, 1979.
66. Hayes, H.M., Milne, K.L., and Mandell, C.P.: Epidemiological features of feline mammary carcinoma. Vet. Rec., 108:476, 1981.
67. Hayes, H.M., Jr., and Young, J.L., Jr.: Epidemiologic features of canine ovarian neoplasms. Gynecol. Oncol., 6:348, 1978.
68. Hernandez, F.J., et al.: Feline mammary carcinoma and progestagens. Feline Pract., 5:45, 1975.
69. Hinton, M., and Gaskell, C.J.: Non-neoplastic mammary hypertrophy in the cat associated either with pregnancy or with oral progestagen therapy. Vet. Rec., 100:277, 1977.
70. Inaba, T., et al.: Estrogen and progesterone receptors and progesterone metabolism in canine mammary tumours. Jpn. J. Vet. Sci., 46:797, 1984.
71. Jabara, A.G.: Canine ovarian tumours following stilboestrol administration. Aust. J. Exp. Biol. Med. Sci., 37:549, 1959.
72. Jabara, A.G.: Induction of canine ovarian tumours by diethylstilboestrol and progesterone. Aust. J. Exp. Biol. Med. Sci., 40:139, 1962.
73. Jabara, A.G.: Two cases of mammary neoplasms arising in male dogs. Aust. Vet. J., 45:476, 1969.
74. Johnston, S.D.: Diagnostic and therapeutic approach to infertility in the bitch. J. Am. Vet. Med. Assoc., 176:1335, 1980.
75. Johnston, S.D., et al.: Progesterone receptors in feline mammary adenocarcinomas. Am. J. Vet. Res., 45:379, 1984.
76. Joshua, J.O.: Feline reproduction: the problem of infertility in purebred queens. Feline Pract., 5:52, 1975.
77. Kaddatz, L.A.: Ovarian papillary adenocarcinoma and pyometra in a bitch. Canine Pract., 8:14, 1981.
78. Kaufer, V.I., and Czernicki, B.: Ein Fall von vollstandiger fibroadenomatoser Veranderung der Mamma (Fibroadenomatose). Kleintier-Praxis, 27:283, 1982.
79. Lein, D.H., and Concannon, P.W.: Infertility and fertility treatments and management in the queen and tom cat. In Current Therapy VIII. Edited by R.W. Kirk. Philadelphia, W.B. Saunders, 1983, pp. 936–942.
80. MacVean, D.W., et al.: Frequency of canine and feline tumors in a defined population. Vet. Pathol., 15:700, 1978.
81. Mandel, M.: Spontaneous remission of feline benign mammary hypertrophy. Vet. Med. Small Anim. Clin., 70:846, 1975.
82. Mann, F.A.: Canine mammary gland neoplasia. Canine Pract., 11:22, 1984.
83. McCandlish, I.A.P., et al.: Hormone producing ovarian tumours in the dog. Vet. Rec., 105:9, 1979.
84. Meagher, D.M., et al.: Granulosa cell tumors in mares—a review of 78 cases. Proceedings of the Am. Assoc. Equine Pract. Assoc., 23:133, 1977.
85. Mills, J.H.L., et al.: Arrhenoblastoma in a mare. J. Am. Vet. Med. Assoc., 171:754, 1977.
86. Misdorp, W., et al.: Canine malignant mammary tumours. I. Sarcomas. Vet. Pathol., 8:99, 1971.
87. Misdorp, W., et al.: Canine malignant mammary tumours. II. Adenocarcinomas, solid carcinomas, and spindle cell carcinomas. Vet. Pathol., 9:447, 1972.
88. Misdorp, W., et al.: Canine malignant mammary tumours. III. Special types of carcinomas, malignant mixed tumours. Vet. Pathol., 10:241, 1973.
89. Misdorp, W., and Hart, A.A.M.: Canine mammary cancer. I. Prognosis. J. Small Anim. Pract., 20:385, 1979.
90. Misdorp, W., and Hart, A.A.M.: Canine mammary cancer. II. Therapy and causes of death. J. Small Anim. Pract., 20:395, 1979.
91. Misdorp, W., and Hart, A.A.M.: Prognostic factors in canine mammary cancer. J. Natl. Cancer Inst., 56:779, 1976.
92. Mitchell, L., et al.: Mammary tumor in dogs: survey of clinical and pathological characteristics. Can. Vet. J., 15:131, 1974.
93. Monlux, A.W., et al.: Classification of epithelial canine mammary tumors in a defined population. Vet. Pathol., 14:194, 1977.

94. Monson, K.R., Malbica, J.O., and Hubben, K.: Determination of estrogen receptors in canine mammary tumors. Am. J. Vet. Res., *38:*1937, 1977.
95. Moulton, J.E., et al.: Canine mammary tumors. Vet. Pathol., *7:*289, 1970.
96. Mulligan, R.M.: Mammary cancer in the dog: a study of 120 cases. Am. J. Vet. Res., *36:*1391, 1975.
97. Nelson, L.W., Carlton, W.W., and Weikel, J.H.: Canine mammary neoplasms and progestogens. J. Am. Med. Assoc., *219:*1601, 1972.
98. Nelson, L.W., and Kelly, W.A.: Changes in mammary gland histology during the estrous cycle. Toxicol. Appl. Pharmacol., *27:*113, 1974.
99. Nelson, L.W., Weikel, J.H., Jr., and Reno, F.E.: Mammary nodules in dogs during four years' treatment with megestrol acetate or chlormadinone acetate. J. Natl. Cancer Inst., *51:*1303, 1973.
100. Nimmo, J.S., and Plummer, J.M.: Ultrastructural studies of fibroadenomatous hyperplasia of mammary glands of 2 cats. J. Comp. Pathol., *91:*41, 1981.
101. Norris, P.J., and Blunden, A.: Fibroadenoma of the mammary glands in a kitten. Vet. Rec., *104:*223, 1979.
102. Norris, H.J., Garner, F.M., and Taylor, H.B.: Comparative of ovarian neoplasms. IV. Gonadal stromal tumours of canine species. J. Comp. Pathol., *80:*399, 1970.
103. Norris, H.J., Garner, F.M., and Taylor, H.B.: Pathology of feline ovarian neoplasms. J. Pathol., *97:*138, 1969.
104. Norris, H.J., Taylor, H.B., and Garner, F.M.: Equine ovarian granulosa tumours. Vet. Rec., *82:*419, 1968.
105. Ogilvie, G.K.: Feline mammary neoplasia. Compendium on Continuing Educ. for the Practicing Vet., *5:*384, 1983.
106. Owen, L., et al.: The role of spontaneous canine tumors in the evaluation of the etiology and therapy of human cancer. J. Small Anim. Pract., *16:*155, 1975.
107. Panko, W.B., Patnaik, A.K., and MacEwen, E.G.: Canine mammary tumors. Cancer Res., *42:*2255, 1982.
108. Patnaik, A.K.: Metastasizing ovarian teratocarcinoma in dogs: a report of two cases and a review of the literature. J. Small Anim. Pract., *17:*235, 1976.
109. Priester, W.A.: Occurrence of mammary neoplasms in bitches in relation to breed, age, tumour type, and geographical region from which reported. J. Small Anim. Pract., *20:*1, 1979.
110. Pukay, B.P., and Stevenson, D.A.: Mammary hypertrophy in an ovariohysterectomized cat. Can. Vet. J., *24:*143, 1983.
111. Raflo, C.P., and Diamond, S.S.: Neoplasm of the mammary papilla in a male dog. Am. J. Vet. Res., *41:*953, 1980.
112. Raynaud, J.P., et al.: Spontaneous canine mammary tumors: a model for human endocrine therapy? J. Steroid Biochem. *15:*201, 1981.
113. Rowley, J.: Cystic ovary in a dog. Vet. Med., Small Anim. Clin., *75:*1888, 1980.
114. Schneider, R.: Comparison of age, sex, and incidence rates in human and canine breast cancer. Cancer, *26:*419, 1970.
115. Schneider, R., Dorn, R.C., and Taylor, D.O.N.: Factors influencing canine mammary cancer development and postsurgical survival. J. Natl. Cancer Inst., *43:*1249, 1974.
116. Seiler, R.J., et al.: Total fibroadenomatous change of the mammary glands of two spayed cats. Feline Pract., *9:*25, 1979.
117. Shille, V.M., Calderwood-Mays, M.B., and Thatcher, M.J.: Infertility in a bitch associated with short interestrous intervals and cystic follicles: a case report. J. Am. Anim. Hosp. Assoc., *20:*171, 1984.
118. Shille, V.M., Thatcher, M.J., and Simmons, K.J.: Efforts to induce estrus in the bitch, using pituitary gonadotropins. J. Am. Vet. Med. Assoc., *184:*1469, 1984.
119. Smith, E.K.: Canine ovarian imbalance. Canine Pract., *8:*41, 1981.
120. Stabenfeldt, G.H., et al.: Clinical findings, pathological changes and endocrinological secretory patterns in mares with ovarian tumors. J. Reprod. Fertil. [Suppl.], *27:*277, 1979.
121. Stabenfeldt, G.H., and Hughes, J.P.: Diagnostic endocrinology of the horse. Vet. Clin. North Am., *2:*253, 1980.
122. Stickle, R.L., et al.: Equine granulosa cell tumors. J. Am. Vet. Med. Assoc., *167:*148, 1975.
123. Strandberg, J.D.: Animal model of human disease. Canine Mammary Neoplasia. Am. J. Pathol., *75:*225, 1974.

124. Taylor, G.N., et al.: Mammary neoplasia in a closed beagle colony. Cancer Res., *36:*2740, 1976.
125. Tomlinson, M.J., et al.: Feline mammary carcinoma: a retrospective evaluation of 17 cases. Can. Vet. J., *25:*435, 1984.
126. Turner, T.A., and Manno, M.: Bilateral granulosa cell tumor in a mare. J. Am. Vet. Med. Assoc., *182:*713, 1983.
127. Vaden, P.: Surgical treatment of polycystic ovaries in the dog. Vet Med. Small Anim. Clin., *73:*1160, 1978.
128. Walker, D.: Mammary adenomas in a male dog—probable oestrogenic neoplasms. J. Small Anim. Pract., *9:*15, 1968.
129. Warner, M.R.: Age incidence and site distribution of mammary dysplasia in young beagle bitches. J. Natl. Cancer Inst., *57:*57, 1976.
130. Weijer, K.: Feline mammary tumours and dysplasias. Vet. Q., *2:*69, 1980.
131. Weijer, K., et al.: Feline malignant mammary tumors. I. Morphology and biology: some comparisons with human and canine mammary carcinomas. J. Natl. Cancer Inst., *49:*1697, 1972.
132. Weijer K., et al.: Feline malignant mammary tumors. II. Immunologic and electron microscopic investigations into a possible viral etiology. J. Natl. Cancer Inst., *52:*673, 1974.
133. Wildt, D.E., Kinney, G.M., and Seager, S.W.J.: Gonadotropin induced reproductive cyclicity in the domestic cat. Lab. Anim. Sci., *28:*301, 1978.
134. Wilson, R.B., et al.: Ovarian teratoma in two dogs. J. Am. Anim. Hosp. Assoc., *21:*249, 1985.

25

Clinical Pharmacology of Gonadal Hormones

Gonadal hormones are steroids with a cyclopentanoperhydrophenanthrene nucleus. Those hormones with an additional carbon at C-18 are estrogens. Androgens have additional carbons at C-19, and progestins (progestogens) have additional carbons at C-21, similar to glucocorticoids and mineralocorticoids. Sources of gonadal hormones used in clinical medicine are natural or synthetic.

ESTROGENS

Preparations

Commercially available estrogens and examples of common trade names are listed in Table 25–1. Sources of estrogens are natural or synthetic. Natural estrogens are extracted from the urine of pregnant mares. These are conjugated estrogens containing 50% to 65% sodium estrone sulfate and 20% to 25% sodium equilin sulfate. Other estrone preparations are esterified estrogens. Esterified estrogens are 75% to 85% sodium estrone sulfate and 6% to 15% sodium equilin sulfate. Estropipate is crystalline estrone solubilized as the sulfate and stabilized with piperazine. Estrone is also available as the free hormone.

Synthetic estrogens are steroidal or nonsteroidal. Estradiol exerts more estrogenic effects than does estrone. It is available in the form of micronized free hormone or bound to esters in oil to delay absorption from the intramuscular injection. The valerate ester with estradiol slows the absorption and prolongs estradiol's effects for 2 to 3 weeks. Estradiol cypionate in oil prolongs estradiol's effects 3 to 4 weeks. Ethinyl estradiol is a potent synthetic steroidal derivative of estradiol available for oral administration. Quinestrol is a lipid soluble 3-cyclopentylether of ethinyl estradiol that is stored in body fat and slowly released over a period of about 1 week.

Nonsteroidal estrogens are diethylstilbestrol and chlorotrianisene. Diethylstilbestrol first gained popularity because it is absorbed intact from the digestive tract and can be inexpensively manufactured. Chlorotrianisene has about one eighth the activity of diethylstilbestrol. It is stored in body fat and slowly released.

Table 25–1. Estrogenic Preparations

Generic Name	Trade Name Examples
Conjugated estrogens	Premarin
Esterified estrogens	Estratab, Menest, Evex
Estropipate	Ogen
Estrone	Theelin, Kestrin
Estradiol	Estrace
Estradiol valerate	Delestrogen
Estradiol cypionate	ECP, Depo-estradiol cypionate, Estra, E-cypionate, Estra-cyp-V
Ethinyl estradiol	Estinyl, Feminone
Quinestrol	Estrovis
Diethylstilbestrol dipropionate	Stilphostrol
Chlorotrianisene	TACE

Indications and Dosages

Estrogen therapy is indicated in bitches to prevent unwanted pregnancy, to correct estrogen-responsive dermatosis, and to correct estrogen-responsive urinary incontinence.

MISMATING. The administration of estrogen after coitus should be the option considered last in the prevention of an unwanted pregnancy. Generally safer alternatives for the bitch are ovariohysterectomy or carrying the pregnancy to term. In many cases in which the owner requests treatment for mismating, the mating was not seen, and the request is given only out of concern for a possible fertile mating. Many of these bitches are probably not pregnant and needlessly receive estrogens.

Recommended mismating treatment has traditionally been the intramuscular injection of a long-acting estrogen in concentrations that far exceed physiologic levels. The most popular preparations have been estradiol cypionate in oil (ECP) or diethylstilbestrol in oil; however, diethylstilbestrol in oil is no longer available. The currently recommended dosage for estradiol cypionate in oil is 0.25 to 1.0 mg (44 μg/kg body weight) for dogs and 0.25 mg/kg body weight for cats. This dosage has caused 25% of the dogs treated to develop pyometra; therefore, it may be unduly risky. If used, the most effective time of administration is during estrus or early metestrus. Vaginal smears should be done beforehand to detect sperm and to assess the necessity of mismating treatment.

See also references 14 and 28.

ESTROGEN-RESPONSIVE DERMATOSIS (OVARIAN IMBALANCE II). An estrogen-responsive alopecia has been described in some bitches ovariectomized before their first estrus. The alopecia first appears in the perineal and genital areas. The ventral abdomen, thorax, neck, and ears may be later affected. This disorder is not a deficiency of estrogen because estrogen is not a requirement for normal hair growth. There is no present explanation why the hair coat would become denser in response to therapy with estrogen. Recommended therapy is 0.1 to 1 mg of diethylstilbestrol given orally on a daily basis for 3 weeks. Administration of estrogen is discontinued for 1 week, then repeated for 3 weeks. A response should be evident in 3 months. Thereafter, diethylstilbestrol is administered once or twice per week for maintenance of the hair coat.

ESTROGEN-RESPONSIVE URINARY INCONTINENCE. Older ovariectomized bitches may have senile atrophy of the urogenital mucosa and musculature. Urinary incontinence can also occur. Therapy with estrogen is a successful and appropriate form of treatment for this condition, which has also been reported in a Shetland pony mare. Unfortunately, estrogen is often used without concern about other causes of urinary incontinence, such as bacterial cystitis, cystic calculi, urethral calculi, and neurogenic disorders. Some of these other causes of urinary incontinence may improve with high doses of estrogens because estrogens cause turgidity of the urethra, increase the thickness of the urethral mucosa, and sensitize the urethral sphincters to alpha-adrenergic stimulation. In other words, apparent response of urinary incontinence is not synonymous with a diagnosis of estrogen-deficient urinary incontinence. A thorough urogenital examination should precede the decision to use estrogen for the rest of the animal's life. An effective oral dosage of diethylstilbestrol for canine estrogen-responsive urinary incontinence is 0.1 mg/5 kg body weight/day for 5 days then once or twice per week as necessary.

See also references 33, 75, and 90.

OTHER USES FOR ESTROGENS. Estrogens have also been used to treat vaginitis and as an adjuvant to antibiotics for the treatment of chronic endometritis.

Adverse Effects

Possible adverse effects of estrogen therapy are listed in Table 25–2. Vaginal hyperplasia and prolapse, cystic endometritis-mucometra-pyometra, enhanced mammary or uterine tumor growth, alopecia, and myelosuppression are hazards associated with treatment using estrogen. Prolonged exposure to diethylstilbestrol has induced ovarian carcinomas in bitches and bile duct toxicity in cats. The risk of endometrial carcinoma and thromboembolism is increased in women treated with estrogens. It is not known if increased risks of endometrial carcinoma and thromboembolism exist in companion animals treated with estrogens. Abortion and teratogenicity are adverse effects that can occur in all species if treated with estrogens during pregnancy.

See also references 6, 9, 12, 20, 31, 32, 35, 36, 38, 45, 63–65, 69, 72, 73, 77, 78, 87, 91, 92, 105, 109, and 111.

ANTIESTROGENS

Antiestrogens bind to estradiol receptors, inhibiting estradiol's more potent effects. Tamoxifen citrate (Nolvadex) is a nonsteroidal antiestrogen

Table 25–2. Possible Adverse Effects From Estrogen Therapy

Alopecia
Canine vaginal hyperplasia or prolapse
Cystic endometritis-mucometra-pyometra
Enhanced growth of some mammary tumors or uterine tumors
Induced ovarian carcinoma
Induced uterine carcinoma
Bile duct toxicity
Canine myelosuppression
Thromboembolism
Abortion and teratogenicity

used to inhibit the estrogen-enhanced growth of metastatic mammary neoplasms possessing estrogen receptors. It may cause nausea, anorexia, vomiting, and leukopenia. Clomiphene citrate (Clomid) is a weak estrogen, a synthetic analogue of chlorotrianisene, that competitively blocks the estradiol receptors inhibiting estradiol's negative feedback on the release of gonadotropin. Clomiphene citrate is a fertility agent used in women without ovarian or pituitary failure. It has also been used successfully to induce estrus in the mare.[89]

ANDROGENS

Preparations

Several androgenic steroid preparations are available for oral or intramuscular administration, or as subcutaneous pellets (Table 25–3). Others are available for sublingual administration, a route of administration not applicable for use in companion animals. Anabolic steroids (Table 25–4) are synthetic derivatives of testosterone that have the potential to promote the retention of nitrogen; moreover, these steroids have some of the virilizing effects of testosterone removed. Mibolerone (Cheque) and danazol (Danocrine) are relatively weak androgens used to block the release of gonadotropins. Dromostanolone proprionate (Drolban) and testolactone (Teslac) are synthetic steroids with antineoplastic effects in some advanced or disseminated mammary cancers.

Table 25–3. Androgenic Preparations

Generic Name	Trade Name
Testosterone	Bay Testone
Testosterone propionate	Repotest, Testex
Testosterone enanthate	Delatestryl
Testosterone cypionate	Depo-testosterone, T-Cypionate
Methyltestosterone	Android, Metandren, Oreton-M, Testred, Virilon
Fluoxymesterone	Halotestin, Ora-Testryl, Android-F

Table 25—4.   Anabolic Steroid Preparations

Generic Name	Examples of Trade Names
Oxymetholone	Anadrol
Ethylestrenol	Maxibolin
Stanozolol	Winstrol, Winstrol-V
Nandrolone phenpropionate	Durabolin
Nandrolone decanoate	Deca-Durabolin, Hybolin decanoate
Boldenone undecylenate	Equipoise, Anapoise
Oxandrolone	Anavar
Methandriol	Andriol
Methandriol dipropionate	Probolik, Steribolic, Cellubolic

Testosterone is inactivated to a large extent by the liver when given orally. Parenteral preparations of testosterone are more effective in reaching desired levels in the systemic circulation. Short-acting aqueous preparations or longer-acting, oil-based preparations of testosterone are available. Esters of testosterone in oil prolong testosterone's rate of absorption when administered by intramuscular injection. Testosterone proprionate is effective for 2 to 3 days, and enanthate and cypionate esters of testosterone prolong the effects of testosterone 2 to 4 weeks. Methyltestosterone and fluoxymesterone are 17α-methylated androgens that are less efficiently metabolized by the liver than is testosterone. This results in the more potent effects seen during oral administration and prolonged metabolic half-lives.

Anabolic steroids have been compared with regard to their anabolic and androgenic effects by comparing the changes in the levator ani muscle relative to the seminal vesicle in castrated rats. For oral products, changes are compared to those produced by methyltestosterone, and for injectable products, the changes produced are compared to the changes produced with testosterone phenylpropionate. Dividing the anabolic value by the androgenic value yields the anabolic quotient. Anabolic quotients range from 1 to 20, with 20 being the most anabolic and least androgenic drug. Androgenicity is often reduced by removing the carbon at the 19 position. Esters in oil used for delayed absorption of anabolic steroids include phenpropionate and dipropionate, which slow absorption for about 1 week. Absorption is delayed for 3 to 4 weeks with the decanoate and undecylenate esters.

See also references 1 and 94.

Indications and Dosages

ANDROGENIC STEROIDS.   Androgenic drugs are used to improve libido and maintain male secondary sex characteristics in cases of male hypogonadism, to treat oligospermia (by rebound), to suppress the growth of certain mammary tumors, and to suppress lactation. Testosterone-responsive urinary incontinence is a reported indication for androgenic steroid therapy in some castrated male dogs. Intramuscular injections of testosterone enanthate

(Delatestryl) or testosterone cypionate (Depo-Testosterone) are the most conveniently administered preparations. They can completely virilize patients without the risk of hepatotoxicity inherent with the 17α-methylated preparations for oral use. The dose for either is empirical and should be adjusted with clinical effects. Initial doses for both preparations may begin with 2 mg/kg body weight every 4 weeks.

See also references 5 and 116.

ANABOLIC STEROIDS. Anabolic steroids are indicated to promote a positive nitrogen balance in patients with catabolic diseases by activating enzymes necessary for the uptake of amino acids by transfer RNA. They are an adjunct to the treatment of chronic renal failure (not nephrosis or the nephrotic syndrome), glucocorticoid debilitation, physical exhaustion from work or exercise, and parasitism. Besides promoting the retention of nitrogen, anabolic steroids cause retention of sodium, chloride, calcium, potassium, sulfate, and phosphorus. The net effects are stimulation of appetite, increased muscle mass, retention of intracellular water, increased skin thickness, increased skeletal mass, premature closure of the growth plates, and increased production of red blood cells.

Anabolic steroids, except nandrolone, are alkylated at the 17-α position and are potentially hepatotoxic. Nandrolone decanoate (Deca-Durabolin) can be administered in a dose of 2 mg/kg body weight every 4 weeks for anabolic purposes with relatively minimal adverse effects to the liver.

Anabolic steroids that are alkylated at the 17-α position are more effective stimulants of bone marrow. They have been effectively used to treat aplastic anemia and pure red blood cell aplasia—satisfactory results were noted in 40% to 70% of patients treated. The proposed mechanisms of action are increased production of erythropoietin, potentiated erythropoietin effects, and a direct effect on erythroid proliferating tissues. Oxygen delivery to the tissues is further aided by stimulation of 2,3 diphosphoglycerate in the red blood cells. The bone marrow stimulus produced by anabolic steroids is nonselective. The order of effects is as follows: red cell mass is increased first, followed by granulocytes, and finally, platelets. Nandrolone phenpropionate (Durabolin) may also be used to treat anemia in a dose of 2 mg/kg body weight/wk (this dosage is the one we prefer). Blood cell counts should be monitored for 3 to 6 months. If red blood cell counts indicate a response, treatment should be continued until platelet counts become normal.

See also references 10, 13, 29, 43, 84, and 93.

MIBOLERONE. Mibolerone (Cheque) is an inhibitor of the release of LH. Secondary follicles form, but they do not ovulate. When administered at 3 μg/kg body weight/day for at least 1 month, it prevents estrus in bitches. All German shepherd dogs must be given 180 μg/day regardless of size. Bitches should not be treated before their first estrus. There is approval for 2 years' continuous use, but safety trials have lasted 6 years without causing detectable harm to treated dogs. After the discontinuation of mibolerone, estrus resumes within 7 to 224 days. Fertility is unaffected by prior treatment with mibolerone, but statistics suggest that litter size may be reduced. Mibolerone is also recommended for the treatment of canine pseudopregnancy at 16 μg/kg body weight for 5 days.

Mibolerone is not recommended in the queen because of its low margin of safety in cats. In queens, doses of mibolerone adequate to inhibit estrus cause thyroid dysfunction, thickening of cervical dermis, a greasy hair coat, and clitoral hypertrophy.

See also references 16, 19, 21, 70, 96–98, 100, and 101.

Adverse Effects

Possible adverse effects of androgen and anabolic steroid therapy are listed (Table 25–5). Enhanced growth of benign prostatic hypertrophy, prostatic carcinoma, hypogonadotropic hypogonadism, canine perianal gland adenoma, premature closure of the epiphyseal plates, seborrhea, polycythemia, and decreased thyroxine-binding globulin and corticosteroid-binding globulin are adverse effects common to both androgens and anabolic steroids. Gynecomastia from aromatization to estrogens, virilization of females and female fetuses, overaggression, and priapism are risks more associated with androgen administration. The 17α-alkylated anabolic steroids may cause cholestatic icterus and, possibly, predispose the patient to hepatic carcinoma. The cause for epiphora in some dogs treated with mibolerone is not known.

See also references 4, 58, 66, 76, 82, and 107.

PROGESTINS

Preparations

Examples of currently available progestins are listed in Table 25–6. The effective oral administration of progesterone is prevented by rapid transfor-

Table 25–5. Possible Adverse Effects From Androgen or Anabolic Steroid Therapy

Cholestatic icterus
Enhanced growth of benign prostatic hypertrophy or prostatic carcinoma
Enhanced growth of canine perianal gland adenomas
Gynecomastia
Polycythemia
Hypogonadotropic hypogonadism
Virilization of females and female fetuses
Hepatic carcinoma
Premature closure of epiphyseal plates
Overaggressiveness
Epiphora
Seborrhea
Alterations in thyroid and adrenal function tests
Priapism

Table 25-6. Progestin Preparations

Generic Name	Examples of Trade Names
Progesterone	Gesterol, Repogest
Medroxyprogesterone acetate	Provera, Depo-Provera
Hydroxyprogesterone caproate	Delalutin
Megestrol acetate	Ovaban, Pallace, Megace
Norethindrone	Norlutin, Micronor
Norethindrone acetate	Norlutate, Aygestin
Altrenogest	Regu-mate
Norgestrel	Ovrette

mation of the drug by the liver; however, progesterone is available in aqueous solution or in oil for intramuscular use. Synthetic progestins are derivatives of 17α-hydroxyprogesterone or 19-nortestosterone (ethinyl testosterone).

Medroxyprogesterone acetate, hydroxyprogesterone caproate, and megestrol acetate are derivatives of 17α-hydroxyprogesterone. Medroxyprogesterone acetate and megestrol acetate, 6-methylated 17α-hydroxyprogesterone derivatives, are effective by oral administration. Medroxyprogesterone acetate and hydroxyprogesterone caproate are available in oil or aqueous medium for intramuscular injection and prolonged duration of effect. Derivatives of 17α-hydroxyprogesterone have anti-androgenic effects by competing for dihydrotestosterone receptors and competitively inhibiting the activity of 5 α-reductase.

Norethindrone, norethindrone acetate, norgestrel, and altrenogest are 19-nortestosterone derivatives. All are available as oral preparations. They have weak estrogenic, androgenic, and anabolic effects. Derivatives of 19-nortestosterone are more effective inhibitors of the secretion of gonadotropins than are 17α-hydroxyprogesterone derivatives. Derivatives of 19-nortestosterone do not maintain pregnancy.

See also references 15, 30, 57, 67, 79, 83, and 108.

Indications and Doses

Progestins are used to inhibit or suppress estrus, to maintain pregnancy, to modify undesirable behavior, to treat canine pseudopregnancy, to delay or suppress estrus, and to synchronize estrous cycles among mares.

See also references 22, 24, 42, 102–104, and 114.

INHIBITION AND SUPPRESSION OF ESTRUS IN DOGS AND CATS. Megestrol acetate (Ovaban) is approved for estrous inhibition or suppression and treatment of pseudopregnancy in bitches. To inhibit an anticipated estrus, a dose of 0.55 mg/kg body weight is administered daily for 32 days. Treatment should begin at least 1 week before the desired effect. The time required to return to estrus after treatment is highly variable (1 to 9 months in most cases). Megestrol acetate should not be administered before or during the first estrous cycle and not more than two consecutive estrous cycles. It is contraindicated in the presence of mammary tumors, uterine disease, or pregnancy. Mating is not advisable if estrus occurs within 30 days of treatment with megestrol acetate. For the treatment of behavioral signs of overt pseudopregnancy or the suppression of an estrous period, 2.2 mg/kg body weight/day is given for 8 days.

Although megestrol acetate is unapproved for estrous inhibition in cats, it has successfully postponed estrus in queens when given in a dose of 5 mg/day for 3 days and maintained on a dose of 2.5 to 5 mg/wk, or when given in a dose of 5 mg/wk for 1 month and then maintained on a dose of 2.5 mg/wk. Medroxyprogesterone acetate in oil is not recommended for inhibition or suppression of estrus because of its long duration of effects and the inability to adjust the dosage after injection.

See also references 8, 11, 17, 18, 25, 28, 34, 60, 68, 85, 88, 99, 112, and 117.

INHIBITION, SUPPRESSION, AND SYNCHRONIZATION OF ESTRUS IN MARES.   Progesterone in oil can inhibit or suppress estrus in mares. At 100 mg/day the behavior seen during estrus, as well as ovulation, can be inhibited. If estrus has begun, it can be suppressed with a dose of 200 mg/day. The purpose of inhibiting or suppressing estrus in mares is to manage irregular estrous cycles during the transitional season, to delay foal heat, and to synchronize estrous cycles among several mares.

An oral progestin, altrenogest (Regu-mate) is available for estrous synchronization in mares. When given in a dose of 0.044 mg/kg body weight/day for 15 days, altrenogest suppresses estrous cycles within 3 days in 95% of treated mares. Estrus usually occurs 4 to 5 days after the 15-day treatment is completed.

MAINTENANCE OF PREGNANCY.   Progestins have been advocated as therapy for threatened or habitual abortion. Insufficient progesterone is a theoretical, but unproven, cause of abortion. Low serum progesterone levels are the inevitable result of all abortions. Administration of progesterone can masculinize female fetuses and possibly cause other congenital anomalies.

BEHAVIOR MODIFICATION.   Progestins have a sedative effect on brain activity and are antiandrogenic. If serum estrogen concentrations are declining, the administration of progestin could initially promote coital behavior in bitches. Megestrol acetate and medroxyprogesterone acetate have been used more than other progestins to modify behavior, especially male behavior in the form of secondary sex characteristics. Among the undesirable behavioral characteristics that have responded favorably to progestins are urine spraying, male roaming, inappropriate urination, aggressive behavior, overgrooming, and neurodermatitis in some cats. Mounting, roaming, urine marking, and aggression have been suppressed in some dogs with progestins. It also seems that progestins have anticonvulsant properties. Megestrol acetate (Ovaban) has been recommended in a dose of 2.2 mg/kg body weight/day for 8 days, followed by a dose of 2.2 mg/kg body weight once weekly to control sexual aggression in male dogs. Cats with behavioral problems are treated with doses of 2.5 to 5.0 mg/day for 2 weeks, then 2.5 to 5.0 mg once weekly, if necessary.

See also references 7, 47, 51–56.

SUPPRESSION OF DERMATOSES IN CATS. Miliary dermatitis, eosinophilic granuloma complex, feline acne, hyperplasia of the tail gland, and flea allergy dermatitis may be controlled with progestins, particularly megestrol acetate. Suppression of acne may be due to the antiandrogenic effects of progestins, since dihydrotestosterone is at least part of the pathophysiology of acne. Experimentally, it has been difficult to show the inhibition of immune responses by treatment with progestin. However, each of the skin disorders that respond to progestins is inflammatory. Furthermore, derivatives of 17α-hydroxyprogesterone cause sequestration of eosinophils and inhibit the production of adrenocorticotropic hormone, as do glucocorticoids. One treatment schedule that has been effective in the cat has been the administration of 2.5 mg of megestrol acetate/day (Ovaban) for 2 weeks, to be followed by 2.5 to 5.0 mg once per week if a maintenance dose is necessary.

See also references 2, 61, 62, and 110.

CANINE PSEUDOPREGNANCY. Canine pseudopregnancy is a disorder of metestrus. Overt canine pseudopregnancy is believed to result from falling serum progesterone levels and increasing serum prolactin levels. Progestins in pharmacologic doses inhibit the secretion of prolactin and produce sedation. Androgens can also effectively suppress clinical signs of overt canine pseudopregnancy and are preferable to progestins. The administration of progestin during metestrus increases the risk of inducing cystic endometrial hyperplasia, whereas the administration of androgens does not.

OTHER USES OF PROGESTINS. Progestins (megestrol acetate) produce temporary regression in the size of the canine prostate with benign prostatic hypertrophy and the size of perianal gland adenomas. However, castration is preferable to treatment with progestins.

Megestrol acetate (Megace) is approved for use in the management of human metastatic breast and endometrial carcinomas. Its use in the management of mammary carcinomas of dogs and cats cannot be currently recommended, because mammary tumors have been induced in bitches and queens with megestrol acetate. Its usefulness in treating metastatic uterine carcinoma in companion animals is unevaluated. Megestrol acetate has also been successfully used in the management of chronic eosinophilic keratitis and feline plasma cell gingivitis-pharyngitis syndrome.

See also references 46 and 71.

Adverse Effects

Potential adverse effects of progestins are numerous (Table 25–7). The incidence of adverse effects depends on the type of progestin used, the dose, the means of administration, the species treated, the time of the

Table 25–7.   Possible Adverse Effects From Progestins

Mammary enlargement
Lactation
Increased appetite
Diabetes mellitus
Cystic hyperplasia of the gallbladder in dogs
Endometritis
Enhanced growth of some mammary tumors
Hypogonadotropic hypogonadism
Hypercholesterolemia in dogs
Acromegaly in dogs
Hypoadrenocorticism
Glomerulopathy
Lethargy
Feline mammary adenocarcinoma
Feline fibroadenomatous hyperplasia of the mammary glands
Diarrhea
Polyuria-polydipsia
Change in hair color in cats

---

estrous cycle when administered, and the duration of treatment. A repositol progestin given intramuscularly and possessing prolonged effects, medroxyprogesterone acetate (Depo-Provera) has the least margin of safety. When approved for inhibition of estrus in bitches in 1963 to 1966, there was a 15% to 20% occurrence of cystic endometrial hyperplasia after its use. In contrast, the reported incidence of endometritis after the oral administration of megestrol acetate in bitches is 0.6%.

Derivatives of 17α-hydroxyprogesterone have been investigated in dogs and cats to a greater extent than progestin derivatives of 19-nortestosterone. For this reason, most of the observed adverse effects of progestins have been associated with megestrol acetate, medroxyprogesterone acetate, and other 17α-hydroxyprogesterone derivatives. All the possible adverse effects listed in Table 25–7 have been noted in dogs or cats treated with megestrol acetate, medroxyprogesterone acetate, or progesterone. Enlargement of the clitoris and masculinization of fetuses may occur with progestin derivatives of 19-nortestosterone. Other adverse effects such as acromegaly, diabetes mellitus, hypoadrenocorticism, and induced mammary gland tumors apparently do not occur with 19-nortestosterone derivatives as they may with 17α-hydroxyprogesterone derivatives.

See also references 3, 23, 26, 27, 37, 39, 41, 44, 48–50, 59, 80, 81, 86, 95, 106, 115, 116, and 118.

REFERENCES

1. Ahn, Y.S., et al.: Danazol for the treatment of idiopathic thrombocytopenic purpura. N. Engl. J. Med., *308:*1396, 1983.
2. Aspinall, K.W., and Evans, J.M.: The use of megestrol acetate in the treatment of miliary eczema in the cat. Vet. Rec., *88:*374, 1971.
3. Attia, M.A., and Zayed, I.: Cytological study on the anterior pituitary of beagle bitches treated subcutaneously with progesterone for 13 weeks. Arch. Toxicol., *42:*147, 1979.

4. Baba, S., et al.: Antiandrogenic effects of spironolactone: hormonal and ultrastructural studies in dogs and men. J. Urol., *119:*375, 1978.
5. Marsanti, J.A., Edwards, P.D., and Losonsky, J.: Testosterone responsive urinary incontinence in a castrated male dog. J. Am. Anim. Hosp. Assoc., *17:*117, 1981.
6. Barsanti, J.A., Medleau, L., and Latimer, K.: Diethylstilbestrol-induced alopecia in a dog. J. Am. Vet. Med. Assoc., *182:*63, 1983.
7. Beach, F.A., and Merari, A.: Coital behavior in dogs. IV. Effects of progesterone in the bitch. Proc. Natl. Acad. Sci., *61:*442, 1968.
8. Bell, E.T., and Christie, D.W.: The use of progestagens in the control of the canine oestrous cycle. J. Small Anim. Pract., *12:*375, 1971.
9. Bernard, S.L., et al.: Estrogen-induced bone marrow depression in ferrets. Am. J. Vet. Res., *44:*657, 1983.
10. Beroza, G.A.: Anabolic steroids in the horse. J. Am. Vet. Med. Assoc., *179:*278, 1981.
11. Bigbee, H.G., and Hennessey, P.W.: Megestrol acetate for postponing estrus in first-heat bitches. Vet. Med. Small Anim. Clin., *72:*1727, 1977.
12. Bland-van den Berg, P., Bomzon, L., and Lurie, A.: Oestrogen-induced bone marrow aplasia in a dog. J. S. Afr. Vet. Assoc., *49:*363, 1978.
13. Boebel, F.W., and Ehrenford, F.A.: Boldenone undecylenate in treatment of debilitation in cats: five clinical cases. Vet. Med. Small Anim. Clin., *73:*149, 1978.
14. Bowen, R.A., et al.: Efficacy and toxicity of estrogens commonly used to terminate canine pregnancy. J. Am. Vet. Med. Assoc., *186:*783, 1985.
15. Britt, J.H., and Ulberg, L.C.: The therapeutics of progestogens. Vet. Scope, *16:*1, 1971.
16. Brown, J.: Efficacy and dosage titration study of mibolerone for treatment of pseudopregnancy in the bitch. J. Am. Vet. Med. Assoc., *184:*1467, 1984.
17. Bryan, H.S.: Parenteral use of medroxyprogesterone acetate as an antifertility agent in the bitch. Am. J. Vet. Res., *34:*659, 1973.
18. Burke, T.J., and Reynolds, H.A.: Megestrol acetate for estrus postponement in the bitch. J. Am. Vet. Med. Assoc., *4:*285, 1975.
19. Burke, T.J., Reynolds, H.A., and Sokolowski, J.H.: A 180-day tolerance-efficacy study with mibolerone for suppression of estrus in the cat. Am. J. Vet. Res., *38:*469, 1977.
20. Capel-Edwards, K., Hall, D.E., and Samson, A.G.: Hematological changes observed in female beagle dogs given ethynylestradiol. Toxicol. Appl. Pharmacol., *20:*319, 1971.
21. Catton, D.G.: Use of mibolerone to prevent estrus in bitches. J. S. Afr. Vet. Assoc., *51:*4, 1980.
22. Chainey, D., McCoubrey, A., and Evans, J.A.: The excretion of megestrol acetate by beagle bitches. Vet. Rec., *86:*278, 1970.
23. Chastain, C.B., Graham, C.L., and Nichols, C.E.: Adrenocortical suppression in cats given megestrol acetate. Am. J. Vet. Res., *42:*2029, 1981.
24. Chesney, C.J.: The response to progestogen treatment of some diseases of cats. J. Small Anim. Pract., *17:*35, 1976.
25. Christie, D.W., and Bell, E.T.: The use of progestogens to control reproductive function in the bitch (Abstract). Anim. Breed, *38:*1, 1970.
26. Coleman, M.E., Murchison, T.E., and Frank, D.: Mammary nodules in dogs receiving Depo-Provera and progesterone: an interim progress report. Toxicol. Appl. Pharmacol., *37:*1, 1976.
27. Concannon, P., et al.: Growth hormone, prolactin, and cortisol in dogs developing mammary nodules and an acromegaly-like appearance during treatment with medroxyprogesterone acetate. Endocrinology, *106:*1173, 1980.
28. Concannon, P.W.: Fertility regulation in the bitch: contraception, sterilization and pregnancy termination. *In* Current Veterinary Therapy VIII. Edited by R.W. Kirk. Philadelphia, W.B. Saunders, 1983, pp. 901–909.
29. Couto, C.G., and Feldman, B.F.: Therapy for abnormal erythropoiesis. J. Am. Vet. Med. Assoc., *181:*501, 1982.
30. Cox, J.E.: Progestagens in bitches: a review. J. Small Anim. Pract., *11:*759, 1970.
31. Crafts, R.C.: The effect of endocrines on the formed elements of the blood. II. The effects of estrogens in the dog and monkey. Endocrinology, *29:*606, 1941.
32. Crafts, R.C.: The effects of estrogens on the bone marrow of adult female dogs. Blood, *3:*276, 1948.
33. Creed, K.E.: Effect of hormones on urethral sensitivity to phenylephrine in normal and incontinent dogs. Res. Vet. Sci., *34:*177, 1983.

34. David, A., et al.: Anti-ovulatory and other biological properties of megestrol acetate. J. Reprod. Fertil., *5*:331, 1963.
35. Dow, C.: Oestrogen-induced atrophy of the skin in dogs. J. Pathol. Bacteriol., *80*:434, 1960.
36. Dow, C.: The pathology of stilbestrol poisoning in the domestic cat. J. Pathol. Bacteriol., *75*:151, 1958.
37. Eigenmann, J.E.: Progestagen-induced and spontaneous canine acromegaly due to reversible growth hormone overproduction: clinical picture and pathogenesis. J. Am. Anim. Hosp. Assoc., *17*:813, 1981.
38. Eigenmann, J.E., Poortman, J., and Koeman, J.P.: Estrogen-induced flank alopecia in the female dog: evidence for local rather than systemic hyperestrogenism. J. Am. Anim. Hosp. Assoc., *20*:621, 1984.
39. El Etreby, M.F.: Effect of cyproterone acetate, levonorgestrel and progesterone on adrenal glands and reproductive organs in the beagle bitch. Cell Tissue Res., *200*:229, 1979.
40. El Etreby, M.F., and Fath El Bab, M.R.: Effect of cyproterone acetate, d-norgestrel and progesterone on cells of the pars distalis of the adenhypophysis in the beagle bitch. Cell Tissue Res., *191*:205, 1978.
41. El Etreby, M.F., and Wrobel, K.H.: Effect of cyproterone acetate, d-norgestrel and progesterone on the canine mammary gland. Cell Tissue Res., *194*:245, 1978.
42. Ellis, C.P.: Oral progestagens in cats. Vet. Rec., *96*:513, 1975.
43. Finco, D.R., Barsanti, J.A., and Adams, D.D.: Effects of an anabolic steroid on acute uremia in the dog. Am. J. Vet. Res., *45*:2285, 1984.
44. Frank, D.W., et al.: Mammary tumors and serum hormones in the bitch treated with medroxyprogesterone acetate or progesterone for four years. Fertil. Steril., *31*:340, 1979.
45. Gardner, W.U., and DeVita, J.: Inhibition of hair growth in dogs receiving estrogens. Yale J. Biol. Med., *13*:213, 1940.
46. Geller, J., Albert, J., and Yen, S.S.: Treatment of advanced cancer of prostate with megestrol acetate. Urology, *12*:537, 1978.
47. Gerber, H.A., Jochle, W., and Sulman, F.G.: Control of reproduction and of undesirable social and sexual behavior in dogs and cats. J. Small Anim. Pract., *14*:151, 1973.
48. Giles, R.C., et al.: Mammary nodules in beagle dogs administered investigational oral contraceptive steroids. J. Natl. Cancer Inst., *60*:1351, 1978.
49. Graf, K.J.: The role of the anterior pituitary gland in progestogen induced proliferative mammary gland changes in the beagle. Drug Res., *28*:54, 1978.
50. Guthrie, G.P., and John, W.J.: The *in vivo* glucocorticoid and antiglucocorticoid actions of medroxyprogesterone acetate. Endocrinology, *107*:1393, 1980.
51. Hart, B.L.: Behavioral effects of long-acting progestins. Feline Pract., *4*:8, 1974.
52. Hart, B.L.: Evaluation of progestin therapy for behavioral problems. Feline Pract., *9*:11, 1979.
53. Hart, B.L.: Indications for progestin therapy for problem behavior in dogs. Canine Pract., *6*:10, 1979.
54. Hart, B.L.: Objectionable urine spraying and urine marking in cats: evaluation of progestin treatment in gonadectomized males and females. J. Am. Vet. Med. Assoc., *177*:529, 1980.
55. Hart, B.L.: Problems with objectionable sociosexual behavior of dogs and cats: therapeutic use of castration and progestins. Compendium on Continuing Educ. for the Practicing Vet., *1*:461, 1979.
56. Hart, B.L.: Progestin therapy for aggressive behavior in male dogs. J. Am. Vet. Med. Assoc., *178*:1070, 1981.
57. Henik, R.A., Olson, P.N., and Rosychuk, R.A.: Progestogen therapy in cats. Compendium on Continuing Educ. for the Practicing Vet., *7*:132, 1985.
58. Heywood, R., et al.: Toxicity of methyl testosterone in the beagle dog. Toxicology, *7*:357, 1977.
59. Hill, R., et al.: Progestational potency of chlormadinone acetate in the immature beagle bitch: preliminary report. Contraception, *2*:381, 1970.
60. Houdeshell, J.W., and Hennessey, P.W.: Megestrol acetate for control of estrus in the cat. Vet. Med. Small Anim. Clin., *72*:1013, 1977.
61. Houdeshell, J.W., Hennessey, P.W., and Bigbee, H.B.: Treatment of feline miliary dermatitis with megestrol acetate. Vet. Med. Small Anim. Clin., *72*:573, 1977.

62. Hutchinson, J.A.: Progestogen therapy for certain skin diseases of cats. Can. Vet. J., *19:*324, 1978.
63. Jabara, A.G.: Canine ovarian tumours following stilboestrol administration. Aust. J. Exp. Biol. Med. Sci., *37:*549, 1959.
64. Jabara, A.G.: Induction of canine ovarian tumours by diethylstilboestrol and progesterone. Aust. J. Exp. Biol. Med. Sci., *40:*139, 1962.
65. Jabara, A.G.: Some tissue changes in the dog following stilbesterol administration. Aust. J. Exp. Biol. Med. Sci., *40:*293, 1962.
66. James, R.W., Crook, D., and Heywood, R.: Canine pituitary-testicular function in relation to toxicity testing. Toxicology *13:*237, 1979.
67. Jochle, W.: Hormones in canine gynecology: a review. Theriogenology, *3:*152, 1975.
68. Jochle, W., and Jochle, M.: Reproductive and behavioral control in the male and female cat with progestins: long-term field observations in individual animals. Theriogenology, *3:*179, 1975.
69. Kociba, G.J., and Caputo, C.A.: Aplastic anemia associated with estrus in pet ferrets. J. Am. Vet. Med. Assoc., *178:*1293, 1981.
70. Krzeminski, L.F., et al.: Serum concentrations of mibolerone in beagle bitches as influenced by time, dosage form, and geographic location. Am. J. Vet. Res., *39:*567, 1978.
71. Lebech, P.E., and Nordentoft, E.L.: A study of endocrine function in the treatment of benign prostatic hypertrophy with megestrol acetate. Acta Obstet. Gynceol. Scand., *48:*25, 1967.
72. Legendre, A.M.: Estrogen-induced bone marrow hypoplasia in a dog. J. Am. Anim. Hosp. Assoc., *12:*525, 1976.
73. Lowenstein, L.J., Ling, G.V., and Schalm, O.W.: Exogenous estrogen toxicity in the dog. Calif. Vet., *26:*14, 1972.
74. Maddux, J.M., and Shaw, S.E.: Possible beneficial effect of lithium therapy in a case of estrogen-induced bone marrow hypoplasia in a dog: a case report. J. Am. Anim. Hosp. Assoc., *19:*242, 1983.
75. Madism, J.B.: Estrogen-responsive urinary incontinence in an aged pony mare. Compendium on Continuing Educ for the Practicing Vet., *6:*S390, 1984.
76. Menard, R.H., et al.: The effect of the administration of spironolactone on the concentration of plasma testosterone, estradiol and cortisol in male dogs. Steroids, *31:*771, 1978.
77. Mills, J.N., and Slatter, D.H.: Stilbestrol toxicity in a dog. Aust. Vet. J., *57:*39, 1981.
78. Mulligan, R.M.: Some effects of chronic doses of stilbesterol in female dogs. Expl. Med. Surg., *5:*196, 1947.
79. Nash, H.A.: Depo-provera: a review. Contraception, *12:*377, 1975.
80. Nelson, L.W., and Kelly, W.A.: Progestogen-related gross and microscopic changes in female beagles. Vet. Pathol., *13:*143, 1976.
81. Nelson, L.W., Weikel, J.H., and Reno, F.E.: Mammary nodules in dogs during four years' treatment with megestrol acetate or chlormadinone acetate. J. Natl. Cancer Inst., *51:*1303, 1973.
82. Neri, R.O., et al.: Effects of an anti-androgen, SH714 (6-chlor 6-1, 2-alpha-methylen-17-alpha-hydroxyprogesterone acetate, cyproterone acetate) on canine prostatic hyperplasia. Endocrinology, *82:*311, 1968.
83. Nimmo-Wilke, J.S.: Progesterone therapy for cats. Can. Vet. J., *20:*164, 1979.
84. O'Connor, J.J., et al.: Evaluation of boldenone undecylenate as an anabolic agent in horses. Can. Vet. J., *14:*154, 1973.
85. Oen, E.O.: The oral administration of megestrol acetate to postpone oestrus in cats. Nord. Vet. Med., *29:*287, 1977.
86. Pukay, B.P.: A hyperglycemia-glucosuria syndrome in cats following megestrol acetate therapy. Can. Vet. J., *20:*117, 1979.
87. Pyle, R.L., Hill, B.L., and Johnson, J.K.: Estrogen toxicity in a dog. Canine Pract., *3:*39, 1976.
88. Remfry, J.: Control of feral cat populations by long-term administration of megestrol acetate. Vet. Rec., *103:*403, 1978.
89. Robinson, J.R.: Use of clomiphene citrate to induce estrus in anestrous mares. Vet. Med. Small Anim. Clin., *72:*605, 1977.
90. Rosin, A.H., and Ross, L.: Diagnosis and pharmacological management of disorders of urinary continence in the dog. Compendium on Continuing Educ. for the Practicing Vet., *3:*601, 1981.

91. Ryland, L.M., and Gorham, J.R.: The ferret and its diseases. J. Am. Vet. Med. Assoc., *173:*1154, 1978.
92. Schalm, O.W.: Exogenous estrogen toxicity in the dog. Canine Pract., *5:*57, 1978.
93. Shahidi, N.T.: Androgens and erythropoiesis. N. Engl. J. Med., *289:*72, 1973.
94. Simmons, J.G., and Hamner, C.E.: Inhibition of estrus in the dog with testosterone implants. Am. J. Vet. Res., *34:*1409, 1973.
95. Sloan, J.M., and Oliver, I.M.: Progestogen-induced diabetes in the dog. Diabetes, *24:*337, 1975.
96. Sokolowski, J.H.: Evaluation of estrous activity in bitches treated with mibolerone and exposed to adult male dogs. J. Am. Vet. Med. Assoc., *173:*983, 1978.
97. Sokolowski, J.H.: Mibolerone for treatment of canine pseudopregnancy and galactorrhea. Canine Pract., *9:*6, 1982.
98. Sokolowski, J.H., and Geng; S.: Biological evaluation of mibolerone in the female beagle. Am. J. Vet. Res., *38:*1371, 1977.
99. Sokolowski, J.H., and Van Ravenswaay, F.: Effects of melengestrol acetate on reproduction in the Beagle bitch. Am. J. Vet. Res., *37:*943, 1976.
100. Sokolowski, J.H., and Kasson, C.W.: Effects of mibolerone on contraception, pregnancy, parturition, and offspring in the beagle. Am. J. Vet. Res., *39:*837, 1978.
101. Sokolowski, J.H., and Van Ravenswaay, F.: Summary of studies evaluating the efficacy of mibolerone in the mature female beagle. Canine Pract., *5:*53, 1978.
102. Sokolowski, J.H., and Zimbelman, R.G.: Canine reproduction. Effects of a single injection of medroxyprogesterone acetate on the reproductive organs of intact and ovariectomized bitches. Am. J. Vet. Res., *34:*1501, 1973.
103. Sokolowski, J.H., and Zimbelman, R.G.: Canine reproduction. Effects of multiple treatments of medroxyprogesterone acetate on reproductive organs of the bitch. Am. J. Vet. Res., *35:*1285, 1974.
104. Sokolowski, J.H., and Zimbelman, R.G.: Evaluation of selected compounds for estrous control in the bitch. Am. J. Vet. Res., *37:*939, 1976.
105. Spano, J.W.: A case of estrogen toxicity in the dog. Auburn Vet., *31:*11, 1974.
106. Spellacy, W.N., et al.: Carbohydrate and lipid studies during six months' treatment with megestrol acetate. Am. J. Obstet. Gynecol., *116:*1074, 1973.
107. Squires, E.L., et al.: Fertility of young mares after long-term anabolic steroid treatment. J. Am. Vet. Med. Assoc., *186:*583, 1985.
108. Stabenfeldt, G.H.: Physiologic and therapeutic roles of progestins in domestic animals. J. Am. Vet. Med. Assoc., *164:*311, 1974.
109. Steinberg, S.: Aplastic anemia in a dog. J. Am. Vet. Med. Assoc., *157:*966, 1970.
110. Turner, W.T.: Use of megestrol acetate in the treatment of miliary eczema in the cat. Vet. Rec., *88:*315, 1971.
111. Tyslowitz, R., and Dinglmanse, E.: Effect of large doses of estrogens on the blood picture of dogs. Endocrinology, *29:*817, 1941.
112. Vecchio, T.J.: Injectable medroxyprogesterone acetate contraception: metabolic and endocrine effects. J. Reprod. Med., *10:*193, 1973.
113. Vincent, D.L., et al.: Maintenance of physiologic concentrations of plasma testosterone in the castrated male dog, using testosterone-filled polydimethylsiloxane capsules. Am. J. Vet. Res., *40:*705, 1979.
114. Walker, C.E.: Oral progestagens in cats. Vet. Rec., *96:*458, 1975.
115. Weikel, J.H., and Nelson, L.W.: Problems in evaluating chronic toxicity of contraceptive steroids in dogs. J. Toxicol. Environ. Health, *3:*167, 1977.
116. Weikel, J.H., Nelson, L.W., and Reno, F.E.: A four-year evaluation of the chronic toxicity of megestrol acetate in dogs. Toxicol. Appl. Pharmacol., *33:*414, 1975.
117. Wildt, D.E., Kinney, G.M., and Seager, S.W.J.: Reproduction control in the dog and cat: an examination and evaluation of current and proposed methods. J. Am. Anim. Hosp. Assoc., *13:*223, 1977.
118. Wright, P.J., et al.: Medroxyprogesterone acetate and reproductive processes in male dogs. Aust. Vet. J., *55:*437, 1979.

Appendix 1. Glossary of Abbreviations and Synonyms

A	Alpha cell (of pancreatic islets)
ACTH	Adrenocorticotropic hormone (corticotropin)
ADH	Antidiuretic hormone
APUD	Amine precursor uptake and decarboxylation
B	Beta cell (of pancreatic islets)
BPH	Canine benign prostatic hypertrophy
BUN	Blood urea nitrogen
C-cell	Calcitonin-secreting cell, parafollicular cells of the thyroid
Ca	Calcium
cAMP	Cyclic 3′, 5′-adenosine monophosphate
cGMP	Cyclic guanosine monophosphate
CBG	Corticosteroid-binding globulin (transcortin)
CCK	Cholecystokinin
CEH	Cystic endometrial hyperplasia
Ci	Curie
CL	Corpus luteum
CLIP	Corticotropin-like intermediate lobe peptide
CPB	Competitive protein-binding assay
CPK	Creatinine phosphokinase
CRH	Corticotropin-releasing hormone
CT scan	Computer-assisted tomography
D_2	Ergocalciferol (a vitamin)
D_3	Cholecalciferol (a vitamin)
DHEA	Dehydroepiandrosterone
DHT	Dihydrotestosterone
DIT	Diiodotyrosine (T_2)
dl	Deciliter
DOC	Deoxycorticosterone
DOCA	Deoxycorticosterone acetate
E_1	Estrone
E_2	Estradiol (17 β-estradiol)
E_3	Estriol
ECG	Electrocardiogram
EEG	Electroencephalogram
ELISA	Enzyme-linked immunoabsorbent assay
EMG	Electromyogram
EMIT	Enzyme-multiplied immunoassay
ER	Estrogen receptor
FFAH	Feline fibroadenomatous hyperplasia of the mammary glands
FSH	Follicle-stimulating hormone (follitropin)
FT_4	Free (unbound) thyroxine
GFR	Glomerular filtration rate
GH	Growth hormone (somatotropic hormone [STH])
GHb	Glycohemoglobin
GIP	Gastric inhibitory polypeptide
GLI	Glucagon-like immunoreactivity
g	Gram
GnRH	Gonadotropin-releasing hormone
GRH	GH-releasing hormone
GTT	Glucose tolerance test
HCG	Human chorionic gonadotropin
H-P-A	Hypothalamic-pituitary-adrenal
H-P-O	Hypothalamic-pituitary-ovarian
H-P-T	Hypothalamic-pituitary-testicular
ICSH	Interstitial-cell-stimulating hormone (LH)
ICT	Interstitial cell tumor
IDDM	Insulin-dependent diabetes mellitus
IGF	Insulin-like growth factor
IRI	Immunoreactive insulin

IU	International unit
K	Potassium
kg	Kilogram
L	Liter
LH	Luteinizing hormone (ICSH, lutropin)
MAIA	Magnetic antibody immunoassay
MEN	Multiple endocrine neoplasia
mEq	Milliequivalent
mg	Milligram
MIT	Monoiodotyrosine (T_1)
ml	Milliliter
mOsm	Milliosmole
MRF	Mullerian duct regression factor
MSH	Melanocyte-stimulating hormone
MW	Molecular weight
Na	Sodium
ng	Nanogram
NIDDM	Noninsulin-dependent diabetes mellitus
NPH	Neutral protamine Hagedorn (an intermediate-acting insulin)
NSILA	Nonsuppressible insulin-like activity
17-OHCS	17-hydroxycorticosteroids
P	Phosphorus
pg	Picogram
PBI	Protein-bound iodine
PCOS	Polycystic ovarian syndrome
PMSG	Pregnant mare serum gonadotropin
POMC	Pro-opiomelanocortin
PP	Pancreatic polypeptide
PR	Progesterone receptor
PRL	Prolactin
PTH	Parathyroid hormone (parathyrin)
PTU	Propylthiouracil
rT_3	Reverse T_3
RIA	Radioimmunoassay
RNA	Ribonucleic acid
RTU	Resin T_3 uptake
SAP	Serum alkaline phosphatase
SCT	Sertoli's cell tumor
SEM	Seminoma
SHBG	Sex-hormone-binding globulin
SIADH	Syndrome of inappropriate antidiuretic hormone
STH	Somatotropic hormone (GH)
T_1	Monoiodotyrosine
T_2	Diiodotyrosine
T_3	Triiodothyronine
T_3U	RTU, T_3 uptake
T_4	Thyroxine
TBG	Thyroxine-binding globulin
TBP	Thyroxine-binding proteins
Tc	Technetium
TER	Teratoma
TRH	Thyrotropin-releasing hormone
TSH	Thyroid-stimulating hormone (thyrotropin)
U	Unit
VIP	Vasoactive intestinal polypeptide
VMA	Vanillylmandelic acid
>	Greater than
<	Less than
≥	Greater than or equal to
≤	Less than or equal to
μg	Microgram

Appendix 2. Units and Weights

kg	Kilogram (1000 g)
g	Gram
mg	Milligram (1/1000 g)
μg	Microgram (1/1000 mg)
ng	Nanogram (1/1000 μg)
pg	Picogram (1/1000 ng)
fg	Femtogram (1/1000 pg)
IU	International unit
U	Unit
μU	Microunit (1/1000 units)
μCi	Microcurie (1/1000 mCi)
L	Liter
dl	Deciliter (1/100 L)
ml	Milliliter (1/1000 L)
mCi	Millicurie (1/1000 Ci)
mEq	Milliequivalent

Appendix 3. Common Guidelines for the Collection, Storage, and Transport of Laboratory Samples for Hormone- or Endocrine-Related Determinations

Determination*	Specimen†	Sample Quantity (ml)	Sample Care‡
ACTH	P	5	A (Do not use glass syringes or tubes)
Aldosterone	P,S	2	B (Ship frozen)
Angiotensin I	P	3	A
Calcium	S	1	B
	U	10	D
Catecholamines	P	1	A
	U	25	D
Cholesterol	S	1	B
Cortisol	P,S	2	C
	U	10	C (Protect from light; ship frozen)
DHEA	P,S	1	B
DHEA-S	P,S	1	B
Dihydrotestosterone	P,S	1	B
Erythropoietin	S	2	B
Estradiol	P,S	3	B (Send frozen)
Estriol	P,S	3	B
Estrone	P,S	3	B
FSH	P,S	2	B (Species specific)
Gastrin	S	1	A (Collect during fasting)
Glycohemoglobin	B	5	B (Use fluoride tube)
Growth hormone	P	3	A (Species specific)
Hydroxyproline	U	25	D
Insulin	S	1	A (Sample during fasting or hypoglycemia)

LH	P,S	2	B (Species specific)
Magnesium	S	1	B
Osmolality	P,S	1	B
	U	25	E
Parathyroid hormone	P	5	A (Request only C-terminal assay)
Phosphorus	S	1	B
	U	10	C
Potassium	S	1	B (Avoid hemolysis)
	U	10	C
Prolactin	P	1	A (Species specific)
Progesterone	P,S	2	B
Renin	P	3	A (Use EDTA, not heparin)
Sodium	S	1	B (Avoid hemolysis)
	U	10	C
Testosterone	P,S	2	B
T_3	S	1	B
T_4	S	1	B
T_4 (free)	S	1	B
Vitamin D (25-hydroxy)	S	1	B
Vitamin D (1,25-dihydrox)	S	5	B (Ship frozen)

* ACTH = adrenocorticotropic hormone; DHEA = dehydroepiandrosterone; FSH = follicle-stimulating hormone; LH = luteinizing hormone; T_3 = triiodothyronine; T_4 = thyroxine.
† P = plasma; S = serum; U = urine; B = whole blood.
‡ A. Collect in cold heparinized tube. Place in ice water bath. Separate from blood cells within 15 minutes. Freeze and ship frozen with dry ice. B. Collect serum in red-top clot tube or plasma in heparinized tube. Separate from cells within 15 minutes. Avoid hemolysis. Ship with cold packs. C. Collect sample from well-mixed aliquot of urine collected over 24-hour period. Record 24-hour volume of urine. D. Same as C, but add 25 ml of 6 N HCl to 24-hour collection of urine. E. Collect urine during dehydration or water deprivation.

Appendix 4. Normal Serum or Plasma Hormone Levels*

Endocrine System	Hormone	Units	Normal Dog	Normal Cat
Hypothalamus/ Pituitary				
	ADH	pg/ml	<1–4	
	ACTH	pg/ml	20–100	30–100
	β LPH	pg/ml	20–80	
	Prolactin	ng/ml	<1–4	<1–4
	GH	ng/ml	<1–4	<1–4
	TSH	ng/ml	3–8	2–4
	FSH (female)	ng/ml	40–70	
	LH†	ng/ml	<1–3	
	Somatomedin C‡	ng/ml	5–300	

Thyroid

T$_4$	μg/dl	1–4	1.5–5
T$_3$	ng/dl	50–150	15–60
T$_3$U	%	40–60	
Post-TSH T$_4$	μg/dl	$\geq$5	$\geq$5
rT$_3$	ng/dl	50–150	
TSH	ng/ml	3–8	2–4
Free T$_4$	ng/dl	0.7–2	
Calcitonin	pg/eq/ml	<2.5	

Parathyroid

PTH (C-terminal)	μl/Eq/ml	10–400	10–400
Total serum calcium	mg/dl	9–11.5	9–11.5
Ionized serum calcium	mg/dl	4–5	4–5
Urine calcium	mg/kg/24 h	0.5–1	
Urine phosphorus	mg/kg/24 h	10–30	
Urine total cAMP	μM/L	5–7	
Urine hydroxyproline	mg/kg/24 h	0.25–0.75	

Pancreatic Islets

Insulin (fasting)	μU/ml	5–30	5–30
Glycosylated plasma proteins	%	9–12	
Glycosylated plasma albumin	%	8–14	
Glycohemoglobin	%	6–8	
Gastrin	pg/ml	30–100	30–100

Adrenal

Cortisol	μg/dl	1–4	1–4
Cortisol levels after the administration of ACTH	μg/dl	$\geq$7–20	$\geq$6–20
Cortisol levels after the administration of dexamethasone	μg/dl	<1.5	<1.5
Aldosterone	ng/dl	1–6	1–6
Androstenedione	ng/dl	50–150	
Renin	ng/ml/h	2–3	
Urine VMA	mg/24 h	0.6–15	

Testes

Testosterone (noncastrated)	ng/ml	0.5–6	0.5–3

Ovaries

Estradiol (anestrus or spayed)	pg/ml	<15	<15
Progesterone (anestrus or spayed)	ng/ml	<1	<1
Testosterone (anestrus or spayed)	ng/ml	<0.3	<0.3

* Levels are only approximate. Normal values vary among assays used and laboratories. Normal values for blood and urine constituents whose concentrations are frequently affected by hormones are also listed. ADH = antidiuretic hormone; ACTH = adrenocorticotropic hormone; LPH= lipotropin hormone; GH= growth hormone, TSH= thyroid-stimulating hormone; FSH= follicle-stimulating hormone; LH= luteinizing hormone; T$_4$= thyroxine; T$_3$ = triiodothyronine; T$_3$U = triiodothyronine uptake; rT$_3$ = reverse triiodothyronine; PTH= parathyroid hormone; cAMP= cyclic adenosine monophosphate; VMA= vanillymandelic acid.

† Normal values vary widely among laboratories.

‡ Depends on breed.

INDEX

Numerals in *italics* indicate figures; "t" following a page number indicates a table.

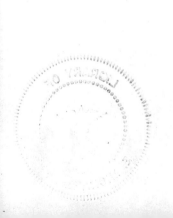